# Tropical Diseases in Travelers

# Tropical Diseases in Travelers

EDITED BY

## Eli Schwartz MD DTMH

Chaim Sheba Medical Center
Tel Hashomer, Israel
and
Sackler School of Medicine
Tel Aviv University
Tel Aviv, Israel

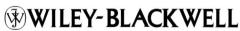
**WILEY-BLACKWELL**
A John Wiley & Sons, Ltd., Publication

This edition first published 2009, © 2009 by Blackwell Publishing

Blackwell Publishing was acquired by John Wiley & Sons in February 2007. Blackwell's publishing programme has been merged with Wiley's global Scientific, Technical and Medical business to form Wiley-Blackwell.

*Registered office:* John Wiley & Sons Ltd, The Atrium, Southern Gate, Chichester, West Sussex, PO19 8SQ, UK

*Editorial offices:* 9600 Garsington Road, Oxford, OX4 2DQ, UK
      The Atrium, Southern Gate, Chichester, West Sussex, PO19 8SQ, UK
      111 River Street, Hoboken, NJ 07030-5774, USA

For details of our global editorial offices, for customer services and for information about how to apply for permission to reuse the copyright material in this book please see our website at www.wiley.com/wiley-blackwell

Wiley also publishes its books in a variety of electronic formats. Some content that appears in print may not be available in electronic books.

Designations used by companies to distinguish their products are often claimed as trademarks. All brand names and product names used in this book are trade names, service marks, trademarks or registered trademarks of their respective owners. The publisher is not associated with any product or vendor mentioned in this book. This publication is designed to provide accurate and authoritative information in regard to the subject matter covered. It is sold on the understanding that the publisher is not engaged in rendering professional services. If professional advice or other expert assistance is required, the services of a competent professional should be sought.

The contents of this work are intended to further general scientific research, understanding, and discussion only and are not intended and should not be relied upon as recommending or promoting a specific method, diagnosis, or treatment by physicians for any particular patient. The publisher and the author make no representations or warranties with respect to the accuracy or completeness of the contents of this work and specifically disclaim all warranties, including without limitation any implied warranties of fitness for a particular purpose. In view of ongoing research, equipment modifications, changes in governmental regulations, and the constant flow of information relating to the use of medicines, equipment, and devices, the reader is urged to review and evaluate the information provided in the package insert or instructions for each medicine, equipment, or device for, among other things, any changes in the instructions or indication of usage and for added warnings and precautions. Readers should consult with a specialist where appropriate. The fact that an organization or Website is referred to in this work as a citation and/or a potential source of further information does not mean that the author or the publisher endorses the information the organization or Website may provide or recommendations it may make. Further, readers should be aware that Internet Websites listed in this work may have changed or disappeared between when this work was written and when it is read. No warranty may be created or extended by any promotional statements for this work. Neither the publisher nor the author shall be liable for any damages arising herefrom.

*Library of Congress Cataloging-in-Publication Data*

Tropical diseases in travelers / edited by Eli Schwartz.
   p. ; cm.
  Includes index.
  ISBN 978-1-4051-8441-0
  1. Tropical medicine. 2. Travel—Health aspects. I. Schwartz, Eli, Dr.
  [DNLM: 1. Tropical Medicine—methods. 2. Communicable Disease Control—methods. 3. Travel. WC 680 T8557 2009]
  RC961.T736 2009
  616.9′993—dc22

                                                     2008055877

A catalogue record for this book is available from the British Library.

Set in 9.25/11.5pt Minion by Aptara® Inc., New Delhi, India
Printed and bound in Singapore by Fabulous Printers Pte Ltd

1   2009

*Dedicated with love*
*to my wife Carmela and our children, Miriam, Aviad, and Naama*

# Contents

# Contributors

**Henry Abramovitch PhD**
Department of Medical Education,
Sackler School of Medicine,
Tel Aviv University,
Tel Aviv, Israel

**Elizabeth D. Barnett MD**
Maxwell Finland Laboratory for Infectious
Diseases,
Boston Medical Center,
Boston, Massachusetts, USA

**Johannes A. Blum MD**
Swiss Tropical Institute,
Basel, Switzerland

**Enrico Brunetti MD**
 University of Pavia
and
IRCCS S. Matteo Hospital Foundation,
Pavia, Italy

**Eric Caumes MD**
Département des Maladies Infectieuses
et Tropicales,
Hôpital Pitié-Salpêtrière,
University Pierre et Marie Curie,
Paris, France

**Peter L. Chiodini MD**
Department of Parasitology,
Hospital for Tropical Diseases
and
London School of Hygiene and
Tropical Medicine,
London, UK

**Michal Chowers MD**
Sakler School of Medicine,
Tel Aviv University,
Tel Aviv, Israel
and
Infectious Disease Unit,

Meir Medical Center,
Kfar Saba, Israel

**Bradley A. Connor MD**
Division of Gastroenterology and
Hepatology,
Weill Medical College of Cornell University,
New York, USA

**Herbert L. DuPont MD**
The University of Texas–Houston School
of Public Health and Medical School,
and
Baylor College of Medicine
and
St. Luke's Episcopal Hospital,
Houston, Texas, USA

**Michael Ehrenfeld MD**
Chaim Sheba Medical Center,
Tel-Hashomer
and
Tel Aviv University Faculty of Medicine,
Tel Aviv, Israel

**David O. Freedman MD**
Division of Infectious Diseases,
University of Alabama at Birmingham,
Birmingham, Alabama, USA

**Thiravat Hemachudha MD**
Faculty of Medicine,
Chulalongkorn University,
Bangkok, Thailand

**Joanna S. Herman MD**
Department of Parasitology,
Hospital for Tropical Diseases,
London, UK

**Nancy Piper Jenks CFNP**
Hudson River Healthcare,
Peekskill, New York, USA

**Mogens Jensenius MD**
Ullevål University Hospital,
Oslo, Norway

**Jay S. Keystone MD**
Division of Infectious Disease,
Toronto General Hospital,
University of Toronto,
Toronto, Ontario, Canada

**Phyllis E. Kozarsky MD**
Division of Infectious Diseases,
Emory University School of Medicine,
Atlanta, Georgia, USA

**Karin Leder MD**
Royal Melbourne Hospital,
University of Melbourne
and
Monash University,
Victoria, Australia

**Eyal Leshem MD**
Chaim Sheba Medical Center,
Tel Hashomer, Israel
and
Sackler School of Medicine,
Tel Aviv University,
Tel Aviv, Israel

**Eyal Meltzer MD**
Chaim Sheba Medical Center,
Tel Hashomer, Israel
and
Sackler School of Medicine,
Tel Aviv University,
Tel Aviv, Israel

**R. Scott Miller**
Walter Reed Army Institute of Research,
Silver Spring, Maryland, USA

**Thomas B. Nutman MD**
Laboratory of Parasitic Diseases,
National Institutes of Health,
Bethesda, Maryland, USA

**Philippe Parola MD**
Hôpital d'Instruction des Armées, Laveran
and
Institut de Médecine Tropicale de Service de
Sante des Armées, Le Pharo,
Marseille, France

**Pamela Rendi-Wagner MD**
Department of Epidemiology and
Preventive Medicine,
Tel Aviv University,
Tel Aviv, Israel
and
Department of Specific Prophylaxis and
Tropical Medicine,
Medical University Vienna,
Vienna, Austria

**Eli Schwartz MD**
Chaim Sheba Medical Center,
Tel Hashomer, Israel
and

Sackler School of Medicine,
Tel Aviv University,
Tel Aviv, Israel

**Michael J. Segel MD**
Chaim Sheba Medical Center,
Tel Hashomer, Israel

**Gil Sidi MD**
Department of Infectious Diseases,
Memorial Sloan Kettering Cancer Center,
New York, USA

**Fabrice Simon MD**
Hôpital d'Instruction des Armées, Laveran
and
Institut de Médecine Tropicale du Service de
Santé des Armées, Le Pharo,
Marseille, France

**John Simon MD**
University of Hong Kong,
Hong Kong, China

**Joseph Torresi MD**
Department of Infectious Diseases,
Austin Hospital,
The University of Melbourne,
Heidelberg, Victoria, Australia

**Elodie Vivier MD**
Hôpital d'Instruction des Armées Laveran,
Marseille, France

**Henry Wilde MD**
Faculty of Medicine,
Chulalongkorn University,
Bangkok, Thailand

**Annelies Wilder-Smith MD**
Division of Infectious Diseases,
National University of Singapore
and
Duke-NUS,
Singapore

**Einar P. Wilder-Smith MD**
Division of Neurology,
National University of Singapore
Singapore

# Foreword

It is with great pleasure that I write this preface to a new and valuable book, *Tropical Diseases in Travelers*, edited by Professor Eli Schwartz. Professor Schwartz has assembled a diverse, international, and very talented team of contributors to address an important, yet underappreciated, concept in tropical and travel medicine. The clinical presentations of infectious disease may be different in the non-immune, infrequently exposed traveler than the immune and multiply exposed inhabitant in a tropical environment.

The classic descriptions of the great tropical diseases began to appear in the 1800s as the Western powers began their imperial era in the Indian subcontinent, China, Southeast Asia, and, finally, in Sub-Saharan Africa. Suddenly, soldiers, businessmen, missionaries, and settlers needed to run the Western empires became casualties of infectious diseases of the tropics. Even in those early days, clinicians recognized that clinical presentations in otherwise healthy, non-immune, well-nourished adults were different from those seen in the native populations. The reasons for this difference included the size and frequency of the infectious inoculum, the lack of any prior immunity from past exposures or maternal immunity, and the fact that local populations often had a complex background of malnutrition, multiple co-infections, and far advanced diseases.

Symptoms in travelers are caused by far fewer organisms, leading to acute presentations with exuberant immune reactions in the non-immune. Symptoms in local populations may be manifest after years of multiple infections, with a large organism burden, organ system damage from years of inflammation, and chronic disability. Finally, the genetic background of travelers is distinctly different than the local population that have co-evolved with infections, such as malaria.

Acute and chronic schistosomiasis are excellent examples. The acute syndrome can be seen following a single exposure to fresh water and is caused by only a few adult worms, leading to an immune-mediated acute syndrome (Katayama fever). In travelers, subsequent clinical disease is often related to sporadic ectopic egg deposition that leads to catastrophic neurologic involvement, dermatologic presentations, or other bizarre syndromes. Chronic schistosomiasis occurs after years of exposure, the presence of hundreds of adult worms, and the near continuous deposition of eggs into the portal circulation leading to cirrhosis and portal hypertension. These are two very different diseases that occur in the local population or the returning traveler.

This book also includes historically important diseases such as typhoid fever, which used to be more common in the developed world, and leptospirosis, which has a cosmopolitan distribution, but is more commonly encountered in the developing world. Providers of travel medicine may be the first to encounter these patients.

Information on how tropical diseases present in travelers has never before been captured in a single, easy-to-access publication. Professor Schwartz, as book editor and co-author of numerous chapters, is eminently qualified for this task. He has been an original thinker in travel medicine, always pushing the discipline to question dogma and to consider new approaches. The other contributors are also all experts in their field.

Travel medicine is a relatively new discipline that has focused on the pre-travel aspect of traveler needs. This new book is the first to summarize the knowledge of post-travel presentations in the otherwise non-immune and non-endemic population. With such focus, this book will be useful to all practitioners, including primary care and infectious disease clinicians, who encounter the post-travel patient. .

*Tropical Diseases in Travelers* is presented in four sections. Following a useful general introduction is a detailed discussion of multiple viral, bacterial, and parasitic infections. The third clinically relevant section on the syndromic approach to patients will be useful in evaluating returning travelers with symptoms. The book concludes with two helpful appendixes.

In the globally connected world of the twenty-first century, the lines of travel and tropical medicine are blurred. Immigrants and refugees, displaced and discarded in their own world, may turn up at your first-world doorstep as tropical medicine patients, whereas soldiers and humanitarian workers may present with clinical presentations in the developing world, confusing those used to caring for local populations. The same infectious agent can lead to dramatically different diseases, depending on the background immunity of the host, access to timely care, and the pathogen load in the body. This book will help us all to see the differences.

*Alan Magill MD, FACP, FIDSA*
*Director, Division of Experimental Therapeutics,*
*Walter Reed Army Institute of Research*
*President, International Society of Travel Medicine*
*(ISTM), 2009–2011*

# Acknowledgments

I would like to begin by thanking the publisher, Blackwell-Wiley, for recognizing the value of a special volume on tropical diseases in travelers and for helping to bring this book to fruition. Special thanks go to Robin Bonner and Eleanor Umali of Aptara, for their dedication to the book's production and their commitment to meeting our target date for publication.

My gratitude goes to all of the contributors for their efforts and for sharing their experience and expertise to produce such high-quality chapters. My special thanks to Nancy Piper-Jenks for her invaluable assistance during the writing of this book. I would also like to thank my colleagues at the Center of Geographic Medicine and at the Department of Medicine C at Sheba Medical Center, Tel Hashomer, for engaging in constant dialogue with me over the years concerning these topics and for their support during the writing of *Tropical Diseases in Travelers*.

I end with our ancient verse: "Much have I learnt from my masters, more from my colleagues, but the most from my own students" [*Talmud of Babylon*, Tractate Taanit, 6].

By the same token, I would like to thank all of my teachers and colleagues, in Israel and abroad, from whom I have learned a great deal. However, a special thanks is dedicated to my patients, from whom I have learned the most.

# Tropical Diseases in Travelers—General Aspects

# 1

# Introduction

## Eli Schwartz

Chaim Sheba Medical Center, Tel Hashomer, Israel and Sackler School of Medicine, Tel Aviv University, Tel Aviv, Israel

The explosion of global travel during recent decades has been well documented, and it has become common to see travelers from the developed world venturing to more and more remote corners of our planet. Exotic travel exposes people to exotic diseases, which they subsequently take with them to other places. The SARS (severe acute respiratory syndrome) epidemic illustrates how one person, who journeyed from an endemic area of China to Hong Kong, was able to infect several people at a hotel, who themselves became infected transporters of SARS, allowing its worldwide spread. A more recent example is the Chikungunia outbreak that began in the regions of the Indian Ocean and spread to Africa and India. Travelers then carried the disease into Europe, thus causing its documented autochthonous outbreak in Italy. Therefore, tropical diseases are no longer confined to the tropics.

The term *tropical diseases* is not limited to ailments acquired from a particular tropical geographic area of the world. Indeed, tropical diseases such as yellow fever and malaria were once a very important cause of morbidity and mortality in regions as far north as Boston, USA. Instead, we are referring to diseases acquired in the developing world, where public health standards are lower and hygiene and sanitation are not customary. For this reason, we are encountering numerous infectious diseases that were at one point endemic worldwide and had been controlled or eradicated in industrialized countries during the twentieth century.

As physicians who encounter returning travelers with various tropical diseases, we see a clear picture of these so-called "exotic diseases" presenting in a unique fashion in travelers. In fact, these diseases tend to manifest very differently in nonimmune travelers than in indigenous populations of the tropics. Textbooks focusing on tropical diseases understandably limit their descriptions to the classical presentation of such tropical diseases, with descriptions of these diseases in indigenous populations, not in travelers.

The significant distinctions between travelers to developing countries and local residents are apparent through differences in the types of infections commonly seen in the two populations, as well as in the clinical presentations and management of these diseases.

*Epidemiologically,* these distinctions reflect differences in the likelihood of exposure to the infections, as well as intensity of exposure, which is typically higher among indigenous populations. For example, melioidosis (caused by the gram-negative soil- and water-associated bacterium *Burkholderia pseudomallei*) is a common cause of community-acquired sepsis in northern Thailand, yet the disease is rarely seen in travelers. The same is true for trypanosomiasis (sleeping sickness), filarial infections, and cholera, which are rarely seen in travelers.

Outbreaks of yellow fever are commonly reported among local residents in endemic regions, but are virtually never seen in travelers—in this case, most likely because of their high uptake of the efficacious yellow fever vaccine.

Disparate *background immunity* also affects the way in which some diseases manifest. For example, malaria in adult populations in endemic countries may not cause life-threatening disease, whereas in traveler populations, even low-grade parasitemia may cause a severe and life-threatening condition.

In many developing countries, hepatitis A is not viewed as an important problem because most children are infected at a young age, when infection is mild and often unrecognized. Older children and adults are therefore immune to the disease. However, the virus regularly contaminates food and water and poses a significant threat to nonimmune travelers who enter the area.

*Clinical manifestations* are also often different. These manifestations may be based on previous immunity and/or other not-yet-defined immunological causes. Excellent examples are the manifestations of infection with the various species of schistosome worms. This disease,

*Tropical Diseases in Travelers*, 1st edition. Edited by E. Schwartz.
© 2009 by Blackwell Publishing, ISBN: 978-1-4051-8441-0.

which is one of the most common infections in the tropics, is a leading cause of morbidity due to late and chronic stages of infection (i.e., hematuria, urinary retention, in *Schistosoma hematobium* infection, and portal hypertension with *S. mansoni*). These manifestations, however, are rarely seen in travelers. They most commonly present with acute schistosomiasis, which occurs several weeks after exposure and leads to Katayama syndrome, a hypersensitivity reaction to the helminth antigen. Katayama syndrome is in fact the principal presentation of schistosomiasis in travelers, causing significant morbidity, whereas among local residents, it is virtually nonexistent, and therefore barely discussed in tropical disease textbooks.

Malaria is another example, in that it always presents as a significant febrile disease among nonimmune travelers and yet it can often occur without fever among local populations.

*Methods of diagnosis* may differ. For example, in endemic countries, diagnosing helminth infections among the indigenous population is done by finding ova in the stool. Serology is usually inadequate because it cannot differentiate between current and past infection and, therefore, will almost always be positive.

In the case of travelers, however, the situation is the contrary; due to low worm burden, ova are infrequently found in stool. Moreover, because travelers can present with illness during the helminthic migration phase, detection of ova in stool is biologically unlikely. Therefore, the most important diagnostic tools in travelers are serological methods.

There are also variations in *treatment*. There are common misconceptions that the best available treatments and most knowledgeable approaches to the treatment of tropical diseases are found in endemic countries. In tropical countries, the most accessible drugs are low-cost medicine, rather than the best available. Thus, malaria may still be treated in local populations with older drugs to which resistance has developed; however, for the nonimmune traveler, this treatment may be fatal.

As another example, we have shown that the most effective (albeit expensive) treatment of *Leishmania braziliensis* is liposomal amphotericin B; yet, antimonial drugs, which are older and more toxic drugs, are used in endemic countries because of their lower costs. Thus, choosing the correct drug and dosage should be tailored to nonimmune travelers.

The study of tropical diseases in travelers offers the advantage of exploring the natural history of these diseases in a clearer light. First of all, these tropical diseases present in nonimmune travelers, resulting in a more accurate picture of their natural history. In addition, there are generally fewer confounders or additional infections (e.g., malnutrition, HIV, or other tropical disease infections) that might impact the natural history of the disease.

The fact that there is usually more thorough patient follow-up in industrialized countries offers an opportunity for further assessment of the outcomes of infectious diseases over the long term. For example, assessing the efficacy of malaria prophylaxis for *Plasmodium vivax* infection can hardly be done in an endemic area because late infection cannot be differentiated from re-infection. However, there are opportunities for long-term follow-up in travelers who return to nonendemic countries. Indeed, observing returning travelers from vivax endemic areas has allowed us to conclude that current malaria prophylaxis is actually inadequate for vivax prevention.

The study of infectious diseases in travelers may also elucidate the natural history of many cosmopolitan diseases, such as leptospirosis, that are seen less frequently these days in industrialized countries. Sporadic cases and outbreaks do occur in industrialized countries, although they tend to be missed by clinicians. The understanding of diseases in travelers can contribute to the clinician's knowledge and awareness of disease when it occurs at home.

Practicing travel medicine may also help in managing patients who have not traveled, such as those with diarrheal diseases. The evaluation of patients with diarrheal diseases in the travel clinic is a large part of everyday practice and can teach non-travel-medicine practitioners about differential diagnosis and methods of detection and management, so that lengthy and expensive evaluations may not be necessary.

Travel medicine is a relatively new discipline and is a subspecialty that has continued to evolve over recent years. A number of textbooks that focus on pretravel health issues and the prevention of illness in travelers are now available.

This book is a first attempt at drawing together knowledge accumulated in recent years in the area of "posttravel"—those issues concerning the manifestation of tropical diseases and their diagnosis and treatment in travelers. The traveler, as a sentinel, has given us the opportunity to observe these diseases from another perspective. This knowledge can help us to understand better the morbidity and mortality of these diseases and, more important, to appropriately evaluate and treat the traveler who may be ill upon returning home.

# 2

# The Art of Travel Medicine a Century Ago

Eli Schwartz

Chaim Sheba Medical Center, Tel Hashomer, Israel and Sackler School of Medicine, Tel Aviv University, Tel Aviv, Israel

In a lecture given about one hundred years ago, Sir Patrick Manson addressed an issue that remains highly relevant today. The title of his lecture was "Diagnosis of Fever in Patients from the Tropics."

As a reminder, Dr. Patrick Manson (1844–1922) was a British parasitologist (born in Scotland) and founder of the field of tropical medicine. He was the first to discover (1877–1879) that filariasis (*Filaria bancrofti*) is a mosquito-borne disease; transmission of a disease by an insect was a revolutionary idea at the time. He hypothesized that malaria could also be transmitted by mosquitoes, which was subsequently proven to be correct through the research of Sir Ronald Ross in India.

In 1890, Dr. Manson settled in London, where he organized the London School of Tropical Medicine (1899). He was knighted in 1903 and continued to practice medicine until his death. His fieldwork in several tropical regions of the world led him to his pioneer observations on tropical diseases, which were then also used to treat colonists and soldiers who encountered infectious diseases unknown in the temperate European climate. His book *Tropical Diseases* (1898) became the classic textbook on this subject.

The British Empire at this time ruled over a vast and expansive domain, encompassing about a quarter of Earth's total land area; as was often said, "The sun never sets on the British Empire." From a medical point of view, this meant that repatriating soldiers or other British officials back to the UK took several weeks, which is a long period of time, exceeding the incubation time of many diseases.

Dr. Manson's lecture (Appendix, this chapter), which was published in the *British Medical Journal* in 1909 [1], may shed some light on the common diseases among travelers of that time, as well as highlight some of the

changes that have occurred both in the tropics and in industrialized countries since then (Table 2.1).

The major points that I would like to highlight include the following.

## The common mistakes among clinicians who see the returned traveler from the tropics

The most important mistake, according to Manson, was the overdiagnosis of "tropical disease" among those who returned to the UK. He called on the diagnostician to "disabuse his mind" of thinking that any fever occurring in a patient from the tropics must be a tropical fever. He was concerned that cosmopolitan diseases, which were the common diseases of his time, would be ignored by physicians. The significant mundane diseases of his time were tuberculosis, syphilis, typhoid, sepsis, and malignant diseases.

In our era, there are two major changes. First and foremost is that the ordinary infectious diseases that Manson mentioned no longer occur routinely in industrialized countries, which corresponds to the changes in epidemiology of diseases throughout the twentieth century. Although, at the beginning of the twentieth century, infectious diseases continued to be the leading cause of morbidity and mortality, with improved hygienic conditions, followed by the introduction of vaccines and antibiotics, there was a progressive decline of infectious diseases [2]. The current situation is that cardiovascular and malignant diseases are the major causes of mortality, whereas infectious diseases account for only about 5% of mortality, in contrast to the current situation in developing countries, where infectious diseases are still the major cause of death (Figures 2.1a and 2.1b) [3].

*Tropical Diseases in Travelers*, 1st edition. Edited by E. Schwartz.
© 2009 by Blackwell Publishing, ISBN: 978-1-4051-8441-0.

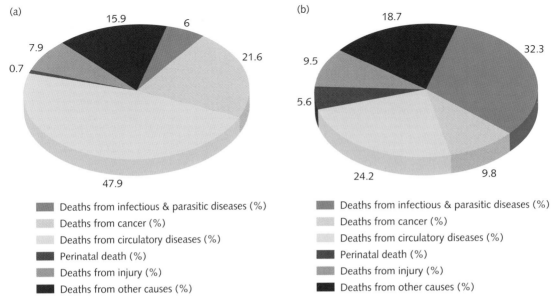

(a)

15.9 6

7.9

0.7

21.6

47.9

(b)

18.7

32.3

9.5

5.6

24.2 9.8

Deaths from infectious & parasitic diseases (%)
Deaths from cancer (%)
Deaths from circulatory diseases (%)
Perinatal death (%)
Deaths from injury (%)
Deaths from other causes (%)

Deaths from infectious & parasitic diseases (%)
Deaths from cancer (%)
Deaths from circulatory diseases (%)
Perinatal death (%)
Deaths from injury (%)
Deaths from other causes (%)

**Figure 2.1** Causes of mortality. (a) Developed world. (b) Developing world.

The second development, which followed the first, is that the principal question of differential diagnosis in returning travelers today is not between tropical infectious diseases and ordinary infectious diseases but rather between tropical infectious diseases and chronic, often incurable Western diseases. Our role in dealing with the health of returning travelers therefore is to re-emphasize to physicians who practice medicine in the industrialized world that infectious diseases still exist in the world. Travelers returning from endemic areas may carry with them an infectious disease that could be either life-threatening, or associated with intolerable symptoms, and which, in either case, may have the potential of a simple and rapid cure. An example of the latter is a returned traveler with a few weeks of diarrhea. A Western physician may tend to think about chronic conditions such as inflammatory bowel disease or malignancy and may fail to consider the possibility of parasitic infections such as giardiasis that can be cured within a few days of treatment.

## The importance of malaria

One of the issues that appears to be constant throughout this period of a century is the importance of malaria. Malaria was the commonest of all tropical febrile infections in Manson's time. This remains unchanged in our era and in almost all case series of febrile ill returned travelers, malaria is the leading cause (see Chapter 3).

However, he stated that "there is no disease so easily and so surely recognized as malaria." He made this statement in spite of the fact that a laboratory diagnosis of malaria was not easily made as compared to this day and age. A malaria diagnosis one hundred years ago was based on one of three options, in the following order of importance:

One was the *periodic character of fever*, demonstrating a rise in fever every 2–3 days.

The second option was the result of a *therapeutic trial of quinine*, a successful trial showing a response within 48–72 hours.

Last, diagnosis was made with the use of a *microscope*. To have a reliable microscopic test, the patient could not be under quinine treatment, but just as important, the microscopist "should know his business." According to Manson, extensive training was needed to make an accurate diagnosis and to avoid "comic" mistakes.

Currently, in travelers with malaria who present usually within a few days after the onset of their fever, the synchronous pattern of the fever with a periodicity of 2–3 days (tertian malaria) is rarely seen (see Chapter 21). Thus, diagnosis must be based on the malaria smear. The lack of experience of microscopists continues to be an important issue, particularly because most laboratory technicians have not seen many cases of malaria. Therefore, there are ongoing attempts to find easier, friendlier methods for

**Table 2.1** Comparison of the status of diseases during Manson period and our time.

| Travel-related diseases in the 1900s | Status of diseases in 1900s | Status of the diseases in the 2000s |
| --- | --- | --- |
| Malaria—leading cause | Common | Malaria—leading cause |
| Hepatitis | | Hepatitis is almost never seen in travelers owing to vaccine |
| | | Hepatitis E—on the rise |
| Liver abscess | | Liver abscess—occasionally seen |
| Brucellosis | | Brucellosis—hardly seen |
| Visceral leishmaniasis (Kala-Azar) | Less common | Seen as co-infection in HIV patients |
| Trypanosoma | | Rarely seen |
| Filaria | | Rarely seen |
| Relapsing fever | | Rarely seen, and mainly from recreational activities in *developed* countries |
| Dengue fever | Not seen | Very common |
| Yellow fever | | Very rare owing to vaccine effect |
| Typhoid, tuberculosis, syphilis | Cosmopolitan | Now mostly tropical diseases |
| Endocarditis, sepsis | | Cosmopolitan diseases, but rarely seen |
| Malignancy | | Not a common cause for fever |

malaria diagnosis. In recent years the antigen-detection rapid test has become a helpful tool, although it cannot replace malaria smears (see Chapter 22). Further development of the polymerase chain reaction (PCR) method for commercial use may significantly improve our ability to diagnose malaria and more accurately identify the malaria species.

However, the most common and the most important problem we encounter these days in malaria diagnosis in industrialized countries is the lack of physician awareness of the risk of malaria exposure in returning travelers and their failure to consider malaria as a potential cause of fever. The mortality rate from malaria in Western countries is high, reaching about 2–3% of all falciparum cases, and about 10–15% among patients with severe malaria. An important factor in this poor outcome is the delay of diagnosis by physicians [4].

Malaria was a common disease in Dr. Manson's time, but it seemed to be, as it currently is in the hyperendemic countries, a "background" disease. Therefore, another important message he wanted to convey was not to miss other diagnoses due to a self-proclaimed malaria diagnosis. As he described at that time, when the patient came in and told the doctor that he had malaria, the reason for his visit was principally to get treatment for his own diagnosis. Under the name of "malaria fever," the patient might in fact have tuberculosis, endocarditis, a liver abscess, or

other illnesses. This is not the case today with returning travelers, but this situation reminds us of scenarios in endemic countries (mainly in Sub-Saharan Africa), where many illnesses are attributed to malaria without a thorough examination and definitive diagnosis, thus missing many other treatable diseases [5].

## The incubation time

Although Dr. Manson did not mention the term "incubation period" directly, he clearly mentioned several diseases that were not relevant to the practitioner seeing the returning patient. The two major examples he gave were dengue fever and yellow fever; these diseases "need not to be considered." These diseases belong to the flaviviruses and were well known at that time. Yellow fever was a major killer during the period (e.g., it was one of the major foes during the Panama Canal construction). However, these viral infections have short incubation periods of about 1 week. Transportation during that era was mainly by sea, which meant that the travel time from most areas in the British empire back to London was lengthy, eliminating diseases with short incubation times. (Around the world even in 80 days was an illusion, as illustrated by the classic science fiction novel written by Jules Verne, who lived during the same period.)

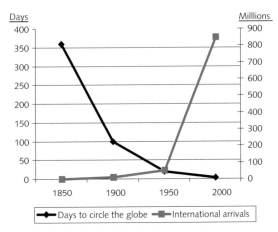

**Figure 2.2** Around the world in 80 days?

One of the major changes that began during the second part of the twentieth century was the public aviation service, which today enables us to circumnavigate the globe within 36 hours (Figure 2.2). The idea corresponding to this change, that "the world has become a global village," assumes medical significance in that the incubation time is no longer a barrier in transmitting disease from one side of the globe to the other. Add to this the fact that traveling outside country borders is no longer confined to a select group of people but instead has become a popular trend (approximately 900 million travelers annually), and the public health significance is obvious.

In relation to the diseases mentioned above, dengue is widespread worldwide and has become the most prevalent arbovirus. For travelers, it is a major threat and is seen very often. According to the GeoSentinel data, dengue is now the second most common disease in returning travelers and is the first cause of fever outside Sub-Saharan Africa (see Chapter 7).

Yellow fever is rarely seen in travelers, but this is a result of another change that has occurred since Dr. Manson's time—the development of a highly effective vaccine, which has dramatically changed the morbidity map of the disease.

### The vigilance needed for the clinician who sees these patients

In Western medicine, we are taught that we should try to find one disease that will explain or encompass all of the patient's symptoms. In tropical medicine, we should be alert to the possibility of multiple infections. The "zoo phenomenon," which refers to a patient's acquiring several pathogens, is not uncommon, especially in dealing with intestinal infections. Additionally, febrile infections can be caused by simultaneous infections (see Chapter 37).

Manson urges his audience not to fall into the trap of limiting findings to one diagnosis, and if there is just one diagnosis, to be sure that it fully explains the case. During this time, he stated, "In tropical disease, malaria is apt to complicate everything, so that multiple infection is rather the rule rather than the exception." In our time, that might be the rule in the malaria-endemic countries, but it is not the rule among travelers. However, vigilance is needed, and whenever the course of the disease does not correspond with the specific diagnosis, a search for another pathogen should be made.

The shrinking world, a process that has progressed rapidly since the time of Manson, has led to the border crossing of many diseases. Thus, physicians now must be familiar with many diseases, irrespective of their geographic locations and incubation time. In addition, there is a substantial increase in the number of travelers, who are mostly short-term travelers, not the long-term expatriates as seen by Manson, and therefore not immune to diseases from outside of their own environment. These conditions of the twenty-first century have shed new light on and revealed new aspects of the old tropical diseases. Physicians in the West are thus further challenged to understand and manage this vast array of travel and tropical diseases.

### References

1 Manson P. An address on the diagnosis of fever in patients from the tropics: delivered at a meeting of the Westminster Division of the Metropolitan Counties Branch. *Br Med J* 1909;1:704–6.
2 Armstrong GL, Conn LA, Pinner RW. Trends in infectious disease mortality in the United States during the 20th century. *JAMA* 1999;281:61–6.
3 WHO (2002) 2nd ed. National Cancer Control Programme, Policies and Managerial Guidelines. World Health Organization, Geneva.
4 Kain KC, Harrington MA, Tennyson S, Keystone JS. Imported malaria: prospective analysis of problems in diagnosis and management. *Clin Infect Dis* 1998;27:142–9.
5 Amexo M, Tolhurst R, Barnish G, Bates I. Malaria misdiagnosis: effects on the poor and vulnerable. *Lancet* 2004; 364:1896–8.

## Appendix: "Diagnosis of Fever in Patients from the Tropics," by Sir Patrick Manson (1909) [1]

### An Address
#### ON THE
## DIAGNOSIS OF FEVER IN PATIENTS FROM THE TROPICS.

DELIVERED AT A MEETING OF THE WESTMINSTER DIVISION OF THE METROPOLITAN COUNTIES BRANCH.

BY

SIR PATRICK MANSON, K.C.M.G., M.D., LL.D., F.R.S.

I HAVE twenty minutes in which to speak about certain points which have to be attended to in attempting the diagnosis of fevers in patients coming from the tropics. The time is very short. I shall not waste it, therefore, in preliminaries, but proceed at once to my subject.

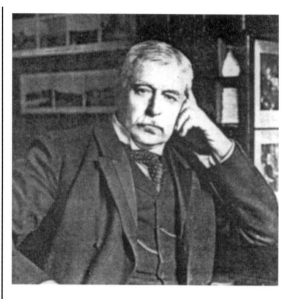

#### Sources of Fallacy.

The first point I shall urge is a very important one. It is the necessity for the diagnostician to disabuse his mind of the very natural idea that because a fever has been contracted in or is occurring in a patient from the tropics it must necessarily be a tropical fever, symptomatic of some infection or condition peculiar to the tropics. This in my experience is one of the commonest and most misleading diagnostic fallacies. It so happens that my line of practice lies in great measure among patients from the tropics; but I am bound to say that half the patients from the tropics sent to me for an opinion or who come to me under the idea that they are suffering from tropical disease are not so suffering, although very likely they have fallen sick in the tropics or soon after return from the tropics. When you have dealings with a Scotsman you are apt to be obsessed with the preconceived idea of the national reputation for canniness, forgetting that, in the main, Scotsmen are very like other men, having the same physical, moral, and mental attributes. Just so, and perhaps even more so, in our contemplation of disease from the tropics. The major portion of a Scotsman's attributes is that of other men; only a very minor portion is peculiar. The major portion of disease in and from the tropics is ordinary disease; the minor portion special. Therefore when you encounter a fever in a patient from the tropics, think last and least (unless the diagnosis be glaringly obvious) of a tropical fever. Think first of and carefully test for these great and pandemic conditions—tuberculosis, syphilis, typhoid, malignant disease, and sepsis. If the seat and nature of the disease are not at once obvious, make it an inflexible rule to go over all the organs systematically, one after the other, beginning at the vertex and ending at the soles of the feet. I could tell many a story illustrative of the wisdom and necessity for this precaution—so obvious when stated thus pointedly, but, like so many other obvious things, so frequently overlooked or ignored. This is the first and perhaps the most important point I would make.

The next and equally obvious point I would impress on you is not to be misled by the diagnosis of malaria which in many instances the patient is nearly sure to volunteer. Patients' statements in this respect are apt to be very positive and correspondingly impressive. Such tropical cases come to you not so much with the idea of your diagnosing their fever as with the idea of getting you to treat them on their own diagnosis. I have seen many cases of tuberculosis, of endocarditis, of liver abscess, of pyelitis, of syphilis overlooked for this reason. It should be an axiom with us never, without a thorough and independent examination, to accept another man's diagnosis, least of all a patient's diagnosis.

Having excluded as far as you can these sources of fallacy, then, and only then, you may conclude that the fever, let us suppose, you are trying to diagnose is probably a tropical one. Your next step should be to put to yourself the question, What are the tropical diseases likely to be brought to this country and which are associated with fever? Of course, we may safely exclude such acute and short fevers as yellow fever, dengue, and so forth; these need not be considered.

#### Tropical Fevers.

Let me enumerate what I might designate the important tropical fevers in the approximate order of the frequency with which they present themselves in practice here. First of all, of course, comes malaria; next, perhaps, hepatitis and liver abscess; then Mediterranean or Malta fever; next, and at a long interval, kala-azar, trypanosomiasis and sleeping sickness, relapsing fever, elephantoid fever, and probably other infections about which we as yet know nothing, but only suspect their existence. Each of the fevers I have mentioned has some feature or features by which it may be recognized, or, at all events, suspected.

*Tests of Malaria.*

Manifestly our first duty is to recognize or to exclude the commonest of them all—namely, malaria. Fortunately, this is easily done. Provided we set about it in the proper way and have a little time allowed us there is no disease so easily and so surely recognizable as malaria, for of this infection we have not one or two, but three absolutely pathognomonic tests. I am in the habit of describing these tests as, *first*, the clinical test of periodicity; *secondly*, the therapeutical test of the action of quinine; and *thirdly*, the microscopical test, the determination of the presence or absence of the malaria parasite or of its product, malarial pigment, in the blood.

There are other indications of malarial infection, such as leucopenia with relative increase of the large mononuclear leucocytes, enlargement of the spleen, and anaemia. These are only of relative value. Their absence is strong evidence against malaria, but their presence, seeing that they occur in other tropical diseases, does not prove the presence of malaria. They are not absolutely diagnostic in the same sense as are the three tests I have just mentioned, and need not be further considered.

The most important clinical test of malaria is *periodicity* —the periodic recurrence of the febrile or other phenomena. Practically all fevers, whether malarial or not, exhibit a periodicity. In tuberculosis, in typhoid, in sepsis, and so forth, there is a regular evening rise and morning fall of temperature, often quite as marked as in malaria. There is very definite quotidian periodicity. Quotidian periodicity is therefore not peculiar to, is no diagnostic mark of, malaria. We do meet with quotidian malarial fevers, especially in malarial countries. But quotidian periodicity, if taken alone, does not justify a diagnosis of malaria. So far from doing so, it is actually misleading. It is perhaps the most frequent cause of erroneous diagnosis in tropical patients. This you can readily understand. A patient from India, for example, comes to you with a story that every afternoon he has a shivering fit followed by a rise of temperature to 103°, and this again after some hours by a drenching sweat. He may mention no other symptoms. You may be in a hurry. You plump for malaria, and you prescribe quinine. The patient does not improve. You make a careful physical examination, and you discover signs of tuberculosis, or of liver abscess, or of some other form of visceral disease.

Quotidian periodicity, therefore, should be absolutely ignored in most cases as an indication of malaria. The periodicity characteristic of malaria, and absolutely diagnostic of that infection, is either a *tertian* or a *quartan periodicity*. These you find in no other condition, and are sure indication of malaria. The only circumstance in which quotidian periodicity may be a help in diagnosis is when the recurring fever sets in very late in the night, say after midnight, or before 12 or 1 o'clock during the day. Such a time for the commencement of a daily fever is almost peculiar to malaria.

The quinine test for malaria has usually been applied more or less intelligently before the case comes under the observation of the consultant. It is reliable if properly applied. Rarely does a malarial fever, in this country at all events, resist adequate dosing with quinine. Ten grains two or three times a day is almost sure in forty-eight to seventy-two hours to tell us whether we are dealing with malaria or not. But in employing this test we must be sure that the quinine is given properly, and that it is absorbed. Very often the quinine is given in adequate dose, but in some insoluble form, as in coated pill, flinty tabloid, or insoluble sulphate. In catarrhal conditions of the stomach given in any of these forms the drug may not be dissolved, much less absorbed, and cannot therefore be regarded as efficiently testing for malaria. When it is of importance that we should be certain of its action, quinine should be given in solution, or, in highly catarrhal or irritable conditions of the stomach, intramuscularly in doses of 7 to 10 grains. If no impression is made on a fever by quinine given in this way, do not blame the drug; revise the diagnosis.

Even more reliable than the clinical or the therapeutical tests of malaria is the microscopical test. If the malaria parasite or its product—haemozoin, or melanin, as it is usually called—is found in the blood, diagnosis is sure. The parasite of malaria is necessarily present at one time or another in the course of all malarial infections; it is always present in the visceral blood, nearly always in the peripheral blood, and, given certain conditions, can be readily demonstrated in the latter. It is necessary, however, to secure these conditions. In the first place the patient must not be under the influence of quinine, in the second place the person who searches for the parasite must know his business. Even a small dose of quinine—one, perhaps, quite insufficient to check the fever—may cause the parasite to disappear temporarily from the peripheral circulation. The possession of a microscope, and even skill in other departments of microscopy, do not always imply ability to recognise the malaria parasite. To do so satisfactorily requires experience—special experience—and long training. It is not a difficult matter, but, as with everything else, you must know how to set about it, and be familiar with the fallacies. It would be a comical list were I to enumerate all the various objects that have been brought to me as specimens of the malaria parasite.

I would warn you, therefore, to be careful about accepting a diagnosis of malaria from an inexperienced microscopist, but I would encourage you to have absolute confidence in the positive diagnosis, and in ninety-nine cases out of a hundred in the negative diagnosis of malaria from an experienced and conscientious microscopist.

*Liver Abscess.*

Assuming that we have to deal with a tropical fever and that by one or all of the tests I have enumerated we have excluded malaria, the question comes to be, which of the several tropical fevers I have mentioned are we dealing with?

Is the case one of liver abscess? The first and all-important question we put is—has the patient had dysentery or diarrhoea? If so there is, to say the least, strong presumption in favour of such diagnosis. We search, therefore, for local signs, for enlargement of the hepatic area, especially upwards, for local pain, oedema, or even redness. We inquire as to anaemia, progressive emaciation, for irritability and depression of mind; we look for a muddy complexion; we inspect the stools, looking for slime or other indications of a former or an existing dysentery; we inquire for a dorsal or right dorsal decubitis, for shoulder pain, and we make a count for the white corpuscles in the blood—a leucopenia being against, a leucocytosis being in favour of, liver abscess. Finally, if the symptoms are reasonably suggestive we explore the liver under chloroform, being prepared to operate at once if abscess is discovered.

### Mediterranean Fever.

We may suspect Mediterranean fever, more especially if the patient has come from Malta, although this disease is by no means unknown elsewhere—as in India, China, and even in Central Africa. The points in favour of a Mediterranean fever diagnosis are an undulant type of the fever, profuse sweats, the occurrence of marked rheumatic pains or of orchitis, and the absence of indications of other disease.

Apart from the symptoms mentioned the evidence for this fever is principally of a negative nature. The fever may assume all sorts of characters. Often it is undulant in type, but as often it is distinctly intermittent and quotidian, often of a low continued type, often a medley of all of these. The serum test is reliable under ideal conditions, but my experience of it in London is the reverse of favourable. When I employ it I usually send the blood to two different laboratories; as often as not I get " positive " from one and " negative " from the other. So I do not trust it here, although, where fresh cultures are obtainable, it is quite as trustworthy as the corresponding test for typhoid, and even more delicate.

### Kala-azar.

We have a patient from India, from China, from the Soudan, or from North Africa. He has a chronic fever, his spleen reaches to near his umbilicus, and his liver is very much enlarged. He has been ill for months; he is anaemic; his tongue is clean and his appetite and digestion are good; he has taken quinine by the pound, and he is gradually going downhill. Probably that patient is suffering from kala-azar—the disease produced by the Leishman body. To make sure of the diagnosis we study the fever chart—a four-hourly one; very likely we note that there are two distinct rises of temperature in the twenty-four hours. We examine the blood; there is a very marked leucopenia, more marked even than in malaria, and there is a relative increase in the large mononuclears. Possibly, though this is not likely, we may find a Leishman body or two, if we search long enough, in the white blood corpuscles. In the presence of such a fever and such a history we are entitled to puncture the spleen or liver and to search for the Leishman body in the juice or fragments of pulp so obtained. Such a procedure is not free from risk and must be done carefully, aseptically, and with a dry needle and syringe. I say " dry needle and syringe," for if a trace of moisture be present in these it will, by endosmosis, so distort the parasites that, though present, they may be hard to recognize. Of course, one must be familiar with the technique for their demonstration and also with the details of the structure of the parasite, for it is exceedingly minute and might be mistaken for a micrococcus or a blood platelet.

### Trypanosomiasis.

The patient comes from tropical Africa. He complains of irregular fever, of great physical and mental lassitude, headache perhaps, tenderness of the limbs when he knocks them against any hard body. You suspect trypanosomiasis. You strip him and inspect his skin. You see great patches of erythema, many inches in diameter, usually having a ringed appearance and looking slightly puffy; you palpate the glands in his neck, axilla, or groin, and you find that some or all of them are enlarged—perhaps only slightly enlarged. The pulse, as a rule, is abnormally quick, and easily excited. That patient is almost surely the subject of trypanosomiasis, and may die of sleeping sickness. Examine his blood with a sixth objective, examining it especially during one of the recurring attacks of fever, and you are almost sure to find the trypanosome. It will not be found in every field of the microscope, and you may have to return to the hunt several times, but in the end you are almost sure to find it. If you fail to find it in the blood, puncture with a hypodermic needle one of the enlarged cervical glands, and examine the lymph so obtained; in it you have even a better chance of finding the parasite. The blood count is very similar to that of kala-azar.

### Relapsing Fever.

The patient comes from India, from tropical Africa, from North Africa, or even from Gibraltar. He tells you that he has attacks of fever, perhaps violent fever, regularly about once a fortnight; that the individual attacks last from three to five or six days, that they subside nearly as suddenly as they begin, and that he is quite free in the interval. He may have had three or four or even eight or nine such attacks. What are they? The blood is negative for malaria; there is no marked leucopenia. Examine the blood during one of the fever paroxysms, and probably you will find the spirochaete of relapsing fever. In the African variety it takes some looking for. If you find it diagnosis is established. Such cases I have seen more than once in recent years in London. They were imported from Africa, from Gibraltar, and from India.

### Elephantoid Fever.

Another patient may tell you he has attacks of violent fever coming on at irregular intervals of weeks, months, or years, that the attacks last for two or three days, and may be attended with severe rigor, delirium, high temperature, and be followed by profuse sweating. If he comes from the West Indies, particularly from Barbados, he will call this disease "fever and ague," but it is not fever and ague as we understand it. It is not malaria, but elephantoid fever for the most part, and if we inquire as to the occurrence of inflammation and cellulitis of limb, scrotum, or acute lymphangitis, we are sure to find that such is the case. The patient is suffering from elephantoid fever, and is or has been the subject of filarial invasion.

The possibility of these various and very different infections should always be present to the diagnostician when he is called on to treat a tropical fever in this country.

### Multiple Infections.

I began with a word of warning; I shall conclude with another word of warning, and it is this: Do not infer because you have found in your patient's blood or elsewhere the malaria or some other parasite, that you have the complete and full explanation of the case. In tropical disease malaria is apt to complicate everything, so that multiple infection of patients is ra r the rule than the exception.

When you find the malaria parasite the patient has certainly got malaria, but that does not exclude other infections. I have sometimes been " caught " in consequence of ignoring this obvious precaution. Some years ago I was asked to see a patient just returned from Portuguese West Africa. He was said to be suffering from fever and dysentery. He had dysentery sure enough, and his spleen was enormously enlarged. He had taken much quinine; as it seemed to irritate his bowels I stopped it. At my first visit he had no fever. I found nothing in his blood. I left instructions that I was to be sent for should he have an attack of fever.

Some days afterwards I was sent for, his temperature being over 103°. I took a slide of his blood, expecting to find in it the parasite of malaria. Judge, however, of my horror when, instead of the malaria parasite, there was an unquestionable trypanosome staring me in the face! After a few days the fever disappeared, and, with the fever, the trypanosome also.

A fortnight later there was again a return of fever, and I again examined the blood, expecting to find the trypanosome. I found no trypanosome, but I found plenty of tertian malaria parasites. And so the case went on, every now and again a fever spell with trypanosomes in the blood, and every now and again a fever spell with malaria parasites in the blood. By the persistent use of atoxyl and of quinine both infections were finally expelled from the circulation. The patient is now, I believe, quite well.

Last year I had in hospital a patient from an African colony who carried about with him the malaria parasite, the trypanosome, the *Spirochaeta pallida*, the filaria, besides an assortment of intestinal parasites, including *Ascaris lumbricoides, Trichiurus trichiurus*, and *Ankylostoma duodenale*—a veritable museum, which, as long as it remained with us, we appreciated very highly at the Tropical School. He could always supply us with a subject for demonstration or for a clinical lecture.

I fear my exposition of the subject has been very sketchy and inadequate; it is necessarily so in consequence of the time limit imposed on me. I trust, however, I have given you the leading points for reliable diagnosis.

# 3 Epidemiology of Post-Travel Illnesses

Pamela Rendi-Wagner[1] and Eli Schwartz[2]

[1]Tel Aviv University, Tel Aviv, Israel and Medical University Vienna, Vienna, Austria
[2]Chaim Sheba Medical Center, Tel Hashomer, Israel and Sackler School of Medicine, Tel Aviv University, Tel Aviv, Israel

## Introduction

Disease surveillance is a prerequisite for the assessment of health risks and the evaluation of established preventive measures. It enables us to identify changing epidemiological patterns and groups of high-risk travelers possibly requiring modifications and optimal targeting of existing intervention concepts or the introduction of novel strategies. Moreover, information on the epidemiology of specific infections also provides guidance for differential diagnoses in ill returned travelers, facilitating the assessment and quantification of disease risks.

International travel is becoming increasingly popular. The current estimate of 846 million international arrivals represents an average growth of 4.2% between 1995 and 2006, with Sub-Saharan Africa being one of the major contributors to this rise. The leading travel destination is Europe, with more than 460 million travelers, followed by Asia, the Americas, the Middle East, and Africa. With regard to long-term prospects, the number of international travelers is expected to reach nearly 1.6 billion by the year 2020 (Figure 3.1) [1].

Undoubtedly, travel is related to enhanced health risks, most notably when travelers visit areas where the communicable disease burden is high, sanitation is poor, and the quality of medical care is limited. Each year, about 50 million people travel from industrialized to developing countries [2]. About 20–70% of international travelers report travel-related illnesses, usually dependent on destination and other travel conditions, including season,

itinerary, duration, and purpose of travel [3, 4]. However, the majority of health problems reported by travelers are mild conditions, such as diarrhea, respiratory infections, and skin disorders [5].

Traveling to endemic countries has become increasingly popular for all age groups. In recent years, the numbers of senior, pregnant, and pediatric travelers have steadily increased. In a population that visited a travel clinic prior to travel, 14% were above 55 years of age [6]. According to an airport survey, 30% of US travelers were 50 years of age or older. Elderly people represent a growing group of travelers with a considerable rate of comorbidity [7]. Also, Stauffer et al. estimated that 4% of overseas travelers are infants and children [8]. This is confirmed by an Israeli study reporting a proportion of more than 5% for the age group below 18 years of age [9]. This varying demography of travelers increasingly needs to be taken into consideration in dealing with post-travel illness.

This lack of surveillance data for imported cases of infectious diseases prompted the establishment of various travel-related surveillance systems.

The GeoSentinel Surveillance Network started in 1995 through a collaborative agreement between the International Society of Travel Medicine (ISTM) and the Centers for Disease Control and Prevention (CDC) and consists of specialized travel/tropical medicine clinics on six continents recording information on ill travelers [10]. The main aims of the GeoSentinel Surveillance Network are to monitor global trends in disease occurrence among travelers and to ascertain risk factors and morbidity in groups of travelers categorized by travel purpose and type of traveler.

A few years later, in 1999, the European Network on Imported Infectious Disease Surveillance (TropNetEurop) was founded, serving as a European electronic network

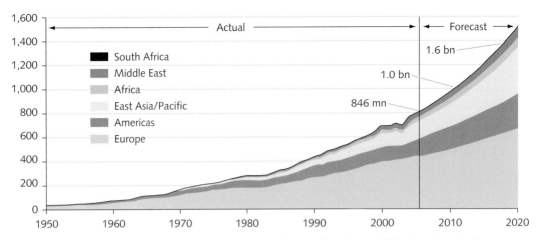

**Figure 3.1** Trend of international tourist arrivals, 1950–2020. (From the United Nations World Tourism Organization, http://www.unwto.org/pub/rights.htm.)

of 37 clinical sites related to importation of the major tropical diseases.

For the first time, these novel sentinel surveillance systems allow the identification of temporal and geographic trends in infectious disease occurrence in traveling populations worldwide. Through the global surveillance of infectious diseases in travelers, refugees, and immigrants, valuable persuasive science-based information about important aspects of post-travel morbidity is generated to guide post-travel diagnosis, develop adequate pretravel prevention strategies, and hopefully lead to travelers' improved health.

This chapter summarizes results of available systematic studies investigating the epidemiology of post-travel illnesses, including data on the above-mentioned large-scale surveillance systems. In-depth epidemiology of specific diseases, however, is covered in the specific chapters.

## Methods of investigations for post-travel morbidity

Generally, two different categories of post-travel disease epidemiology data exist.

### Disease attack rate

Attack rates of specific diseases is calculated by dividing the number of ill travelers (numerator) by the number of all people who traveled to the same destination during the same observation period (denominator). Data of this kind, however, are rare.

### Population-based risk

Only a few studies have supplied such specific population-based risk figures, which provide a useful pretravel tool for travelers for assessment and rating of disease-specific geographic risks. The data are limited to selected traveling population groups and/or geographic areas, such as Israeli travelers in Bolivia contracting cutaneous leishmaniasis (attack rate, 1 in 300 travelers) [11] or sufferers from myiasis in the Amazon basin (attack rate 1 in 190 travelers) [12].

In a recent survey, the rabies exposure risk among long-term travelers was estimated to be 2.66 per 1000 travelers per month [13].

### Serosurveys

Serosurveys performed pre- and post-travel may likewise provide estimates of disease attack rates. This approach has been used, for instance, to evaluate the incidence of dengue fever in populations traveling to selected geographic regions. Dutch travelers to Asia (with a median stay of 1 month) had a seroconversion rate of 2.9% [14]. An Israeli survey performed among travelers who had spent at least 3 months in a tropical area observed a seroconversion rate of 6.7% [15]. A survey of tuberculin skin-test conversion among Dutch long-term travelers revealed an overall incidence rate of 3.5 per 1000 person-months of travel [16].

## Proportion of morbidity

The majority of available data on the epidemiology of post-travel illness, including the worldwide GeoSentinel database, address the proportion of morbidity, providing information exclusively on ill returned travelers. Proportionate morbidity data pose an adjuvant reference for clinicians in the diagnostic evaluation of ill returned travelers, as well as providing estimates for common diseases that might be seen in returning travelers based on their travel destination.

Until recently, systematic scientific data on the epidemiology of travel-associated diseases and health risks have been rather meager, relying mostly on case reports, case series, or single-center cohort or cross-sectional studies. Today, various approaches are in use.

### Case series and chart reviews

Case series and chart reviews collect information on ill travelers who present for medical care to identify the spectrum and relative frequency of particular health problems.

### Cross-sectional studies

Cross-sectional studies usually use questionnaires, mostly airport surveys, to investigate both ill and well travelers' attitudes, knowledge, and practices regarding preventive measures to identify potential risk factors.

### Cohort studies

Cohort studies usually are based on travelers who seek pretravel health advice; they are then followed up on their return to determine the frequency and types of health outcomes during or after travel. This method provides estimates of disease incidence because the numerator and denominator are given.

### Case reports

Case reports are particularly useful for the observation and identification of rare diseases and outcomes in travelers.

### Sentinel surveillance networks

Sentinel surveillance networks collect in a prospective and systematic manner data on large samples of ill returned travelers, but are missing external denominator data. This approach enables the calculation of proportionate morbidity, allowing the development of a hierarchy of risk according to travel destination.

## Limitations of investigation in ill returned travelers

The major limitations of travel health surveys are retrospective design, bias due to the study population's specific travel habits, and limited post-travel follow-up periods, as well as selection bias because case detection depends on the medical specialization of the reporting physicians (e.g., tropical medicine specialists, dermatologists, pediatricians) or the type of patients (inpatients versus outpatients). Hence, in interpreting study results, one should be aware that most epidemiological data merely reflect a subset of the true number of ill returned travelers. Also, the majority of current studies focus on the epidemiology of travel-associated illness occurring during travel, whereas only a small number investigate the epidemiology of post-travel illness. As a matter of fact, the disease frequency and the spectrum of reported medical conditions originating from these two distinct sources may differ substantially. In a survey analyzing post-travel health problems in a large cohort of American travelers, illness during travel was reported by 64%, including 8% who sought medical care, whereas only 26% of this cohort became ill upon return (during 2 months post-travel), 12% of whom consulted doctors after their trips [17]. One of the pioneer surveys of travelers' morbidity revealed that 15% reported health problems upon return and 8% consulted doctors [3].

## Post-travel morbidity data

Generally, data on post-travel morbidity can be divided into outpatient morbidity data in hospitalized ill returned travelers, for whom more information is available. However, these two cohorts must be linked for a clearer understanding of post-travel morbidity.

The large-scale GeoSentinel database combined these two patient cohorts, although the proportion of each was not precisely known and was not scientifically selected. Yet, the GeoSentinel data provide clear evidence that the major group of post-travel illnesses is gastrointestinal disease, followed by fever, dermatological problems, and respiratory illness (Figure 3.2). Table 3.1 presents a comparison between ill returned in- and outpatients with

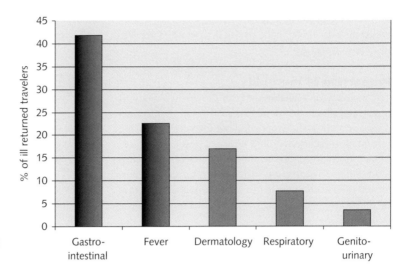

**Figure 3.2** The proportion of morbidity per 100 patients (%), in travelers presenting post-travel at GeoSentinel sites. All regions are combined. (Adapted from [32].)

regard to the relative frequencies of the main illness categories.

## Post-travel hospitalization data

Hospitalization of ill returned travelers could be due to an acute disease with a potentially severe outcome or to a subacute debilitating condition that could not be resolved in an outpatient setting.

The interval between return from travel and medical evaluation varies widely by diagnosis. Several hurdles constrain surveillance of post-travel hospitalization. Morbidity data on hospitalized patients represent only a very small selection of cases at the severe end of the scale. Moreover, in interpreting disease frequency data, one needs to be aware that in most studies case detection is performed at tertiary care facilities such as highly specialized travel or tropical medicine clinics rather than at primary health care levels. However, it may be assumed that the vast majority of ill travelers consult their family physicians rather than tropical medicine clinics. Another limitation is posed by differing hospitalization practices between various countries, which make comparisons rather difficult.

A study of hospitalized Israeli travelers showed that the majority (77%) were hospitalized due to febrile diseases, with malaria, unidentified febrile diseases, and dengue fever being the most common. The other causes for hospital admission were dermatologic problems, gastrointestinal illnesses, and respiratory diseases [18]. Because fever poses the major challenge of post-travel hospitalization, several studies have focused specifically on febrile patients (Table 3.2).

## Post-travel outpatient data

The current understanding of the morbidity profile among post-travel outpatients is, with the exception of GeoSentinel data, mostly based on data from single-site studies that examine individual diseases, specific destinations, or defined groups of travelers. Importantly, morbidity rates of ill returned outpatients calculated from present surveillance data constitute a extensive underestimate because case detection misses patients with self-limiting or mild illnesses, who usually consult nonspecialized primary care practices. Hence, in interpreting outpatient data, one has to assume that systemically reported morbidity of ill travelers is only the tip of the iceberg.

**Table 3.1** Relative frequencies of post-travel health conditions (%), comparing in- and outpatient populations.

|  | Percentage of patients | |
|---|---|---|
|  | Outpatients [19] | Inpatients [18] |
| Gastrointestinal illness | 23 | 11 |
| Dermatologic illness[a] | 26 | 14 |
| Fever | 14 | 59 |
| Respiratory illness | 3 | 4 |

[a] Including animal bites.

**Table 3.2** Causes of fever recognized after travel as reported in various published studies (%).

| Population | Doherty et al./ 1995/UK [20] Adults/ hospitalized | Klein et al./ 1998/UK [21] Children/ hospitalized | O'Brien et al./2001/ Australia [23] Adults/ hospitalized | Casalino et al./ 2002/France [24] Adults/ in- and outpatients | D'Acremont et al./2002/ Switzerland [25] Adults/ outpatients | West et al./ 2003/UK [22] Children/ hospitalized | Antinori et al./ 2004/Italy [26] Adults/ hospitalized | Stienlauf et al./ 2005/Israel [18] Adults/ hospitalized | Wilson et al./ 2007/ GeoSentinel [27] All ages/ in- and outpatients |
|---|---|---|---|---|---|---|---|---|---|
| Total number | 195 | 31 | 232 | 783 | 336 | 153 | 147 | 163 | 6957 |
| % | | | | | | | | | |
| Malaria | 42 | 13 | 27 | 18.5 | 29 | 14 | 48 | 33 | 35 |
| Gastroenteritis | 7 | 3 | 4 | 12.5 | NA | 27 | 4.8 | 6 | 15 |
| Dengue | 6 | 6.4 | 8 | NA | 1 | | 3.4 | | 6 |
| Typhoid | 2 | 6.4 | 3.5 | NA | 2 | 3 | 4.1 | 17 | 2 |
| Viral hepatitis | 3 | 3.2 | 3 | 2.8 | 2 | 5 | 8.8 | 3 | 1 |
| Pneumonia bacterial | 2.5 | 3.2 | 6 | 9.6 | 3 | 8.5 | NA | 2 | 1 |
| Upper respiratory tract infection | 3 | 3.2 | 12 | 6.8 | 8 | 6 | NA | 4 | 9.6 |
| Urinary tract infection | 2.5 | NA | 2 | 9.6 | 3 | 4 | 1.4 | 0 | 2 |
| Rickettiosis | 0.5 | NA | 2 | NA | 1 | 0.6 | 0.7 | 0.2 | |
| Non-specific/ undiagnosed | 24.5 | 45 | 9 | 55.3 | 32 | 34 | 4.8 | 21 | 22 |

NA = not available.

Of 205 ill, New Zealander returned travelers presenting in an outpatient setting, most suffered from diarrheal diseases, followed by dermatologic conditions and febrile illnesses. Tropical diseases were uncommon in this group. As a matter of fact, the specific etiology was not always defined. Usually, one-third of illnesses in returned outpatients remain unspecified [19]. In contrast to the New Zealand study, dermatoses and tropical infections were the chief complaints among a cohort of French post-travel outpatients. This discrepancy clearly reflects the large variety of single-site observations, due mostly to population-specific travel patterns in combination with destination-dependent differences of morbidity profiles. Imported tropical diseases accounted for 36% of the diagnoses in this cohort of ill returned French travelers; malaria, schistosomiasis, intestinal nematodiasis, amebiasis, and dengue fever being the most frequent. This observation is most likely explained by the relatively large number of immigrants among this specific study population.

Generally, the most important difference between in- and outpatient groups in post-travel morbidity profiles is that fever is the major condition in hospitalized patients, whereas in outpatients, gastrointestinal and dermatologic illnesses are the most common causes reported for consulting a doctor.

The four following major syndrome categories of post-travel health problems are discussed in this chapter:
- Systemic febrile diseases
- Gastrointestinal illnesses
- Dermatologic disorders
- Respiratory diseases.

### Systemic febrile diseases

Fever is a relatively common cause for seeking medical advice after tropical travel and, because of increasing international mobility, it will be observed even more frequently in the future. Indeed, this may pose a diagnostic challenge to Western physicians, because fever serves as an important marker of potentially serious conditions in persons who have recently traveled.

The majority of ill returned travelers with fever present within 1–2 weeks after their return (Figure 3.3).

Surveys consistently show that the majority of febrile patients who return from Africa present less than a week after return, reflecting the short incubation time of *Plasmodium falciparum* malaria. Immigrants who visited their countries of origin and who traveled to Sub-Saharan Africa, South Central Asia, and Latin America were more likely to experience fever than any other group of travelers.

Whatever the setting or population considered (i.e., tourists or migrants, adults or children), malaria poses by far the most frequent cause of febrile illness in hospitalized patients diagnosed after travel to the tropics, with a prevalence ranging between 13% and 48% (Table 3.2) [18–26]. Moreover, the majority of ill returned malaria patients require inpatient care. Importantly, *P. falciparum*, which causes the most severe form of malaria, was identified in 23–74% of all returned travelers with malaria. In fact, according to reports to the GeoSentinel Surveillance Network, falciparum malaria is listed as a contributory cause in 33% of deaths in febrile travelers [27]. Hence, the presence of malaria in febrile travelers poses a crucial diagnostic consideration, regardless of previous use of antimalarial agents. Of all cases of malaria, persons visiting friends and relatives (VFRs) while traveling are at particular risk and account for approximately 40% of reported cases of malaria in the United States [29].

Similarly, the majority of hospital admissions in Israelis following travel were of febrile diseases [18]. The most common specific diagnosis leading to post-travel hospitalization due to fever for this specific travel population was malaria (26%), followed by dengue fever (13%). In contrast, according to record data for outpatients presenting at travel clinics in New Zealand, febrile illness ranked only third in the list of diagnoses, after diarrheal and dermatologic illnesses [19].

Table 3.2 summarizes the relative frequencies of fever causes in ill returned travelers in several published studies, including in- and outpatient data.

Male ill returned travelers were more likely than female travelers to seek medical care because of fever [26].

Comparison of the travel destinations of the general population and post-travel hospital patients revealed that the risk of contracting severe disease is higher in Sub-Saharan Africa than in any other region. Although malaria, mainly falciparum malaria, was the most common condition in travelers returning from Africa, dengue fever was the most common cause for hospitalization in travelers returning from Asia. Hospitalization due to malaria, as well as dengue fever, showed a clear seasonal pattern, mostly corresponding to the rainy seasons in the respective destinations and to a lesser extent to seasonal travel activity to each region.

Notably, a significant proportion of hospitalized patients have fever that resolves spontaneously without any specific diagnosis or treatment. The proportion of undetermined febrile illness among ill returned inpatients ranges 5–45% (see Table 3.2). Surprisingly, this figure has hardly changed for a long time despite the increased

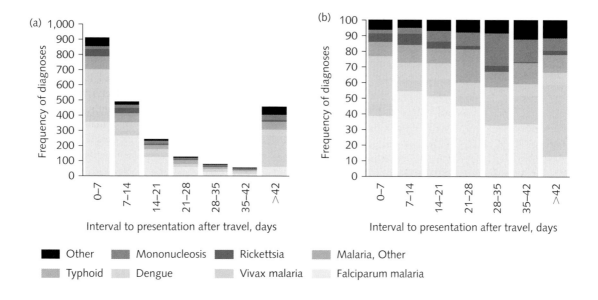

**Figure 3.3** Interval from return from travel to clinic presentation for patients who had fevers, by specific febrile illness. (a) Frequency of systemic febrile illnesses based on the duration of the interval to presentation. (b) Proportion of systemic febrile illnesses based on the duration of the interval to presentation. (Reproduced with permission from The University of Chicago Press. Wilson et al. *Clin Infect Dis* 2007;44:1560–8.)

availability of improved diagnostic tools and facilities. According to the worldwide GeoSentinel database, no specific diagnosis could be made in 22% of 4500 febrile travelers (27). However, high hospital admission rates of travelers with systemic febrile illness and a 5-day mean duration of hospitalization suggest that ill returned travelers may consume substantial medical resources [18].

## Gastrointestinal illnesses

Gastrointestinal (GI) illnesses pose the most common disorders in travelers [3, 29, 30], with up to 70% of travelers affected by diarrhea during travel [31]. Bacterial diarrhea was reported as the main cause for diarrhea during travel.

GI complaints are also the most common cause for seeking medical advice post-travel, accounting for about 40% of all referrals (Figure 3.2). Diarrheal diseases are still the most common complaint. However, there are differences between the "during" and "post"-travel presentations.

In post-travel referrals, chronic diarrhea is the major reason for seeking medical care. Interestingly, with the exception of Sub-Saharan Africa, where malaria is the predominant pathogen, in all other regions chronic diarrhea is the most common, with a rate of 10–17% of all referrals. The chronic diarrhea group might encompass

unrecognized parasitic pathogens or "postinfectious irritable bowel syndrome" (see Chapter 36). The other change between "during" and "post"-travel diarrhea is that bacterial pathogens are the main cause of travelers' diarrhea; whereas parasitic diseases are more common, with giardiasis and amebiasis being the leading identifiable causes, in post-travel diarrhea, even in those who present shortly after travel (Figure 3.4a).

The explanation for this discrepancy is that bacterial diarrhea has a relatively short incubation period and is usually mild and self-limiting, whereas parasitic infections have longer incubation periods and tend to be more chronic. In fact, it is estimated that up to 1.8% of all travelers will develop post-travel chronic diarrhea [3], which is ranked second in causing inability to work among returning travelers [32].

Travelers returning from the Indian subcontinent and from Central America most commonly present with GI illnesses [32].

It should be remembered that infectious GI pathogens may cause nondiarrheal diseases as well, such as viral hepatitis A and E and typhoid and paratyphoid fever.

Between 3% and 14% of adult hospital admissions after travel are reported to be due to febrile gastroenteritis

(a)

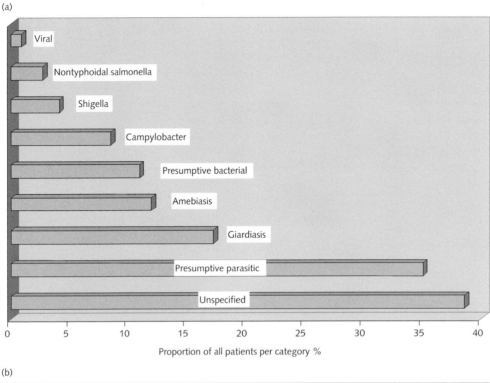

Proportion of all patients per category %

(b)

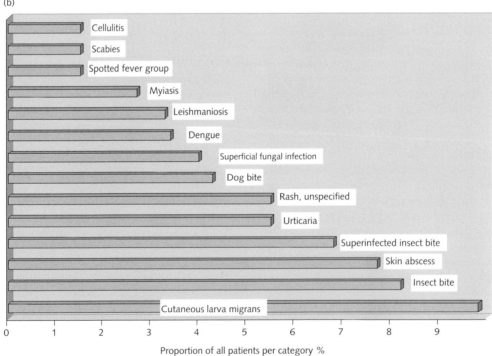

Proportion of all patients per category %

**Figure 3.4** Proportions of etiologic diagnoses (%) within selected syndrome categories according to data collected by the GeoSentinel surveillance network. (a) Acute diarrhea (adapted from [32]). (b) Dermatologic disorders (adapted from [33]). (c) Respiratory illnesses (adapted from [39]).

(c)

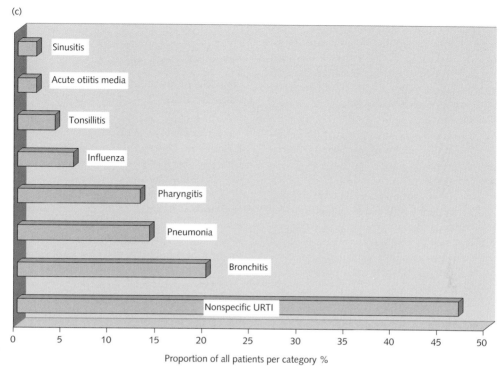

Proportion of all patients per category %

**Figure 3.4** (*Continued*)

(Table 3.2). Other causes of hospitalization may be nondiarrheal GI infections presenting as systemic febrile infections. The protracted and sometimes debilitating course of chronic diarrhea may lead to hospitalization as well. Among post-travel hospitalized Israeli travelers, 4% were hospitalized with prolonged, nonfebrile GI diseases [18].

In small children, diarrheal diseases often have a particularly severe and longer lasting course, which explains the higher pediatric post-travel hospitalization rate for diarrhea [21].

In post-travel bacterial diarrhea, the most common isolated pathogens were *Campylobacter* species, followed by *Shigella* and nontyphoidal *Salmonella* [22, 32] (Figure 3.4a).

## Dermatologic disorders

Skin disorders are among the six most common reasons for returned travelers to seek medical care [17, 22, 33]. Of all post-travel dermatologic illness self-reported by a cohort of American travelers, 11% needed medical care for their skin problems [17]. The most common complaints are cutaneous larva migrans, arthropod bites, skin abscesses, myiasis, urticaria, tinea, and leishmaniasis

[33–35]. Moreover, skin conditions may be associated with the length of stay and environmental risk factors. The frequency of reported skin diseases, however, is highly dependent on the geographical destination, explaining the differences between various traveling populations with different destination preferences. In hospitalized ill returned Israeli travelers, who commonly travel to Latin America, for instance, skin diseases, mostly infections with *Leishmania braziliensis*, account for up to 14% of all diagnoses among hospitalized travelers (due to the need for systemic treatment) and account for the majority of nonfebrile diagnoses [18]. Other studies focusing on febrile inpatients report far lower rates (5%) of skin lesions among ill returned travelers [22, 26].

According to the GeoSentinel database, including in- and outpatients, skin-related diagnoses were reported for 18% of all patients seen in GeoSentinel clinics after travel, mainly imported from the Caribbean. Only 24% of patients had classical tropical skin diseases (e.g., CLM, myiasis, leishmaniasis, dengue); children had a greater likelihood of presenting with dog bites [33]. The GeoSentinel-based proportions of the most common diagnoses within this category are presented in Figure 3.4b.

## Respiratory diseases

Respiratory illnesses are among the most common infections affecting human beings, but little information has been published on them in relation to travel. The possible public health significance of imported infections includes the introduction and transmission of new strains of respiratory pathogens into susceptible populations on a traveler's return home.

However, post-travel data on respiratory illness most likely underestimate the number of travelers who develop respiratory tract infections. Studies have documented that respiratory tract symptoms occur in about 26% of persons during travel, but only in 10% post-travel [36]. Respiratory tract infections accounted for about 8% of all infections in returned travelers reported to GeoSentinel, with nonspecific upper respiratory infection being the most common diagnosis [36]. Figure 3.4c summarizes the major causes of respiratory complaints reported to the GeoSentinel network clinics.

A review of admissions to an Australian tertiary care hospital following travel showed respiratory tract infections to be the second most common cause of febrile illness after malaria [22]. About a quarter of patients with post-travel respiratory illness and fever require hospitalization. Diagnoses of pneumonia (odds ratio [OR], 9.92; 95% confidence interval [CI], 6.77–14.57), influenza (OR, 5.88; 95% CI, 3.60–9.59), and lower respiratory tract infection (OR, 6.49; 95% CI, 4.22–9.99) showed far higher risk for hospital admission compared with other diagnoses such as bronchitis and upper respiratory infections [36].

Among outpatients, between 3% and 12% are diagnosed with respiratory tract infections [19, 36, 37], the majority of which are infections of the upper respiratory tract.

Generally, the most significant predictors for developing specific categories of respiratory infections while abroad were age, sex, season of travel, trip duration, and type of traveler. Long-term travel was associated with an increased risk of influenza and lower respiratory tract infection. Furthermore, increasing age and male sex are associated with a greater risk of lower respiratory tract infection, particularly pneumonia and bronchitis. Importantly, persons visiting friends and relatives are more likely to acquire influenza than any other group of travelers [38]. This is most likely explained by the close contact between these travelers and the local populations. Undoubtedly, this group should be specifically considered for pretravel influenza vaccination, regardless of age, because it may

significantly reduce morbidity associated with this infection [39].

## Profile of post-travel illness according to destination

The probabilities of specific diagnoses among ill returned travelers are closely associated with travel destination. Based on the worldwide GeoSentinel surveillance data [32], including more than 17,000 reports of a broad range of ill travelers returning from developing regions on all continents, a summary of the proportions of specific diagnoses or diagnosis groups is given in Figure 3.5. Shown is the proportion of morbidity per 100 patients (%), not the incidence rate, of each of the leading five diagnoses among travelers returning from each of these regions.

As can be seen, fever is the most common cause for seeking care after trips to Africa, due to overpresentation of falciparum infection, whereas in the other regions dengue supersedes malaria as a cause of fever in returning travelers presenting at the GeoSentinel sites [32]. Skin diseases are more frequently seen in travelers from Latin America, where tropical skin diseases are common, and the overwhelming majority of leishmaniasis cases are from there. In Sub-Saharan Africa, schistosomiasis is very close in frequency to dermatologic and respiratory diseases.

## Rare diagnoses in post-travel illnesses

Rare diagnoses in returning travelers (e.g., Japanese encephalitis, Ebola virus disease, plague, anthrax, or yellow fever) are usually reported in sporadic case reports. It is comforting to know that among more then 17,000 diagnoses of ill returned patients reported to the GeoSentinel surveillance network, no such exotic condition has been reported [32].

However, according to Internet-based disease monitoring and reporting systems such as Program for Monitoring Emerging Diseases (ProMED-mail), established in 1994, or GIDEON, founded in 1992 as a global infectious diseases database, sporadic cases of Japanese encephalitis, yellow fever, Lassa fever, and rabies have been reported in travelers. These reports stress that these often fatal diagnoses may be rare but pose a serious health risk to travelers in areas where they are endemic, and even a large

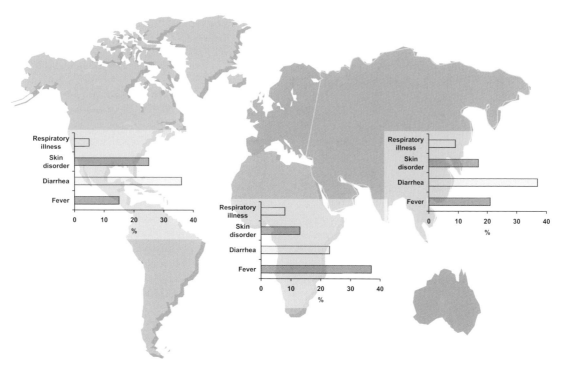

**Figure 3.5** Proportion of morbidity among ill returned travelers (%) by continent visited, according to the GeoSentinel database, including in- and outpatients. (Adapted from [32].)

international system such as GeoSentinel may not capture them. Some of these diseases are vaccine-preventable, which emphasizes the role of pretravel consultation.

## Risk in special populations

Generally, VFRs, as well as adventure travelers, are at increased risk of becoming ill while traveling because they have an increased risk of exposure, may less perceive travel-associated risks, and may forgo recommended vaccinations and chemoprophylactic measures [39] (see Chapter 5).

Furthermore, both age and travel duration are potential risk factors for post-travel illness and hospitalization and may explain the varying frequencies of illness in different study populations.

### Gender-related morbidity

Over the past decade, it has become increasingly apparent that differences in the prevalence and severity of a broad range of diseases, disorders, and conditions exist between genders.

With regard to travel-related morbidity, a higher proportion of males, relative to healthy travelers, experience all major imported diseases. Surveys show clear male preponderance among ill returned outpatients (50% vs 42%) [19], as well as among febrile hospitalized travelers [18, 20, 27].

Males represented 71% of Israeli hospitalized ill returned patients, whereas they represented only 55% of the population of healthy travelers [18]. Data collected by the GeoSentinel surveillance network revealed that one of the most significant predictors for developing specific categories of respiratory infections while abroad was sex. Male sex was associated with a greater risk of lower respiratory tract infection, particularly pneumonia and bronchitis, but a lower risk of upper respiratory tract infection [36]. According to an Indian study, male travelers also revealed a higher rate of attack by hepatitis E virus [40]. The preponderance of men among malaria patients has been documented extensively among both travelers and local populations [41, 42]. Moreover, Canadian male travelers had a higher risk of dying [71% vs 22%] and were also more likely to be arrested or detained while abroad [42].

Interestingly, no such observation has been made for dengue fever. Studies from various countries showed that the risk of acquiring dengue fever in travelers is not affected by gender [14, 18, 43, 44].

The reasons for gender differences in major illnesses are not yet clear. Some authors have argued that men follow riskier itineraries, or take fewer precautions, thus putting them at higher risk for febrile illnesses, such as malaria. One case-control study, however, did not find any major differences between men and women in terms of compliance with chemoprophylaxis and the use of protective measures. It has been concluded that males are generally more susceptible to malaria or infections [45]. However, to date, the biological causes of the suspected vulnerability of men are poorly understood. X-linked immunoregulatory genes appear to contribute to greater female resistance to infectious diseases [46].

On the other hand, women may have a lower threshold than men for seeking pre- and post-travel advice and may be more likely to present to health care facilities for nonfebrile illnesses [47]. This observation is most likely to be explained by the fact that women worry more than men about travel-related stressors such as infected food, contaminated water, and illness [48].

## Post-travel morbidity in children

Over recent years, families with children have traveled increasingly to tropical destinations, exposing themselves to numerous infectious agents and tropical illnesses not encountered at home. However, there exist only a very limited number of published data on the subject of imported infections in children. Generally, it is assumed that children are more at risk of falling ill while traveling than adults. For this reason, traveling to tropical destinations with small children is mostly discouraged by pediatricians. Yet, there is no science-based evidence to support this presumption.

According to a prospective controlled study of 157 Swiss children and their parents, which included reports during as well as after travel, no major differences between children and adults in the incidence of illnesses apart from febrile episodes were observed. Age seems not to be a major determinant of travel-related morbidity. The chief complaint reported during and following travel was diarrhea, followed by febrile illness [49]. Similarly, the primary diagnosis of febrile hospitalized children from the UK who had returned from a tropical country within 4 weeks prior to hospital admission was unspecified fever,

self-limiting illnesses of presumed viral origin, followed by malaria, bacillary dysentery, and dengue fever [21].

Like other retrospective reviews of imported malaria [50], most of these cases were reported among children of former immigrants who had visited their families' countries of origin [21]. Many people from this particular group of travelers do not feel that they need prophylaxis when returning home. Hence, the proportion of cases of imported pediatric malaria in children who received any form of malaria chemoprophylaxis was less than 50% [50].

More important, children are particularly at risk from malaria because symptoms may be very severe and usually develop more rapidly than in adult malaria patients. In addition, symptoms may differ from those in adults and, as children often suffer febrile diseases, malaria may not be suspected in the first place. As likewise observed for adults, most cases of officially reported pediatric malaria in travelers are caused by *P. falciparum* [50]. With regard to the time interval between return from travel and medical evaluation, 88% of pediatric cases of falciparum malaria but only 30% of *P. vivax* infections were diagnosed within a month of return [42]. Vivax malaria can occur late because of the dormancy of hypnozoites in the liver, which are not affected by the chemoprophylactic agents commonly used [51].

## Air evacuation from abroad

Data on medical repatriation offer a portrait of serious medical problems for travelers while abroad. According to Steffen et al., about 50 per 100,000 travelers require air evacuation [52]. Based on another analysis, male travelers accounted for more than 65% of all medical escorts. In European countries, the majority of evacuations [53] were for medical reasons, mainly cardiovascular; in developing countries trauma and medical conditions accounted for 50%. Interestingly, infectious diseases were the reason for only 7% of all repatriations from developing countries [53].

## Death

In terms of the hundreds of millions of international journeys completed annually, international travel is generally a safe undertaking. However, a number of travelers do experience serious injury, illness, and death. In a Canadian study tracking death notification data abroad, male travelers accounted for more than twice as many deaths as female travelers. Most were due to natural causes (73%), followed by accidents (17%), murder (4%), and suicide (4%) [54].

Referring to the GeoSentinel database, diagnoses contributing to death were reported in 1 per 1000 ill returned travelers and consisted of severe and complicated malaria, pulmonary embolism, pneumonia, and pyogenic abscesses. The death rate was highest in travelers to of South Central Asia (3/1000) [32]. However, death is certainly under-reported to the GeoSentinel database because it may be assumed that many cases occur while travelers are abroad.

## Summary

With continuing worldwide growth in travel, timely information about the epidemiology of post-travel illness provides an adjuvant reference for likely diagnoses in returned travelers, with stratification according to destination, seasonality, purpose of travel, and host characteristics, including sex. Assessment of post-travel morbidity, however, differs from "during travel" surveys. A population-based assessment of returning travelers has never been performed systematically because many travelers seek medical advice long after their trips, making short prospective post-travel studies inappropriate. Consequently, assessment of the proportion of morbidity in ill returned travelers appears more feasible and may provide valuable information for guiding post-travel diagnosis and empirical therapy as well as for prioritizing pretravel intervention strategies.

## References

1 UNWTO. *Tourism Highlights* 2007 ed. [Online]. 2007. Available from http://www.unwto.org.

2 Ryan ET, Wilson ME, Kain CK. Illness after international travel. *N Engl J Med* 2002;347:505–16.

3 Steffen R, Rickenbach M, Wilhelm U, et al. Health problems after travel to developing countries. *J Infect Dis* 1987;156:84–91.

4 Steffen R, Jong EC. Travelers' and immigrants' health. In: Guerrant RL, Walker DH, Wyler PF, eds. *Tropical Infectious Diseases: Principles, Pathogens, and Practice.* Philadelphia: Churchill-Livingstone; 1999. p. 106–14.

5 Steffen R, Lobel HO. Epidemiologic basis for the basis of travel medicine. *J Wilderness Med* 1987;5:56–66.

6 Duval B, De Serre G, Shadmani R. A population-based comparison between travelers who consulted travel clinics and those who did not. *J Travel Med* 2003;10:6–7.

7 Hamer DH, Connor BA. Travel health knowledge, attitudes and practices among United States travelers. *J Travel Med* 2004;11:23–6.

8 Stauffer WM, Konop RJ, Kamat D. Traveling with infants and young children. Part I: Anticipatory guidance: travel preparation and preventive health advice. *J Travel Med* 2001;8:254–9.

9 Steinlauf S, Meltzer E, Leshem E, Schwartz E. The profile of Israeli travelers—Travel clinic perspective. Presented at the Annual Meeting of the Israel Society for Parasitology, Protozoology, and Tropical Diseases, 2007 Dec 10–11; Tel Aviv, Israel.

10 Freedman DO, Kozarsky PE, Weld LH, Cetron MS. GeoSentinel: The global emerging infections sentinel network of the International Society of Travel Medicine. *J Travel Med* 1999;6:94–8.

11 Scope A, Trau H, Anders G, Barzilai A, Confino Y, Schwartz E. Experience with New World cutaneous leishmaniasis in travelers. *J Am Acad Dermatol* 2003;49(4):672–8.

12 Schwartz E, Gur H. *Dermatobia hominis* myiasis: an emerging disease among travelers to the Amazon Basin of Bolivia. *J Travel Med* 2002;9:97–9.

13 Menachem M, Grupper M, Paz A, Potasman I. Assessment of rabies exposure risk among Israeli travelers. *Travel Med Infect Dis* 2008;6(1–2):12–16.

14 Cobelens FG, Groen J, Osterhaus AD, Leentvaar-Kuipers A, Wertheim-Van Dillen PM, Kager PA. Incidence and risk factors of probable dengue virus infection among Dutch travellers to Asia. *Trop Med Int Health* 2002;7:331–8.

15 Potasman I, Ssrugo I, Schwartz E. Dengue seroconversion among Israeli travellers to tropical countries. *Emerg Infect Dis* 1999;5(6):824–7.

16 Cobelens FG, Van Deutekom H, Draaver-Jansen JW, et al. Risk of infection with *Mycobacterium tuberculosis* in travellers to areas of high tuberculosis endemicity. *Lancet* 2000;356:461–5.

17 Hill DR. Health problems in a large cohort of Americans traveling to developing countries. *J Travel Med* 2000;7:259–66.

18 Steinlauf S, Segal G, Sidi Y, Schwartz E. Epidemiology of travel-related hospitalization. *J Travel Med* 2005;12:136–41.

19 Shaw MTM, Leggat PA, Weld LH, Williams LM, Cetron Ms. Illness in returned travellers presenting at GeoSentinel sites in New Zealand. *Aust N Z J Public Health* 2003;27:82–6.

20 Doherty JF, Grant AD, Bryceson ADM. Fever as the presenting complaint of travellers returning from the tropics. *Q J Med* 1995;88:277–81.

21 Klein JL, Millman GC. Prospective, hospital based study of fever in children in the United Kingdom who had recently spent time in the tropics. *BMJ* 1998;316:1425–6.

22 West NS, Riordan FAI. Fever in returned travellers: a prospective review of hospital admissions for a 2 1/2 year period. *Arch Dis Child* 2003;88:432–4.

23 O'Brien D, Tobin S, Brown GV, Torresi J. Fever in returned travelers: review of hospital admissions for a 3-year period. *Clin Infect Dis* 2001;33:603–9.

24 Casalino E, Le Bras J, Chaussin F, et al. Predictive factors of malaria in travelers to areas where malaria is endemic. *Arch Intern Med* 2002;162:1625–30.

25 D'Acremont V, Landry P, Mueller I, et al. Clinical and laboratory predictors of imported malaria in an outpatient setting: an aid to medical decision making in returning travellers with fever. *Am J Trop Med Hyg* 2002;66:481–6.

26 Antinori S, Galimberti L, Granelli E, et al. Prospective observational study of fever in hospitalized returning travelers and migrants from tropical areas, 1997–2001. *J Travel Med* 2004;11:135–42.

27 Wilson ME, Weld LH, Boggild A, et al. Fever in returned travelers: results from the GeoSentinel surveillance network. *Clin Infect Dis* 2007;44:1560–68.

28 Newman RD, Barber AM, Roberts J, Holtz T, Steketee RW, Parise ME. Malaria surveillance—United States, 1999. *MMWR CDC Surveill Summ* 2002;51(SS-1):15–28.

29 Bruni M, Steffen R. Impact of travel-related health impairments. *J Travel Med* 1997;4:61–4.

30 Steffen R, van der Linde F, Gyr K, Schar M. Epidemiology of diarrhea in travelers. *JAMA* 1983;249:1176–80.

31 Gorbach SL. Travellers' diarrhea. *N Engl J Med* 1982;307:881–3.

32 Freedman DO, Weld LH, Phyllis E. Kozarsky PE, et al. Spectrum of disease and relation to place of exposure among ill returned travelers. *N Engl J Med* 2006;354(2):119–30.

33 Lederman ER, Weld LH, Elyazar IRF, et al. Dermatologic conditions of the ill returned traveler: an analysis from the GeoSentinel surveillance network. *Int J Infect Dis* 2008;12(6):593–602.

34 Kain KC. Skin lesions in returned travelers. *Med Clin North Am* 1999;83:1077–1102.

35 Wilson ME. Skin problems in the traveler. *Infect Dis Clin N Am* 1998;12:471–88.

36 Leder K, Sundararajan V, Weld L. Respiratory tract infections in travelers: a review of the GeoSentinel surveillance network. *Clin Infect Dis* 2003;36:399–406.

37 Ansart S, Perez L, Vergely O, et al. Illness in travelers returning from the tropics: a prospective study of 622 patients. *J Travel Med* 2005;12:312–18.

38 Zuckerman JN. Imported tropical respiratory tract infections. *Curr Opin Pulm Med* 1999;5:164–7.

39 Leder K, Tong S, Leisa Weld L, et al. Illness in travelers visiting friends and relatives: a review of the GeoSentinel surveillance network. *Clin Infect Dis* 2006;43:1185–93.

40 Aggarwal R, Kumar R, Pal R, Naik S, Semwal SN, Naik SR. Role of travel as a risk factor for hepatitis E virus infection in a disease-endemic area. *Indian J Gastroenterol* 2002;21(1):14–18.

41 Askling HH, Nilsson J, Tegnell A, Janzon R, Ekdahl K. Malaria risk in travelers. *Emerg Infect Dis* 2005;11(3):436–41.

42 Boggild AK, Yohanna S, Keystone JS, Kain KC. Prospective analysis of parasitic infections in Canadian travelers and immigrants. *J Travel Med* 2006;13(3):138–44.

43 Jelinek T, Dobler G, Hölscher M, Löscher T, Nothdurft H. Prevalence of infection with dengue virus among international travelers. *Arch Intern Med* 1997;157:2367–70.

44 Lindback H, Lindback J, Tegnell A, et al. Dengue fever in travellers to the tropics, 1998 and 1999. *Emerg Infect Dis* 2003;9:438–42.

45 Genton B, D'Acremont V. Clinical features of malaria in returning travelers and migrants. In: Schlagenhauf-Lawlor P, editor. *Travelers' Malaria.* Hamilton (ON): BC Decker; 2001. p. 371–92.

46 Waldron I. Sex differences in illness incidence, prognosis and mortality: issues and evidence. *Soc Sci Med* 1983;17(16):1107–23.

47 Cabada MM, Maldonado F, Quispe W, Serrano E, Mozo K, Gonzales E, et al. Pretravel health advice among international travelers visiting Cuzco, Peru. *J Travel Med* 2005;12(2):61–5.

48 McIntosh IB, Power KG, Reed JM. Prevalence, intensity, and sex differences in travel related stressors. *J Travel Med* 1996;3(2):96–102.

49 Newman-Klee C, D'Acremont V, Newman CJ, et al. Incidence and types of illness when traveling to the tropics: A prospective controlled study of children and their parents. *Am J Trop Med Hyg* 2007;77:764–9.

50 Brabin BJ, Ganley Y. Imported malaria in children in the UK. *Arch Dis Child* 1997;77:76–81.

51 Schwartz E, Parise M, Kozarsky P, Cetron M. Delayed onset of malaria—implication for chemoprophylaxis in travellers. *N Engl J Med* 2003;349:1510–16.

52 Steffen R, Bernardis C, Banos A, et al. Travel epidemiology—a global perspective. *Int J Antimicrob Agents* 2003;21:89–95.

53 Ish-Tov E, Attias D, Schwartz E. Air-evacuation of Israeli travellers—analysis of 7 years. Presented at the Annual Meeting of the Israeli Society of Parasitology, Protozoology, and Tropical Diseases, 2007 Dec; Tel Aviv, Israel.

54 MacPherson DW, Gushulak BD, Sandhu J. Death and international travel—the Canadian experience: 1996 to 2004. *J Travel Med* 2007;14(2):77–84.

# 4

# Travelers as Sentinels for Disease Occurrence in Destination Countries

David O. Freedman[1] and Eli Schwartz[2]

[1]University of Alabama at Birmingham, Birmingham, AL, USA
[2]Chaim Sheba Medical Center, Tel Hashomer, Israel and Sackler School of Medicine, Tel Aviv University, Tel Aviv, Israel

## Introduction

Eighty million people from industrialized nations travel to the developing world each year for commerce, research, education, aid/voluntary missions, and military purposes. These travelers are ideally suited to effectively detect and monitor endemic and emerging infections of potential global impact at their points of entry into domestic populations and to track ongoing trends in travel-related morbidity. Travelers seen at relatively few sentinel sites after or during their trips provide a sample of disease agents in over 230 different countries. Real-time data may be captured at the clinical point of service.

A sentinel is defined as "one who gives a warning or indicates danger." Pathogens frequently emerge first in resource-poor countries but are then first identified and characterized in developed countries. Human immunodeficiency virus (HIV), which has been identified as having occurred in humans in Africa in the 1950s, is perhaps the best example. This is because resources for surveillance of ill persons and adequate subsequent diagnostic capabilities are lacking. Because travelers are exposed to infectious diseases while traveling and are usually able to seek medical attention rapidly upon return to settings with sophisticated technology, monitoring illnesses among travelers can provide information on the distribution and transmission of disease among local populations in the locations visited. Disease surveillance among travelers may also be the mechanism for detection of emerging resistance patterns among microorganisms.

On a basic level is the increasingly frequent scenario where a traveler returns home with an unusual disease and serves as the first clue to a new outbreak. Astute clinicians may make seminal observations and are able to disseminate the information rapidly through emerging online infectious diseases communities such as Program for Monitoring Emerging Diseases (ProMED-mail) (www.promedmail.org).

Over the past decade, both global and regional provider-based surveillance networks have emerged that have provided, for the first time, systematic and robust data that define the spectrum of illness and the places of exposure to the most significant health risks that face travelers. Clinicians record the travel itineraries, travel dates, and diagnoses of their patients on standardized electronic forms and submit these via the Internet to a central database. Investigators, including epidemiologists and statisticians, regularly examine the data to detect anomalies that might indicate a new outbreak. When facing an acute outbreak or global health emergency, these organized groups or networks of clinicians are able to track a fast-moving disease outbreak quickly by being linked by sophisticated communications infrastructures. Networks such as GeoSentinel [1, 2], the largest global network monitoring sentinel travelers, with 41 sites in 19 countries, provides a system for almost instant sharing of information among networks of travel and tropical medicine clinics. Ill travelers are monitored mostly after their return home, but at a few locations, notably in Asia, they can be monitored during their trips as well.

*Tropical Diseases in Travelers*, 1st edition. Edited by E. Schwartz.
© 2009 by Blackwell Publishing, ISBN: 978-1-4051-8441-0.

To elaborate on the ways in which travelers can serve as effective and timely sentinels of disease occurrence in many parts of the world, illustrative examples will be given below. In some cases, travelers' illnesses herald the emergence of novel pathogens that will have the greatest impact upon populations resident in the area of acquisition. At other times, the travelers will serve as sentinels for diseases or trends that will impact both the local population and future travelers to the same country or region. Finally, travelers' illnesses may provide a sentinel indication of an infection, either newly emergent or not, that has the potential to cause an explosive international outbreak as it moves from place to place with the traveler as its vector.

## Pre-Internet sentinel surveillance

Prior to the advent of e-mail, the Internet, and wired communities of reference laboratories and front-line providers, there were already many examples of travelers serving as sentinels for emerging new infections. In the 1960s, the first outbreak of Lassa fever was described because of its infection of several American missionaries in Nigeria and subsequent transmission to a laboratory technician in the United States processing specimens from a case that had been evacuated [3].

In the 1970s and 1980s, the US Centers for Disease Control and Prevention (CDC) surveillance reports on dengue occurrence in the Caribbean and in the Pacific Islands were restricted to data from returning tourists. Because no reports from national ministries of health were available or published at the time, alerts to travelers and physicians that appeared in the *MMWR* (*Morbidity and Mortality Weekly Report*) were based only on cases reported in returning tourists [4, 5]. The lack of epidemiological reporting in local populations was likely caused by a combination of lack of laboratory capabilities and concern over the protection of the local tourist industry.

In the 1990s, the emergence of schistosomiasis as a public health problem in Lake Malawi was recognized subsequent to two cases of neuroschistosomiasis among Peace Corps volunteers in 1992. Later, retrospective epidemiological and serological studies among US and non-US foreign nationals, many of whom had swum for less than 30 minutes in the lake, established for the first time that such brief exposures could lead to infection rates as high as 30% and that the estimated risk increased to as high as 90% for a 10-day exposure [6].

## Modern sentinel surveillance of travelers

The advent of the Internet and e-mail and their widespread adoption in the 1990s in many clinical practices at the direct interface with ill patients allowed a constant interchange of clinical observations in close to real time. This led to the establishment of several international communication networks, beginning with ProMED-mail in 1994. ProMED-mail is an Internet-based reporting system dedicated to rapid global dissemination of information on outbreaks of infectious diseases and acute exposures to toxins that affect human health. Open electronic submission by e-mail with rapid selection of electronic postings by an editorial board for same-day Web posting enables ProMED-mail to provide up-to-date and reliable news to a worldwide audience. GeoSentinel relies on 40 major clinical referral centers in 23 countries that monitor sentinel travelers with a full spectrum of diseases upon their return home from destinations in over 230 countries. Regional networks such as the European Network on Surveillance of Imported Infectious Diseases (TropNetEurop) report on travelers with a small set of key indicator diseases.

By providing early warning of outbreaks of emerging and re-emerging diseases, public health precautions at all levels can be taken in a timely manner to prevent further spread to local populations or export to new countries. The first powerful example of the utility of these methods for identifying an outbreak in real time was detection of leptospirosis in participants in the EcoChallenge adventure race in 2000. Other examples of ways in which travelers can act as sentinels for emerging infectious diseases are then described.

## Leptospirosis—detection of a point source outbreak with global spread of affected travelers

The GeoSentinel network was able to recognize the extent of the global spread of an outbreak of leptospirosis in participants in an adventure race (EcoChallenge) held in Borneo in August 2000. An electronic network query to all participating surveillance sites following an initial report from a site in London disclosed within 6 hours nearly simultaneous cases presenting in New York and Toronto. An e-mail alert issued by GeoSentinel within 14 hours of the initial report on September 11, 2000 in collaboration with ISTM, ASTMH, IDSA, CANTROPMED, and ProMED-Mail was immediately disseminated to an estimated 10,000 clinicians in over 100 countries [7]. This included all 26 countries known to have participants in the race. Leptospirosis is a treatable disease and some participants would still have been in the incubation phase at that point in time. GeoSentinel sites in other countries then assisted the US CDC in contacting national public health authorities to carry out and publish in *MMWR* and the *Emerging Infectious Diseases Journal* a comprehensive analysis of morbidity and risk factors [7–9].

This outbreak demonstrates the usefulness of real-time reporting of clinical data to quickly track a fast-moving disease outbreak—in contrast to epidemiological or laboratory data, which are more time-consuming to acquire. When one member site sees an unusual case, it immediately notifies the rest of the network. If any other sites have had similar cases, a pattern can be found, and the location where and date when the disease originated can be pinpointed.

## Dengue

In many ways, dengue is the prototypical travelers' disease [10–12] and, in recent years, monitoring of sentinel travelers has provided important and timely data about its distribution, its seasonality, and the onset of outbreaks in endemic areas. Dengue is currently the most frequent cause of fever in returned travelers from all parts of the world outside of Africa [2]. No vaccine and no chemoprophylaxis are available, and pretravel advice seems to have a minimal impact on dengue acquisition. In April 2002, GeoSentinel alerted the international community when it reported on ProMED-Mail a dramatic increase in dengue in travelers returning home from Thailand [13]. Official surveillance data from local populations were not immediately available to the international community. Data reported later to the World Health Organization (WHO) by Thai authorities confirmed the observation. Based on this and other data from two outbreak years (1998 and 2002), excess dengue cases in returned travelers from Southeast Asia and in particular from Thailand, beginning in February of a particular year, may have been an early marker of epidemic dengue in local populations [14]. An increase in dengue cases in returned travelers from South Central Asia (India and Bangladesh) in 2003 was also evident before official surveillance data were internationally available. Thus, information gathered from travelers' illnesses may complement local surveillance and assist local authorities in areas where public health resources are limited. Even in endemic areas with significant surveillance protocols in place, resources may limit year-round surveillance and local cases occurring outside the usual season

may not be immediately detected. Because the number of travelers to areas with epidemics may be small and some epidemics may occur in parts of a country that are not visited by travelers, sentinel surveillance is not a definitive and uniquely sensitive tool for detection of all disease outbreaks.

In Africa, dengue is uncommon. Reports of epidemic or endemic dengue activity have usually been from East Africa, and dengue 2 (DENV-2) has usually been isolated [15]. In August 2008, DENV-3 was isolated in France from an ill French citizen resident in Abidjan, Ivory Coast, who had become ill while visiting France [16]. DENV-3 had never previously been identified anywhere in West Africa. DENV-3 had recently caused unexpected outbreaks of dengue hemorrhagic fever (DHF) in Sri Lanka, East Africa, and Latin America. This report highlights the use of travelers as sentinels and the importance of this population in predicting dengue fever in inhabitants of the endemic areas. In addition, travelers can provide specimens to sophisticated laboratories in their home countries for use in the isolation and identification of emerging pathogens acquired many thousands of miles away.

## Malaria

Place of exposure for travelers' malaria diagnosed in the home country can provide valuable information for future travelers who will potentially be exposed to malaria, as well as for affected populations in endemic countries [17]. Because malaria parasites may be isolated from human blood and cultured for drug sensitivity testing, malaria resistance patterns in endemic areas have been recognized by assessing malaria isolates in ill returned travelers. This testing results in ongoing changes to recommended chemoprophylaxis regimens for future travelers to specific destinations. In addition, development of emerging resistance in traveler's malaria parasites during a treatment course of atovaquone/proguanil, which is currently frequently used to treat malaria in returned travelers, has resulted in both closer monitoring of such patients and the identification of a specific parasite mutation responsible for this resistance pattern [18–21].

Cases of malaria imported to Germany, Canada, and the USA, beginning in 1999, have identified new foci of infection in frequently visited resort areas in the Dominican Republic and in the Bahamas [22–27]. Over subsequent years, recurring cases in returned travelers even after the malaria foci were declared quiescent by local authorities on several occasions have guided ongoing revisions to chemoprophylaxis guidelines.

## Schistosomiasis

Because of earlier lessons from popular destinations such as Lake Malawi, the Omo River in Ethiopia, and Mali, which indicated the likelihood that there is really no safe fresh water in Africa [6, 28, 29], the advice of most travel medicine advisors is to avoid fresh water exposure in Africa. Nevertheless, schistosomiasis is still frequently diagnosed in returning travelers. Concurrent with the widespread risk, hotspots and point source outbreaks still occur and sentinel travelers can be helpful in identifying potential clusters that may warrant further active surveillance or case finding. For example, in 2007, a travel-related schistosomiasis cluster occurred that was apparently localized to an artificial swimming pond at a small tented camp hotel near Lake Eyasi, Tanzania [30]. The cluster of 22/27 (81%) Israeli travelers were found to be seropositive for schistosomiasis, with 19/22 (86%) being symptomatic [31].

Upon dissemination of the information and its publication on ProMED-Mail, further cases were reported from Germany, and a further cluster of four cases with the same exposure were reported from the USA. As the small artificial pool at a single busy resort seemed heavily contaminated, with a high attack rate, notification of still undiagnosed returned travelers by all available means, including postings on the Travelers' Health Web site of the US CDC, was undertaken based on the cases in sentinel travelers.

## Chikungunya

The emergence of chikungunya virus provides another example of travelers tracking a disease outbreak. Since 2005, there have been millions of cases of chikungunya in the Indian Ocean region and in India, and over 1000 travelers returning to Europe and the USA have been affected [32, 33]. Sequence analysis performed in France on blood samples from four infected travelers demonstrated the emergence of a new virus variant [34]. In addition, better descriptions of the clinical manifestations and evolution of the chronic persistent arthritis associated with this infection were possible because of the large numbers of cases that could be investigated and followed over time in well-resourced European medical facilities [35–37].

## African trypanosomiasis

In 2000, GeoSentinel Surveillance Network and a regional traveler surveillance network, the European Network on Surveillance of Imported Infectious Diseases (TropNet-Europ), noted two cases of African trypanosomiasis in travelers returning from Tanzania [38]. Affiliated surveillance sites quickly recognized nine additional cases among tourists to the Tarangire and Serengeti National Parks. When presented with information on this unusual cluster, national health authorities were proactive in instituting control measures and limiting the outbreak.

## SARS—a pathogen with explosive potential

According to the WHO bulletin initially issued on March 13, 2003 regarding an atypical pneumonia later found to be SARS (severe acute respiratory syndrome), the disease was a regional Asian condition. SARS was caused by a novel agent, which apparently had originated in November 2002 in the Guangdong Province of southern China. The infection was later found to have been transmitted to the outside by a physician from mainland China who traveled to Hong Kong and stayed in a local hotel, where he infected travelers from other countries. Because of the direct air connection from Hong Kong to Toronto, Canada, clinicians there were the first to alert the world that SARS "had boarded an airplane" and was now a global problem. The travelers infected in the Hong Kong hotel subsequently spread the virus as they returned to their respective countries, thereby initiating a global SARS epidemic that, over a 7-month period, ultimately involved 27 countries and over 8000 cases. At the time, there were no published data on the expected occurrence or frequency of respiratory illness in travelers to Asia. The GeoSentinel network had been collecting such data on sentinel travelers for a number of years by this time, and its database was accessed to provide baseline data for respiratory illness in travelers for the first *MMWR* issue published during the SARS epidemic [39]. Trend graphs following respiratory illness in travelers could then be monitored daily for the duration of the outbreak, looking for anomalies that might indicate increased rates in returning travelers heralding a further and disastrous spread of the outbreak. The laboratory isolation of the coronavirus that causes SARS and its complete genomic sequencing in only a few weeks by a laboratory in Germany were a scientific achievement of unprecedented magnitude [40]. This was made possible by the availability of virus from the sputum of a traveler transiting Frankfurt who became ill and had to be hospitalized there.

## Avian influenza

Fortunately, as of August 2008, no travel-related cases of H5N1 or other potentially pandemic strains of influenza have occurred. The current strains of H5N1 are poorly transmitted from human to human, but with the emergence of a highly infectious pandemic strain of influenza, travelers will be key determinants of the pattern of global spread. In the absence of specific laboratory diagnostics in the early stages of a pandemic, existing surveillance systems need to be in place to track occurrences of avian flu in travelers. GeoSentinel, in particular, is in a good position to, because it has collected data on flulike illnesses in travelers returning to their home countries since its creation and now has a firm understanding of where, when, and how frequently flu normally occurs. An avian influenza outbreak would cause a significant deviation from this pattern, which GeoSentinel could identify well before a laboratory could make the diagnosis. Using the Internet-based worldwide data entry system, existing analytic methods used to track morbidity over time can be modified within hours to better track an illness or syndrome of concern. During the 2003 SARS outbreak, visual review of the geographic extent of every suspected respiratory illness submitted to GeoSentinel and weekly examination of monthly trends in all presenting respiratory complaints were implemented. Protocols for immediate implementation of similar enhanced surveillance are currently in place.

## Paratyphoid fever

The incidence of typhoid fever worldwide has been increasing since the 1990s and it now causes 13 million cases annually in Asia, the most affected area [41]. Routine childhood immunization programs in highly affected areas are now being advocated.

*Salmonella paratyphi* A, considered of minor epidemiological importance, has now emerged as an increasingly important etiological agent. However, among travelers, the incidence of disease caused by *S. paratyphi* A was found more than a decade ago to be high. In a report from a major travel clinic in Nepal in 1990, the ratio of *S. paratyphi* A to *S. typhi* was 70:30 among travelers, who were mostly vaccinated, whereas this ratio was reversed, as expected, in the local population or in unvaccinated travelers [42]. This phenomenon was again clearly shown in a nationwide study among Israeli travelers with enteric fever [43]. Because the vaccinated travelers were protected against *S. typhi* by the current vaccine, this trend indicated the wide circulation of *S. paratyphi* in the community. *S. paratyphi* emergence also occurs in vaccinated local populations and calls into question the effectiveness of the existing typhoid vaccine alone in controlling enteric fevers [44]. Thus, travelers were the sentinels that sounded the call for

*S. paratyphi* A vaccine for the benefit of travelers and of local populations.

## Hepatitis A

Hepatitis A is the most common vaccine-preventable disease in travelers to endemic regions of the world. In the 1980s and 1990s, prospective studies of European and American travelers who had not received immune globulin had a risk of infection of 3–5/1000 per month of stay. Persons eating and drinking under poor hygienic conditions were estimated to have a rate of 20/1000 per month. More recent epidemiological data have been analyzed looking at the risk of hepatitis A virus (HAV) in nonimmune travelers to destinations with high or intermediate risk of transmission. These estimates are significantly lower than previously thought, with a risk of 3–11/100,000 per month in all travelers to high or intermediate endemic areas and 6–30/100,000 per month in those presumed to be nonimmune [45].

Thus, the risk of hepatitis A virus infections has decreased by a factor of 10- to 50-fold during about the last 2 decades, which reflects the improvement of hygiene in many endemic countries. In this case, travelers proved to be sensitive sentinels to show improvements in endemic countries. In fact, studies in India have shown reduced anti-HAV antibodies in the general population, which probably reflects improved sanitation [46].

## Long-term trend analysis by sentinel networks

In addition to the capability for rapid surveillance response to alarming sentinel events, systematic and ongoing collection of aggregated data from these collaborative networks provides surveillance of ongoing trends in imported diseases. This aids clinicians in diagnosing ill returnees, in advising prospective travelers, and in defining associations between patient characteristics and disease. Participation across all continents allows standardized, aggregate multinational description of the full spectrum of disease acquired by a broad range of travelers returning from diverse global destinations, provides a large sample of ill travelers, and allows a focus on the destination of exposure and not on inherent biases due to specific patient populations reported in single-center studies of ill returnees. Diagnoses are physician-verified and not self-reported.

For example, in 2006, GeoSentinel published a detailed study describing which diseases travelers are most likely to acquire in different parts of the tropical world [2]. Earlier studies had treated all returning travelers as a homogenous group. The GeoSentinel database was used to verify for the first time the assumption that the destination of travel is associated with the probability of each diagnosis among travelers returning from the developing world. In this study, specific travel destinations were clearly associated with the probability of the diagnosis of certain diseases. Diagnostic approaches and empirical therapies can thus be guided by these destination-specific differences. Specific findings from this sentinel sample of 17,000 ill returned travelers included the following: febrile illness is more likely to be from Africa and southeast Asia; malaria is one of the top three diagnoses from every region in the tropics, but dengue is the most common febrile illness from every region except Sub-Saharan Africa; in Sub-Saharan Africa, where dengue is uncommon, rickettsial disease is second only to malaria as a cause of fever; respiratory illness is more common from Southeast Asia; and acute diarrhea occurs disproportionately from South Central Asia (India, Nepal, Bangladesh).

At the same time, provider-based networks have several limitations. They do not describe all illnesses in all travelers; the focus is on medically important, not mild or self-limited illness. The emphasis is often on illness presenting at specialized centers, and attribution of place of exposure is not possible for all ill travelers, many of whom are on multicountry itineraries. The perceived risky destinations may be overrepresented in those who seek medical care, as the same relatively minor symptom is more likely to lead to a medical consultation in a traveler returned from rural Africa than from a beach resort in the Caribbean. The denominator of all travelers at risk is often elusive.

## The politics of traveler-based surveillance

Public health officials and ministries of health in many countries have traditionally expressed concern that using travelers as sentinels implies that local officials are not fully competent to do their own surveillance, or even that any reliance on internationally acquired data may threaten their own budget allocations for surveillance. Reinforcement that sentinel data from travelers is complementary to local systems is still necessary. Even with a robust local surveillance program in place, the increasingly sophisticated diagnostic technology that is accessible in developed countries can be the source of rapid identification of new outbreaks or emerging foci of infections, which will benefit the diagnosis and treatment of the local populations. Not to be discounted is pressure on health authorities to suppress information about diseases that may impact trade, commerce, or tourist influx from other countries.

## The need for increased use of travelers as sentinels

For many years, it was necessary to use local disease information from endemic populations to infer health risks for travelers. For some more uncommon or focal diseases, consideration of the reported rates of incidence among local populations is still integral to the assessment of risk. However, the behavior and living conditions of travelers may result in levels of risk different from those among native populations. Now, many robust studies that have been discussed here have focused explicitly on health outcomes among travelers. Some examples of disease hotspots identified by sentinel travelers are shown in Table 4.1.

**Table 4.1** "Hot spots" for some common travel-related diseases.

| Disease | High-risk destination |
| --- | --- |
| Malaria due to *Plasmodium vivax* | Omo River, Ethiopia; Papua, New Guinea; Rural India; Amazonia |
| Leishmaniasis | Madidi National Park, Bolivia; Manu National Park, Peru; Costa Rica, Surinam |
| Dengue fever | The islands of the Gulf of Siam, Thailand (mainly Koh Phangan) |
| Typhoid fever | India; Nepal |
| Tick-borne rickettsiosis (*R. Africae*) | South Africa |
| African trypanosomiasis | Tanzania |
| Schistosomiasis | Lake Malawi; Lake Victoria; Dogon-Mali; Mekong River, Laos |

In their role as surveillance tools for imported diseases, travelers have many advantages. They travel to every country and expose themselves to widely diverse environments and pathogens. They often return home during or just after the incubation period to an advanced medical care system that can accurately diagnose known diseases and is poised to identify new pathogens or new variants. Sentinel surveillance of travelers is not a stand-alone tool but complements traditional surveillance of notifiable and non-notifiable diseases in endemic areas. Partnerships between surveillance programs in disease-endemic areas and the newer traveler-based networks can provide mutual benefits to local populations and travelers.

# References

1 Freedman DO, Kozarsky PE, Weld LH, Cetron MS. GeoSentinel: the global emerging infections sentinel network of the International Society of Travel Medicine. *J Travel Med* 1999;6(2):94–8.

2 Freedman DO, Weld LH, Kozarsky PE, Fisk T, Robins R, von Sonnenburg F, et al. Spectrum of disease and relation to place of exposure among ill returned travelers. *N Engl J Med* 2006;354(2):119–30.

3 Carey DE, Kemp GE, White HA, Pinneo L, Addy RF, Fom AL, et al. Lassa fever. Epidemiological aspects of the 1970 epidemic, Jos, Nigeria. *Trans R Soc Trop Med Hyg* 1972;66(3):402–8.

4 Dengue type 4 infections in U.S. travelers to the Caribbean. *MMWR Morb Mortal Wkly Rep* 1981;30(21):249–50.

5 Imported dengue fever—United States, 1982. *MMWR Morb Mortal Wkly Rep* 1983;32(11):145–6.

6 Cetron MS, Chitsulo L, Sullivan JJ, Pilcher J, Wilson M, Noh J, et al. Schistosomiasis in Lake Malawi. *Lancet* 1996;348(9037):1274–8.

7 Update: outbreak of acute febrile illness among athletes participating in Eco-Challenge-Sabah 2000—Borneo, Malaysia, 2000. *MMWR Morb Mortal Wkly Rep* 2001;50(2): 21–4.

8 Centers for Disease Control and Prevention. Update: outbreak of acute febrile illness among athletes participating in Eco-Challenge-Sabah 2000—Borneo, Malaysia, 2000. *JAMA* 2001;285(6):728–30.

9 Sejvar J, Bancroft E, Winthrop K, Bettinger J, Bajani M, Bragg S, et al. Leptospirosis in "Eco-Challenge" athletes, Malaysian Borneo, 2000. *Emerg Infect Dis* 2003;9(6):702–7.

10 Wichmann O, Jelinek T. Dengue in travelers: a review. *J Travel Med* 2004;11(3):161–70.

11 Travel-associated dengue—United States, 2005. *MMWR Morb Mortal Wkly Rep* 2006;55(25):700–702.

12 Travel-associated dengue infections—United States, 2001–2004. *MMWR Morb Mortal Wkly Rep* 2005;54(22):556–8.

13 Freedman DO. Thailand: out of season dengue outbreak in travellers to Koh Phangan. ProMedMail 2002; Archive Number:20020426.4039.

14 Schwartz E, Weld LH, Wilder-Smith A, von Sonnenburg F, Keystone JS, Kain KC, et al. Seasonality, annual trends, and characteristics of dengue among ill returned travelers, 1997–2006. *Emerg Infect Dis* 2008;14(7):1081–8.

15 Dengue type 2 virus in East Africa. *MMWR Morb Mortal Wkly Rep* 1982;31(30):407–8, 413.

16 Parola P, Gautret P, Freedman DO. Dengue/DHF Update 2008 (32): France e Cote d'Ivoire. ProMedMail 2008; Archive Number: 20080808.2446

17 Jelinek T, Behrens R, Bisoffi Z, Bjorkmann A, Gascon J, Hellgren U, et al. Recent cases of falciparum malaria imported to Europe from Goa, India, December 2006–January 2007. *Euro Surveill* 2007;12(1):E070111 1.

18 Parola P, Pradines B, Simon F, Carlotti MP, Minodier P, Ranjeva MP, et al. Antimalarial drug susceptibility and point mutations associated with drug resistance in 248 *Plasmodium falciparum* isolates imported from Comoros to Marseille, France in 2004–2006. *Am J Trop Med Hyg* 2007;77(3):431–7.

19 Schwartz E, Bujanover S, Kain KC. Genetic confirmation of atovaquone-proguanil-resistant *Plasmodium falciparum* malaria acquired by a nonimmune traveler to East Africa. *Clin Infect Dis* 2003;37(3):450–51.

20 Wichmann O, Muehlberger N, Jelinek T, Alifrangis M, Peyerl-Hoffmann G, Muhlen M, et al. Screening for mutations related to atovaquone/proguanil resistance in treatment failures and other imported isolates of *Plasmodium falciparum* in Europe. *J Infect Dis* 2004;190(9):1541–6.

21 Wichmann O, Muehlen M, Gruss H, Mockenhaupt FP, Suttorp N, Jelinek T. Malarone treatment failure not associated with previously described mutations in the cytochrome b gene. *Malar J* 2004;3:14.

22 Malaria in Mexico and the Dominican Republic. *Commun Dis Rep CDR Wkly* 2000;10(6):49, 52.

23 Transmission of malaria in resort areas—Dominican Republic, 2004. *MMWR Morb Mortal Wkly Rep* 2005;53(51): 1195–8.

24 Malaria—Great Exuma, Bahamas, May–June 2006. *MMWR Morb Mortal Wkly Rep* 2006;55(37):1013–16.

25 Malaria, Bahamas. *Wkly Epidemiol Rec* 2008;83(17):156.

26 Haro-Gonza JL, Bernabeu-Wittel M, Canas E, Regordan C. Malaria and travel to the Dominican Republic. *Emerg Infect Dis* 2005;11(3):499–500.

27 Jelinek T, Grobusch M, Harms-Zwingenberger G, Kollaritsch H, Richter J, Zieger B. Falciparum malaria in European tourists to the Dominican Republic. *Emerg Infect Dis* 2000;6(5):537–8.

28 Schwartz E, Kozarsky P, Wilson M, Cetron M. Schistosome infection among river rafters on Omo River, Ethiopia. *J Travel Med* 2005;12(1):3–8.

29 Visser LG, Polderman AM, Stuiver PC. Outbreak of schisto-somiasis among travelers returning from Mali, West Africa. *Clin Infect Dis* 1995;20(2):280–85.

30 ProMED-mail. Schistosomiasis—Tanzania (Lake Eyasi). ProMED-mail 2007;20070904.2912 [cited 2008 July 8]. Available from http://www.promedmail.org.

31 Leshem E, Maor Y, Meltzer E, Assous M, Schwartz E, Acute schistosomiasis outbreak: morbidity and economic impact. *Clin Infect Dis* 2008;47:1499–506.

32 Panning M, Grywna K, van Esbroeck M, Emmerich P, Drosten C. Chikungunya fever in travelers returning to Europe from the Indian Ocean region, 2006. *Emerg Infect Dis* 2008;14(3):416–22.

33 Lanciotti RS, Kosoy OL, Laven JJ, Panella AJ, Velez JO, Lambert AJ, et al. Chikungunya virus in US travelers returning from India, 2006. *Emerg Infect Dis* 2007;13(5):764–7.

34 Parola P, de Lamballerie X, Jourdan J, Rovery C, Vaillant V, Minodier P, et al. Novel chikungunya virus variant in travelers returning from Indian Ocean islands. *Emerg Infect Dis* 2006;12(10):1493–9.

35 Taubitz W, Cramer JP, Kapaun A, Pfeffer M, Drosten C, Dobler G, et al. Chikungunya fever in travelers: clinical presentation and course. *Clin Infect Dis* 2007;45(1):e1–e4.

36 Parola P, Simon F, Oliver M. Tenosynovitis and vascular disorders associated with chikungunya virus-related rheumatism. *Clin Infect Dis* 2007;45(6):801–2.

37 Simon F, Parola P, Grandadam M, Fourcade S, Oliver M, Brouqui P, et al. Chikungunya infection: an emerging rheumatism among travelers returned from Indian Ocean islands. Report of 47 cases. *Medicine (Baltimore)* 2007;86(3):123–37.

38 Jelinek T, Bisoffi Z, Bonazzi L, van Thiel P, Bronner U, de Frey A, et al. Cluster of African trypanosomiasis in travelers to Tanzanian national parks. *Emerg Infect Dis* 2002;8(6):634–5.

39 Outbreak of severe acute respiratory syndrome—worldwide, 2003. *MMWR Morb Mortal Wkly Rep* 2003;52(11):226–8.

40 Drosten C, Gunther S, Preiser W, van der Werf S, Brodt HR, Becker S, et al. Identification of a novel coronavirus in patients with severe acute respiratory syndrome. *N Engl J Med* 2003;348(20):1967–76.

41 Crump JA, Luby SP, Mintz ED. The global burden of typhoid fever. *Bull World Health Organ* 2004;82(5):346–53.

42 Schwartz E, Shlim DR, Eaton M, Jenks N, Houston R. The effect of oral and parenteral typhoid vaccination on the rate of infection with *Salmonella typhi* and *Salmonella paratyphi* A among foreigners in Nepal. *Arch Intern Med* 1990;150(2):349–51.

43 Meltzer E, Sadik C, Schwartz E. Enteric fever in Israeli travelers: a nationwide study. *J Travel Med* 2005;12(5):275–81.

44 Ochiai RL, Wang X, von Seidlein L, Yang J, Bhutta ZA, Bhattacharya SK, et al. *Salmonella paratyphi* A rates, Asia. *Emerg Infect Dis* 2005;11(11):1764–6.

45 Mutsch M, Spicher VM, Gut C, Steffen R. Hepatitis A virus infections in travelers, 1988–2004. *Clin Infect Dis* 2006;42(4):490–97.

46 Gadgil PS, Fadnis RS, Joshi MS, Rao PS, Chitambar SD. Seroepidemiology of hepatitis A in voluntary blood donors from Pune, western India (2002 and 2004–2005). *Epidemiol Infect* 2008;136(3):406–9.

# 5 VFR (Visiting Friends and Relatives) Travelers

Phyllis E. Kozarsky[1] and Jay S. Keystone[2]

[1] Emory University School of Medicine, Atlanta, GA, USA
[2] Toronto General Hospital, University of Toronto, Toronto, ON, Canada

## Introduction and definitions

In studying health risks in travelers and illness following travel, it is important to note special groups with low rates of accessing preventive advice and high rates of important health problems. Groups visiting friends and relatives (VFRs) are at the top of this list.

That VFRs have a greater likelihood of acquiring certain infections has been suggested for a number of years, but more recently, authors have been more careful to be specific about their definition of the VFR traveler. In examining data, it is important always to use the same definition. A useful one was coined by Keystone in 2003: "A VFR is an immigrant, ethnically and racially distinct from the country of residence who returns to his/her homeland to Visit Friends and/or Relatives."

The key elements of the definition of a VFR are as follow:
1 The traveler has family in the destination country (and tends to live with them at the local standard).
2 The destination country is one of lower income than the current country of residence.

Of note is that the VFR can be either an immigrant who was born in the destination country (immigrant VFR) or someone not born in the destination country but with close ties, such as an immigrant's child or other close family member (traveler VFR).

For the most part, this chapter can be summarized by noting that many infections occur in VFR travelers with a greater frequency than in other groups of travelers. The extent to which these infections manifest themselves

differently from those in native populations depends upon how long the VFR traveler has been outside the country of birth and when he or she first acquired the infection. For example, a VFR who acquired malaria on a first trip back to his or her native Nigeria within a year following initial emigration is likely to present differently, and with milder symptoms, than if he or she were to acquire malaria 10 years after emigration on a trip back to the homeland. Thus, there is a spectrum of "semi-immunity" that the VFR traveler may retain after leaving his or her country of birth. Other elements of the individual's health would also play a role in how one might manifest an infection, such as nutritional level or whether other chronic or immunocompromising diseases are present.

## Characteristics of VFR travel

The rise in international travel has been paralleled by the rise in immigrants in many Western countries and thus the rise in VFR travel. Survey data from the United Kingdom in 2003 revealed that ethnic groups accounted for 8% of the population and yet, 14% of visits abroad were made by VFRs, with Africa and India being prime destinations [1]. Of almost 300 million people in the USA in 2006, roughly 37 million, or 12% of the population, are foreign-born [2]. Fifty-six million, or one-fifth of the population, either are foreign-born or are children of foreign-born parents [3]. In the early and mid-twentieth century, most immigrants to the USA came from Europe; however, now the majority come from Asia, Latin America, and Sub-Saharan Africa (Figures 5.1 and 5.2). These new Americans travel home frequently for occasions such as family illnesses, weddings, and funerals. Data from the Office of Travel and Tourism Industries in the USA show that in 2007, the percentage of international travelers reporting VFR as their primary

*Tropical Diseases in Travelers*, 1st edition. Edited by E. Schwartz.
© 2009 by Blackwell Publishing, ISBN: 978-1-4051-8441-0.

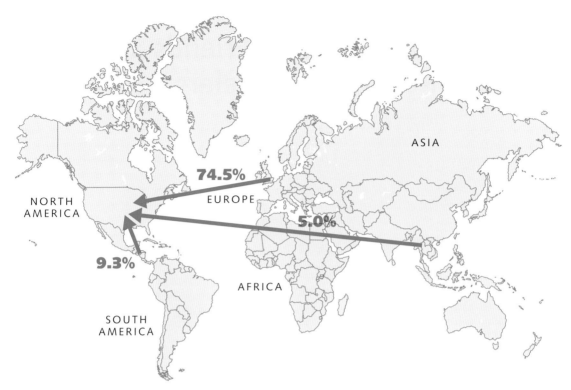

**Figure 5.1 US 1960**: 5.4% foreign-born. Population: $N = 9.7$ million. Profile of selected foreign-born populations in the USA. (From US Census Bureau, December 2001.)

reason for international travel was 38%, compared to 25% in 1996 [4] (Table 5.1). One example is that travel to India among US residents increased about 150% from 1994 to 2004, and 55% listed VFR as their primary reason for travel [5]. In addition to the striking increase in VFR travel is the ongoing immigration into Western countries, primarily from developing nations. In the USA, there are about 350,000 immigrants per year and another 30,000 refugees [6].

There are many reasons why VFR travelers are considered to be at high risk. First, studies repeatedly show that VFRs seek pretravel health advice far less than tourists or business travelers, with some studies showing 30% or fewer having had a pretravel encounter [7–12]. There are a number of reasons for this occurrence. There is a lack of awareness of the importance of health advice for travel as well as a lack of awareness by health care providers regarding the importance of pretravel counseling. In addition, there is a misconception about their level of risk. VFR travelers tend to believe that they are immune to illnesses that are endemic in their countries of origin because they often lived there for many years and either may not have

experienced life-threatening illnesses or do not recall any illnesses during that time. Their providers may also have originated from the same countries and express the opinion that there is little risk to such travel. Alternatively, family members in the home countries, who may in fact be semi-immune to some illnesses, share information with the travelers that there is little or no risk. Some do not seek pretravel advice because the travel clinic environment is not culturally suitable or easily accessible to their homes. Also, in many countries, the cost of the consultation, the vaccines for travel, and the preventive medications are not covered by health insurance and can be quite expensive, even when there is national health insurance for routine care [7, 12, 13–15]. Unfortunately, data also show that even with pretravel counseling, VFRs are often not likely to follow recommendations [16–19].

Another reason that VFRs are at greater risk is that they tend to travel for longer periods of time. Behrens recently showed that the length of stay in malaria-endemic areas for UK residents was in general greater for VFRs than for non-VFRs [1]. In addition, VFRs travel not only to major cities where most tourists and business people congregate, but

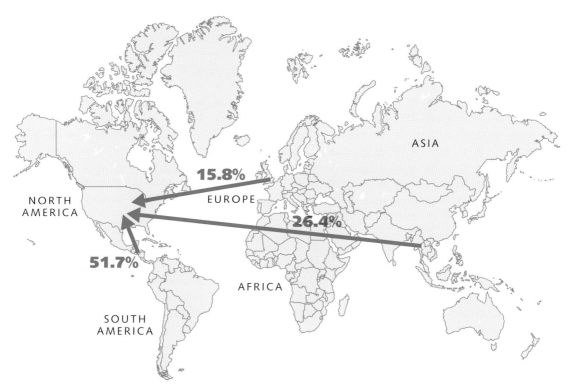

**Figure 5.2 US 2000**: 10.4% foreign-born. Population $N = 28.4$ million. Profile of selected foreign-born populations in the USA. (From US Census Bureau, December 2001.)

also to more remote and rural areas where their families live. Their exposures are different than those of typical tourists; they eat at home with family, drink from local water supplies, and, in malarious areas, may sleep without air-conditioning and in unscreened quarters.

**Table 5.1** Purpose of international travel from the USA.

| Main purpose of travel | 1996% | 2001% | 2006% |
| --- | --- | --- | --- |
| Leisure/holiday | 37 | 39 | 42 |
| VFF | 25 | 29 | 31 |
| Business | 30 | 25 | 21 |
| Convention/conference | 3 | 2 | 2 |
| Study/teaching | | 2 | 2 |

*Source:* From Elizabeth Barnett, MD. Used with permission.
Office of Travel and Tourism Industries data. Available from http://tinet_ita.doc.gov/cat/f-2006-101-001/html.

## Specific illnesses

Although this text contains sections dedicated to specific diseases, it is worth pointing out that there are special risks for VFR travelers as such. According to data from the international surveillance group GeoSentinel, the immigrant VFR group presents with more serious, potentially preventable travel-related illnesses than tourists [11]. In addition, VFRs who return from Sub-Saharan Africa, South Central Asia, and Latin America are more likely to experience fever than any other group [20]. However, for cultural reasons, the VFR traveler may be more reluctant to seek medical care on return to the country of residence. Clinical presentation may be late as a result of lack of attention paid to the risk of travel and the fact that a fever or other illness may not be associated with recent travel. Ill patients may lack the knowledge, language, and communicative skills to effectively convey their symptoms and may fear and distrust the medical system, especially when they feel sick and vulnerable. The cost of the evaluation,

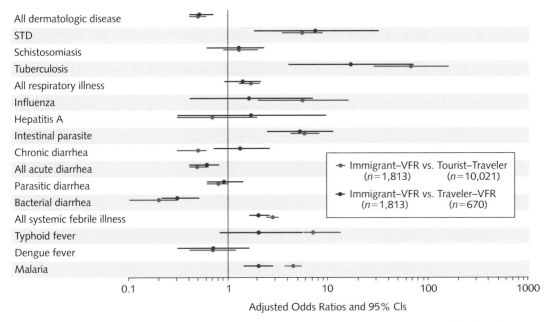

**Figure 5.3** Differing disease diagnosis profiles in immigrant VFRs versus traveler VFRs (1997–2004). (Reproduced with permission from the University of Chicago Press. Leder K, Tong S, Weld L, Kain KC, Wilder-Smith A, von Sonnenburg F, et al.; GeoSentinel Surveillance Network. Illness in travelers visiting friends and relatives: a review of the GeoSentinel Surveillance Network. *Clin Infect Dis* 2006;43:1185–93.)

the care, and medications may also be prohibitive. And, finally, this marginalized group may not receive the same level of care as others.

Of interest are GeoSentinel data showing that immigrant and traveler VFRs have slightly different profiles with regard to diagnoses [11] (Figure 5.3). VFR groups are not all alike. Disease rates depend not only on whether the traveler is an immigrant or traveler VFR, but also on the home country destination. For example, whereas travelers to West Africa have the highest incidence of malaria, those to the Indian subcontinent have the highest rate of typhoid. On the whole, immigrant VFRs are more likely to require hospitalization following travel than are other groups [11].

A summary of these diseases, reasons for risk variance, and recommendations to reduce the risks are found in Table 5.2.

## Malaria

Studies in the last 20 years have shown that VFR travelers of African ethnicity are most likely to be responsible for imported malaria [21–25]. An interesting predeparture study assessing VFR perception and knowledge about malaria at travel agencies and at travel clinics in Paris re-

vealed that although 49% considered themselves at risk, 26% failed to mention that mosquitoes transmitted the illness, instead citing such items as water or poor personal hygiene. Thirty-five percent thought there was a preventive vaccine and most thought they had been vaccinated [25].

Chemoprophylaxis use is low in VFR travelers. Surveys consistently show that VFR travelers are unaware of their malaria risk and even if aware, they continue to travel without prophylaxis [7, 24–28]. Also, data show that although some may begin their chemoprophylaxis, the rates of completion of the regimens are poor, as noted in a study from Barcelona, where almost 97% of VFRs did not complete their regimens [29]. As well, a survey done in the Roissy Charles de Gaulle Airport over a period of 12 months revealed that VFRs are twice as likely to be carrying an inappropriate antimalarial medication as those who travel on organized tours [29–31].

Indeed, returned VFR travelers make up a high proportion of malaria cases in developed countries. The proportion of malaria cases diagnosed in Europe in VFRs is consistently high [21, 22, 26, 27, 29, 32]. Even in areas where there has been a relative decrease in malaria cases, such as the Netherlands, the number of malaria cases in

**Table 5.2** Specific diseases risk, proposed reasons for risk variance, and recommendations to reduce risk specific to travelers visiting friends and relatives.

| Specific diseases | VFR vs traditional traveler risk of exposure | Reason for risk variance | Recommendations to stress with VFR travelers |
|---|---|---|---|
| Food and waterborne illness | Increased | Social and cultural pressure (i.e., eat the meal of hosts) Less likely to obtain potable water Less pretravel advice | Frequent handwashing Avoid high-risk foods (e.g., dairy products, undercooked foods). Simplify treatment regimens(i.e., single-antibiotic dose such as azithromycin, 1000 mg or ciprofloxacin, 500 mg) Discuss food preparation (i.e., cleaning vegetables) |
| Fish-related toxins and infections | Increased | Ingestion of high-risk foods [27, 52] Less pretravel advice | Avoidance counseling of specific cultural foods (e.g., raw freshwater fish) |
| Malaria | Increased | Longer stays Higher-risk destinations Less pretravel advice leading to less use of chemoprophylaxis [23] and fewer personal protection measures Belief that already immune | Education on maleria, mosquito avoidance, and the need for chemoprophylaxis Consider cost in chemoprophylaxis Use of insecticide-treated bednets |
| Tuberculosis (particularly multidrug resistant) | Increased | Increased close contact with local population Increased contact with HIV-coinfected persons | Check PPD 3–6 months after return if history of prior negative PPD and long stay (>3 months) Educate about tuberculosis signs, symptoms, and avoidance |
| Blood and body fluid for sexually transmitted diseases | Increased | More likely to seek substandard, local care (e.g., dental) Cultural practices (e.g., tattoos, female genital mutilation) Longer stays and increased chance of blood transfusion Higher likelihood of sexual encounters with local population | Discuss high-risk behaviors including tattoos, piercings, dental work, sexual encounters Purchase condoms prior to travel Consider providing syringes, needles, and intravenous catheters for long-term travel |
| Schistosomiasis and helminths | Increased | Limited access to pipe-borne water in rural areas for bathing and washing clothes | Avoid freshwater exposure Use liposomal DEET preparation with freshwater exposures[l] Discourage child from playing in dirt Use ground cover Use protective footwear |

*(Continued)*

**Table 5.2** (*Continued*)

| Specific diseases | VFR vs traditional traveler risk of exposure | Reason for risk variance | Recommendations to stress with VFR travelers |
|---|---|---|---|
| Respiratory problems | Increased | Increased close exposure to fires, smoking, or pollution | Prepare for asthma exacerbations by considering stand-by steroids |
| Zoonotic diseases (e.g., rickettsial, leptospirosis, viral fevers, leishmaniasis, anthrax) | Increased | Rural destinations Stays with family where animals are kept, and increased exposure to insects Increased exposure to mice and rats Sleeping of floors | Avoid animals Wash hands Wear protective clothing Perform daily tick checks Avoid thatched roofs, mud walls in Latin America Avoid sleeping at floor level |
| Envenomations (e.g., snakes, spiders, scorpions) | Increased | Sleeping on floors | Avoid sleeping at floor level Use footwear out-of-doors at night |
| Toxin ingestion (e.g., medication adverse events, heavy metal ingestion) | Increased | Purchasing of local medications Use of traditional therapies Use of contaminated products (e.g., Mexican pottery with lead glaze) Ingestion of contaminated food items (e.g., large reef fish, mercury-contaminated freshwater fish) | Anticipate and purchase medications prior to travel Counsel avoidance of known traditional medications (e.g., Hmong bark tea with aspirin) and high-risk items (e.g., large reef fish) |
| Yellow fever and Japanese encephalitis | Decreased in adults | Unclear, partial immunity due to previous exposure or vaccination | Avoid mosquitoes by taking protective measures and receiving vaccination when appropriate |
| Dengue fever | Increased (especially risk of DHF and DSS) | DHF and DSS occur on repeat exposure to a second serotype of dengue. VFRs more likely to have had previous exposure. | Avoid mosquitoes by taking protective measures |

Abbreviations: DEET, N,N-diethyl-m-toluamide; DHF, dengue hemorrhagic fever; DSS, dengue shock syndrome; HN, human immunodeficiency virus; PPD, purified protein derivative; VFR, visiting friends and relatives.
Hypothesis unless reference cited to support assertions.
†DEET (liposomal preparations) has been demonstrated in animal models to prevent skin penetration of *Schistosomiasis cercariae*.
*Source:* Copyright 2004 American Medical Association. All rights reserved. From *JAMA* 2004 June 1;291(23):2859.

VFR travelers has not decreased [33]. The GeoSentinel network reported that VFR travelers have an eight times greater likelihood of acquiring malaria than tourists [31], and reports from the UK as early as 1990 showed that travelers to West Africa were 10 times more likely to develop malaria than were tourists [34]. The most recent malaria surveillance in the USA shows that malaria is more common in VFR travelers than in any other category of travelers [32], accounting for >50% of cases (Table 5.3). Similar percentages have been reported in France and in the UK

**Table 5.3** Malaria in Europe.

| Country/source | Proportion of cases in VFRs/immigrants |
|---|---|
| TropNetEurope (CID 2002) | 50% |
| France, 2000 | 63% |
| UK 1987–2004 | 64% |
| Italy 1985–1998 | 32% |

[21, 26, 30]. Data from Italy show that the majority of malaria-affected children were those of immigrants from Sub-Saharan Africa [29].

Unfortunately, even those who choose to take chemoprophylaxis may think that purchasing an antimalarial such as chloroquine in their home village in Sub-Saharan Africa or in India will protect them; it may have served them adequately in years gone by. Unfortunately, the intensity of malaria may be greater than it had been previously and the resistance of the organisms may be higher as well, both contributing to the lack of protection. In addition, data show that counterfeit medications now represent a significant number of those sold in many developing countries where malaria is endemic. For example, WHO reported that 20% of medications sold in India are counterfeit; in Nigeria there are estimates that up to 70% of drugs in circulation are either fake or adulterated. Similar reports have been found in other Sub-Saharan African countries, as well as in Southeast Asia [35–38].

On the positive side, immunity to severe and fatal malaria seems to be long-standing. Nonetheless, of the six deaths due to malaria in the USA in 2006, three were in immigrants and one was in a VFR who had returned from Uganda [32, 39]. Clearly, the illness may be more severe if ignored by the traveler and by the clinician.

## Typhoid and paratyphoid fever

Although rates of enteric fever have dropped substantially in developed countries such as Israel and the USA, rates remain extremely high in many areas of the world [40]. Typically, there are >100 cases per 100,000 persons per year in South Central Asia and Southeast Asia, although in areas such as the Mekong Delta of Vietnam, the rate is 198 per 100,000, and it can be as high as 980 per 100,000 in Delhi, India. In the USA, travel to the Indian subcontinent is associated with an incidence rate about 18 times higher than for travel to any other destination; further-

more, the VFR population has a greater likelihood than tourists of acquiring typhoid [11, 41–43]. In the USA, 77% of typhoid cases occur in VFRs, mostly from South Asia and Latin America, and most of those with paratyphoid are also returnees from South Asia. A recent study from Quebec, Canada, confirmed these data, showing that 86% of the imported typhoid cases in the province occurred in VFRs [44]. Worldwide GeoSentinel data from a 10-year period between 1997 and 2006 support the increased risk of enteric fever in VFRs returning from South Central Asia [20].

## Hepatitis A

It was previously assumed that immigrant VFRs, because of birth in developing countries where hepatitis A is an endemic disease, would be immune and thus not require vaccination for protection [45]. Recent data suggest that one cannot assume immunity in the VFR population; it is best to check hepatitis A IgG or vaccinate (whichever is more cost-effective given the circumstances). One study revealed that, although there was only 2% susceptibility in New Delhi residents in those older than 45 years, almost 50% between the ages of 15 and 24 years were susceptible. Van Herck et al., in a European airport study, asked travelers about protection against food-borne illness. The VFRs planned fewer food restrictions and reported far less hepatitis A coverage than did tourists [12]. Furthermore, Behrens reported that VFR children in the UK are at very high risk [46]; travel accounts for about 10% of cases, mainly related to travel to the Indian subcontinent. In the USA, travel is also a risk factor in a similar percentage of cases [39]. In addition to those directly affected by travel, infected VFRs bring hepatitis A back to the country of residence and can transmit the infection to siblings, grandparents, schoolmates, and others [47, 48].

## Tuberculosis

Although the immigrant populations in many Western countries are diagnosed with tuberculosis (TB) with greater frequency than those native to the developed world [49], it is difficult to know how much TB is acquired prior to immigration and how much is acquired when these travelers visit their homelands [39]. An early British study estimated that over a 5-year period in one sector in London about 20% of Asian immigrants who had developed TB had likely acquired the illness after recent travel to Asia [50, 51]. Data also suggest that VFR children who traveled within the previous year had a greater likelihood of a positive tuberculin skin test [52].

## Other infections

Varicella is an unusual infection because in certain tropical areas the age of infection tends to be greater. It is also known that the risk of serious complications such as encephalitis and pneumonia is greater in adulthood. Although no literature documents outbreaks among the VFR population in particular, this is a group that is underimmunized against standard childhood illnesses and, thus, would be expected to suffer greater morbidity from this infection [53].

Cholera is a rare illness in developed countries and in tourist travelers. In the USA between January 1995 and December 2000, 61 cases of cholera were reported. Travel accounted for 37 of these. Of 27 who reported a reason for travel, 16 (59%) were VFRs and 4 (15%) were immigrants. Data such as these have been relatively stable [54].

The incidence of sexually transmitted infections (STIs) and blood-borne infections such as hepatitis B has also been reported to be high in VFRs [11, 39]. The predominance of human immunodeficiency virus-1 (HIV-1) non-B subtypes and other concurrent STIs increases the risk of HIV transmission. Education of travelers regarding the use of condoms is difficult and condoms found in certain regions may not be as effective.

Although it has repeatedly been noted that acute diarrhea is reported with less frequency in the VFR population following travel, the rates of gastrointestinal parasites are notable [55, 56]. However, similarly to tuberculosis, it is often difficult to ascertain in this group if the infections were acquired on the recent trip to the homeland or prior to initial emigration. Risk behavior that may continue with each would includes walking barefoot, thus risking strongyloidiasis and hookworm, and eating fruits and vegetables fertilized with human feces, which increases the risk of acquiring helminthic infections [57, 58].

Also scattered throughout the literature are reports of other illnesses occurring in VFRs, such as brucellosis occurring from consumption of contaminated unpasteurized milk products, or respiratory illnesses and pneumonias due to coxiella, mycoplasma, legionella, and other causes [59, 60].

## Summary and conclusions

VFR travelers are at greater risk for many infectious diseases because they are more likely to visit rural areas for long periods of time, to consume contaminated food and beverages, and to have prolonged intimate contact with local populations. They are less likely to seek pretravel advice or take antimalarial chemoprophylaxis. Many of the illnesses they acquire are preventable, such as the routine vaccine-preventable diseases, hepatitis A and B, typhoid, and malaria.

The removal of barriers to VFR pretravel health care is challenging. First of all, VFRs represent many diverse groups. For example, some VFRs from India are college educated and have the funds available to access pretravel health care, understand the issues, and take appropriate measures to prevent illness; yet this does not always happen. On the other hand, many other groups do not have the same resources. The problem is not merely financial; in countries with universal access to health care, the VFR population still has a higher risk. As Angell and Cetron have noted, there are tremendous cultural barriers—lack of understanding of risk and lack of trust of health care practiced in settings where people may not feel comfortable [16]. In fact, ethnicity may play a role in the ways in which individuals think about risk and protection; the problem may not be just whether or not someone is a VFR. Unpublished work from the CDC demonstrates that travelers of South Asian ethnicity going to India are less likely than travelers of other ethnic groups to be protected against preventable travel-related infections, regardless of their VFR status.

Suggestions have been made in recent years to improve cross-cultural competency within the health care provider sector; this is happening slowly. Language barriers can be aided by interpreters. Providing clinics with travel and tropical medicine expertise in communities where the foreign-born live and providing handouts in multiple languages (e.g., available from http://www.tropical.umn.edu/vfr/index.htm) are useful. Focusing during the pretravel consult on behaviors that are helpful in reducing risk may be productive. Educating the children of VFRs in schools, religious facilities, and other venues is one good strategy, as children often take messages home to their families [39]. Community outreach using local newspapers and flyers may reach some.

Unfortunately, much of what has been stated here has been noted previously and has been reported and published since the 1980s. Solutions are difficult to develop and implement because of the fact that the greater numbers of immigrants to developed countries from the developing world will continue to increase the number of VFR travelers. Health care providers need to be innovative regarding how to better reach the VFR population and this will require a multidisciplinary approach, probably with some subsidization. These are challenging problems, both for the medical communities and for those who are most affected by their marginalized status.

# References

1  Travel Trends 2003. A report on the International Passenger Survey. 2004. Available from URL: http://www.statistics.gov.uk.

2  U.S. Census Bureau. American factfinder. 2008 [cited 2008 July 6]. Available from URL: http://factfinder.census.gov.

3  Bacaner N, Stauffer B, Boulware DR, Walker PF, Keystone JS. Travel medicine considerations for North American immigrants visiting friends and relatives. *JAMA* 2004;291(23):2856–64.

4  Office of Travel and Tourism Industries. 2008 [cited 2008 July 6]. Available from URL: http://www.tinet.ita.doc.gov.

5  Office of Travel and Tourism Industries. Available from URL: http://www.tinet.ita.doc.gov.

6  Maloney SA, Ortega LS, Cetron MS. Overseas medical screening for immigrants and refugees. In: Walker PF, Barnett ED, editors. *Immigrant Medicine 2007*. Philadelphia, PA: Elsevier; 2007. p. 111–21.

7  Dos Santos CC, Anvar A, Keystone JS, Kain KC. Survey of use of malaria prevention measures by Canadians visiting India. *CMAJ* 1999;160:195–200.

8  Leonard L, VanLandingham M. Adherence to travel health guidelines: the experience of Nigerian immigrants in Houston, Texas. *J Immigr Health* 2001;3:31–45.

9  Chatterjee S. Compliance of malaria chemoprophylaxis among travelers to India. *J Travel Med* 1999;6:7–11.

10  Scolari C, Tedoldi S, Casalini C, Scarcella C, Matteelli A, Casari S, et al. Knowledge, attitudes, and practices on malaria preventive measures of migrants attending a public health clinic in northern Italy. *J Travel Med* 2002;9:160–62.

11  Leder K, Tong S, Weld L, Kain KC, Wilder-Smith A, von Sonnenburg F, et al.; GeoSentinel Surveillance Network. Illness in travelers visiting friends and relatives: a review of the GeoSentinel Surveillance Network. *Clin Infect Dis* 2006;43:1185–93.

12  Van Herck K, Van Damme P, Castelli F, Zuckerman J, Nothdurft H, Dahlgren AL, et al. Knowledge, attitudes and practices in travel-related infectious diseases: the European airport survey. *J Travel Med* 2004;11:3–8.

13  Keystone JS, Hébert PC, Stanbrook MB, Sibbald B, Flegel K, MacDonald N, et al. Protecting Canadian travellers: prevention is better than cure. *CMAJ* 2008;178:373.

14  Badrinath P, Ejidokun OO, Barnes N, Ramaiah S. Change in NHS regulations may have caused increase in malaria. *BMJ* 1998;316:1746–7.

15  Schilthuis HJ, Goossens I, Ligthelm RJ, de Vlas SJ, Varkevisser C, Richardus JH. Factors determining use of pre-travel preventive health services by West African immigrants in the Netherlands. *Trop Med Int Health* 2007;12:990–98.

16  Angell SY, Cetron MS. Health disparities among travelers visiting friends and relatives abroad. *Ann Intern Med* 2005;142:67–72.

17  Casalino E, Le Bras J, Chaussin F, Fichelle A, Bouvet E. Predictive factors of malaria in travelers to areas where malaria is endemic. *Arch Intern Med*. 2002;162:1625–30.

18  Duval B, De Serre G, Shadmani R, et al. A population-based comparison between travelers who consulted travel clinics and those who did not. *J Travel Med* 2003;10:4–10.

19  Laver SM, Wetzels J, Behrens RH. Knowledge of malaria, risk perception, and compliance with prophylaxis and personal and environmental preventive measures in travelers exiting Zimbabwe from Harare and Victoria Falls International airport. *J Travel Med* 2001;8:298–303.

20  Wilson ME, Weld LH, Boggild A, Keystone JS, Kain KC, von Sonnenburg F, et al.; GeoSentinel Surveillance Network. Fever in returned travelers: results from the GeoSentinel Surveillance Network. *Clin Infect Dis* 2007;44:1560–68.

21  Smith AD, Bradley DJ, Smith V, Blaze M, Behrens RH, Chiodini PL, et al. Imported malaria and high risk groups: observational study using UK surveillance data 1987–2006. *BMJ* 2008;337:a120.

22  Fenner L, Weber R, Steffen R, Schlagenhauf P. Imported infectious disease and purpose of travel, Switzerland. *Emerg Infect Dis* 2007;13:217–22.

23  Ladhani S, Aibara RJ, Riordan FA, Shingadia D. Imported malaria in children: a review of clinical studies. *Lancet Infect Dis* 2007;7:349–57.

24  Castelli F, Matteelli A, Caligaris S, Gulletta M, el-Hamad I, Scolari C, et al. Malaria in migrants. *Parassitologia* 1999;41:261–5.

25  Pistone T, Guibert P, Gay F, Malvy D, Ezzedine K, Receveur MC, et al. Malaria risk perception, knowledge and prophylaxis practices among travellers of African ethnicity living in Paris and visiting their country of origin in Sub-Saharan Africa. *Trans Royal Soc Tropical Hed & Hygiene* 2007;101(10):990–5.

26  Schlagenhauf P, Steffen R, Loutan L. Migrants as a major risk group for imported malaria in European countries. *J Trav Med* 2003;10:106–7.

27  Jelinek T, Schulte C, Behrens R, Grobusch MP, Coulaud JP, Bisoffi Z, et al. Imported falciparum malaria in Europe: sentinel surveillance data from the European network on surveillance of imported infectious diseases. *Clin Infect Dis* 2002;34:572–6.

28  Matteelli A, Colombini P, Gulletta M, Castelli F, Carosi G. Epidemiological features and case management practices of imported malaria in northern Italy 1991–1995. *Trop Med Int Health* 1999;4:653–7.

29  Millet JP, Garcia de Olalla P, Carrillo-Santisteve P, Gascón J, Treviño B, Muñoz J, et al. Caylà JA. Imported malaria in a cosmopolitan European city: a mirror image of the world epidemiological situation. *Malar J* 2008;7:56.

30 Semaille C, Santin A, Prazuck T, Bargain P, Lafaix C, Fisch A. Malaria chemoprophylaxis of 3,446 French travelers departing from Paris to eight tropical countries. *J Travel Med* 1999;6:3–6.

31 Leder K, Black J, O'Brien D, Greenwood Z, Kain KC, Schwartz E, et al. Malaria in travelers: a review of the GeoSentinel surveillance network. *Clin Infect Dis* 2004;39:1104–12.

32 Mali S, Steele S, Slutsker L, Arguin PM; Centers for Disease Control and Prevention (CDC). Malaria surveillance—United States, 2006. *MMWR Surveill Summ* 2008;57:24–39.

33 Baas MC, Wetsteyn JCFM, van Gool T. Patterns of imported malaria at the Academic Medical Center, Amsterdam, the Netherlands. *J Travel Med* 2006:13:2–7.

34 Phillips-Howard PA, Radalowicz A, Mitchell J, et al. Risk of malaria in British residents returning home from malarious areas. *BMJ* 1990;300:499–503.

35 Counterfeit medicines: an update on estimates [news release]. WHO/7.13;March 2007.

36 Dondorp AM, Newton PN, Mayxay M, Van Damme W, Smithuis FM, Yeung S, et al. Fake antimalarials in Southeast Asia are a major impediment to malaria control: multinational cross-sectional survey on the prevalence of fake antimalarials. *Trop Med Int Health* 2004;9:1241–6.

37 Amin AA, Kokwaro GO. Antimalarial drug quality in Africa. *J Clin Pharm Ther* 2007;32:429–40.

38 Bate R, Coticelli P, Tren R, Attaran A. Antimalarial drug quality in the most severely malarious parts of Africa—a six country study. *PLoS ONE* May 7 2008;3(5):e2132.

39 Angell SY, Behrens RH. Risk assessment and disease prevention in travelers visiting friends and relatives. *Infect Dis Clin North Am* 2005;19:49–65.

40 Connor B, Schwartz E. Typhoid and paratyphoid fever in travelers. *Lancet Infect Dis* 2005;5:623–8.

41 Ackers ML, Puhr ND, Tauxe RV, Mintz ED. Laboratory-based surveillance of *Salmonella* serotype Typhi infections in the United States: antimicrobial resistance on the rise. *JAMA* 2000;283:2668–73.

42 Basnyat B, Maskey AP, Zimmerman MD, Murdoch DR. Enteric (typhoid) fever in travelers. *Clin Infect Dis* 2005; 41:1467–72.

43 Steinberg EB, Bishop R, Haber P, Dempsey AF, Hoekstra RM, Nelson JM, et al. Typhoid fever in travelers: who should be targeted for prevention? *Clin Infect Dis* 2004;39(2): 186–91.

44 Provost S, Gagnon S, Lonergan G, Bui YG, Labbé AC. Hepatitis A, typhoid and malaria among travelers—surveillance data from Québec (Canada). *J Travel Med* 2006;13:219–26.

45 Das K, Jain A, Gupta S, Kapoor S, Gupta RK, Chakravorty A, et al. The changing epidemiological pattern of hepatitis A in an urban population of India: emergence of a trend similar to the European countries. *Eur J Epidemiol* 2000;16: 507–10.

46 Behrens RH, Collins M, Boho B, et al. Risk for British travelers of acquiring hepatitis A. *BMJ* 1995;311:193.

47 Gervelmeyer A, Nielsen MS, Frey LC, Sckerl H, Damberg E, Mølbak K. An outbreak of hepatitis A among children and adults in Denmark, August 2002 to February 2003. *Epidemiol Infect* 2006;134:485–91.

48 Jong EC. United States epidemiology of hepatitis A: influenced by immigrants visiting friends and relatives in Mexico? *Am J Med* 2005;118 Suppl 10A:50S–57S.

49 CDC trends in tuberculosis morbidity—US 1999–2002. *MMWR Morb Mortal Wkly Rep* 2003;52:217–224.

50 McCarthy BJ. Asian immigrant tuberculosis effect of visiting Asia. *Dis Chest* 1984;78:248–52.

51 Shah S, Tanowitz HB, Wittner M. The ethnic minority traveler. *Infect Dis Clin North Am* 1998;12:523–41.

52 Lobato MN, Hopewell PC. Mycobacterium tuberculosis infection after travel to or contact with visitors from countries with a high prevalence of tuberculosis. *Am J Respir Crit Care Med* 1998;158:1871–5.

53 Lee BW. Review of varicella zoster seroepidemiology in India and Southeast Asia. *Trop Med Int Health* 1998;3:886–90.

54 Mahon BE, Mintz ED, Greene KD, Wells JG, Tauxe RV. Reported cholera in the United States, 1992–1994: a reflection of global changes in cholera epidemiology. *JAMA* 1996;276: 307–12.

55 Boggild AK, Yohanna S, Keystone JS, Kain KC. Prospective analysis of parasitic infections in Canadian travelers and immigrants. *J Travel Med* 2006;13(3):138–44.

56 Freedman DO, Kozarsky PE et al. GeoS: the global emerging infections sentinel network of the ISTM. *J Travel Med* 1999;6:94–8.

57 Stauffer WM, Rothenberger M. Hearing hoofbeats, thinking zebras: five diseases common among refugees that Minnesota physicians need to know about. *Minn Med* 2007;90:42–6.

58 Stauffer WM, Sellman JS, Walker PF. Biliary liver flukes (opisthorchiasis and clonorchiasis) in immigrants in the United States: often subtle and diagnosed years after arrival. *J Travel Med* 2004 11:157–9.

59 Ansart S, Pajot O, Grivois JP, Zeller V, Klement E, Perez L, et al. Pneumonia among travelers returning from abroad. *J Travel Med* 2004;11:87–91.

60 Matteelli A, Beltrame A, Saleri N, Bisoffi Z, Allegri R, Volonterio A, et al. Respiratory syndrome and respiratory tract infections in foreign–born and national travelers hospitalized with fever in Italy. *J Travel Med* 2005;12(4):190–96.

# 6 Post-Tropical Screening

### Joanna S. Herman[1] and Peter L. Chiodini[1,2]

[1]Hospital for Tropical Diseases, London, UK
[2]London School of Hygiene and Tropical Medicine, London, UK

## Introduction

In this era of frequent international travel, an estimated 50 million residents of industrialized countries travel annually to the tropics [1, 2]. Such travel brings exposure to a broad range of pathogens rarely, if ever, encountered at home. The risk of morbidity during travel has been shown to vary between 20% and 70% [3]. Accurate data on tropical infections contracted abroad are limited, and many studies have been designed to examine individual diseases or particular groups of travelers.

The majority of infections acquired tend to be short-lived and easily detected and treatable, whereas the more exotic tropical infections, such as filarial and helminth infections, tend to be limited to those who spend prolonged periods in rural endemic areas. Risk of infection depends on behavior, duration of stay, preventative measures taken, and degree of endemicity in the area visited.

## Post-tropical screening of the asymptomatic traveler

Post-tropical screening is aimed at detecting occult infections in asymptomatic individuals, or uncovering potential health risk exposures that may in future years lead to serious morbidity. Screening practices vary widely in different centers and different countries and are dependent on both local expertise and economics.

The value of screening depends to a large extent on the risk of exposure of the individual traveler to potential infections. Two groups of asymptomatic travelers will commonly request screening: those concerned that they may have a latent infection—the "worried well," and those

who want a retrospective diagnosis of an illness (usually febrile) that they experienced while abroad. However, the investigation of a febrile illness that has already resolved is of very little value. Screening of asymptomatic individuals should be reserved for those who have had definite exposure risk and who have been back from the tropics for at least 3 months, to allow adequate time for schistosomiasis and other serology (where relevant) to become positive. Not all travelers from the tropics need screening, and average package holidaymakers who have only been abroad for 2 weeks do not warrant post-tropical screening, unless they have had definite exposure risk. Screening can also provide an opportunity to raise other important, but frequently neglected, concerns for long-term travelers, such as human immunodeficiency virus (HIV) testing and psychological well-being.

Few studies have been done on screening of asymptomatic travelers, and therefore data are limited. One of the earliest studies done (published in 1980) was on ex-servicemen who were prisoners of war in Southeast Asia during 1942–1945; they were screened for infection with *Strongyloides stercoralis* [4]. Despite having left the tropics on average 35 years earlier, 27% of men were found to be infected. At the time, the only method of diagnosis available was stool examination and culture, which is notoriously insensitive compared with the serological tests now available, particularly if the parasite load is low. Therefore, this figure was probably an underestimation of the true prevalence. More recent studies have examined the utility of screening, but few have looked at its cost-effectiveness [5, 6]. This remains controversial and practitioners are divided in opinion about its usefulness [7].

Evidence from some studies suggests that screening does give a reasonable yield of occult infections (particularly schistosomiasis, strongyloidiasis, and gastrointestinal infections such as *Giardia lamblia* and *Entamoeba histolytica*) if the appropriate individuals are targeted [5, 6]. These should be people who have spent a significant

**45**

length of time abroad in more rural areas, such as back-packers, missionaries, employees of nongovernmental organizations, or armed forces personnel. A study by Carroll et al. found that 25% of asymptomatic individuals who were screened had an abnormal result when investigations were targeted according to assessment of exposure risk [5]. In the same study, stool microscopy was found to be abnormal in 18.7% (the most common abnormality being cysts of *G. lamblia, E. histolytica,* or *E. dispar*), and 16% had eosinophilia. Of this last group, over a third were found to have a parasitosis, most often schistosomiasis (10%), but also filariasis, hookworm, strongyloidiasis, and trichiuriasis.

Some would argue that most infections detected by post-travel screening are not life-threatening and pose little threat to either the individual or public health. The important exceptions to these are HIV and strongyloidiasis. Furthermore, some protozoan or helminth infections detected by screening will clear untreated with time [7]. However, on an individual level, screening is useful in allaying anxiety, and importantly, it can detect certain infections that have the potential to cause serious morbidity years later if left untreated. These include strongyloidiasis (hyperinfestation syndrome), schistosomiasis (acute tetraplegia, bladder carcinoma), and *E. histolytica* (abscesses). Therefore, given the large number of travelers, screening can only be justified on a cost-benefit analysis if there is an acceptable pickup rate for treatable, but potentially pathogenic disease. From a public health point of view, HIV and sexually transmitted infections (STIs) pose the greatest problem, but these are not always included in basic post-tropical screening, and therefore it could be argued that screening in the interest of public health is of little cost-benefit.

Several studies have set out to evaluate the usefulness of different elements of screening strategies [6, 7]. The usual approach is detailed history taking and examination, which then guide laboratory investigations. But this can be time-consuming and is not necessarily appropriate for returning travelers, who often have no symptoms or signs of the parasites they are harboring. The best approach is a structured and targeted questionnaire that identifies potential exposure risks. Physical examination has been shown to add little to the management of these individuals [5, 6].

The individuals who should be considered for screening include the following:
• Those who have had specific exposure risks, such as freshwater exposure;

• Long-term travelers or backpackers who have traveled for at least 3 months;
• Expatriates or missionaries who return home after living in the tropics;
• Military personnel or employees of nongovernmental organizations deployed to the tropics.

Generally, there is no benefit in screening those who have had a short self-limiting illness while abroad, unless it can alleviate fear of having acquired some persistent exotic disease. Travelers who are visiting friends and relatives (VFRs) are a specific subgroup who present particular exposure risks, and are discussed in Chapter 5.

## The screening consultation

Structured history taking (with particular questions about specific locations visited, type of accommodation, freshwater exposure, and timing of possible exposure) and relevant laboratory tests are the most important part of screening. Physical examination adds little to the management of these patients [5, 6].

Initial screening tests can be chosen according to three broad geographical areas visited, based upon in-country prevalence data: West Africa, the rest of Africa, and the rest of the world. All travelers returning from any part of the tropics should have a full blood count, stool examination for ova, cysts, and parasites, and serology for strongyloidiasis. In addition, those returning from any part of Africa should have terminal urine examination for schistosomal ova and serology for schistosomiasis. Investigation for schistosomiasis from parts of the world other than Africa has a very low yield, and so should be very carefully targeted if undertaken on travelers to those areas [6]. Travelers to West Africa should additionally have filarial serology, and if there is a high index of suspicion, day and night blood tests should be performed, as they may be positive despite negative filarial serology (see Figure 6.1).

Examination of stool and urine for strongyloides and schistosomiasis has low sensitivity, and therefore serological testing is recommended as well [8]. It is also prudent to screen for schistosomiasis in those who have been in endemic areas even if they deny relevant exposure, as data have shown that schistosomiasis serology may be positive in those who deny freshwater exposure [9]. In interpreting serological results, it is important to remember that some assays will cross-react, particularly those for strongyloides and filarial antibodies.

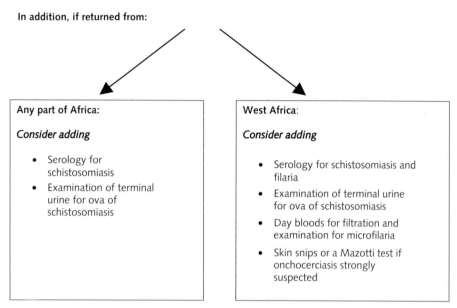

**Figure 6.1** Post-tropical screening tests according to geographical area visited.

Many travelers are worried about the possibility of malaria, but screening for this is of no value. Instead, they should be advised that if they develop a fever within 12 months of returning home from a malaria-endemic area, a malaria film should be performed.

People who have had unprotected sexual exposure should routinely be offered screening for HIV and STIs, and travelers should be directed toward appropriate clinics. The diagnosis of such infections has important implications for public health as well as for the individual. Mental health should also be part of screening for those who have spent extended periods in the tropics, but is often neglected. Although screening refers to asymptomatic individuals, it is important to ask key questions that might reveal an underlying mental health problem. Such problems may manifest as a variety of symptoms, including exhaustion, depression, anxiety, and excess alcohol or drug use [10].

## Specific screening investigations for eosinophilia

Screening of the asymptomatic traveler for eosinophilia is one of the most basic and easily available investigations. Eosinophilia is usually defined as a peripheral eosinophil count of $>0.45 \times 10^9$/L. Its prevalence varies from 5% to 8% (UK series of 852 asymptomatic individuals) to 10% (Canadian series of 1605 patients) [6, 8, 11]. The most frequently identified cause of eosinophilia is helminth infection, particularly schistosomiasis and strongyloidiasis. However, it is often transient and usually occurs in the tissue migration phase of the parasite (during the prepatent period), when both serology and stool examination may be negative. Noninfectious causes of eosinophilia should also be considered, and include autoimmune conditions, connective tissue disease, malignancy, atopy, and allergic drug reactions (see Chapter 39).

Many helminth infections in travelers are asymptomatic, but some may cause serious problems, such as paraparesis due to schistosomiasis, or may present much later with complications, such as strongyloidiasis hyperinfection. All helminth infections are treatable. However, it should also be remembered that helminth infection may occur in the absence of eosinophilia, so investigations other than a full blood count are required for reliable exclusion.

Like any screening test, investigations for eosinophilia should be tailored according to geographical location visited and risk exposure behavior. Timing of tests is also important, as many serological tests do not become positive until some weeks after exposure. Therefore, for asymptomatic individuals, it is worth deferring screening tests until at least 12 weeks after return. A large number of cases of eosinophilia, however, will resolve spontaneously and their cause will remain undetermined.

Blind treatment of eosinophilia in a returning traveler is not recommended if facilities permit detailed investigation for the presence of parasites. As for initial screening, in the choice of investigations to ascertain the cause of eosinophilia, the world can be divided into three broad geographical areas, based on both in-country prevalence data and other study data, and tests for eosinophilia selected accordingly [8]:

1 Africa, excluding West Africa: Feco-orally acquired helminths with worldwide distribution associated with limited sanitation. *Schistosoma mansoni* and *haematobium*, *S. stercoralis*, and hookworm are common. *Wuchereria bancrofti* is widespread but rare in travelers.

2 West Africa: Filaria, especially *Onchocerca volvulus* and *Loa loa*.

3 The rest of the world: *strongyloides* and hookworm.

Some would advocate treating eosinophilia empirically with albendazole and monitoring the response to treatment by resolution of eosinophilia [12]. Where investigative resources are limited this may be appropriate, and it has been suggested for mass treatment of immigrants [13]. However, although albendazole may be effective for a number of geohelminths, particularly the ones that tend to cause the least morbidity (e.g., hookworm, *Ascaris*, and *Trichuris*, as well as the protozoan *Giardia* frequently acquired by travelers), it is not the best treatment for those that cause the more serious pathology (e.g., *S. stercoralis*, *Gnathostoma spinigerum*, *Echinococcus* sp., filariae, and cystercicosis). In the case of strongyloides, the cure rate with albendazole varies from 45% to 75%, and ivermectin is the treatment of choice [14]. Therefore, if empiric treatment is contemplated, albendazole and ivermectin should be prescribed rather than albendazole alone.

## Stool examination

Examination of the stool for parasitic infection should be routinely carried out in all travelers being screened. It is easy and cost-effective, and the yield is high for the common geohelminths such as *Ascaris lumbricoides*, *Trichuris trichiura*, and hookworm species. When results are positive, appropriate treatment should be offered, even if the patient is asymptomatic, as untreated infections can cause serious problems later. However, the yield from stool can be low because of the low burden of infection in travelers, and for some organisms serology provides greater sensitivity. Because the yield for strongyloides and schistosomiasis is relatively low, serology for these should be offered in addition to stool microscopy.

## Screening for schistosomiasis

Schistosomiasis can be acquired by anyone who swims, washes, or bathes in infected water. Adult flukes may survive as long as 30 years. Most cases of schistosomiasis in travelers are acquired in Africa, according to data from the European Network on Surveillance of Imported Infectious Diseases (TropNetEurop) surveillance network and the GeoSentinel group [15, 16]. Other studies have found that 18% of asymptomatic travelers with freshwater exposure who were screened had positive schistosomiasis serology [6, 17], and chronic schistosomiasis developed in 26% of patients who were asymptomatic when initially screened [18]. This supports the policy of treating asymptomatic patients with positive screening tests [18].

Diagnosis of schistosomiasis is made either by finding eggs in a terminal urine sample or stool or by detecting positive serology. Looking for eggs is more useful as a screening tool in the immigrant population than for lightly infected travelers with limited exposure. In this latter group, serology is more sensitive. However, eosinophilia is a poor predictor of schistosomiasis (especially in chronic infections), and even if it is normal in people who have been in an endemic area, serology should still be performed.

The most sensitive test for diagnosis is serology done 3 months or more after last exposure (the time taken to develop an antibody response to the egg antigens). The schistosomal enzyme-linked immunosorbant assay (ELISA) used in UK (based on egg antigen) has a published sensitivity of 96% with *Sch. mansoni* and 92% with *Sch. haematobium* and a specificity of 97% [19]. Whitty et al. found that if serology by ELISA is used alone, 14% of cases will be missed; they, therefore, advocate the use of stool and urine in addition to serology to increase the yield of screening [9]. Serology may remain positive for years, and therefore positive results may represent old treated infections or infections that are no longer active.

## Screening for tuberculosis

The risk of a traveler to the tropics acquiring tuberculosis (TB) depends on various factors, but generally is thought to be very low [20]. These factors include the prevalence of infection in the area visited, the time spent there, and the closeness of contact with individuals who have smear positive pulmonary TB. Risk is minimal in short-term travelers, but may be higher in those who spend longer periods in the tropics and have prolonged contact with infected individuals in confined spaces, such as health care workers. For long-term travelers, incidence is thought to be comparable to that in the indigenous population [21].

Screening of travelers for TB is a contentious issue, and an evidence-based practice is lacking. Acquisition of TB is usually defined as conversion from a negative to a positive tuberculin skin test (TST)—either a Mantoux or a Heaf test. This usually occurs within 6 weeks after exposure to an individual with active pulmonary TB, but may take longer. Interpretation of these tests can be complicated, and the development of a response to TST will be influenced by various factors including previous bacille Calmette-Guérin (BCG) vaccination (when the test may be strongly positive) and immune status (when the test may be falsely negative if the subject is immunodeficient). To detect acquisition of TB during travel, pre- and post-travel TSTs must be performed, and each test requires two clinic visits—one to administer the test and one to read it. This practice is highly time intensive for both traveler and physician, and may be impractical. Screening with a chest X-ray is often performed in those who suspect they have had recent exposure, but this is an insensitive test for newly acquired infection and should not be used. Routine administration of BCG to travelers going to the tropics for prolonged periods is not recommended, as its efficacy is limited in adults.

As a general principle, if active TB is suspected during a screening consultation, referral should be made to a specialist clinic (usually infectious disease or respiratory) for further investigation.

Other screening tests may also need to be done, and will be guided by initial consultation. As a result of studies on screening of travelers at the Hospital for Tropical Diseases in London, a nurse-led screening clinic was set up in 2006. In this setting, a structured questionnaire guides the relevant laboratory tests, and if this yields positive results the traveler is then referred for follow-up to a consultant clinic.

## Conclusions

In summary, the key to screening is structured history taking, including a sexual history, followed by relevant laboratory tests based on the geographical area visited and risk exposure. Short-term package tourists will rarely warrant screening unless they have well-defined exposure, and screening should be reserved for longer-term, more adventurous travelers. Mental health should not be ignored. Screening practices will be based on both local expertise and economics, but can be effectively carried out in nurse-led clinics.

## References

1 Ryan ET, Wilson ME, Kain KC. Illness after international travel. *N Eng J Med* 2002;347:505–16.

2 Steffen R, deBarnardis C, Banos A. Travel epidemiology—a global perspective. *Int J Antimicrob Agents* 2003;21:89–95.

3 Steffen R, Rickenbach M, Wilhelm U, Helminger A, Schar M. Health problems after travel to developing countries. *J Infect Dis* 1987;156:84–91.

4 Grove DI. Strongyloidiasis in Allied ex-prisoners of war in South-east Asia. *BMJ* 1980;280(6214):598–601.

5 Carroll B, Dow C, Snashall D, Marshall T, Chiodini PL. Post-tropical screening: how useful is it? *BMJ* 1993;307:541.

6 Whitty CJM, Carroll B, Armstrong M, et al. Utility of history, examination and laboratory tests in screening those returning to Europe from the tropics for parasitic infection. *Trop Med Int Health* 2000;11:818–23.

7 Conlon CP, Peto T. Post-tropical screening is of little value. *BMJ* 1993;307:1008.

8 Whetham J, Day JN, Armstrong M, Chiodini PL, Whitty CJ. Investigation of tropical eosinophilia: assessing a strategy based on geographical area. *J Infect* 2003;46;(3):180–85.

9 Whitty CJ, Mabey DC, Armstrong M, Wright SG, Chiodini PL. Presentation and outcome of 1107 cases of schistosomiasis from Africa diagnosed in a non-endemic country. *Trans R Soc Trop Med Hyg* 2000;94(5):531–4.

10 Lankester T. Health screening and psychological considerations in the returned traveller. In: *Travel Medicine and Migrant Health*. Churchill Livingstone. p. 443–52.

11 Libman MD, MacLean JD, Gyorkos TW. Screening for schistosomiasis, filariasis, and strongyloidiasis among

expatriates returning from the tropics. *Clin Infect Dis* 1993;17(3):353–9.

12 Meltzer E, Percik R, Shatzkes J, et al. Eosinophilia among returning travelers: a practical approach. *Am J Trop Med Hyg* 2008;78(5):702–9.

13 Muennig P, Pallin D, Sell R, Chan M-S. The cost effectiveness of strategies for the treatment of intestinal parasites in immigrants. *N Engl J Med* 1999;340(10):773–9.

14 Marti H, Haji HJ, Savioli L, Chwaya HM, Mgeni AF, Ameir JS, et al. A comparative trial of a single-dose ivermectin versus three days of albendazole for treatment of *Strongyloides stercoralis* and other soil-transmitted helminth infections in children *Am J Trop Med Hyg* 1996;55(5):477–81.

15 Grobusch MP, Mühlberger N, Jelinek T, et al. Imported schistosomiasis in Europe: sentinel surveillance data from Trop-NetEurop. *J Travel Med* 2003 10;(3):164–9.

16 Nicolls D, Weld L, Reed C, et al. for the GeoSentinel Survey Group. Schistosomiasis in travelers: a review of patients seen through the Geosentinel Surveillance. *Am J Trop Med Hyg*, in press.

17 Bierman WF, Wetsteyn JC, van Gool T. Presentation and diagnosis of imported schistosomiasis: relevance of eosinophilia, microscopy for ova, and serology. *J Travel Med* 2005; 12(1):9–13.

18 Meltzer E, Artom G, Marva E, et al. Schistosomiasis among travelers: new aspects of an old disease. *Emerg Inf Dis* 2006;12(11):1696–1700.

19 Tosswill JH, Ridley DS. An evaluation of the ELISA for schistosomiasis in a hospital population. *Tran R Soc Med Hyg* 1986;80(3):435–8.

20 Rieder HL. Risk of travel-associated tuberculosis. *Clin Infect Dis* 2001; 33(8):1393–6.

21 Cobelens FG, van Deutekom H, Draayer-Jansen IW, et al. Risk of infection with *Mycobacterium tuberculosis* infection in travelers to areas of high tuberculosis endemicity. *Lancet* 2000;356:442–3.

# II Specific Infections

# 7 Dengue Fever

Eli Schwartz

Chaim Sheba Medical Center, Tel Hashomer, Israel and Sackler School of Medicine, Tel Aviv University, Tel Aviv, Israel

## Introduction

Dengue virus infection has become one of the world's major emerging infectious diseases. About 100 million cases of dengue fever (DF) are estimated to occur annually [1]. Over the past 20 years, epidemic DF and dengue hemorrhagic fever (DHF) have dramatically expanded geographically in endemic areas. Corresponding to the changes in epidemiology of dengue in endemic populations are an increasing number of reports of dengue fever among travelers to dengue-infected areas [2–5]. Therefore, medical practitioners, especially those who deal with travelers pre- and post-travel, should be knowledgeable about the epidemiology, risk, clinical spectrum, diagnosis, management, and prevention of dengue in travelers.

## Epidemiology of dengue

Dengue viruses are now the most common cause of arboviral diseases in the world, with an estimated 100 million annual cases of DF, 250,000 annual cases of DHF, and an annual mortality rate of 25,000. Dengue virus infections have been reported in over 100 countries, with 2.5 billion people living in areas where dengue is endemic [6] (Figure 7.1). The majority of DHF cases are reported from Asia, where it is a leading cause of hospitalization and death among children. In the American tropics, DHF was a rare disease before 1981. The 1980s and 1990s saw a dramatic geographical expansion of epidemic DF and DHF from Southeast Asia to the South Pacific islands, the Caribbean, and the Americas, with regions changing from nonendemic to hyperendemic, with multiple serotypes present. Due to the expanding geographical distribution of both the virus and the mosquito

vector, increased frequency of epidemics, co-circulation of multiple virus serotypes, and the emergence of DHF in new areas, the World Health Organization (WHO) now classifies dengue as a major international public health concern [1]. The reasons for this resurgence include increasing urbanization with substandard living conditions, lack of vector control, climatic change, virus evolution, and international travel [6].

*The vector:* Dengue viruses are transmitted by mosquitoes of the genus *Aedes* (e.g., *A. aegypti* and *A. albopticus*). The principal vector, *A. aegypti*, is found worldwide in the tropics and subtropics (see Figure 7.1) and is an efficient vector for several reasons: it is highly susceptible to dengue virus, feeds preferentially on human blood, is a daytime feeder, has an almost imperceptible bite, and is capable of biting several people in a short period for one blood meal. As a peridomiciliary mosquito, it is well adapted to urban life. It typically breeds in clean, stagnant water in a wide variety of artificial containers that collect rainwater, such as tires, tin cans, pots, and buckets [1].

*A. albopticus* is a less efficient vector. However, its resurgence in new regions such as the southern US and Southern Europe increases the risk of travel-associated autochthonous dengue in these regions (as happened with chikungunia virus in Italy—see Chapter 11).

## Epidemiology of dengue in travelers

Dengue fever is diagnosed in an increasing proportion of febrile travelers returning from the tropics, ranging from 2% in the early 1990s to 16% more recently [2]. In some case series, DF now presents as the second most frequent cause of hospitalization (after malaria) in travelers returning from the tropics [7, 8].

The true incidence of DF in travelers is very difficult to estimate, because the denominator (the number of travelers to a specific region) is not always known, and the

*Tropical Diseases in Travelers*, 1st edition. Edited by E. Schwartz.
© 2009 by Blackwell Publishing, ISBN: 978-1-4051-8441-0.

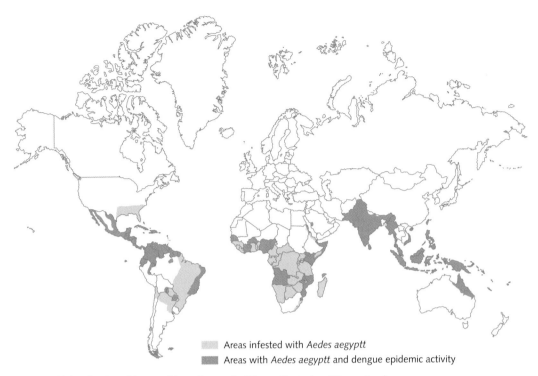

Areas infested with *Aedes aegyptt*

Areas with *Aedes aegyptt* and dengue epidemic activity

**Figure 7.1** World distribution of dengue. (From Centers for Disease Control and Prevention.)

number of dengue cases is underestimated for several reasons: dengue is not notifiable in many countries, is often underreported because travelers may fall ill during travel, and is underdiagnosed because of the nonspecific nature of the majority of dengue viral infections and the lack of diagnostic methods in many medical facilities in nonendemic regions.

An attempt to estimate the rate of DF in Israeli travelers to Thailand was made in 1998 (which happened to be a year of dengue epidemic in Thailand) and an attack rate of 3.4 per 1000 clinically ill travelers who sought medical care was calculated [9]. Prospective studies on seroconversion rates based on dengue IgM in travelers (which include asymptomatic and symptomatic cases) revealed the incidence of dengue to be 2.9% among Dutch travelers (traveling for a mean of 1 month) [5] and 6.7% among Israeli travelers (traveling for a mean of 6 months) [10]. Serological data have to be interpreted with caution because of cross-reactivity of enzyme-linked immunosorbant assay (ELISA)-based assays between DF and other flaviviruses and with other flavivirus vaccines that travelers may have received, such as YF and JE vaccine [11].

It is apparent, therefore, that DF has become a major threat to travelers, with an attack rate as high as that of malaria (without chemoprophylaxis), and higher than that of other travel-related diseases such as hepatitis A or typhoid fever [12]. In fact, according to the GeoSentinel database, dengue morbidity exceeds malaria in almost all regions except Sub-Saharan Africa [13]. The highest rate of dengue cases is seen among travelers returning from Asia (mainly Thailand), followed by the Americas; for unexplained reasons, lower rates are seen in returning travelers from Africa, despite the fact that the vector is abundant there.

Scattered reports exist that returning travelers have transmitted dengue virus infection to health care workers in nonendemic countries via needle stick injuries [14, 15] or mucocutaneous exposure to blood [16]. However, these modes of nonvector transmission of dengue are rarely reported.

## Characteristics of travelers with dengue

The mean age of travelers with dengue was 33.8 years and the male:female ratio was 1.17:1 in 522 dengue cases reported to GeoSentinel during a 10-year period. Of the patients studied, about 70% were traveling only for tourism, and the median trip duration was <28 days.

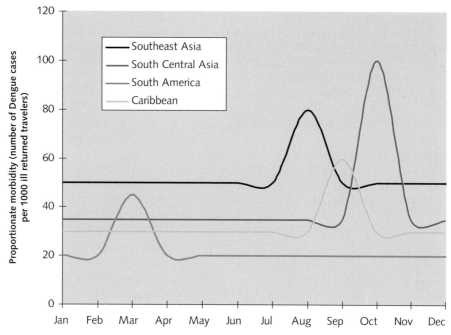

**Figure 7.2** Seasonality of dengue in returned travelers according to geographic area. (From [13].)

As expected, due to the short incubation period, >75% of dengue patients sought treatment within 2 weeks after return. Significantly more dengue patients were hospitalized than patients with other diagnoses in the GeoSentinel database (24% vs 6%, $p < 0.001$) [13].

A comparison of the characteristics of travelers with dengue and of those with malaria, which is the important mosquito-borne disease in travelers, shows some important differences. Unlike dengue, which affects both sexes almost equally, malaria is more common in male travelers [7]. Patients with malaria are less likely to have had a recorded pretravel encounter. Malaria is much more common in first- or second-generation immigrants visiting friends and relatives (VFRs), whereas dengue is mostly a disease of routine tourism. Overall, DF is the prototypical travelers' disease, as it is a threat to anyone who travels to dengue-infected areas, even those with short stays in luxury hotels (because the mosquito is a daytime feeder).

## Seasonality of dengue

Based on the GeoSentinel data, travel-related dengue cases showed typical seasonality with region-specific peaks for Southeast Asia (June, September), South Central Asia (October), South America (March), and the Caribbean (August, October) [13] (Figure 7.2). In addition, travel-related dengue exhibited annual oscillations, with several epidemics occurring during the 10 years of the study period, such as in 1998 and 2002 in Thailand. The annual proportionate morbidity increased from 50 dengue cases per 1000 ill returned travelers in nonepidemic years to an average of 159 cases per 1000 travelers during epidemic years [13]. During the epidemic years, at least in Thailand, the season of the disease was expanded. An outbreak was heralded initially by an excess of cases beginning in February, with a dramatic upsurge in April, well ahead of the usual initial peak month of June both temporally and in magnitude.

## The virus and immunity

Dengue virus is a single-stranded, nonsegmented ribonucleic acid (RNA) virus belonging to the family of flaviviridae. Dengue has four serologically distinct dengue virus serotypes (DEN-1, DEN-2, DEN-3, DEN-4) [1]. Infection with one serotype confers long-term immunity to that specific serotype but not to the other types, and individuals may, therefore, be infected up to four

**Table 7.1** Symptoms of dengue infection in travelers.

| Countries (years) | Europe (1999–2001) | Sweden (1998–1999) | USA (1993–2000) | Europe (2003–2005) |
|---|---|---|---|---|
| Reference | [3] | [4] | [29–33] | [21] |
| Number of travelers diagnosed with dengue | 250 | 74 | 266 | 219 |
| Fever | 86% | 100% | 95% | 93% |
| Headache | 60% | 78% | 62% | 69% |
| Rash | 29% | 62% | 53% | 53% |
| Myalgia/arthralgia | 42% | 73% | 50% | 50% |
| Vomiting/nausea | 8% | 16% | 25% | 13% |
| Hemorrhagic manifestations | Not reported | 28% | 13% | 26% |
| DHF/DSS | 2% | Uncertain | 1.8% | 0.9% |
| Death | 0 | 0 | 2 | 0 |

times [6]. Humans are the main reservoir for the dengue virus, although nonhuman primates are also infected in Asia and Africa.

## Clinical aspects of dengue virus infections

The incubation period is 3–14 days, usually 4–7 days. After the bite of an infected mosquito, the virus replicates in regional lymph nodes and is disseminated via the lymph and blood to other tissues. Replication in the reticuloendothelial system and skin produces a viremia. The infection of all four virus serotypes causes a spectrum of illness ranging from asymptomatic or mild febrile illness to severe and fatal hemorrhagic disease.

## Asymptomatic infection and acute febrile illness

The vast majority of dengue infections in endemic areas are asymptomatic. In travelers, the information is scarce and was examined in only two studies [5, 10]. In these studies the ratios of clinical to subclinical infection were reported to be 1:0.75 and 1:3.3.

## Classic dengue fever

### Symptoms

Classic DF is characterized by a sudden onset of high fever, accompanied by a significant headache, usually a frontal headache with retro-orbital pain, and incapacitating fatigue (see Table 7.1). It is often associated with severe myalgia and arthralgia, from which the name "breakbone

fever" was derived. Fever usually lasts 5–7 days, and the pattern of two peaks ("saddleback") of fever is usually not seen. Rash, typically macular or maculopapular, often becoming confluent and sparing small islands of normal skin (Figure 7.3), has been reported in about half of infected people, and usually appears around the time of defervescence, often involving the palms and feet. The rash lasts 2–4 days and may be accompanied by scaling and pruritus, which usually does not respond to antihistamines or corticosteroids [3, 17]. Thus, although DF is included in the differential diagnosis of febrile illness with rash, the fact that the rash usually appears toward the end of the febrile disease prevents its use as a sign during the initial stage of the febrile illness.

Other signs and symptoms include a flushed face (usually during the first 24–48 hours) or a whole body flush, blanching with pressure (often mistaken for sunburn during a vacation in the tropics). Gastrointestinal symptoms (diarrhea, vomiting, nausea, and metallic taste), injected conjunctivae (as in leptospirosis), inflamed pharynx, lymphadenopathy, and mild respiratory symptoms may occur.

Mild hemorrhagic manifestations in DF patients may occur, such as purpuric rash, gum bleeding, epistaxis, menorrhagia, and, rarely, gastrointestinal hemorrhage. Blurred vision due to ophthalmic complications, including retinal hemorrhage, usually correlates with low platelet count [18]. These manifestations do not establish a diagnosis of DHF (see below). Very rare complications of DF include myocarditis, severe hepatitis [19], and neurological abnormalities such as encephalopathy and neuropathies [20].

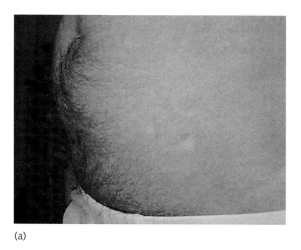
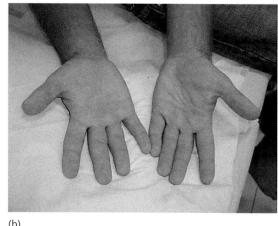

(a)                                                                  (b)

**Figure 7.3** Dengue rash (a) with island sparing and (b) involving the palms.

## Laboratory findings

Blood count reveals thrombocytopenia, leukopenia (with initial lymphopenia), and normal hemoglobin level. The nadir of the leukopenia and thrombocytopenia is usually at days 3–4 from onset of fever, and may be well below $100,000 \times 10^9/L$ thrombocytes and $3000 \times 10^9L$ of leucocytes (Figure 7.4). Mild to moderately elevated liver transaminases and lactate dehydrogenase and mild hyponatremia are common [17, 21]. Coagulation studies are usually within normal limits, with elevated D-dimers as a sign of endothelial damage. There are studies that show correlation between increased levels of D-dimer and disease severity [22].

Classic DF in travelers, although it is a self-limiting disease and rarely fatal, can be incapacitating, halt travel, and end with hospitalization and evacuation back home. The GeoSentinel database shows that about 25% of dengue cases were hospitalized back home, and a similar rate was reported in a study of European travelers [3, 13]. Among Israeli travelers who contracted DF, 30% were evacuated, and 66% were hospitalized either at the travel destination or back home [17].

Convalescence may be prolonged for weeks with asthenia and rarely depression.

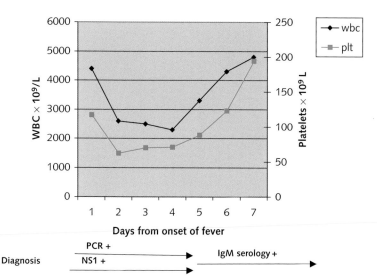

**Figure 7.4** A typical curve of blood count of a dengue patient. Note the relevant diagnostic tests during this period.

## Dengue hemorrhagic fever and dengue shock syndrome

The hallmark of dengue shock syndrome (DSS) is a *capillary leakage syndrome*, accompanied by hemorrhagic manifestations.

Patients present in the first days similarly to those with DF, but then plasma leakage develops at the time of defervescence, around 4–7 days after the onset of disease. Abdominal pain and vomiting, restlessness, change in level of consciousness, and a sudden change from fever to hypothermia may be the first clinical warning signs, associated with a significant decrease in platelets [6].

According to WHO criteria, the diagnosis of DHF is made based on the combination of hemorrhagic manifestations, with platelet count <100,000/mm$^3$, and objective evidence of plasma leakage, shown by either increased packed cell volume >20% during the course of illness or hematocrit >45% and clinical signs of plasma leakage, such as pleural effusion, ascites, or hypoproteinemia [6]. Hemorrhagic manifestations without capillary leakage do not constitute DHF.

The *tourniquet test*, which assesses capillary fragility, is defined as positive if 20 or more petechiae appear in a 1-inch-square patch (6.25 cm$^2$) on the forearm after the blood pressure cuff is deflated (Figure 7.5). A positive tourniquet test is incorporated into the WHO clinical case definition of DHF, but differentiates poorly between DF and DHF and does not seem to be very specific [23].

Mortality of DHF can be up to 10–20%, but it is as low as 0.2% in hospitals with staff experienced in the management of the disease [24]. DSS is characterized by profound hypotension (defined as systolic pressure <90 mmHg for those ≥5 years) or a rapid weak pulse with narrowing pulse pressure <20 mmHg, regardless of the blood pressure. The duration of shock is short; typically, the patient dies within 12–24 hours (mortality rate is up to 40%) or recovers rapidly following appropriate volume replacement therapy.

### Risk factors for dengue hemorrhagic fever and dengue shock syndrome

Although the mechanisms for developing severe hemorrhagic disease are not fully understood, the main risk factor for developing DHF and DSS is thought to be secondary infection with another serotype [6, 25].

The pathophysiology that is proposed is that non-neutralizing antidengue antibodies from the previous infection bind to the new infecting serotype and enhance viral uptake on monocytes and macrophages. This antibody-dependent enhancement results in an amplified cascade of cytokines and complement activation, causing endothelial dysfunction, platelet destruction, and consumption of coagulation factors, which result in plasma leakage and hemorrhagic manifestations [26, 27].

It is important to note that authorities in this field believe that classical DF and DHF are two distinct diseases

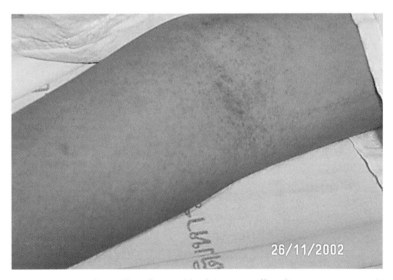

**Figure 7.5** Tourniquet test. The test is performed by inflating a blood pressure cuff on the upper arm to a point midway between systolic and diastolic blood pressures for 5 minutes. A test is considered positive when 20 or more petechiae per square inch are observed. (Courtesy of Dr. Ann McCarthy, Tropical Medicine and International Health Clinic, Ottawa Hospital, Canada.)

based on their pathogenesis. Whereas DF is due to the direct effect of the virus, DHF is due to enhanced antibodies. As mentioned by Cardosa: "It is important to recognize that DHF is not merely a febrile disease with hemorrhagic manifestations, however severe, but is qualitatively distinct, potentially life-threatening leaky capillary syndrome" [25].

This theory, which is currently the dominant theory, was first proposed by Halstead to explain the rapid increase of DHF in several regions of the world. The theory was opposed by Rosen [28], but this opposition did not garner much attention.

The data accumulated in travelers do not seem to support the Halstead theory.

## Dengue hemorrhagic fever and dengue shock syndrome in travelers

### Epidemiology

Historically, DHF/DSS was rarely reported in travelers, which was consistent with the antibody enhancement theory, because most travelers with DF had not been exposed previously to dengue viruses and contracted DF as a first-time infection. However, with growth in travel and an increase in the number of dengue cases in travelers, more reports of DHF have been published. Within the European Network on Imported Infectious Disease Surveillance (Trop NeTEurope), DHF was reported in 2.7% of 483 dengue cases [3]. A similar rate was described in the GeoSentinel database, where 12 (2.2%) out of 522 cases were diagnosed as DHF [13], although without verification that all imported cases met the strict WHO criteria for DHF. Published data by the Centers for Disease Control and Prevention (CDC) concerning cases of dengue imported to the US between 1993 and 2000 reported 1.8% DHF out of 266 cases. In these case series, two deaths were reported (0.7%) [29–33]. Recent study from the European Network reported 0.9% (2 out of 219) who met the criteria for DHF [21].

In addition to this report, one case of mortality among travelers has also been reported each year for the last 4 years. In some cases, it was well documented as primary dengue infection [34–37].

Thus, from the epidemiological point of view, the rate of about 1–2% of DHF in travelers is not less than estimates in local populations (250,000 cases of DHF out of 100 million cases of dengue fever), despite the fact that among the traveler population, significant numbers receive their first exposure to dengue.

### Capillary leakage in travelers

The WHO criteria for capillary leakage are either indirect, such as increased hematocrit (which is rarely seen in an ill traveler receiving intravenous [IV] fluids), or a measurement of a very large volume of leakage, such as accumulation of pleural fluid, which can be seen on chest X-rays.

A more sensitive method of detection of even a small amount of fluid in the pleural or abdominal cavity is ultrasonography. Therefore, an ultrasound study on sequential hospitalized dengue cases after travel was initiated in our center. For each case, ultrasonography was done on days 6–8 after the onset of fever and included the abdomen and pleura. In total, 25% of the cases (8 out of 31 cases) showed evidence of free fluids in the abdomen or in the pleura, whereas none of them had DHF according to the WHO criteria and, for all of them, the disease was clinically the first dengue infection [E. Schwartz, manuscript in preparation].

This simple study demonstrated that when a more sensitive method is used to detect capillary leakage (one that is not easily available in many endemic countries), there are approximately 10 times more "DHF" cases in travelers than found solely through clinical presentations.

Thus, based on experience with travelers, dengue fever, including DHF/DSS, is a disease with a spectrum of clinical manifestations ranging from asymptomatic infection to febrile disease. About 25% of those infected will have capillary leakage, but only 1–2% may develop severe clinical disease. Fatality is less than 1% (Figure 7.6).

In fact, reports from endemic countries in recent years mention that the severity of the disease also depends on the strain and serotype of the infecting virus, the age and genetic background of the patient, and the degree of viremia [6, 28, 38].

The dispute about the pathophysiology and risk factors of DHF/DSS is not merely academic but rather has significant implications for vaccine production. According to the current theory, a dengue vaccine should provide full protective immunity to the four serotypes to avoid the phenomenon of antibody-dependent enhancement;

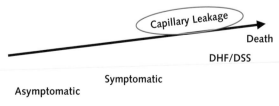

**Figure 7.6** The clinical spectrum of dengue fever.

otherwise, the vaccine may put the recipients in danger of severe disease.

This fear has stopped vaccine manufacturers from delivering a vaccine with less than 100% protection, but if the theory of secondary infection is incorrect, a vaccine with partial coverage (only three serotypes) for dengue could have been marketed years ago and reduced the dengue burden.

## Diagnosis and differential diagnosis

A confirmed diagnosis is established by virus culture, PCR (polymerase chain reaction), or serological assays (Table 7.2). All of these tests have limitations. PCR is not available in many settings, and is sensitive early in the course of the disease (during the first week) (Figure 7.4). Serology tests must have a fourfold or greater increase in dengue IgG titers as a confirmatory test, which means they require a convalescent serum.

The most commonly used and most practical test for dengue is the IgM capture enzyme-linked immunosorbent assay (ELISA), which is also available commercially. The limitations of its use are that this test is negative early in the illness and should only be done at least 4–5 days after the onset of fever [11]. In addition, a positive IgM result is considered only a "probable" diagnosis (see Table 7.2). False positive dengue IgM may be caused by rheumatoid factor in serum [39] or by other flavivirus infections. (We observed it in Israel with West Nile infection.)

In travelers, a particular issue is possible cross-reactions with other flavivirus vaccines (e.g., yellow fever, Japanese encephalitis, and tick-borne encephalitis) that travelers may have had. In fact, it was found that cross-reaction occurs in up to 40% of cases, although only with ELISA IgG [11].

**Table 7.2** Laboratory diagnosis of dengue.

| Type of diagnosis | Advantages and limitations |
| --- | --- |
| Confirmed diagnosis | |
| • Fourfold or greater increase in serum IgG and IgM (by hemagglutination inhibition test) specific to dengue virus | Requires convalescent serum<br>Cross-reactivity to other flaviviruses (including previous vaccinations against Japanese encephalitis and yellow fever). |
| • Isolation of dengue virus from serum or autopsy samples | Less than 50% sensitive; only early in disease.<br>Test is not commonly available. |
| • Detection of dengue virus genomic sequences by reverse transcription-PCR | Sensitivity >90% in the first few days of illness, rapidly declines and usually <10% sensitivity 7 days after onset of symptoms.<br>High specificity.<br>Test is not commercially available. |
| • Detection of dengue virus in tissue, serum, or cerebrospinal fluid by immunohistochemistry, immunofluorescence, or enzyme-linked immunosorbent assay | Less than 50% sensitive; only early in disease. Test is not commonly available. |
| Probable diagnosis | |
| • Positive dengue IgM antibody test | Most commonly used test; sensitivity 89–99%, specificity 92%, commercially available.<br>Negative early in disease; only positive from 4–5 days after onset of symptoms. |
| • Single serum sample: titer ≥1280 with hemagglutination inhibition test, comparable IgG titer with enzyme-linked immunosorbent assay | Cross-reactivity to other flaviviruses (including previous vaccinations against Japanese encephalitis and yellow fever) |

*Source*: Adapted from Wilder-Smith A, Schwartz E. Dengue in travelers. *N Engl J Med* 2005 Sep 1;353(9):924–32.

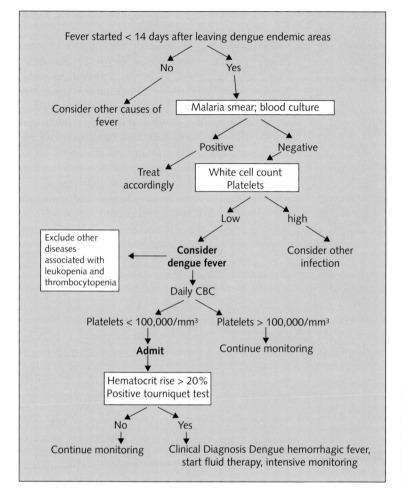

**Figure 7.7** Flow diagram for the clinical diagnosis of dengue in returning travelers. (From Wilder-Smith A, Schwartz E. Dengue in travelers. *N Engl J Med* 2005 Sep 1;353(9):924–32. © 2005 Massachusetts Medical Society. All rights reserved.)

In primary infections, there is an increase in dengue-specific IgM first, followed by IgG antibodies about 7–10 days after the onset of fever. The IgM remains detectable for 3–6 months, whereas IgG remains for life. In secondary infections, early titers of IgG are present; however, in travelers, that level might be due to a previous flavivirus vaccine.

As a laboratory-based diagnosis of dengue is, therefore, often not available at the time of care, the diagnosis is initially only clinical, based on the development of clinical manifestations and laboratory features over time, and excluding other potentially life-threatening diseases such as malaria (Figure 7.7).

Thus, dengue antigen detection tests should help clinicians make diagnoses in real time. The detection of secreted NS1 protein (one of seven nonstructural proteins of dengue membrane) represents a new approach to the diagnosis of acute dengue infection. A recently developed commercially available diagnostic test based on dengue NS1 antigen-capture ELISA showed overall sensitivity of 88.7% and 93.4% in two studies, with 100% specificity. The sensitivity of NS1 detection rapidly decreases on day 5, requiring NS1 detection between days 0 and 4 for accurate diagnosis [40]. More experience with travelers should be gained with this new promising method.

The travel history is an important clue because the incubation period is less than 2 weeks, and dengue can be ruled out if symptoms begin more than 2 weeks after the traveler or immigrant has left an endemic area (Figure 7.7). Fever for more than 10 days also practically excludes dengue.

The differential diagnosis includes malaria, typhoid fever, leptospirosis, chikungunya, West Nile virus infection, measles, rubella, acute HIV conversion illness,

Epstein–Barr virus infection, viral hemorrhagic fevers, rickettsial diseases, and any other disease that may present in the acute phase as an undifferentiated febrile syndrome.

The combination of laboratory parameters of low platelets, low leukocyte count, and increased liver transaminases is characteristic of dengue but may exist in many of these diseases.

## Management

No specific therapeutic agents exist for dengue. Steroids, carbazochrome (which decreases capillary permeability), and antiviral agents (although ribavirin, interferon alpha, and 6-azauridine have showed antiviral activity in vitro) have no proven role [41, 42]. Treatment is therefore symptomatic and supportive, with the primary aim of preventing mortality from severe DHF/DSS. Mild or classic dengue is treated with antipyretics (i.e., paracetamol), bed rest, and fluid replacement. Most cases can be managed on an outpatient basis. Aspirin, nonsteroidal anti-inflammatory drugs, and intramuscular injections are best avoided because of bleeding tendencies. Platelet and hematocrit determinations should be repeated at least every 24 hours to promptly recognize the development of DHF and institute fluid replacement. Patients with a platelet count less than 100,000 should be admitted, as they are at highest risk of developing DHF (see Figure 7.7). The critical period is usually on the day of defervescence, typically 4–7 days after onset of the illness. A decrease in the platelet count is of prognostic value for the development of DHF. A rise in hematocrit of 20% indicates significant plasma loss, and the patient requires intensive care with intravenous fluid replacement with normal saline. Specific WHO guidelines have been published concerning the IV infusion rate and specific time periods of infusion [43], which are more relevant for the endemic population.

## Prevention of dengue infections in travelers

Effective control of dengue remains elusive. Public health efforts must focus on vector control and community-based programs to keep the environment free of potential breeding sources. A dengue vaccine that provides effective, long-term immunity against all four serotypes is urgently needed. Live attenuated tetravalent dengue vaccines have been shown to be immunogenic and safe and are undergoing further clinical trials [44].

The current dengue preventive measure for travelers to endemic areas is taking precautions to avoid mosquito bites, such as using mosquito repellents (based on DEET), protective clothing (permethrin-impregnated is best), and insecticides. Protection from dengue is more difficult than for malaria because *Aedes* are daytime biting mosquitoes, and therefore these measures must be taken during the day, in particular in the morning and late afternoon. In addition, the main risk of exposure for travelers is in urban and peridomestic areas, whereas for malaria, the risk is in more rural areas. *Aedes* are also indoor feeders and are often found in dark areas (inside closets and bathrooms, behind curtains, and under beds), and it is advisable to spray these areas with insecticides. Care should be taken not to leave trash, pots, or any other containers that could fill with rainwater and become breeding grounds.

Pretravel advice should include information about the potential risks of acquiring dengue fever, destinations of high risk, and symptoms of dengue infection. There is no actual "safe" season, although there seems to be a rise in cases during the rainy season in several regions (see Figure 7.2). It is also important to remind travelers that the symptoms of dengue may resemble those of malaria and that malaria needs to be excluded first.

## Reinfection

A common concern among previously dengue-infected travelers is the issue of traveling again to dengue-infected areas, because reinfection with another serotype of dengue virus is considered to be a predisposing factor for the development of DHF/DSS, with a high mortality risk. Data on the extent of this risk in travelers are lacking. However, taking into account the data on risk of dengue in travelers, the risk of mortality is very low. This estimate is based on the serosurvey studies, which showed a risk of contract clinical DF of about 1% per month of stay in a high-risk area, and out of those cases, about a 1% risk of clinical DHF, with a mortality rate of less than 1%. Overall, the risk of mortality is about 1 case per million.

## Conclusions

Because *Aedes* mosquitoes cannot be effectively controlled in the near future, an effective vaccine is urgently needed.

In the meantime, dengue will continue to escalate, and therefore clinicians in nonendemic areas are expected to encounter and treat increasing numbers of travelers returning from endemic areas with dengue. Thus, clinicians should be acquainted with the clinical picture of the disease and its diagnosis and management.

## References

1 Gubler DJ. The global emergence/resurgence of arboviral diseases as public health problems. *Arch Med Res* 2002;33:330–42.

2 Wilder-Smith A, Schwartz E. Dengue in travelers. *N Engl J Med* 2005 Sep 1;353(9):924–32.

3 Jelinek T, Muhlberger N, Harms G, et al. Epidemiology and clinical features of imported dengue fever in Europe: sentinel surveillance data from TropNetEurope. *Clin Infect Dis* 2002;35:1047–52.

4 Lindback H, Lindback J, Tegnell A, Janzon R, Vene S, Ekdahl K. Dengue fever in travelers to the tropics, 1998 and 1999. *Emerg Infect Dis* 2003;9(4):438–42.

5 Cobelens FG, Groen J, Osterhaus AD, Leentvaar-Kuipers A, Wertheim-van Dillen PM, Kager PA. Incidence and risk factors of probable dengue virus infection among Dutch travellers to Asia. *Trop Med Int Health* 2002;7:331–8.

6 Guzman MG, Kouri G. Dengue: an update. *Lancet Infect Dis* 2002;2:33–42.

7 Steinlauf S, Segall G, Sidi Y, Schwartz E. Post-travel related hospitalization in Israel. *J Travel Med* 2000;12:136–41.

8 O'Brien D, Tobin S, Brown GV, Torresi J. Fever in returned travelers: review of hospital admissions for a 3-year period. *Clin Infect Dis* 2001;33:603–9.

9 Schwartz E, Moskovitz A, Potasman I, Peri G, Grossman Z, Alkan ML. Changing epidemiology of dengue fever in travelers to Thailand. *Eur J Clin Microbiol Infect Dis* 2000;19:784–6.

10 Potasman I, Srugo I, Schwartz E. Dengue seroconversion among Israeli travelers to tropical countries. *Emerg Infect Dis* 1999;5:824–7.

11 Schwartz E, Mileguir F, Grossman Z, Mendelson E. Evaluation of ELISA-based sero-diagnosis of dengue fever in travelers. *J Clin Virol* 2000;19:169–73.

12 Steffen RRM, Wilhelm U, Helminger A, Schär M. Health problems after travel to developing countries. *J Infect Dis* 1987;56:84–91.

13 Schwartz E, Weld LH, Wilder-Smith A, von Sonnenburg F, Keystone JS, Kain KC, et al. Seasonality, annual trends, and characteristics of dengue among ill returned travelers, 1997–2006. *Emerg Infect Dis* 2008;14(7):1081–8.

14 De Wazieres B, Gil H, Vuitton DA, Dupond JL. Nosocomial transmission of dengue from a needlestick injury. *Lancet* 1998;351:498.

15 Wagner D, de With K, Huzly D, et al. Nosocomial acquisition of dengue. *Emerg Infect Dis* 2004;10:1872–3.

16 Chen LH, Wilson ME. Transmission of dengue virus without a mosquito vector: nosocomial mucocutaneous transmission and other routes of transmission. *Clin Infect Dis* 2004;39:e56–60.

17 Schwartz E, Mendelson E, Sidi Y. Dengue fever among travelers. *Am J Med* 1996;101:516–20.

18 Chan DP, Teoh SC, Tan CS, Nah GK, Rajagopalan R, Prabhakaragupta MK, et al.; The Eye Institute Dengue-Related Ophthalmic Complications Workgroup. Ophthalmic complications of dengue. *Emerg Infect Dis* 2006;12:285–9.

19 Lum LC, Lam SK, George R, Devi S. Fulminant hepatitis in dengue infection. *Southeast Asian J Trop Med Public Health* 1993;24:467–71.

20 Sumarmo, Wulur H, Jahja E, Gubler DJ, Sutomenggolo TS, Saroso JS. Encephalopathy associated with dengue infection. *Lancet* 1978;1:449–502.

21 Wichmann O, Gascon J, Schunk M, Puente S, Siikamaki H, Gjørup I, et al.; European Network on Surveillance of Imported Infectious Diseases. Severe dengue virus infection in travelers: risk factors and laboratory indicators. *J Infect Dis* 2007;15(195):1089–96.

22 Setrkraising K, Bongsebandhu-phubhakdi C, Voraphani N, et al. D-dimer as an indicator of dengue severity. *Asian Biomedicine* 2007;1(1):53–7.

23 Phuong CX, Nhan NT, Kneen R, et al. Clinical diagnosis and assessment of severity of confirmed dengue infections in Vietnamese children: is the World Health Organization classification system helpful? *Am J Trop Med Hyg* 2004;70:172–9.

24 Gubler DJ. Dengue and dengue hemorrhagic fever. *Clin Microbiol Rev* 1998;11:480–96.

25 Cardosa M. Dengue haemorrhagic fever: questions of pathogenesis. *Curr Opin Infect Dis* 2000; 13(5)431–3.

26 Halstead SB, O'Rourke EJ. Dengue viruses and mononuclear phagocytes. I. Infection enhancement by non-neutralizing antibody. *J Exp Med* 1977;146:201–17.

27 Halstead SB. In vivo enhancement of dengue virus infection in rhesus monkeys by passively transferred antibody. *J Infect Dis* 1979;140:527–33.

28 Rosen L. The Emperor's New Clothes revisited, or reflections on the pathogenesis of dengue hemorrhagic fever. *Am J Trop Med Hyg* 1977;26:337–43.

29 Centers for Disease Control and Prevention (CDC). Imported dengue—United States, 1993–1994. *MMWR Morb Mortal Wkly Rep* 1995; 44:353–6.

30 Centers for Disease Control and Prevention (CDC). Imported dengue—United States, 1995. *MMWR Morb Mortal Wkly Rep* 1996;45:988–91.

31 Imported dengue—United States, 1996. *Can Commun Dis Rep* 1998;24:164–5, 168.

32 Centers for Disease Control and Prevention (CDC). Imported dengue—United States, 1997 and 1998. *MMWR Morb Mortal Wkly Rep* 2000;49:248–53.

33 Centers for Disease Control and Prevention (CDC). Imported dengue—United States, 1999 and 2000. *MMWR Morb Mortal Wkly Rep* 2002;51:281–3.

34 Centers for Disease Control and Prevention (CDC). Travel-associated dengue infections—United States, 2001–2004. *MMWR Morb Mortal Wkly Rep* 2005 Jun 10;54(22):556–8.

35 Centers for Disease Control and Prevention (CDC). Travel-associated dengue—United States, 2005. *MMWR Morb Mortal Wkly Rep* 2006 Jun 30;55(25):700–702.

36 Huhtamo E, Vuorinen S, Uzcátegui NY, Vapalahti O, Haapasalo H, Lumio J. Fatal dengue virus infection in a Finnish traveler. *J Clin Virol* 2006;37:323–6.

37 Jensenius M, Berild D, Ormaasen V, Maehlen J, Lindegren G, Falk KI. Fatal subarachnoidal haemorrhage in a Norwegian traveller with dengue virus infection. *Scand J Infect Dis* 2007;39:272–4.

38 Vaughn DW, Green S, Kalayanarooj S, et al. Dengue viremia titer, antibody response pattern, and virus serotype correlate with disease severity. *J Infect Dis* 2000;181:2–9.

39 Jelinek T, Wastlhuber J, Proll S, Schattenkirchner M, Loscher T. Influence of rheumatoid factor on the specificity of a rapid immunochromatographic test for diagnosing dengue infection. *Eur J Clin Microbiol Infect Dis* 2000;19:555–6.

40 Dussart P, Petit L, Labeau B, Bremand L, Leduc A, Moua D, et al. Evaluation of two new commercial tests for the diagnosis of acute dengue virus infection using NS1 antigen detection in human serum. *PLoS Negl Trop Dis* 2008;20;2: e280.

41 Crance JM, Scaramozzino N, Jouan A, Garin D. Interferon, ribavirin, 6-azauridine and glycyrrhizin: antiviral compounds active against pathogenic flaviviruses. *Antiviral Res* 2003;58:73–9.

42 Tassniyom S, Vasanawathana S, Chirawatkul A, Rojanasuphot S. Failure of high-dose methylprednisolone in established dengue shock syndrome: a placebo-controlled, double-blind study. *Pediatrics* 1993;92:111–15.

43 http://www.who.int/csr/resources/publications/dengue/en/024-33.pdf.

44 Sun W, Cunningham D, Wasserman SS, Perry J, Putnak JR, Eckels KH, et al. Phase 2 clinical trial of three formulations of tetravalent live-attenuated dengue vaccine in flavivirus-naïve adults. *Hum Vaccin* 2009;5:33–40.

# 8 West Nile Fever

Michal Chowers

Sackler School of Medicine, Tel Aviv University, Tel Aviv, Israel and Meir Medical Center, Kfar Saba, Israel

## Introduction

West Nile virus (WNV) is a mosquito-borne pathogen that belongs to the family Flaviviridae, genus *Flavivirus*. It is a member of the Japanese encephalitis virus subgroup of flaviviruses, which includes Japanese encephalitis in Asia, Murray Valley encephalitis in Australia, and St. Louis encephalitis in the Americas. The virus was first isolated in 1937 from a febrile woman who lived in the West Nile region of Uganda [1]. It was later recognized as endemic in Africa, Europe, and Asia [2]. In the last decade, a change in the epidemiology and the severity of the disease led to increased attention by the medical community and the public. The increased incidence of this disease and the fact that most of the cases appear in the summer months of the northern hemisphere resulted in more travelers being exposed in endemic areas.

## Epidemiology

Mosquitoes are the principal vector of WNV. The virus has been isolated from more than 40 mosquito species, but the predominant genus is *Culex*. Wild birds are the principal host, and the virus has been isolated from both wetland and terrestrial species. Some of those birds suffer from high long-term viremia, which is critical for transmission to the vector mosquito. Humans and horses acquire the virus by mosquito bites, but the ensuing viremia is of low titer and short-lived and is insufficient for infecting other vector mosquitoes. Thus, humans and horses are accidental dead-end hosts.

The occurrence of the disease in humans depends on the intensity of infection in birds, the feeding patterns of affected mosquitoes, and the exposure of humans to those mosquitoes. In contrast to many other infectious diseases, previous outbreaks and the resulting protective immunity cannot account for change in disease activity in humans. In affected countries, even after extensive epidemics, IgM seroprevalence ranges from 2% to 4% [3, 4], and IgG seroprevalence ranges from 13% to 18%, a level that leaves most of the population susceptible to the disease [3].

The disease is seasonal and usually occurs during the summer and early fall (July to October) [5]. Reports from the southern USA suggest that in different climates the transmission season can change; cases of WNV infection have been reported as early as April and as late as December [6].

Since its discovery in 1937 in Uganda and up to the past decade, few outbreaks have been reported. After the first three successive outbreaks from Israel in the 1950s, the only large outbreak was reported in South Africa in 1974, with an estimated 18,000 cases, but with low mortality. Throughout those years, the virus was isolated sporadically either from mosquitoes or from mammals from most of the Old World—Europe, the Middle East, Africa, and India—but morbidity and mortality were low [7].

However, in 1996, a large outbreak resulted in 835 hospitalized patients with many severe encephalitis cases, and high mortality was reported in Romania [8]. This was the first outbreak of many that brought West Nile-associated diseases to the attention of the public and the medical community. Reports followed yearly: Tunisia in 1997 with 173 patients [7], Russia in 1999 with 826 patients [9], and Israel in 2000 with 325 hospitalized patients [5]. Another unexpected observation was the death of geese from West Nile disease in Israel during 1998, an occurrence that changed the view that birds were unaffected hosts. In 1999 WNV was detected for the first time on the American continent. The disease was identified in 62 encephalitis cases from the state of New York [10]. In parallel and similarly to the observation in Israel, this outbreak led to remarkable mortality in infected birds, especially crows

*Tropical Diseases in Travelers*, 1st edition. Edited by E. Schwartz.
© 2009 by Blackwell Publishing, ISBN: 978-1-4051-8441-0.

and blue jays. Interestingly, the virus identified in 1999 in New York was similar to the one identified from a goose in Israel the previous year [11], and probably arrived from the same area via illegal import of an exotic bird, or the arrival of mosquitoes by air transportation. Since its arrival on the American continent, WNV has been identified yearly in birds, mosquitoes, and humans, with annual outbreaks involving thousands of people. What started as a local outbreak in the New York City with 62 diagnosed cases and 7 deaths became a countrywide yearly outbreak that, by the end of 2007, infected more than 24,000 people and caused the deaths of more than 1000 individuals [12].

The virus continued to spread unchecked north and south on the American continent. In Canada, it caused disease similar to that observed in the USA [13]. This was in contrast to Mexico, the Caribbean, and South America, where, although the virus was isolated from mosquitoes and resident birds, it did not cause any significant disease in humans [14–16]. One possible explanation for this discrepancy is the difficulty of identifying WNV infection in the context of the background of the more common dengue infection. Another possibility is that previous dengue infection might confer some immunity to WNV and abrogate or ameliorate severe infection.

## Other modes of transmission

In 2002, the number of WNV cases dramatically expanded in the USA: from 66 cases detected in 14 states during 2001 to 4156 cases detected in 41 states during 2002. Not surprisingly, several new modes of transmission were reported during that year.

### Transmission through blood product transfusion

Twenty-three cases from 16 viremic donors were identified in 2002. Transmission was documented following transfusion of platelets, red cells, and fresh-frozen plasma. None of the donors had antibodies against WNV [17]. Following the recognition of this new mode of transmission, starting in June 2003, US and Canadian blood collection agencies implemented nucleic acid amplification testing for WNV. This screen identified 818 infected blood donors in 2003 alone [18]. Even after donor blood screening, a few cases of transfusion-associated transmission occurred during 2003; they appeared to result from blood con-

taining very low viral titers that escaped the screening procedure.

### Transmission through organ transplantation

An organ donor and four of his recipients were identified as having WNV infection. All four recipients became ill and three of them suffered from subsequent encephalitis [19].

### Transmission transplacentally

Transplacental transmission resulted in one case of chorioretinitis and cystic damage to the cerebral tissue. However, in a follow-up on 74 women infected during pregnancy, it was reported that all of them delivered apparently healthy infants [6, 20]. Transmission via breast feeding was also reported by the Centers for Disease Control and Prevention (CDC), but resulted only in asymptomatic seroconversion of the baby [21].

### Transmission to laboratory workers

Percutaneous inoculation of laboratory workers with infected material is documented. The current recommendation is for biosafety level four for laboratories handling arboviruses [22].

## Epidemiology in travelers

Imported human cases have been reported in tourists returning from an endemic country or following an epidemic. A high level of caution is necessary in diagnosing these cases, given that the signs and symptoms of the disease are not specific. The country of travel, the season, and the clinical presentation, taken together, should serve as clues in properly diagnosing the disease. It is important to note that the disease in tourists is not different from disease in residents of endemic countries.

The reported cases of post-travel West Nile infection are summarized in Table 8.1. The majority of reports are from the developed world and specifically from North America, which is a reflection of significant recurrent outbreaks over the past several years. Several reports describe elderly patients who had febrile illnesses at the end of trips, or shortly after arriving back home, and who subsequently developed signs and symptoms of encephalitis.

Among the cases, at least one had a fatal outcome [26], and many presented with encephalitis. This may reflect a

**Table 8.1** Imported West Nile fever cases.

| Acquired in | Country | No cases | Imported to |
|---|---|---|---|
| North America | USA | 11 | France [23], Germany [24], Czech Republic [25], Mexico [26], Netherlands [26], Uruguay [26], Japan [26], Canada [26] |
| | Canada | 2 | Denmark [27], Netherlands [28] |
| Europe | Portugal | 2 | Ireland [26] |
| Middle East | Israel | 2 | Netherlands [29], Denmark [27] |
| Africa | Senegal | 2 | France [30] |
| | Djibouti | 4 | France [26] |

tendency to report the more severe cases. Many cases were probably either not reported or not diagnosed.

## Clinical manifestations

West Nile virus was first isolated and identified from the blood of a febrile woman in Uganda in 1937 [1]. At that time, no symptomatology other than fever was attributed to the disease associated with WNV. In the early 1950s, however, several reports of outbreaks in Israel were the first to describe the clinical characteristics of WNV infection in detail. The clinical picture that emerged from those reports was of a benign febrile disease in young adults [31]. In a later outbreak in Israel during 1957, a link between WNV infection and severe central nervous system (CNS) disease was first noted [32]. The last decade witnessed large outbreaks that dramatically increased our knowledge of the clinical manifestations of WNV infection.

Based on serological studies [33], it became increasingly clear that the majority (80%) of infected individuals are asymptomatic, that approximately 20% suffer from West Nile fever (WNF), and that less than 1% develop West Nile neuroinvasive disease (WNND) (Figure 8.1). Moreover, most of our knowledge of the clinical manifestations derives from hospitalized patients, and thus even the portrayal of benign WNF illness is biased and describes the more severe forms of the illness.

## West Nile fever

The incubation period of WNV ranges from 3 to 14 days. Common clinical features include the abrupt onset of fever, often accompanied by headache, malaise, myalgia, gastrointestinal symptoms including nausea, vomiting, abdominal pain and diarrhea, and rash. Lymphadenopathy was commonly described in early outbreaks in the 1950s, but is less common in more recent reports [31, 34].

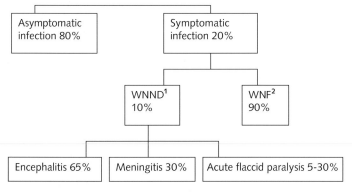

<sup></sup>[1] WNND = West Nile neuroinvasive disease
[2] WNF    = West Nile fever

**Figure 8.1** West Nile infection: clinical manifestations.

The fever tends to be high: in one study, 60% of the patients presented with fevers above 39°C and 20% with fevers above 40°C. The rash is transient, nonpruritic, and maculopapular, and usually appears over the torso and extremities, sparing the palms and soles.

WNF is self-limited and is not mortal. In the study of Watson et al., which was based on all diagnosed WNF cases in Illinois, it was found that 30% of WNF cases resulted in hospitalization [35]. It is important that the less severe cases that presented as mild febrile diseases probably were not diagnosed and thus are not represented. Nonetheless, the disease can be severe enough to result in hospitalization.

## West Nile neuroinvasive disease

West Nile neuroinvasive disease includes meningitis, encephalitis, and acute flaccid paralysis (AFP), similar to poliomyelitis. Patients with headache and abnormal cerebrospinal fluid (CSF) findings, with no changes in mental status, are diagnosed as having meningitis. Patients with altered levels of consciousness or confusion, or who exhibit focal neurological signs, are diagnosed as having encephalitis. The distinction between these entities is clinical and somewhat subjective; some patients may exhibit mixed clinical signs and symptoms, such as nuchal rigidity, altered mental status, and paralysis.

In studies from Europe describing WNND patients, about 65% were diagnosed with encephalitis, 30% with meningitis, and only 2–5% with symptoms of acute flaccid paralysis. In recent reports from North America, AFP was more commonly seen and composed about 13–40% of the WNND spectrum [13]. The reason for this difference is not clear.

The distribution of these different clinical manifestations is highly correlated with age. In the study describing the Israeli outbreak in 2000, encephalitis occurred in 80% of elderly patients (>70 years old), as compared with 47% of younger patients. In contrast, meningitis was more common in the younger age group (27%), compared with only 1% in the elderly [34].

## West Nile meningitis

The clinical presentation of WNV meningitis is similar to that of WNF, with the presence of headache and meningeal signs. CSF characteristics are similar to those in other viral meningitides. As previously mentioned, the affected population is mainly young adults, with a median age of 35 years [36], and the outcome is favorable.

## West Nile encephalitis

West Nile encephalitis (WNE) is a disease that affects mainly the elderly, as was described in the 1950s for an outbreak in a long-term care facility, and validated in recent studies in Israel and North America. The median age of patients with encephalitis is 70 years [8, 34, 36, 37]. A newer population exposed to WNV, and probably more susceptible to encephalitis, is immunocompromised patients. Several reports describe severe WNE in organ transplant patients undergoing immunosuppressive therapy [38, 39].

The most common signs and symptoms are fever and confusion or deteriorating mental status. The exact frequency of other signs is more difficult to assess due to the variable state of consciousness of the patients. Some symptoms are diagnosed only after comatose patients improve and try to ambulate. The frequency of tremor varies from 12% to 80%. The tremor is usually coarse and asymmetric, and is often observed in the upper extremities. Myoclonus, which is reported in about 30% of patients, occurs in the upper extremities and facial muscles (34). The presence of tremors and myoclonus should increase the clinical suspicion of WNND. Parkinsonian features, including rigidity, bradykinesia, and postural instability, are reported in up to 60% of patients [40]. Cerebellar ataxia with gait disturbances has been described, but its frequency varies among studies. Cranial nerve palsies, mainly of the seventh nerve, have been described as well. Seizures are reported less frequently [41]. For example, in the Israeli outbreak, 6.7% of the patients with encephalitis suffered from seizures (unpublished data). WNE is associated with high mortality. In recent studies, mortality from WNV infection was about 8–14%, of which nearly all was attributed to WNE. The outcome is much worse in the elderly population and can approach as much as 30% mortality [8, 10, 34].

## Acute flaccid paralysis/poliomyelitis

Whereas severe fatigue has been a known clinical manifestation of WNF for many years, a remarkable increase in the frequency of AFP has been reported in recent years [42–45]. AFP results from viral infection and damage to motor neurons in the anterior horn of the spinal cord, leading to asymmetric weakness or paralysis in one or more limbs without sensory loss. In severe cases, it can result in quadriplegia [44, 46]. Areflexia or hyporeflexia and loss of bowel and bladder function can also occur. In some cases, involvement of respiratory muscle innervation can result in respiratory failure, which dramatically increases morbidity and mortality. AFP generally develops early in the course of the disease, and can accompany either encephalitis or meningitis.

## Other illnesses associated with WNV infection

Visual problems such as blurry vision and photophobia are increasingly associated with WNV infection. In addition, chorioretinitis, optic neuritis, vitritis, and uveitis have been reported [47–49]. Hepatitis and pancreatitis have been reported in cases of severe WNV infection, in which the virus was identified in those organs at pathology [50].

## Laboratory and imaging findings

### Chemistry and hematology

Anemia and leukocytosis have been described in about 40% of patients, and thrombocytopenia in 15%. Hyponatremia has been described in 35–50% of patients in different studies. Hypokalemia has been detected in 13% of patients and liver function abnormalities have been observed in about 20%.

### Cerebrospinal fluid

CSF findings for 153 patients with neurological symptoms revealed mild leukocytosis with a median of 77 leukocytes/mm$^3$ (range 0–1750, mainly mononuclear), high protein (median 85 mg/dL, range 19–1900), and normal glucose (median 67 mg/dL, range 3–197) [34].

Electroencephalographic (EEG) patterns are characterized by diffuse, nonspecific slow wave abnormalities, consistent with encephalitis. One study suggested that anterior predominance of slow waves is characteristic of WNV infection [51].

Electromyelography and nerve conduction studies in patients with AFP are consistent with motor axonopathy, but with preservation of sensory nerve potentials. Notably, these tests can be normal in the first 2 weeks of the disease [42, 44].

Computed tomography of the head is usually normal, or reflects previous unrelated abnormalities that are expected in this elderly population [13, 34, 36].

Magnetic resonance imaging is also mostly normal in the initial days of the disease, but the frequency of abnormal lesions increases over the first week and even later.

When present, lesions can be found in deep gray matter structures, predominantly the posterior thalami and basal ganglia [36, 52].

## Long-term outcomes

West Nile fever is considered to have good clinical outcomes. However, one study that focused on WNF patients only found that 96% complained of fatigue after a median of 36 days post-illness, and 71% complained of muscle weakness for a median of 28 days. As a note of caution, results were obtained by telephone interviews several months after the onset of acute illness [35]. Another study assessed outcomes for WNV-infected patients from North Dakota (78% with WNF) a year after the acute infection. Surveys and neuropsychological tests found high rates of self-reported fatigue, weakness, and memory problems. Interestingly, there was no correlation with the severity of the acute disease. In fact, higher rates of fatigue and sleepiness were found in the nonhospitalized patients. Neuropsychological testing found abnormalities in motor skills, attention, and executive functions [53].

WNE occurs more often in elderly patients with co-morbidities and in immunocompromised patients. This population suffers high mortality not only during hospitalization for the acute illness, but in the year following the acute disease as well. In a study that followed surviving hospitalized patients from Israel, the age-standardized mortality during the year following the hospitalization was two and a half times the expected rate. As a comparison, this excess risk is similar to that observed a year after hospitalization with acute myocardial infarction [54].

The long-term outcome of West Nile AFP is very heterogeneous and the initial severity of the disease may not predict the final outcome. Some cases of quadriplegia recovered almost completely after 9 months, but others with less severe disease showed no improvement almost 2 years later [46]. The most severe manifestation is respiratory failure, resulting from the involvement of diaphragmatic and respiratory muscle innervation. Respiratory involvement was associated with a high death rate of >50% [41].

## Diagnosis

Suspicion of WNV infection on clinical grounds is only possible in the midst of an outbreak. During an outbreak, the appearance of elderly patients with high fever and encephalitis or AFP is highly suggestive of the diagnosis. Otherwise, the clinical signs and symptoms are not specific and can be attributed to other infectious agents.

Isolation of the virus from the blood by culture is the gold standard. This was previously done during outbreaks back in the 1950s, but it is difficult and not appropriate for routine diagnosis. Viremia after symptom onset is short-lived and may be absent by the time the patient develops CNS signs. Moreover, culture can only be done in laboratories equipped with biosafety containment facilities.

The polymerase chain reaction (PCR) is a very specific test, but it lacks acceptable sensitivity. In a study that compared diagnosis with PCR to serology, PCR had low sensitivity (57–70%) [55]. Real-time (RT)-PCR is rapid and reliable but costly. It has been used since 2003 for the screening of blood donations in the USA [56].

At this time, serological testing remains the primary method of diagnosing WNV infection. Diagnosis is made by detecting IgM antibodies in the blood or CSF or by observing a fourfold increase in IgG or IgM titer between acute and convalescent samples taken 10 to 28 days apart.

IgM antibody titer rises rapidly during the first week of symptoms. In a study of viremic blood donors with negative serology at baseline, 9 days after index blood donations, all serum samples had detectable IgM antibodies. IgG antibodies started to rise 4 days later, but all patients had positive IgG serology by day 16 [57]. Notably, immunocompromised patients might have prolonged viremia associated with a delayed immune response [19]. In one report, serology turned positive in an immunocompromised patient more than 52 days after the onset of illness. However, basing diagnosis on serology is not problem-free. Approximately 50% of patients after an acute WNV infection are expected to have persistent IgM antibodies for more than 8 months, and in a few patients IgM antibodies persisted for over a year [58]. Thus, the presence of IgM antibody alone is not diagnostic of acute WNV infection, and a fourfold rise in antibody titer is required for confirmation. Moreover, cross-reacting antibodies can emerge either from infection or from vaccination with other flaviviruses, such as Saint Louis encephalitis, Japanese encephalitis, dengue, or yellow fever [59]. A detailed history of previous vaccinations is important in overcoming these problems, as is conducting concurrent testing for other indigenous flaviviruses where relevant (e.g., Saint Louis encephalitis in the USA, dengue in Central or South America).

## Treatment

Currently, there is no proven efficacious treatment for WNV infection, and its management remains supportive. Attention to the level of consciousness and airway protection are critical. Usually, diagnosis leads to the discontinuation of unnecessary antibacterial and antiviral therapies that were started empirically.

The antiviral drug ribavirin was found to inhibit WNV grown in tissue culture [60]. However, in the Israeli outbreak, ribavirin was given orally in a nonrandomized manner to patients with WNND and was found to be correlated with higher mortality [34]. Possible explanations for this unexpected finding are that sicker patients were preferentially treated, and that subtherapeutic doses of ribavirin were administered. If the effective doses from the *in vitro* trial are extrapolated to effective levels in the CSF, this would require intravenous (IV) administration of exceptionally high doses that are correlated with increased adverse events.

Interferon (INF) α-2b was found to be effective in murine models when administered before WNV challenge, but not after viral exposure [61]. Currently, a randomized controlled trial of INF-α-2b for the treatment of WNV meningoencephalitis is under way.

Human immunoglobulin (Ig with high titer against WNV) was found to be effective in treating WNV-infected mice when administered before or right after inoculation, during the viremic phase before the virus has entered the brain [62]. It is not clear, however, whether this approach is relevant to humans, who are usually diagnosed after the disappearance of viremia and the beginning of WNND. One case report of a comatose woman with CLL reported improvement after administration of Ig; however, others did not show such an effect. Note that the outcome of WNND is not predictable and some severe cases will resolve spontaneously; thus, the results of a randomized study are awaited.

## Prevention

WNV infection is transmitted by mosquitoes, and thus reduced exposure to mosquitoes is the best method of protection. Because the vectors, the *Culex* mosquitoes, are night feeders, protection is needed from dusk to dawn. Although personal protection by using mosquito repellent and covering exposed skin is feasible and effective, several studies reported very low use of these measures, even in the setting of an established epidemic [3, 33]. Hence, a comprehensive mosquito eradication program should be a priority in endemic countries.

In the absence of effective treatment, vaccination against WNV infection is attractive. Currently, there are commercial vaccines in use for horses and geese, but none for humans. Several candidate vaccines are in the initial phases of trial in humans; the results are expected and may be applicable both during epidemics and for travelers to endemic areas.

## References

1 Smithburn KC, Hughes TP, Burke AW, Paul JH. A neurotropic virus isolated from the blood of a native of Uganda. *Am J Trop Med* 1940;s1–20(4):471–92.

2 Murgue B, Zeller H, Deubel V. The ecology and epidemiology of West Nile virus in Africa, Europe and Asia. *Curr Top Microbiol Immunol* 2002;267:195–221.

3 Chowers MY, Green MS, Bin H, Weinberger M, Schlaeffer F, Pitlik S, et al. Post-epidemic serosurvey of West Nile fever in Israel. *Eur J Clin Microbiol Infect Dis* 2005;24(12):851–3.

4 Tsai TF, Popovici F, Cernescu C, Campbell GL, Nedelcu NI. West Nile encephalitis epidemic in southeastern Romania. *Lancet* 1998;352(9130):767–71.

5 Weinberger M, Pitlik SD, Gandacu D, Lang R, Nassar F, Ben David D, et al. West Nile fever outbreak, Israel, 2000: epidemiologic aspects. *Emerg Infect Dis* 2001;7(4):686–91.

6 Hayes EB, Komar N, Nasci RS, Montgomery SP, O'Leary DR, Campbell GL. Epidemiology and transmission dynamics of West Nile virus disease. *Emerg Infect Dis* 2005;11(8):1167–73.

7 Dauphin G, Zientara S, Zeller H, Murgue B. West Nile: worldwide current situation in animals and humans. *Comp Immunol Microbiol Infect Dis* 2004;27(5):343–55.

8 Cernescu C, Ruta SM, Tardei G, Grancea C, Moldoveanu L, Spulbar E, et al. A high number of severe neurologic clinical forms during an epidemic of West Nile virus infection. *Rom J Virol* 1997;48(1–4):13–25.

9 Platonov AE, Shipulin GA, Shipulina OY, Tyutyunnik EN, Frolochkina TI, Lanciotti RS, et al. Outbreak of West Nile virus infection, Volgograd Region, Russia, 1999. *Emerg Infect Dis* 2001;7(1):128–32.

10 Asnis DS, Conetta R, Teixeira AA, Waldman G, Sampson BA. The West Nile virus outbreak of 1999 in New York: the Flushing Hospital experience. *Clin Infect Dis* 2000;30(3):413–18.

11 Lanciotti RS, Roehrig JT, Deubel V, Smith J, Parker M, Steele K, et al. Origin of the West Nile virus responsible for an outbreak of encephalitis in the northeastern United States. *Science* 1999;286(5448):2333–7.

12 Centers for Disease Control [CDC] [Online]. 2008 [cited 2008 Febuary 20]. Available from URL: http://www.cdc.gov/ncidod/dvbid/westnile/surv&control.htm.

13 Pepperell C, Rau N, Krajden S, Kern R, Humar A, Mederski B, et al. West Nile virus infection in 2002: morbidity and mortality among patients admitted to hospital in southcentral Ontario. *CMAJ* 2003;168(11):1399–1405.

14 Komar O, Robbins MB, Klenk K, Blitvich BJ, Marlenee NL, Burkhalter KL, et al. West Nile virus transmission in resident birds, Dominican Republic. *Emerg Infect Dis* 2003;9(10):1299–1302.

15 Lorono-Pino MA, Blitvich BJ, Farfan-Ale JA, Puerto FI, Blanco JM, Marlenee NL, et al. Serologic evidence of West Nile virus infection in horses, Yucatan State, Mexico. *Emerg Infect Dis* 2003;9(7):857–9.

16 Morales MA, Barrandeguy M, Fabbri C, Garcia JB, Vissani A, Trono K, et al. West Nile virus isolation from equines in Argentina, 2006. *Emerg Infect Dis* 2006;12(10):1559–61.

17 Pealer LN, Marfin AA, Petersen LR, Lanciotti RS, Page PL, Stramer SL, et al. Transmission of West Nile virus through blood transfusion in the United States in 2002. *N Engl J Med* 2003;349(13):1236–45.

18 Montgomery SP, Brown JA, Kuehnert M, Smith TL, Crall N, Lanciotti RS, et al. Transfusion-associated transmission of West Nile virus, United States 2003 through 2005. *Transfusion* 2006;46(12):2038–46.

19 Iwamoto M, Jernigan DB, Guasch A, Trepka MJ, Blackmore CG, Hellinger WC, et al. Transmission of West Nile virus from an organ donor to four transplant recipients. *N Engl J Med* 2003;348(22):2196–2203.

20 Intrauterine West Nile virus infection—New York, 2002. *MMWR Morb Mortal Wkly Rep* 2002;51(50):1135–6.

21 Possible West Nile virus transmission to an infant through breast-feeding—Michigan, 2002. *MMWR Morb Mortal Wkly Rep* 2002;51(39):877–8.

22 Laboratory-acquired West Nile virus infections—United States, 2002. *MMWR Morb Mortal Wkly Rep* 2002;51(50):1133–5.

23 Charles PE, Zeller H, Bonnotte B, Decasimacker AL, Bour JB, Chavanet P, et al. Imported West Nile virus infection in Europe. *Emerg Infect Dis* 2003;9(6):750.

24 Haas W, Krause G, Marcus U, Stark K, Ammon A, Burger R. "Emerging infectious diseases". Dengue-fever, West-Nile-fever, SARS, avian influenza, HIV. *Internist (Berl)* 2004;45(6):684–92.

25 Hubalek Z, Lukacova L, Halouzka J, Sirucek P, Januska J, Precechtelova J, et al. Import of West Nile virus infection in the Czech Republic. *Eur J Epidemiol* 2006;21(4):323–4.

26 ProMED-mail. West Nile virus, human 2008 [Online]. 2008 [cited 2008 April 27]; 20051008.2938. Available from URL: http://www.promedmail.org/.

27 Knudsen TB, Wilcke JT, Andersen O. Two imported cases of West Nile fever in Denmark. *Ugeskr Laeg* 2003;165(19):2003–4.

28  Prick JJ, Kuipers S, Kuipers HD, Vliegen JH, van Doornum GJ. Another case of West Nile fever in the Netherlands: a man with encephalitis following a trip to Canada. Ned Tijdschr Geneeskd 2003;147(20):978–80.

29  Meeuse JJ, ter Borg F, Lohmann HJ, Groen J. Patient with West Nile fever in the Netherlands. Ned Tijdschr Geneeskd 2001;145(43):2084–6.

30  Estival JL, Skowron F, Dupin M, Combemale P. Primary infection with West-Nile virus. *Ann Dermatol Venereol* 2001;128(5):656–8.

31  Goldblum N, Sterk V, Paderski B. West Nile fever: the clinical features of the disease and the isolation of West Nile virus from the blood of nine human cases. *Am J Epidemiol* 1954;59(1):89–103.

32  Mostashari F, Bunning ML, Kitsutani PT, Singer DA, Nash D, Cooper MJ, et al. Epidemic West Nile encephalitis, New York, 1999: results of a household-based seroepidemiological survey. *Lancet* 2001;358(9278):261–4.

33  Chowers MY, Lang R, Nassar F, Ben-David D, Giladi M, Rubinshtein E, et al. Clinical characteristics of the West Nile fever outbreak, Israel, 2000. *Emerg Infect Dis* 2001;7(4): 675–8.

34  Watson JT, Pertel PE, Jones RC, Siston AM, Paul WS, Austin CC, et al. Clinical characteristics and functional outcomes of West Nile Fever. *Ann Intern Med* 2004;141(5): 360–65.

35  Sejvar JJ, Haddad MB, Tierney BC, Campbell GL, Marfin AA, Van Gerpen JA, et al. Neurologic manifestations and outcome of West Nile virus infection. *JAMA* 2003;290(4):511–5.

36  Nash D, Mostashari F, Fine A, Miller J, O'Leary D, Murray K, et al. The outbreak of West Nile virus infection in the New York City area in 1999. *N Engl J Med* 2001;344(24): 1807–14.

37  Kleinschmidt-DeMasters BK, Marder BA, Levi ME, Laird SP, McNutt JT, Escott EJ, et al. Naturally acquired West Nile virus encephalomyelitis in transplant recipients: clinical, laboratory, diagnostic, and neuropathological features. *Arch Neurol* 2004;61(8):1210–20.

38  Ravindra KV, Freifeld AG, Kalil AC, Mercer DF, Grant WJ, Botha JF, et al. West Nile virus-associated encephalitis in recipients of renal and pancreas transplants: case series and literature review. *Clin Infect Dis* 2004;38(9):1257–60.

39  Robinson RL, Shahida S, Madan N, Rao S, Khardori N. Transient parkinsonism in West Nile virus encephalitis. *Am J Med* 2003;115(3):252–3.

40  Sejvar JJ, Marfin AA. Manifestations of West Nile neuro-invasive disease. *Rev Med Virol* 2006;16(4):209–24.

41  Leis AA, Stokic DS, Webb RM, Slavinski SA, Fratkin J. Clinical spectrum of muscle weakness in human West Nile virus infection. *Muscle Nerve* 2003;28(3):302–8.

42  Li J, Loeb JA, Shy ME, Shah AK, Tselis AC, Kupski WJ, et al. Asymmetric flaccid paralysis: a neuromuscular presentation of West Nile virus infection. *Ann Neurol* 2003;53(6):703–10.

43  Saad M, Youssef S, Kirschke D, Shubair M, Haddadin D, Myers J, et al. Acute flaccid paralysis: the spectrum of a newly recognized complication of West Nile virus infection. *J Infect* 2005;51(2):120–27.

44  Sejvar JJ, Bode AV, Marfin AA, Campbell GL, Ewing D, Mazowiecki M, et al. West Nile virus-associated flaccid paralysis. *Emerg Infect Dis* 2005;11(7):1021–7.

45  Cao NJ, Ranganathan C, Kupsky WJ, Li J. Recovery and prognosticators of paralysis in West Nile virus infection. *J Neurol Sci* 2005;236(1–2):73–80.

46  Bains HS, Jampol LM, Caughron MC, Parnell JR. Vitritis and chorioretinitis in a patient with West Nile virus infection. *Arch Ophthalmol* 2003;121(2):205–7.

47  Hershberger VS, Augsburger JJ, Hutchins RK, Miller SA, Horwitz JA, Bergmann M. Chorioretinal lesions in nonfatal cases of West Nile virus infection. *Ophthalmology* 2003;110(9):1732–6.

48  Kuchtey RW, Kosmorsky GS, Martin D, Lee MS. Uveitis associated with West Nile virus infection. *Arch Ophthalmol* 2003;121(11):1648–9.

49  Sampson BA, Ambrosi C, Charlot A, Reiber K, Veress JF, Armbrustmacher V. The pathology of human West Nile Virus infection. *Hum Pathol* 2000;31(5):527–31.

50  Gandelman-Marton R, Kimiagar I, Itzhaki A, Klein C, Theitler J, Rabey JM. Electroencephalography findings in adult patients with West Nile virus-associated meningitis and meningoencephalitis. *Clin Infect Dis* 2003;37(11):1573–8.

51  Ali M, Safriel Y, Sohi J, Llave A, Weathers S. West Nile virus infection: MR imaging findings in the nervous system. *AJNR Am J Neuroradiol* 2005;26(2):289–97.

52  Carson PJ, Konewko P, Wold KS, Mariani P, Goli S, Bergloff P, et al. Long-term clinical and neuropsychological outcomes of West Nile virus infection. *Clin Infect Dis* 2006;43(6):723–30.

53  Green MS, Weinberger M, Ben-Ezer J, Bin H, Mendelson E, Gandacu D, et al. Long-term death rates, West Nile virus epidemic, Israel, 2000. *Emerg Infect Dis* 2005;11(11):1754–7.

54  Lanciotti RS, Kerst AJ, Nasci RS, Godsey MS, Mitchell CJ, Savage HM, et al. Rapid detection of West Nile virus from human clinical specimens, field-collected mosquitoes, and avian samples by a TaqMan reverse transcriptase-PCR assay. *J Clin Microbiol* 2000;38(11):4066–71.

55  Dauphin G, Zientara S. West Nile virus: recent trends in diagnosis and vaccine development. *Vaccine* 2007;25(30): 5563–76.

56  Prince HE, Tobler LH, Lape-Nixon M, Foster GA, Stramer SL, Busch MP. Development and persistence of West Nile virus-specific immunoglobulin M (IgM), IgA, and IgG in viremic blood donors. *J Clin Microbiol* 2005;43(9):4316–20.

57  Roehrig JT, Nash D, Maldin B, Labowitz A, Martin DA, Lanciotti RS, et al. Persistence of virus-reactive serum immunoglobulin m antibody in confirmed West Nile virus encephalitis cases. *Emerg Infect Dis* 2003;9(3):376–9.

58 Shi PY, Wong SJ. Serologic diagnosis of West Nile virus infection. *Expert Rev Mol Diagn* 2003;3(6):733–41.

59 Jordan I, Briese T, Fischer N, Lau JY, Lipkin WI. Ribavirin inhibits West Nile virus replication and cytopathic effect in neural cells. *J Infect Dis* 2000;182(4):1214–17.

60 Morrey JD, Day CW, Julander JG, Blatt LM, Smee DF, Sidwell RW. Effect of interferon-alpha and interferon-inducers on West Nile virus in mouse and hamster animal models. *Antivir Chem Chemother* 2004;15(2):101–9.

61 Ben-Nathan D, Lustig S, Tam G, Robinzon S, Segal S, Rager-Zisman B. Prophylactic and therapeutic efficacy of human intravenous immunoglobulin in treating West Nile virus infection in mice. *J Infect Dis* 2003;188(1): 5–12.

62 Spigland I, Jasinska-Klingberg W, Hofshi E, Goldblum N. Clinical and laboratory observations in an outbreak of West Nile fever in Israel in 1957. *Harefuah* 1958;54(11):275–80; English & French abstracts 280–81.

# 9 Japanese Encephalitis in Travelers

## John Simon
University of Hong Kong, Hong Kong, China

## Introduction

Japanese encephalitis (JE) is a mosquito-borne flaviviral infection of the central nervous system (CNS). The disease has been called "a plague of the Orient." In Nepal, it is known as "the visitation of the Goddess of the Forest." Three billion people are at risk for it. There are 20,000 to 50,000 cases annually with 6000 to 15,000 deaths. These figures probably represent a gross underestimate due to inadequate surveillance. Almost 50% of cases occur in China and 20% in India. The case incidence in endemic areas ranges from 10–100 per 100,000 per year. About 20–33% die, 25–33% completely recover, and 33–50% are left with sequelae, including intellectual impairment and dyskinesia. Mortality probably depends upon the quality of supportive care. Mortality is higher in the elderly. For every clinical case there are 50–1000 inapparent infections. This results in immunity in almost 100% of adults, and JE affects mainly children. In hyperendemic areas, 50% of cases occur in children under 4 years old and most cases are under 10 years old. In countries with well-established immunization programs, most cases occur in adults over 50 years old who have never been immunized nor developed natural immunity.

The JE virus is a single serotype with five genotypes. There is no significant correlation between genotype and virulence or vaccine efficacy. JE is transmitted in an enzootic cycle involving birds, particularly wading ardeids such as herons and egrets. Birds can carry the disease over long distances and may spread it from rural to urban areas. Mosquitoes transmit the virus to pigs, the most important amplifiers of the virus. Humans and horses have low-level transient viremias and are dead-end hosts

that do not transmit the virus. The major vector is *Culex tritaeniorhynchus*, which has a flight range of 3000 meters and bites outdoors from late afternoon to early evening. Other culicine mosquitoes may be vectors and some may bite into the early hours of the morning. Culicines breed in flooded rice fields, marshy areas, shallow ditches, and irrigation channels. Wind-blown mosquitoes may spread JE long distances.

The prevention of JE in humans is best achieved by immunization of humans. Pig vaccination is not successful in controlling JE transmission. Pigs should be kept in bio-secured pig farms at least 3 kilometers away from human habitation. Backyard pig farming should cease. In Singapore, pig farming stopped in the 1980s. However, sporadic cases of JE still occur in Singapore. Stopping pig farming therefore reduces but does not eliminate JE. Vector control, using larvicides and insecticides, has been only marginally successful. Reduction of the avian reservoir is not feasible. The spread of JE to new areas is mainly due to agricultural development, including deforestation, land clearing, and development of new rice paddies, especially when supported by irrigation schemes.

## Epidemiology

JE extended its range in the latter half of the twentieth century. There is now a risk from Pakistan in the west to Oceania in the east (see Figure 9.1). The general epidemiology is shown in the Appendix. Most cases in recent years are reported from India, Sri Lanka, Nepal, and China. The use of vaccine in Vietnam, Sri Lanka, Thailand, and China has significantly decreased the incidence of JE; increasing vaccination use in India and Nepal is beginning to reduce its incidence there. Widespread vaccination programs in Japan, South Korea, and Taiwan

*Tropical Diseases in Travelers*, 1st edition. Edited by E. Schwartz.
© 2009 by Blackwell Publishing, ISBN: 978-1-4051-8441-0.

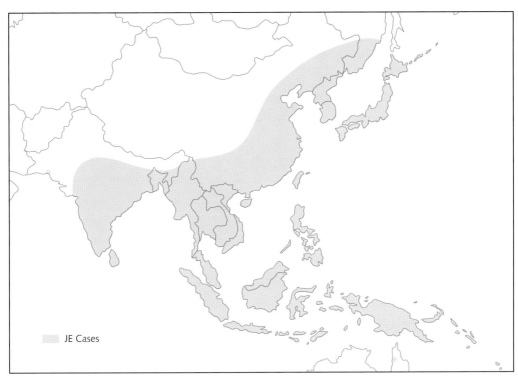

JE Cases

**Figure 9.1** Epidemiology of Japanese encephalitis. (From centers for Disease Control and Prevention table, used in Tsai TR, Chang GW, Yu YX. Japanese encephalitis vaccines. In: Plotkin SA and Orenstein WA, editors, *Vaccines*. 3rd edition. Philadelphia: WB Saunders, Inc., 1999;672–710.)

have effectively eliminated the disease from humans, and fewer than 10 cases/year are reported from each of these countries.

Transmission is usually seasonal, and epidemics usually occur toward the end of the rainy (monsoon) season [1]. In temperate zones of northern China, Japan, Korea, and Taiwan, it is transmitted during the epidemic rainy season, which starts in May or June and ends in September or October. The same is true for the northern parts of Southeast Asia, including northern Vietnam and north Thailand, although there the risk may extend until November and sporadic cases may occur throughout the rest of the year. In northern India and Nepal, the risk may extend up to December. In southern tropical areas, the peak is at the start of the rainy season, but sporadic cases occur throughout the year. Thus, in southern India and Sri Lanka, the risk extends from May to January, with epidemics occurring from September to January. In southern Vietnam and southern Thailand, the highest risk occurs from May to December. In other parts of the tropics, such as Malaysia, Indonesia, and the Philippines, where rain

falls throughout the year or where there is irrigation of the fields, transmission occurs year round.

## Epidemiology in travelers

Travelers, unless vaccinated or previously exposed, are not immune to JE and are as susceptible as unvaccinated children living in endemic areas. Travelers to rural areas of Taiwan, Japan, and Korea should not be misled by the very small number of human cases in these countries. These small numbers are due to immunization of the population; the enzootic cycle of JE remains unchanged—and travelers remain at significant risk. The risk depends on the season, duration, and type of travel. Backpackers are at higher risk than businessmen who stay mostly in urban areas. The risk to a traveler to a rural endemic area in the peak transmission season is 1 in 5000 for a 4-week stay or 1 in 20,000 for a 1-week stay [2]. Cases are reported in travelers who made only a few excursions into rural areas [3]. The risk is greatest in those visiting rural areas,

**Table 9.1** Reported cases of JE in travelers.

| Case number | Nationality | Country acquired | Area | Year | Age | Sex | Vaccine | Outcome | Ref. |
|---|---|---|---|---|---|---|---|---|---|
| 1 | Norway | China | | 1998 | | | | | PC |
| 2 | Finland | China | Beijing | 2001 | 45 | M | No | Recovered* | 6 |
| 3 | New Zealand | China | Yangtze River | 2005 | 49 | F | | | 5 |
| 4 | Hong Kong | China | | 2002 | | | No | | 6 |
| 5 | Hong Kong | China | | 2002 | | | No | | 6 |
| 6 | Hong Kong | China | | 2005 | 54 | M | No | Recovered | 6 |
| 7 | Hong Kong | China | Guangdong | 2007 | 22 | F | No | Recovered | 6 |
| 8 | Hong Kong | China | Guizhou | 2007 | 15 | M | No | Recovered | 6 |
| 9 | Belgium | China | Shanghai | 2004 | 10 | F | No | | |
| 10 | UK | Hong Kong | Hong Kong | 1982 | 35 | F | No | Died | 7 |
| 11 | Nepal | India | | 2007 | | | | | |
| 12 | Australia | Indonesia | Bali | 1989 | 10 | F | No | Recovered | 3 |
| 13 | Sweden | Indonesia | Bali | 1994 | 60 | F | | Recovered | 8 |
| 14 | Denmark | Indonesia | Bali | 1995 | | M | | Died | 9 |
| 15 | Sweden | Indonesia | Java and Bali | 2004 | 80 | M | | Recovered | 10 |
| 16 | Netherlands | Indonesia | | 2005 | 29 | F | No | Recovered* | 11 |
| 17 | USA | Japan | Okinawa | 1991 | | M | No | | 12 |
| 18 | USA | Japan | Okinawa | 1991 | | M | No | | 12 |
| 19 | USA | Japan | Okinawa | 1991 | | M | No | | 12 |
| 20 | USA | Philippines | Manila | 1980s | | M | No | | PC |
| 21 | Norway | Philippines | | 1998 | | | | | |
| 22 | Norway | Philippines | | 1998 | | | | | |
| 23 | Israel | Thailand | | 1989 | | F | No | | 4 |
| 24 | UK | Thailand | | 1994 | | F | | | 13 |
| 25 | USA | Thailand | Chiang Mai | 2004 | 22 | F | No | Recovered | 14 |
| 26 | Netherlands | Thailand | | 2005 | 30 | F | No | Recovered* | 11 |
| 27 | Norway | Thailand | | 1997 | | | | | |
| 28 | Australia | Vietnam | | 1975 | | M | No | | 15 |
| 29 | Italy | Vietnam | North | 2006 | 49 | M | No | Recovered* | 16 |

PC = personal communication.
\* = recovery but with slight intellectual impairment.

especially those who sleep outside at night or who go bicycling, hiking, camping, or golfing. The overall risk of symptomatic disease to travelers visiting countries where there is JE is 1 in 1 million for a 4-week period [1]. However, this was calculated from data on outbound airline travelers from the USA to Asia, of whom some may have been vaccinated against JE, so that the risk for the unvaccinated is underestimated. Asymptomatic seroconversion has been demonstrated in travelers. The risk of acquiring symptomatic JE is low [4]. In hyperendemic areas, <3% of mosquitoes are infected, and the ratio of symptomatic to asymptomatic disease is around 1 in 250. The chances of developing symptomatic JE from a single bite, therefore, are 1 in 33 × 1 in 250, or around 1 in 8250. In areas

where <1% of mosquitoes are infected, the risk of getting symptomatic JE from a single bite is 1 in 100 × 1 in 250, or 1 in 25,000.

Only 24 cases were reported in Western travelers in 1978 to 1992. JE is probably underreported in travelers, as evidenced by at least five proven cases not written up in the literature (Table 9.1). As can be seen in the table, about a third of the cases were acquired in China, followed by Thailand and Indonesia. Details of some of these cases are as follow:

Case #2: A Finnish man from Beijing was evacuated to Hong Kong under the care of the author. He was an expatriate and had rented a house in the outskirts of Beijing on August 1, 2001. In early September, he developed an encephalitic illness and was evacuated to Hong Kong, where he was proven to have JE.

Case #3: A New Zealand woman had traveled in China for 3 weeks.

Case #7: A woman from Hong Kong had traveled to rural areas of Guangdong (Huizhou, Jiangmen, and Zhongshan) in 2007 and developed JE in June 2007. JE was confirmed by a fourfold rise in paired titers.

Case #9: A Belgium girl who developed JE in July 2004 had spent 2 weeks in Shanghai at her parents' accommodation in an urban area, and did not visit rural areas. She was evacuated to Belgium. Diagnosis was made in Belgium by showing JE-specific declining IgM titers and increasing IgG titers, whereas dengue serology remained negative.

Case #12: An Australian girl who developed JE in 1989 4 days after returning to Australia had been in Bali for 2 weeks. She recovered after 3 months.

Case #13: A Swedish woman who developed JE in March 1994 had spent 10 days in Bali. She stayed at a coastal hotel and made only one day trip to the countryside.

Case #14: A Danish man who died of JE in January 1995 had visited Bali for 12 days.

Cases #17, #18, #19: Prior to cases of three US marines stationed in Okinawa who developed JE in 1991, no cases had been reported since 1974 either in Okinawan residents or in US servicemen.

Case #20: A US citizen developed proven JE in the 1980s in Manila. It is uncertain whether this person had visited rural areas in the incubation period.

Case #23: Following the case of an Israeli woman who developed JE after a trip to Thailand in 1989, Israeli public health authorities recommended vaccination for all travelers to Thailand.

Case #25: A woman from Washington, USA, who developed JE after a trip to northern Thailand for 32 days in May 2004 had spent most of the time in the city of Chiang Mai, but had spent one night in a cabin in rural Chiang Mai valley.

Case #28: An Australian who developed JE in 1975 after returning from Vietnam was a soldier.

Case #29: An Italian man who developed JE in 2006 had traveled extensively in the rural north of Thailand for 3 weeks. He became symptomatic in May 2006 on his return flight to Italy.

The outcome is known in 13 of the 29 cases listed: 11 recovered and 2 died (crude fatality rate 18%). Four of those who recovered showed persistent intellectual impairment (36%). This is all in line with typical outcomes. The sex is known for 22 cases, and JE occurred equally in men and women. No case we know of involved a vaccinated person. Of particular note was that several cases involved persons who spent only short periods in the endemic area—suggesting that the 1-month rule for vaccination is incorrect. Moreover, three cases occurred in major cities, again suggesting that the rule for vaccination, when traveling in a rural area, is incorrect.

## Clinical features

The incubation period is 4–15 days and usually is 6–8 days. Most cases are inapparent, subclinical, or mild nonspecific febrile illnesses presenting with sudden onset of fever, chills, aches, malaise, nausea, vomiting, and headache. Children may have gastrointestinal pain. After 3–4 days of prodromal illness with a high swinging fever of up to 40°C or higher, a generalized CNS infection develops. Fever lasts a total of 7 days.

Neurological manifestations depend on the part of the CNS most affected, and there is often overlap. Damage to both upper and lower motor neurons may result in a bizarre mixture of signs. Encephalitis is the major feature of 75–85% of cases, aseptic meningitis the major feature in 5–10%, and myelitis predominates in <10%.

Encephalitic cases have a reduced level of consciousness, confusion, delirium, or stupor, with progression to coma in 40%. Generalized weakness, hypertonia, and hyperreflexia are common. Meningism occurs in 80% of encephalitic cases. Spasticity occurs in 44%, and a further 37% show flaccidity. Hemiplegia occurs in 40% and can be an initial manifestation. Paralysis of the upper extremities is more common than that of the legs. Extensor plantars are seen in 44%. Convulsions occur in 85% of children. Status epilepticus correlates with a poor outcome. A subtle convulsive status, such as twitching of the eyebrow, finger, or mouth, is associated with a poor outcome. Cranial nerve palsies occur in 2%. Disorders of conjugate gaze occur in up to 33%. A Parkinsonian syndrome, due to involvement of basal ganglia, occurs in 27%. In week 2, fever and other neurological manifestations resolve; however, there is a dull, flat, mask-like facies with wide, unblinking eyes, tremor, generalized hypertonia, cogwheel rigidity, and abnormalities of movement, including choreoathetosis, myoclonic jerks, jaw dystonia, and abnormal tongue protrusions. Papilloedema occurs in <10%. A "locked-in" syndrome may occur if there is severe brain stem involvement. Mutism is reported as a presenting symptom.

Myelitis presents as a flaccid paralysis complicating encephalitic cases or as a pure myelitis in fully conscious cases. There is lower motor neuron flaccid paresis mimicking poliomyelitis. Respiratory or bulbar paralysis may occur. Over 55% of cases of acute flaccid paralysis (AFP) in Vietnam were due to JE. Over 50% of 9857 cases of AFP reported to World Health Organization (WHO) in 1996 were due to JE.

Complications include cardiac arrhythmias, fluctuating blood pressure, and, rarely, pericarditis. Recrudescence occurs rarely and is due to viral latency in peripheral lymphocytes. Pregnancy studies in Uttar Pradesh show a high risk of intrauterine death or miscarriage among those infected in the first two trimesters, but not in the third trimester. The clinical features of JE in the presence of acquired immunodeficiency syndrome (AIDS) are not known.

Most patients have peripheral leucocytosis with relative neutrophilia. The opening pressure in the CSF is usually normal. The CSF is normal in 30%. The CSF may show neutrophils in the first few hours. Thereafter, there is a lymphocytic pleocytosis. Moderate lymphocytosis (mean 380 cells/mm$^3$) is seen in 45%. CSF protein is mildly increased in 37% (mean 0.77 g/L). CSF sugar is normal. Imaging findings are nonspecific. However, changes in the thalami and substantia nigra suggest JE. EEGs may show several patterns, including periodic lateralized epileptiform discharges similar to herpes simplex encephalitis. EMGs may show changes suggesting denervation. Nerve conduction studies sometimes suggest Guillain–Barré syndrome.

## Diagnosis

Differential diagnosis is mainly from *Herpes simplex* encephalitis and other forms of locally circulating viral encephalitis, such as Murray valley encephalitis and Chandipura virus. Dengue fever may rarely present with encephalitis. Cerebral malaria should always be considered.

JE is difficult to diagnose serologically in countries where several flaviviruses co-circulate because of an amnestic IgG response to previous flavivirus exposure. A fourfold increase in IgG titer may give a false positive result because of the presence of heterologous flaviral antibodies, for example, to dengue. IgG antibodies appear around days 10–14. If only IgG testing is available, then parallel testing against other flaviviruses improves speci-

ficity. If no rise in IgG titers occurs, there is no need to test for IgM. IgM testing allows early diagnosis. IgM can be detected on days 3–4 in 75% of cases, and almost 100% are positive within 1 week of disease onset. False negative results may occur if IgM is measured too early. Measuring IgM antibody is useful in areas where multiple flaviviruses circulate. A nitrocellulose-membrane-based IgM capture dot enzyme immunoassay (MAC DOT) allows rapid diagnosis and is 95% sensitive and 99.2% specific. Demonstration of specific IgM in the CSF or the serum by IgM-capture ELISA is specific. Diagnosis can also be performed by isolating JE virus from the blood or CSF, but this is difficult and needs to be done during the first week of the illness. RT-PCR is 100% specific but has low sensitivity due to the low level of viremia in humans. PCR is much more sensitive with CSF.

## Treatment

There is no specific treatment for JE. Outcome depends on the quality of supportive care, including mechanical ventilation, anticonvulsants for seizures, and control of increased intracranial pressure using mannitol and invasive monitoring. Limb contractures, deep vein thromboses, pneumonia, urinary tract infections, and bedsores should be prevented or treated. The use of steroids is controversial. Early reports that interferon alpha A is beneficial were not confirmed in a well-controlled Vietnamese trial.

## Prevention

### General measures
Travelers should implement mosquito avoidance measures, especially in the late afternoon and at dusk. These include DEET 30%, impregnated bed nets, knockdown spray, and wearing long-sleeved light-colored clothing.

### Vaccination
The U.S. Advisory Committee on Immunization Practices (ACIP) recommends vaccination for persons planning to reside in areas where JE is endemic. Thus, expatriates posted to any urban area in endemic countries, including Shanghai or Beijing, should consider vaccination. The possibility of unexpected travel to high-risk areas may influence the decision to vaccinate. ACIP recommends vaccination for persons spending a month or more in endemic areas during the transmission season, especially if travel includes rural areas [2]. Vaccination can be

offered for stays of less than a month for high-risk travel to epidemic areas. The Centers for Disease Control and Prevention (CDC) recommends that "JE vaccine should be offered to those visiting areas with epidemic transmission or engaging in extensive outdoor activities in rural settings regardless of the duration of the visit" [17]. A CDC study presented in 2008 showed that only 11% of travelers fulfilling CDC criteria for immunization were vaccinated. The elderly have more risk of acquiring symptomatic disease and their threshold criteria for immunization should be lowered. Most recommendations for vaccination were determined by comparing the relative risk of acquiring symptomatic JE to the risk of developing adverse reactions to currently available vaccines. Recommendations for vaccination will probably increase when safer vaccines appear on the market.

## Vaccines

Inactivated mouse-brain-derived JE vaccine is manufactured by Biken Company, Osaka University, and distributed by Connaught in the USA. Protective efficacy was 94% after three vaccinations given at 0, 7, and 28 days. Most authorities recommend a booster every 3 years. Manufacture was discontinued because of concern over potentially serious reactions including urticaria, erythema multiforme, angioedema, and anaphylaxis. These varied in frequency from 1 to 62 per 10,000 vaccinated. Reactions could be delayed up to 10 days and could occur with the second or third vaccination even if there was no reaction to the first or second vaccination. Severe neurological reactions, including acute disseminated encephalomyelitis (ADEM), occurred in 1–2.3/million vaccinated. When current supplies expire, the Biken vaccine will no longer be available. Similar inactivated mouse-brain-derived vaccines based on the Nakayama strain are manufactured in Korea, Vietnam, India, and Thailand, and Taiwan manufactures a vaccine based on the Zhongshan strain. The Korean Green Cross vaccine has been used in the UK since 1989 on a named patient basis, and import licenses are available in Finland, the Netherlands, Sweden, and Israel. It has the same safety spectrum as the Biken vaccine.

A vaccine is urgently needed to replace the Biken vaccine. The Chengdu Institute of Biological Products makes a live attenuated JE vaccine using the SA14-14-2 strain. It has been in use since 1988. It has high protective efficacy after a single dose. Serious adverse effects have not been reported in large trials in China, Nepal, and South Korea. It has been submitted to the WHO for prequalification, which will allow vaccine procurement by UN agencies. Two companies have developed new vaccines based on the SA14-14-2 strain. The JE Intercell vaccine (IC51) is manufactured by Intercell and will be distributed by Novartis. It is an inactivated vaccine based on the SA14-14-2 strain attenuated in Vero cells. Two doses are given on days 0 and 28. It is more immunogenic than the Biken vaccine and has a better adverse effect profile. It is expected to be licensed late in 2008 by the Food and Drug Administration (FDA) and European Medicines Agency (EMEA) [18]. JE-CV or ChimeriVax-JE is manufactured by Acambis and will be distributed by Sanofi Pasteur. It is a live attenuated vaccine based on the SA14-14-2 strain and the yellow fever17D strain. It is grown in Vero cells. It contains no preservatives or adjuvant. A single dose of 0.5 ml gives 94% seroconversion at 14 days. There is much less erythema, pruritus, and swelling than with the Biken vaccine [19].

## References

1  Monath TP, Tsai TF. Flaviviruses. In: Richman DD, Whitley RJ, Hayden FG, editors. *Clinical Virology*. Washington (DC): ASM Press; 2002. p. 1097–151.

2  Centers for Disease Control [CDC]. Inactivated Japanese encephalitis vaccine. Recommendations of the Advisory Committee on Immunization Practices (ACIP). *MMWRMorb Mortal Wkly Rep* 1993;42(RR-1):1–15.

3  MacDonald WBG, Tink AR, Ouvrier RA, Menser MA, de Silva LM, Maim H, et al. Japanese encephalitis after a two-week holiday in Bali. *Med J Aust* 1989;150(6):334–7, 339.

4  Shlim DR, Solomon T. Japanese encephalitis vaccine for travelers: exploring the limits of risk. *Clin Infect Dis* 2002;35: 183–8.

5  Centre for Health Protection [CHP] Hong Kong. Available from http://www.chp.gov.hk.

6  Cutfield NJ, et al. Japanese encephalitis acquired during travel in China. *Intern Med J* 2005;35(8):497–8.

7  Rose MR, Hughes SM, Gatus BJ. A case of Japanese B encephalitis imported into the United Kingdom. *J Infect* 1983; 6(3):261–5.

8  Wittesjo B, Eitrem R, Niklasson B, Vene S, Mangiafico JA. Japanese encephalitis after a 10-day holiday in Bali. *Lancet* 1995;345:856.

9  Buhl MS, Black FT, Andersen PL, Laursen A. Fatal Japanese encephalitis in a Danish tourist visiting Bali for 12 days. *Scand J Infect Dis* 1996;28(2):189.

10  Ostlund MR, Kan B, Karlsson M, Vene S. Japanese encephalitis in a Swedish tourist after traveling to Java and Bali. *Scand J Infect Dis* 2004;36(6–7):512–13.

11  Delsing CE, Ardesch J, Nihorn J, Mulder L, Kootstra GJ, Hylkerna BS. An unusual cause of meningo-encephalitis: Japanese encephalitis. *Ned Tijdschr Geneeskd* 2005;149(43):2423–7.

12 Saito M, Sunagawa T, Makino Y, Tadano M, Hasegawa H, Kanemura K, et al. Three JE cases in Okinawa, Japan 1991. *Southeast Asian J Trop Med Public Health* 1999;30(2):277–9.

13 Burdon JT, Stanley PJ, Lloyd G, Jones N. A case of Japanese encephalitis. *J Infect* 1994;28:175–9.

14 Japanese encephalitis in a U.S. traveler returning from Thailand, 2004. *MMWR Morb Mortal Wkly Rep* 2005;54(5):123–5.

15 Fleming K. JE in an Australian soldier returned from Vietnam. *Med J Aust* 1975; 5;2(1):19–23.

16 Caramello P, Canta F, Balbiano R, Lipani F, Ariaudo S, De Agostini M, Calleri G, Boglione L, Di Caro A. A case of imported JE acquired during short travel to Vietnam. *J Travel Med* 2007;14(5):346–8.

17 Centers for Disease Control [CDC]. *MMWR Morb Mortal Wkly Rep* 2005;54(05):123–5.

18 Kaltenbock A, Jilma B, Golor G, Klade C, Kollaritsch H, Voicu V, et al. Long term immunogenicity and safety of the Japanese encephalitis vaccine IC51. Interim results of an uncontrolled phase 3 follow-up study until month 12. Presented at the APICTM 2008, Feb 26, 2008, Melbourne, Australia.

19 Monath TP, McCarthy K, Bedford P, et al. Clinical proof of principle for ChimeriVax recombinant live, attenuated vaccines against flavivirus infections. *Vaccine* 2002;20:1004–18.

## Appendix: General epidemiology

*Australia*: Cases have been reported from Badu Island in the Torres Strait and from Cape York.

*Bangladesh*: Transmission probably is widespread and follows the same pattern as in northern India.

*Bhutan*: Little is known about the epidemiology.

*Brunei*: Probably follows the same pattern as Malaysia with presumptive year-round transmission.

*Cambodia*: JE is probably hyperendemic in rural areas, with a high prevalence near Phnom Penh.

*China*: Vaccination programs have resulted in a decrease in cases from 200,000 cases in 1970 to 5,104 cases in 2005. Cases occur in all provinces except Xizang (Tibet), Xinjiang, and Qinghai. It is hyperendemic in southern China. There was a large outbreak in Yuncheng in Shanxi province in 2006. JE is endemic in Shanghai and there are summer outbreaks around Beijing.

*Guam* and *Saipan*: Two epidemics have been reported in the Pacific Islands in the Northern Marianas. It is thought that an enzootic cycle may not be sustainable and that epidemics follow reintroduction of the virus.

*Hong Kong*: Most cases are imported but rare locally acquired cases are reported from the New Territories. In 2004, five local cases were reported, and none have been reported since 2004.

*India:* The CDC "Yellow Book" says that cases have not been reported from Arunachal, Dadra, Daman, Diu, Gujarat, Himachal, Jammu, Kashmir, Lakshadweep, Meghalaya, Nagar Haveli, Rajasthan, and Sikkim. This is incorrect, as cases have been reported from Arunachal Pradesh, Punjab, and Orissa. Cases are reported from all other states. Epidemics have occurred in West Bengal, Bihar, Tamil Nadu, Andhra Pradesh, Assam, Uttar Pradesh, Karnataka, Manipur, and Goa. JE spread into Haryana state in 1993 and into Kerala state in 1996. A large epidemic occurred in Uttar Pradesh in 2005 with spread to Bihar and to Nepal. Urban cases have been reported in Lucknow.

*Indonesia*: Transmission varies from island to island but is probably year-round and depends on rainfall, rice cultivation, and the presence of pigs. Surveillance is poor and the number of reported cases is an underestimate. It is noted that Indonesia is mainly a Muslim country and has, in general, a small pig population. However, Bali, where the majority of the population are Hindu, has a large pig population.

*Japan*: Sporadic cases occur on all islands except Hokkaido. Enzootic transmission occurs on Hokkaido.

*Laos*: JE is probably endemic or hyperendemic in rural areas.

*Malaysia:* JE is the cause of 38.5% of encephalitis cases and of 0.4% of nonspecific febrile illness. Two hundred cases were reported in 2000. Most cases occur in Penang, Perak, Selangor, Johor, and Sarawak, but JE almost certainly exists in all other states, including Sabah. Outbreaks occurred in Pulau Langkawi in 1974, Pulau Pinang in 1988, Serian, Sarawak in 1992, and northern Perak and Negri Sembilan in 2001.

*Myanmar*: Outbreaks have been reported in Shan State in the Chiang Mai valley. The incidence is probably increasing.

*Nepal:* There were 3000 cases in 2000. It is hyperendemic on the Terai (the plains). There was an epidemic in the Kathmandu Valley in 2005. Nepalgani, 500 km west of Kathmandu, was severely affected. There is little risk to travelers visiting only high-altitude areas.

*North Korea*: Little is known about the epidemiology.

*Pakistan*: JE may be transmitted in central deltas. Cases have been reported near Karachi. The Lower Indus Valley may be an endemic area. Areas overlap those for the West Nile Virus.

*Papua New Guinea (PNG):* Cases have been reported in Kiunga in Western province, in Milne Bay province, and in Gulf and South Highland provinces. A 64-year-old European farmer who had lived on a farm 20 km from Port

Moresby since 1970 and who had not traveled for over a month was proven to have JE in January 2004.

*Philippines:* The disease is probably endemic on all islands. Surveillance is poor and the number of reported cases is a gross underestimate. Outbreaks have been described in Nueva Ecija, Luzon, and even in Manila.

*Russia:* The first cases for over 30 years were recently reported in the far eastern maritime areas south of Khabarousk.

*Singapore:* There are rare cases with year-round transmission.

*South Korea:* One thousand cases were reported in 1985. Now only sporadic cases are reported.

*Sri Lanka:* JE is endemic in all areas except mountainous areas. It is periodically epidemic in northern and central provinces. Outbreaks have been reported in central (Anuradhapura) and northwestern provinces.

*Taiwan:* Sporadic cases are reported in and around Taipei and the Kaohsiung–Pingtung river basins.

*Thailand:* A childhood immunization program resulted in a decrease in cases from 2000 cases annually from 1990–2000 to 500 cases annually since 2000. In Northern Thailand, it is hyperendemic. There was a major epidemic in Chiang Mai in 1969, where there are still annual outbreaks. Sporadic cases occur in the Bangkok suburbs and in the south of Thailand. There is little risk in the major seaside resorts.

*Vietnam:* The disease is endemic to hyperendemic in all provinces. The incidence has fallen from 3000 to 5000 cases annually from 1970 to 1990 to 500 cases annually since 2000. The highest rates occur in and near Hanoi. In Ho Chi Minh City transmission occurs in periurban areas.

# 10 Yellow Fever and Yellow Fever Vaccine-Associated Disease

Elizabeth D. Barnett

Boston Medical Center, Boston, MA, USA

## Introduction

Yellow fever is a mosquito-transmitted viral hemorrhagic fever that occurs in parts of Africa and South America. Mosquito control activities and effective vaccines have limited the spread of the disease, but recent circumstances, including climate change, population mobility, and reduction in mosquito control activities, have led to recrudescence in areas where it was once eradicated. Concerns about adverse vaccine-associated events have focused attention on the use of vaccine in both travelers and populations in endemic areas. This chapter focuses on the epidemiology, clinical manifestations, and prevention of YF and on adverse reactions to YF vaccine.

## Epidemiology

Yellow fever (YF) occurs both endemically and epidemically in parts of South America and Africa. In the 20-year period from 1985 to 2004, 28,264 cases and 7880 deaths were reported to the World Health Organization (WHO); 87% of these deaths occurred in Africa. Significant underreporting is likely because of disease occurrence in remote areas, lack of diagnostic capability, and late recognition of outbreaks. Estimates of ratios of actual cases to officially notified cases range as high as 311:1 [1]. Large epidemics, with >100,000 cases, have been recorded repeatedly in Sub-Saharan Africa. Epidemics also occurred in the Americas, likely beginning in the seventeenth century, introduced by ships carrying infected mosquitoes. The mosquito was identified as the vector of transmission of yellow fever through studies carried out by Carlos Findlay in Cuba and Walter Reed and colleagues in Panama. This discovery led to implementation of aggressive vector-control measures, resulting in elimination of the disease from the USA and reduction in the areas in which outbreaks of YF occurred.

YF epidemic activity in the late twentieth century has been described in detail by Monath [2] and Robertson et al. [3]. A dramatic resurgence of YF has occurred since the 1980s in both Sub-Saharan Africa and South America. Although a series of outbreaks throughout West Africa were responsible for most of the increased incidence of YF in Africa, the first epidemic reported in Kenya in more than two decades also signaled a change in the distribution of the disease [4]. Most recent outbreaks have occurred in West Africa (Senegal in 2002–2003, the southern Sudan in 2003 and 2005, Togo in 2006) [1], and Brazil, Argentina, and Paraguay in 2008.

Transmission of YF in Africa is maintained by dense mosquito populations coexisting with human populations with low immunization rates. Thirty-two African countries are now considered at risk of YF, with a total population of 610 million people, more than 219 million of whom live in urban settings. Although some countries have incorporated YF vaccine into childhood immunization programs, vaccine coverage is not optimal. The interruption of regular mass vaccination campaigns has also played a role in the current resurgence of YF.

YF in South America occurs in the Amazon region and surrounding areas. Disease transmission is lower than in Africa because of higher vaccine coverage and lower density of vector mosquitoes, monkeys (which are also carriers of YF virus), and human hosts. The largest outbreak in South America since the 1950s occurred in Peru in 1995, and cases were reported in Bolivia, Brazil, Colombia, Ecuador, and Peru from 1985 to 1994. Mass vaccination campaigns were initiated following resurgence of the

*Tropical Diseases in Travelers*, 1st edition. Edited by E. Schwartz.
© 2009 by Blackwell Publishing, ISBN: 978-1-4051-8441-0.

**Table 10.1** Yellow fever in unvaccinated travelers 1978–2008.

| Year | Country of acquisition | Nature of travel | Sex/age | Country of residence | Outcome |
|------|------------------------|------------------|---------|----------------------|---------|
| 1979 | Senegal | Tourism; near border of The Gambia | M/42 | France | Fatal |
| 1979 | Senegal | Tourism; near border of The Gambia | M/25 | France | Fatal |
| 1985 | West Africa (three countries) | Rural areas | F/27 | The Netherlands | Survived |
| 1996 | Brazil | Tourism; jungle areas | M/53 | Switzerland | Fatal |
| 1996 | Brazil | Tourism; jungle areas | M/45 | USA | Fatal |
| 1999 | Venezuela | 10-day trip to southern Venezuela (Amazonas state) | M/48 | USA | Fatal |
| 1999 | Ivory Coast | 2 weeks, rural areas | M/39 | Germany | Fatal |
| 2001 | The Gambia | Tourism; 1-week trip | F/47 | Belgium | Fatal |
| 2002 | Brazil | 6-day fishing trip on Rio Negro | M/47 | USA | Fatal |

Adapted from [1, 7, 8].

disease in Brazil in the late 1990s and early 2000s. Early in 2008, Paraguay reported the first cases of YF in 30 years (including a few cases of presumed urban transmission) and Brazil reported cases in states previously felt to lack risk of YF [6]. The last urban outbreak of YF in Brazil was in 1942, but the presence of growing and largely unimmunized urban populations living in areas infested with *Aedes aegypti* and *A. albopictus* mosquitoes (able to transmit YF) is cause for concern. Argentina also reported its first confirmed cases in humans in decades in March 2008 [6]. An increasing number of primate deaths from what was thought to be YF occurred before the human cases were noted. Ministry of Health officials in the affected countries have instituted YF vaccination campaigns and strengthened preventive public health measures.

A. *aegypti* is the major mosquito vector for YF in Africa, and *Haemogogus* in South America. Other *Aedes* species are also involved in transmission, some in interhuman transmission. Mosquito control, combined with immunization programs, contributed to significant reduction of the disease in South America and Africa in the first half of the twentieth century. Vector control strategies, although initially highly successful, have faltered in the past several decades. Spread of YF into areas where it had been eradicated or areas where it never appeared could occur as a result of the continued spread of *A. aegypti* vector mosquitoes, the recent increase in human YF infections, the shift of human populations into remote rural areas where transmission can occur, economic development and the growth of air travel, and relaxation of international regulations concerning vaccination certification for travelers [1]. It is unlikely that vector control strate-

gies alone will result in elimination of YF; such strategies must be combined with effective vaccination programs. The disease is unlikely to be eradicable because monkeys are part of the sylvatic cycle of transmission.

## Yellow fever in travelers

Yellow fever has occurred in unvaccinated travelers. Nine cases were reported in unimmunized travelers from the USA and Europe between 1970 and 2002; these cases are listed in Table 10.1. Many of the affected individuals returned to their home countries while ill or while incubating the infection. The mortality rate of unvaccinated travelers who acquired YF was 89% (8 of 9 cases). Another case occurred in 1987 in an immunized traveler from Spain who visited four countries in West Africa; this individual survived [7, 8]. Mortality rates in local populations are difficult to assess because the spectrum of disease includes asymptomatic or mildly symptomatic infection, because all cases may not be identified, especially in remote areas, and because diagnostic tests may not be available in all settings. Case fatality rates of about 20% (in patients with jaundice) in West Africa, 44% in Brazil, and 57.9% in South America have been reported [1]. In Brazil, male sex and age > 40 were associated with higher case fatality rates [9]. Comparison of case fatality rates in travelers with those of local populations is problematic due to incomplete mortality data from many countries, especially in Africa; variability in the availability of accurate diagnostic tests; and incomplete understanding of the prevalence of asymptomatic or mildly symptomatic disease in travelers. The possibility of differences in the virulence of virus strains, racial/genetic differences in

**Table 10.2** Yellow fever- and yellow fever vaccine-associated adverse events, risks, and case fatality rates.

| Disease/adverse event | Group affected | Reference | Case fatality rate | Risk of disease/adverse event |
|---|---|---|---|---|
| Yellow fever | Travelers | [1, 7, 8] | 89% (limited by lack of data on mild or asymptomatic infection) | 3.67/1000 for 2-week trip to Africa during epidemic period; 1.1–2.4/1000 during interepidemic period |
| | West Africa | [1] | ~ 20% (limited by incomplete reporting of deaths) | ~$\frac{1}{10}$ of risk in Africa for 2-week trip to South America |
| | South America | [9] | 57.9% | |
| | Brazil | | 44% | |
| Yellow fever vaccine-associated neurologic disease | First-time vaccine recipients | [1, 26, 27] | <5% | 0.5-4/1000 in very young infants 1:150,000–1:250,000 in all ages |
| Yellow fever vaccine-associated viscevotropic disease | First-time vaccine recipients | [1, 27, 30, 31] | 58% | 1:200,000–1:300,000 in all ages 1:40,000–1:50,000 in ages 60 years or older |

susceptibility to disease, and other factors must continue to be entertained until further data are available. Estimating the risk of YF for a specific traveler is challenging because of the fluctuation of disease by year and season, incomplete surveillance data, and partial vaccine coverage of the local population, making it more difficult to estimate risk to the unimmunized (Table 10.2) [10]. Areas of current YF risk are shown in Figures 10.1 and 10.2.

Risks of illness and death for a two-week trip to an area of Africa experiencing epidemic YF activity have been estimated at 1:267 (3.67/1000) and 1:1333 (0.75/1000), respectively, for an unimmunized individual. During interepidemic periods, risks of illness and death have been estimated at 1.1–2.4 cases/1000 persons and 0.2–0.5 deaths/1000 persons [7]. Risks of illness and death in South America have been estimated to be 10 times lower than in Africa. This may vary by season, local epidemic activity, and location of travel. Estimation of risk is most difficult during interepidemic periods, when transmission may be epidemiologically silent, with incidence of overt disease being below the limits of detection for existing surveillance systems [1].

## Virology

YF virus, a small (40–60 nm) single-stranded RNA flavivirus, is antigenically and evolutionarily distinct from other flaviviruses. A single serotype exists, although wild-type strains have been classified into at least seven geno-

types based on sequence analysis. Entire genomes have been sequenced for two: the Asibi strain, from which the 17D vaccine is derived, and the French viscerotropic virus, from which the French neurotropic vaccines were derived [11, 12]. Virulence of the virus appears to be determined by both structural and nonstructural genes. Mouse models, employed by almost all virulence studies, reveal only neurotropism. Recent development of a hamster model will allow further study of molecular determinants associated with viscerotropism. Neurovirulence and viscerotropism may not be linked at the molecular level, and this may be one explanation for the variation in mortality rates seen in human epidemics of yellow fever [1, 13].

## Clinical description of yellow fever

YF disease ranges from an asymptomatic or nonspecific illness to a potentially fatal systemic disease involving fever, jaundice, hemorrhage, and renal failure. Differences in virus strains and incompletely understood host immune factors are likely responsible for the range of clinical symptoms. A short incubation period (3–6 days) is followed by an acute illness characterized by high fever, headache, malaise, nausea, vomiting, generalized myalgia, irritability, dizziness, and a generally ill appearance. In some cases, the high fever is accompanied by relative bradycardia (Faget's sign). Leukopenia, present at the

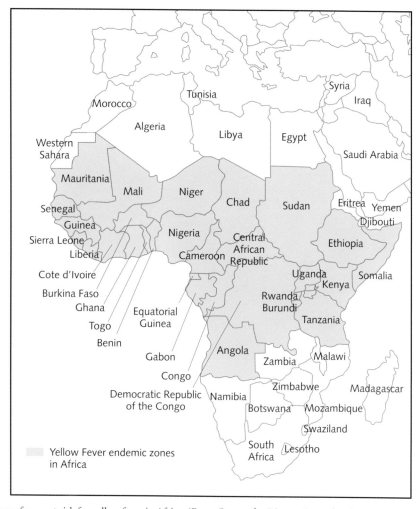

**Figure 10.1** Areas of current risk for yellow fever in Africa. (From Centers for Disease Control and Prevention.)

onset of the illness, and elevation of serum transaminase levels on days 2–3 of the illness, before the onset of jaundice, are noted. Viremia peaks 2–3 days after infection, and continues for 3–5 days; fatal cases have a longer duration of viremia than survivors.

The second phase is characterized by improvement in symptoms and reduction of fever; this may last up to 48 hours, but is not noted in all cases. Some infected individuals recover in this phase without developing jaundice. The third phase, characterized by return of fever, nausea, vomiting, jaundice, and bleeding diathesis, occurs in about 15% of cases. Multi-organ-system involvement is typical. Serum transaminase levels are proportional to

disease severity; they peak early in the second week of illness in patients who recover. Antibodies appear in the blood by 6–7 days after the onset of symptoms and are associated with elimination of the virus.

The highest morbidity and mortality with the YF virus in endemic areas have been reported in infants and persons over 50 years. Genetic factors may also play a role in susceptibility and immune response to YF virus and are the subject of current investigation. Findings that a single nucleotide polymorphism in genes for $2'$–$5'$-oligoadenylate synthetase was associated with susceptibility to severe disease with another flavivirus, West Nile virus, and that a deficiency of CCR5, a monocyte

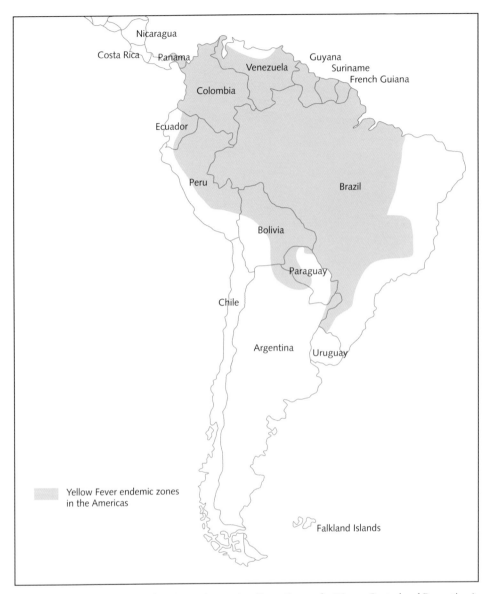

**Figure 10.2** Areas of current risk for yellow fever in South America. (From Centers for Disease Control and Prevention.)

and T lymphocyte chemokine receptor, increased risk of symptomatic West Nile virus infection, support this hypothesis [14, 15].

## Diagnosis

Mild forms of YF are difficult to distinguish from other undifferentiated febrile illnesses in returning travelers. YF should be suspected, however, when an unimmunized traveler who visited a YF endemic area presents with fever and jaundice. Diagnosis of YF is made by detection of virus, virus antigen, or virus genome (by ELISA, PCR, or inoculation of the virus into suckling mice, mosquitoes, or cell cultures) or by serology (IgM capture ELISA), although cross reaction with other flaviviruses may complicate serologic methods of diagnosis. The virus may be detected in serum from 4 to 12 days or, perhaps, even later, after onset of illness. IgM antibodies appear in the first week of illness, peak in the second week, and decline over the next 1–2 months. Neutralizing antibodies persist for many years after YF infection. Testing for YF virus or antibody usually is done in specialized laboratories; in the United States it is done at the Centers for Disease Control and Prevention (CDC) laboratory in Fort Collins, Colorado.

Midzonal necrosis of the liver on post-mortem examination is a pathognomonic feature of YF, and a definitive diagnosis can be made by immunohistochemical staining of tissues (liver, heart, kidneys) for YF antigen. Liver biopsy should never be used for diagnosis during acute YF because of the risk of fatal hemorrhage at the biopsy site [1].

## Treatment

There is no specific therapy for yellow fever; the goal of treatment is to support the patient through the critical part of the illness. Information about potential treatment modalities is available from studies in humans, from animal models, and from retrospective epidemiologic studies of YF vaccine (YFV) adverse events [10]. Rhesus monkeys were protected from YF virus challenge when given YF antiserum; administration of immune serum after onset of clinical disease had no beneficial effect [1]. Treatment with immune globulin in cases of vaccine-induced viscerotropic disease (a rare and severe side effect, described below) has not been promising, but use of the product very early in the clinical illness, when affecting the level of viremia remains possible, has not been studied. Use of interferons for prevention and treatment of YF is limited by the need to use these products before infection or during the incubation period in order to have therapeutic benefit; therefore, there is no practical use for these products at this time [1]. Ribavirin is active against YF in vitro, but high doses are required to achieve a beneficial effect. Ribavirin was ineffective in monkey and mouse models, but did show reduced mortality in a hamster model.

## Prevention of yellow fever

Vector control strategies, initially highly successful in many parts of the world, have foundered in recent decades because of lack of coordinated political will, the shifting balance of human populations and development of rural areas, and global warming, all of which have contributed to reducing barriers to the spread of the mosquito vectors.

## Yellow fever vaccine

### History

Vaccines for YF have been in existence for over 70 years. YF virus was first isolated in 1927 in Dakar, Senegal (French strain) and Lagos, Nigeria (Asibi strain). Development of YFV began soon thereafter in England, the United States, West Africa, and Brazil. After unsuccessful efforts to produce inactivated vaccines early in the twentieth century, subsequent work on vaccine development focused on live virus products. French neurotropic vaccine was used beginning in the 1930s and proved effective, especially in curtailing epidemic disease in West Africa. Use of this vaccine, however, was discontinued in 1982 because of an unacceptably high incidence of adverse events, especially encephalitis.

All current vaccines are derived from the 17D yellow fever virus strain. Two main lineages of the 17D line, 17D-204 and 17DD, were used in the initial phase of YF vaccine production in the USA and Brazil between 1937 and 1941 [1]. The "seed-lot" system of vaccine production was adopted following recognition that continued serial passage could result in substrains with unacceptably high rates of adverse events. Primary and secondary seed lots were prepared and characterized, and all vaccine lots were prepared from a single passage from the secondary seed. *Requirements for Yellow Fever Vaccine*, published by the World Health Organization in 1957, specifies standards for the seed lot and manufacturing process. New seed lots are tested for neurovirulence and viscerotropism before being used for vaccine production. The vaccine contains no antibiotics or preservatives such as thimerosal, but some preparations do contain gelatin, and latex is present in the stopper of the vaccine vial [1].

### Vaccine response

Vaccination against YF produces high levels of protection. Neutralizing antibody develops in >90% of children and adults and the duration of immunity has been described as "almost life-long" [1, 16, 17]. International health regulations recommend revaccination at 10-year intervals for those remaining at risk and the vaccination certificate remains valid for 10 years. Serologic response to YF vaccine is not diminished by co-administration of multiple other vaccines, including other live and inactivated vaccines [1]. Prior infection with Japanese encephalitis (JE) does not interfere with response to YF vaccine; there are no data on response to YF vaccine when it is administered with JE vaccine [18]. Immune globulin did not decrease the antibody response to YF vaccine when given 0–7 days before immunization. Chloroquine does not have an adverse effect on the antibody response to YF vaccine.

Low levels of viremia occur after immunization with 17D YF vaccine, beginning about 3–7 days after immunization and lasting for 1–3 days in first-time vaccinees. Increased levels of interferon alpha, tumor necrosis factor alpha, and markers of T cell activation occur at this time and are likely to have a role in some of the common mild side effects of YF vaccine [19, 20]. The balance of activation events and modulatory pathways involving lymphocyte subpopulations following 17DD YF vaccine administration may also be important in the development of an adequate immune response and the prevention of adverse reactions [21, 22]. Resolution of viremia occurs as neutralizing antibody develops about 8–9 days after first-time immunization. Viremia does not occur with subsequent doses of vaccine, and side effects are milder. No data are available about levels or duration of viremia in children or immunosuppressed individuals [1].

### Common vaccine side effects

Side effects are generally mild, and include headaches, myalgia, and low-grade fever occurring 5–10 days after immunization in < 25% of those participating in clinical trials of YF vaccine.

### Hypersensitivity reactions

Systemic allergic reactions, such as anaphylaxis and urticaria, have been reported in 1 in 58,000–131,000 individuals after YF vaccination. Sensitivity to vaccine components, especially gelatin, but also potentially latex found in the stopper of the vaccine vial, may play a role in these events. YF vaccine is prepared in embryonated eggs; individuals with egg allergies should not receive vaccine, but individuals able to eat eggs or egg products may receive vaccine.

### Yellow fever vaccine-associated neurotropic disease

YF vaccine-associated neurologic disease (YEL-AND), specifically encephalitis, was historically the most common severe adverse reaction, especially in infants. This was noted especially with the French neurotropic vaccine used from the 1930s until its use was discontinued in 1982, largely as a result of these neurologic complications. Age restrictions placed on the use of YF vaccine in infants further decreased this complication [1, 23]. Twenty-nine cases of YEL-AND were reported worldwide between 1991 and 2006, including a fatal case of encephalitis in a man from Thailand with unrecognized HIV infection [24, 25].

U.S. Vaccine Adverse Events Reporting System (VAERS) data were used to estimate rates of YEL-AND at 0.4 per 100,000 doses distributed, with higher rates in individuals over 60 years of age [26, 27]. Rates as high as 0.5 to 4 per 1000 have been estimated in very young infants [1]. The Vaccine Information Statement (VIS) for YF vaccine, prepared by the CDC, states that there is an incidence of 1:150,000–250,000 distributed doses (Available from: URL: http://www.cdc.gov/nip/publications/VIS/vis-yf .pdf).

Onset of YEL-AND has occurred from 4–23 days after immunization, and the signs and symptoms include fever, headache, and focal or generalized neurologic dysfunction. Laboratory findings include cerebrospinal fluid (CSF) pleocytosis (100–500 WBCs per $\mu$L) and elevated protein, indicating inflammation of the central nervous system. Liver function tests are usually normal. Laboratory diagnosis of YEL-AND is made by finding virus, viral genome, or YF-specific IgM in cerebrospinal fluid. The case fatality rate is <5%, and most affected individuals recover without sequelae. Acute disseminated encephalomyelitis (ADEM) and Guillain–Barré syndrome have been reported after YF immunization, and 12 cases of aseptic meningitis were reported in association with the 2001 YF mass immunization campaign in Juiz de Fora, Brazil [24, 28].

### Yellow fever vaccine-associated viscerotropic disease

YF vaccine-associated viscerotropic disease (YEL-AVD) was recognized first in 1996 when a syndrome of fever, jaundice, and multiple organ system failure following YF vaccination was reported. Over the next decade, 36 cases were reported worldwide [26]. This syndrome may have been occurring unnoticed for many years; recently, a 1975 case in Brazil initially thought to be a wild-type strain infection was characterized as a vaccine-derived case [29].

YEL-AVD, initially called febrile multiple organ system failure, ranges in severity from moderate disease with focal organ dysfunction to severe multisystem failure and death, and may include neurotropic disease. Symptoms begin 2–5 days after immunization and include fever, elevated hepatocellular enzymes, respiratory failure, blood dyscrasias, and, in some cases, renal failure. The syndrome resembles severe wild-type yellow fever and laboratory evidence indicates overwhelming infection with vaccine strain yellow fever virus. The case-fatality rate among US cases was 58% [26]. It has occurred only in first-time nonimmune vaccine recipients.

Advanced age is a risk factor for adverse events associated with YF immunization. The US CDC Vaccine Information Statement (VIS) gives the incidence as 1:200,000–300,000 doses for all first-time vaccine recipients, and 1:40,000–50,000 doses for those 60 years of age or older [30]. Two subsequent studies of age-related risk of adverse events report similar increased risk; one of these documented a reporting rate ratio of 5.9 (95% CI 1.6–22.2) for severe adverse events in first-time vaccinees aged ≥ 60 years [27, 31].

Disease of the thymus gland has been identified as another risk factor for severe adverse reactions to YFV. Fifteen percent of 26 individuals with YEL-AVD described in a 2004 paper had a history of thymus disease, including thymoma and myasthenia gravis [32]. The CDC's Health Information for International Travel lists thymus disease as a contraindication to YFV [26].

Widespread inflammatory response and exuberant viral replication are the hallmarks of YEL-AVD. Antibody levels are significantly higher than would be expected after YF vaccination. Examination of tissues from fatal cases of YEL-AVD reveals widespread dissemination of YFV strain virus and active viral replication in multiple organs [1]. Mutations in vaccine virus have not been identified by sequencing studies that could explain these adverse events [33]. It is believed that most likely, host genetic factors, as yet poorly understood, are responsible for susceptibility to severe adverse reactions to YF vaccine. The occurrence of two cases in one family in Brazil (one confirmed) supports this hypothesis [1].

## Treatment of YEL-AND and YEL-AVD

There is no standardized treatment for adverse reactions to YFV. A retrospective study of corticosteroid therapy in 11 cases of YEL-AVD identified a higher rate of survival in patients receiving stress dose steroids (200–300 mg/day) (75%; 3 of 4) than for those who received no steroids, or high (>300 mg/day) or low (<200 mg/day) dose steroids (29%; 2 of 7) [34]. Supportive care remains the mainstay of treatment, and patients should be managed in settings in which intensive care is available.

## Indications, precautions, and contraindications for yellow fever immunization

YFV, administered at least 10 days before departure, is indicated for travelers to countries or regions where there is increased risk of YF, unless there are specific contraindi-

cations. YFV must be given at official yellow fever vaccine centers in some countries, and should be documented in an International Certificate of Vaccination, valid from 10 days through 10 years after the date of immunization. Vaccine is contraindicated absolutely in children <6 months of age, and should be given to infants 6–9 months of age only if risk of disease is significant and other methods of prevention cannot be employed. The single most important step in judicious use of YFV is to immunize only travelers to YF-endemic areas: two of five individuals with multiorgan system failure in one report were traveling to areas where YF had never been described [35]. Travelers should also use personal protective measures to prevent mosquito bites, such as mosquito repellant and protective clothing.

Thymus disease is a contraindication to YFV [26]. Immunocompromised individuals also should not be immunized. Asymptomatic HIV-infected individuals with CD4 counts >200/mm$^3$ who face increased risk of YF infection and cannot avoid potential exposure should be offered the choice of immunization [26]. Such individuals, however, may have impaired response to the vaccine, and if they remain at risk for yellow fever, testing for neutralizing antibody may be advisable. Individuals immunized for the first time after age 60 are at increased risk for adverse events. Relatives of those who have experienced a severe adverse response to YFV may also be at increased risk. Use of YFV in such individuals requires careful review of risk during the travel itinerary and elucidation of information about the likelihood of severe adverse events.

The safety of YF immunization during pregnancy has not been established, as the potential for vaccine-associated virus strains to infect the fetus is incompletely understood [36]. Fetal infection was documented in 1 of 41 infants exposed to maternal vaccination and increased risk of spontaneous abortion found in a Brazilian study of 39 pregnant women immunized with YFV compared with 74 control patients [37]. Inadvertent immunization of 480 pregnant women with 17DD vaccine occurred in Brazil in early 2000 during a mass vaccination campaign. Rates of maternal seroconversion were high, and no infants were found to be infected at birth (no IgM antibodies were detected and no placental or umbilical cord blood was found to contain YFV strain virus by PCR) [38]. Apart from the potential effect on the fetus, immunization during pregnancy may result in antibody concentrations inferior to those obtained following immunization of nonpregnant women [39]. Therefore, YF immunization should be avoided during pregnancy except when there is a clear and unavoidable increased risk of infection. Inadvertent administration of vaccine during pregnancy is not an indication for termination of pregnancy.

There are no reports of transmission of YFV virus from nursing mothers to their infants, and it is not known whether YFV virus is excreted into breast milk. Nursing mothers who travel to YF endemic areas and whose risk of YF infection exceeds the theoretical risk of transmission of vaccine virus to their infants may be immunized [26].

## References

1  Monath TP, Cetron MS, Teuwen DE. Yellow fever vaccine. In: Plotkin S, Orenstein W, Offit P, editors. *Vaccines*. UK: Elsevier; 2008. p. 959–1055.

2  Monath TP. Yellow fever: Victor, Victoria? conqueror, conquest? epidemics and research in the last forty years and prospects for the future. *Am J Trop Med Hyg* 1991;45:1–43.

3  Robertson SE, Hull BP, Tomori O, et al. Yellow fever: a decade of reemergence. *JAMA* 1996;276:1157–62.

4  Sanders EJ, Marfin AA, Tukei PM, et al. First recorded outbreak of yellow fever in Kenya, 1992–1993. I. Epidemiologic investigations. *Am J Trop Med Hyg* 1998;59:644–9.

5  Centers for Disease Control [Online]. Available from URL: http://wwwn.cdc.gov/travel/contentYellowFeverBrazil.aspx (accessed 2009, Jan 21).

6  Centers for Disease Control [Online]. Available from URL: http://wwwn.cdc.gov/travel/contentUpdatedYFMapArgentina.aspx (accessed 2009, Jan 21).

7  Monath TP, Cetron MS. Prevention of yellow fever in persons traveling to the tropics. *Clin Infect Dis* 2002;34:1369–78.

8  Wilson ME, Chen LH, Barnett ED. Yellow fever immunizations: indications and risks. *Curr Infect Dis Rep* 2004;6:34–42.

9  Tuboi SH, Costa ZG, Vasconcelos PFC, Hatch D. Clinical and epidemiological characteristics of yellow fever in Brazil: analysis of reported cases 1998–2002. *Trans R Soc Trop Med Hyg* 2007;101:169–75.

10  Barnett ED. Yellow fever: epidemiology and prevention. *Clin Infect Dis* 2007;44:850–56.

11  Hahn CH, Dalrymple JM, Strauss JH, et al. Comparison of the virulent Asibi strain of yellow fever virus with the 17D vaccine strain derived from it. *Proc Natl Acad Sci USA* 1987;84:2019.

12  Wang E, Ryman KD, Jennings AD, et al. Comparison of the genomes of the wild-type French viscerotropic strain of yellow fever virus with its vaccine derivative French neurotropic vaccine. *J Gen Virol* 1995;76:2749–55.

13  Monath TP, Barrett AD. Pathogenesis and pathophysiology of yellow fever. *Adv Virus Res* 2003;60:343–95.

14  Yakub I, Lillibridge KM, Moran A, et al. Single nucleotide polymorphisms in genes for 2'-5'-oligoadenylate synthetase and RNase L in patients hospitalized with West Nile virus infection. *J Infect Dis* 2005;192:1741–8.

15  Glass WG, McDermott DH, Lim JK, et al. CCR5 deficiency increases risk of symptomatic West Nile virus infection. *J Exp Med* 2006;203:35–40.

16  Rozenzweig EC, Babione RW, Wisseman CJ Jr. Immunological studies with group B arthropod-borne viruses. IV. Persistence of yellow fever antibodies following vaccination with 17D strain yellow fever vaccine. *Am J Trop Med Hyg* 1963;12:230–35.

17  Poland JD, Calisher CH, Monath, TP, Downs WG, Murphy K. Persistence of neutralizing antibody to yellow fever virus 30–35 years following immunization with 17D yellow fever vaccine: a study of World War II veterans in 1975–1976. *Bull World Health Organ* 1981;59:895–900.

18  Sweet BH, Wisseman CJ Jr, Kitaoka M. Immunological studies with group B arthropod-borne viruses. II. Effect of prior infection with Japanese encephalitis virus on the viremia in human subjects following administration of 17D yellow fever vaccine. *Am J Trop Med Hyg* 1962;11:652.

19  Hacker UT, Jelinek T, Erhardt S, et al. In vivo synthesis of tumor necrosis factor-alpha in healthy humans after live yellow fever vaccination. *J Infect Dis* 1998;177:774–8.

20  Reinhardt B, Jaspert R, Niedrig M, et al. Development of viremia and humoral and cellular parameters of immune activation after vaccination with yellow fever virus strain 17D: a model of human flavivirus infection. *J Med Virol* 1998;56:159–67.

21  Martins MA, Silva ML, Marciano AP, et al. Activation/modulation of adaptive immunity emerges simultaneously after 17DD yellow fever first-time vaccination: is this the key to prevent severe adverse reactions following immunization? *Clin Exp Immunol* 2007;148:90–100.

22  Martins MA, Silva ML, Eloi-Santos SM, et al. Innate immunity phenotypic features point toward simultaneous rise of activation and modulation events following 17DD live attenuated yellow fever first-time vaccination. *Vaccine* 2008;26:1173–84.

23  Centers for Disease Control and Prevention. Yellow fever vaccine; recommendations of the Advisory Committee on Immunization Practices (ACIP). *MMWR Morb Mortal Wkly Rep* 2002;51(No. RR–17):4–6.

24  McMahon AW, Eidex RB, Marfin AA, et al. Neurologic disease associated with 17D-204 yellow fever vaccination: a report of 15 cases. *Vaccine* 2007;25:1727–34.

25  Kengsakul K, Sathirapongsasuti K, Punyagupta S. Fatal myeloencephalitis following yellow fever vaccination in a case with HIV infection. *J Med Assoc Thai* 2002;85:131–4.

26  Eidex RB, Hayes EB, Russell M. Yellow Fever. In: Centers for Disease Control and Prevention. *Health Information for International Travel 2008*. Atlanta, GA: US Department of Health and Human Services, Public Health Service; 2007. p. 362–79. Available from URL: http://www.cdc.gov/travel/yellowBookCh4-YellowFever.aspx.

27  Khromava AY, Eidex RB, Weld LH, et al. Yellow fever vaccine: an updated assessment of advanced age as a risk

factor for serious adverse events. *Vaccine* 2005;23:3256–63.

28 Fernandes GC, Camacho LAB, Carvalho MS, Batista M, de Almeida SMR. Neurological adverse events temporally associated to mass vaccination against yellow fever in Juiz de Fora, Brazil, 1999–2005. *Vaccine* 2007;25:3124–8.

29 Engel AR, Vasconcelos PFC, McArthur MA, Barrett ADT. Characterization of a viscerotropic yellow fever vaccine variant from a patient in Brazil. *Vaccine* 2006;24:2803–9.

30 Martin M, Weld LH, Tsai TF, et al. Advanced age a risk factor for illness temporally associated with yellow fever vaccination. *Emerg Infect Dis* 2001;7:945–51.

31 Monath TP, Cetron MS, McCarthy K, et al. Yellow fever 17D vaccine safety and immunogenicity in the elderly. *Hum Vaccin* 2005;1(5):e1–e8. Available from URL: http://www.landesbioscience.com.

32 Barwick RE. History of thymoma and yellow fever vaccination. *Lancet* 2004;364:936.

33 Barban V, Girerd Y, Aguirre M, et al. High stability of yellow fever 17D-204 vaccine: a 12-year retrospective analysis of large-scale production. *Vaccine* 2007;25:2941–50.

34 Vellozzi C, Mitchell T, Miller E, et al. Yellow fever vaccine-associated viscerotropic disease (YEL-AVD) and corticosteroid therapy: eleven United States cases, 1996–2004. *Am J Trop Med Hyg* 2006;75:333–6.

35 Centers for Disease Control and Prevention. Fever, jaundice, and multiple organ system failure associated with 17D-derived yellow fever vaccination, 1996–2001. *MMWR Morb Mortal Wkly Rep* 2001;50:643–5.

36 Tsai T. Congenital arboviral infections: something new, something old. *Pediatrics* 2006;117:936–9.

37 Nishioka Sde A, Nunes-Araujo FR, Pires WP, Silva FA, Costa HL. Yellow fever vaccination during pregnancy and spontaneous abortion: a case-control study. *Trop Med Int Health* 1998;3:29–33.

38 Suzano CE, Amaral E, Sato HK, Papaiordanou PM. The effects of yellow fever immunization (17DD) inadvertently used in early pregnancy during a mass campaign in Brazil. *Vaccine* 2006;24:1421–6.

39 Nasidi A, Monath TP, Vandenberg J, et al. Yellow fever vaccination and pregnancy: a four-year prospective study. *Trans R Soc Trop Med Hyg* 1993;87(3):337–9.

# 11

# Chikungunya: An Emerging Disease in Travelers

Fabrice Simon,[1] Elodie Vivier,[2] and Philippe Parola[3]

[1] Hôpital d'Instruction des Armées, Laveran and Institut de Médecine Tropicale du Service de Santé des Armées, Le Pharo, Marseille, France

[2] Hôpital d'Instruction des Armées Laveran, Marseille, France

[3] Institut de Médecine Tropicale du Service de Santé des Armées, Le Pharo, Université de la Mediterranée and Hôpital Nord, AP-HM, Marseille, France

## Introduction

Chikungunya virus (CHIKV) is an arthropod-borne virus (genus *Alphavirus*, family Togaviridae). The name "chikungunya" means "that which contorts or bends up" in Kimakonde, an East African dialect. It refers to the posture of infected people suffering from disabling polyarthritis. After a short incubation, patients undergo an acute stage with a brutal, febrile, and sometimes eruptive polyarthritis, which is commonly followed by long-lasting rheumatism. This arbovirus, responsible primarily for clustered cases or local outbreaks in rural Africa or Asian towns, had been neglected for many years. Before 2000, only a few benign imported infections were reported in North American and European travelers [1]. CHIKV came to attention in 2005–2006 after five decades of obscurity, with a large-scale outbreak that swept through East Africa, the western Indian Ocean islands, India, and the eastern Indian Ocean Islands [2]. For the first time, CHIKV struck a country with a Western health care system, Reunion Island (a French overseas territory), with unexpected morbidity and mortality. This outbreak and those that followed appeared to be associated with recent changes in the CHIKV genome and its new epidemiological profile, which provided new insights into clinical features and pathophysiology [2]. An exponential increase of reports of CHIKV-infected travelers paralleled these outbreaks. This allowed an improved description of signs and symptoms, in both acute and chronic stages. Some CHIKV-infected travelers were highly viremic soon after

returning to their native countries, where competent vectors are present, raising serious concerns for the spread of disease [3]. This threat turned into reality when a local outbreak occurred in Italy during the summer of 2007. Two hundred individuals were infected after a presumed single index patient returned from an epidemic area in India [4]. Thus, all physicians should be prepared to identify, confirm, and manage CHIKV infection in travelers, with the goal of helping the individual patient as well as protecting the local population from the spread of infection.

## General epidemiology

Like other alphaviruses, CHIKV is a linear single-stranded RNA molecule with a positive polarity. This virus was first isolated in Tanzania in 1952–1953 [5]. From the 1960s to the end of the twentieth century, CHIKV was isolated repeatedly in numerous focal outbreaks and clusters (usually after an unpredictable period of CHIV absence) in numerous countries in Central, South, and West Africa, as well as in Asia [5] (Figure 11.1).

Only two epidemiological profiles of CHIKV infection were known until recently (Table 11.1). In Africa, CHIKV was known to be maintained in a sylvatic cycle, involving wild primates, rodents, and forest-dwelling *Aedes* spp. mosquitoes [5, 6]. On the other hand, in Asian countries, CHIKV was known to be transmitted by the urban mosquito *A. aegypti* (the urban, peridomestic, anthropophilic vector of dengue), with an epidemiologic cycle resembling that of dengue. Other abundant peridomestic species, including *A. albopictus*, which colonize both artificial and natural containers in suburban and rural

*Tropical Diseases in Travelers*, 1st edition. Edited by E. Schwartz.
© 2009 by Blackwell Publishing, ISBN: 978-1-4051-8441-0.

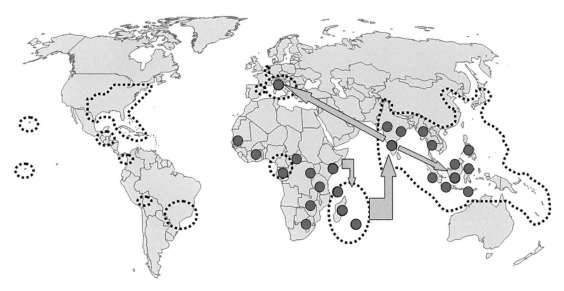

**Figure 11.1** Estimated global distribution of *A. albopictus* (areas enclosed in dotted lines) and distribution of chikungunya virus (●), including the Indian Ocean variants responsible for the 2006 outbreak. Arrows indicate the spread of the recent large-scale outbreak. (Adapted from [3].)

areas, were also suspected to supplement *A. aegypti* in the transmission of CHIKV [5, 6]. At the end of the century, an urban emergence was documented in the Democratic Republic of the Congo, where thousands of persons were infected, after 39 years without any isolation of CHIKV. In 2001–2003, in Indonesia, epidemic re-emergence was also documented after a nearly 20-year absence [1].

In 2004, an ongoing large-scale CHIKV outbreak started in Kenya. It then spread to the Indian Ocean islands, including the Comoros Islands, Reunion and Mayotte (two French territories), Mauritius, the Sey-

chelles, and Madagascar [1, 2] (Figure 11.1). After a period of lower transmission during the Southern Hemisphere winter, a second wave occurred. Reunion Island suffered an explosive outbreak. By the end of September 2006, an estimate of 266,000 residents (out of a population of 770,000) were reportedly infected with CHIKV. This was the first CHIKV epidemic in a country with a Western health care infrastructure [7]. In 2006–2007, CHIKV moved to and spread within India, with several million cases being reported continuously until December 2007 [8]. Continued spread was reported in Sri Lanka,

**Table 11.1** Main epidemiological profiles of chikungunya infection in the world.

|  | Historical African profile | Historical Asian profile | Current global profile (A226-CHIKV) |
|---|---|---|---|
| Epidemic profile | Endemo-epidemic, focal outbreaks, clusters | Focal outbreaks | Explosive outbreaks |
| Localization | Rural (forests) | Urban/suburban | Urban |
| Reservoirs | Wild animals: primates, rodents, birds, forest-dwelling mosquitoes | Humans | Humans |
| Main vectors | Forest dwelling *Aedes* spp., particularly *A. furcifer/taylori* group | *A. aegypti*, possibly supplemented by *A. albopictus* | *A. albopictus* |

Indonesia, and Malaysia [1, 2]. Finally, in 2007, the virus was transmitted within Europe [4].

The CHIKV strains responsible for this massive outbreak are related to Central/East African CHIKV isolates, from which new variants may have evolved [3, 9]. On reaching Reunion and Mauritius, CHIKV encountered a different ecological environment, characterized by the absence or scarcity of *A. aegypti* (present in Kenya, the Comoros, and the Seychelles) and the proliferation of *A. albopictus* around human habitations. Within 1 year, a new mutation (A226V) appeared in CHIKV strains in Reunion and was subsequently found elsewhere [10]. This mutation is associated with improved adaptation of CHIKV to *A. albopictus*, which was previously considered as a secondary vector [11].

A new epidemiological profile of chikungunya fever was born, one of global dissemination (Table 11.1). Indeed, the so-called Asian tiger mosquito, *A. albopictus*, has spread to tropical areas previously occupied predominantly by *A. aegypti* and is now present in the western Pacific, Southeast Asia, and Indian Ocean islands. It reached the United States, Brazil, and Central America in the 1980s and Africa in 1992 (Figure 11.1). The species has been established in several European countries, particularly in Italy, where it is active from February through December, peaking in August and September [12] (Figure 11.1). When introduced, for example as drought-resistant eggs surviving in miscellaneous containers (such as used tires) after long trips around the world, the mosquito has the potential of proliferating in any country, even temperate ones if environmental conditions are favorable (mean winter temperature higher than $0°C$, annual rainfall at least 500 mm, sufficient rainfall during the warm season, and summer temperature around $25–30°C$) [13].

## Epidemiology in travelers

Because of the increasing numbers of international flights and the recent genomic and ecological changes in CHIKV infection, CHIKV has become an emerging vector-borne disease among travelers. Travelers have been of concern since the beginning of the recent large-scale outbreak, because the Indian Ocean islands are popular tourist destinations. According to the World Organization of Tourism, 719,000 tourists arrived in Mauritius, 430,000 in Reunion Island, 229,000 in Madagascar, and 121,000 in the Seychelles in 2004 [14]. Since 2006, CHIKV infection has been identified in an unprecedented number of travelers (more

than 1000) after they returned home from the epidemic areas to European countries, the USA, Australia, and Asia [1]. Many industrialized countries experienced this situation, as imported cases in returned travelers paralleled the spread of the explosive outbreaks [14, 15].

High CHIKV viremia was identified in some of the recently infected travelers, raising concern about the potential globalization of the disease [3, 15]. Travelers and migrants visiting friends and relatives in their countries of origin were seen as sentinels and potential transmitters of infectious diseases [15]. This situation is of major concern because viremic travelers may be bitten in their own countries by local *A. albopictus*, which have been demonstrated to be vectors competent to initiate local outbreaks [12, 17]. This happened in the local outbreak in Italy in 2007 that developed from a recently CHIKV-infected traveler returning from an epidemic area of India [4]. Occupational contamination after needlestick has also been evidenced in a nurse who performed a blood puncture on a symptomatic CHIKV-infected traveler [3].

## Clinical aspects

Most CHIKV-infected adults are symptomatic. Clinical features during the two stages of the disease, specifically in infected travelers, have been described after the recent outbreaks [14, 18].

### Typical acute stage

After an incubation period of 2–6 days, the acute stage starts brutally with high fever, disabling polyarthritis, and skin manifestations (Figure 11.2). These signs can be synchronous or not, and commonly last 5–10 days. A number of general manifestations can occur, such as asthenia, headache, and diffuse myalgia. The clinical burden of this stage is due to constant rheumatic symptoms, that is, disabling polyarthritis with arthritis and/or inflammatory arthralgia involving numerous joint groups. This acute rheumatism is mostly peripheral, bilateral, symmetrical, and cumulative. Hands, wrists, feet, and ankles are characteristically involved, but the disease can reach any other joint and the spine as well. Other features that have recently been identified are periarticular edema, asymmetry of the polyarthritis, atypical arthritis (Baker's cyst), and acute tenosynovitis (intense pain provoked by pressure on the anterior part of the wrists) [3, 14, 19]. Polymorphism of acute skin manifestations was demonstrated in Reunion Island, with manifestations including

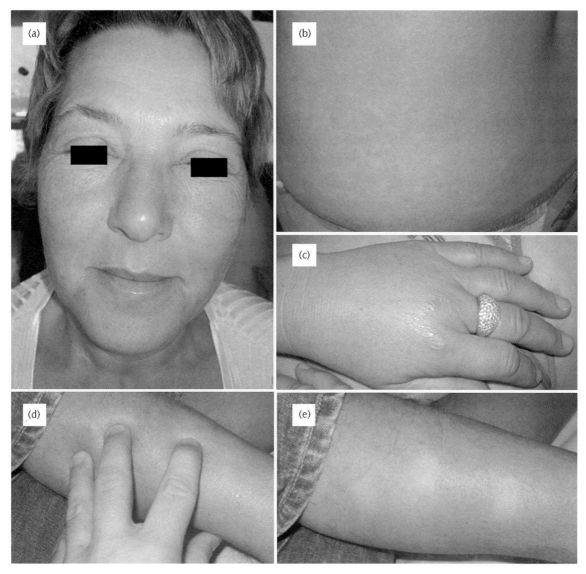

**Figure 11.2** Skin manifestations in patients with CHIKV infection returning from Reunion Island to Marseille in 2006, including a 45-year-old woman with a rash of the face (a) and abdomen (b) and edema of the face (a) and hand (c), and a 36-year-old man with a rash on the right arm that blanches with pressure (d, e). (From [14] with permission.)

maculopapular rash, petechiae, vesicles, epidermolysis bullosa, edema, diffuse hyperemia (face and extremities), and mucosal bleeding. Nonspecific gastrointestinal signs are quite common [20, 21] and neurological signs have been reported, with delirium in older patients [21]. Acute signs improve spontaneously after 7–10 days, but a large proportion of infected patients continue to suffer from joint pain after that initial period.

## Severe to lethal acute forms

Recent outbreaks in developed countries brought attention to forgotten or unexpected complications of the disease. The direct role of CHIKV in severe complications seems to be limited to rare but early acute central neurological (encephalitis/polyradiculonevritis/flaccid paralysis) or cardiac events [22]. In fact, most patients with severe or deadly forms (respiratory failure, cardiovascular

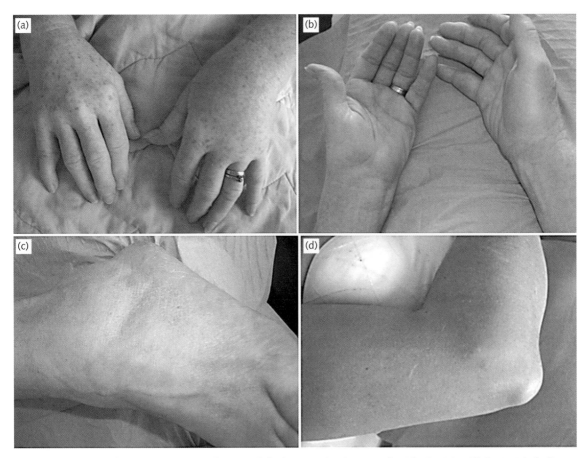

**Figure 11.3** Joint manifestations in patients with CHIKV infection returning from Reunion Island to Marseille in 2006, including bilateral tenosynovitis of extensors of wrists and fingers (a) and of wrist flexors (b), tenosynovitis of peroneus longus and brevis muscles (c), and elbow hygroma (d).

decompensation, hepatitis, kidney failure, pancytopenia, or septicemia) also had underlying diseases that worsened [21] and/or iatrogenic complications. CHIKV infection also increases the risk of spontaneous abortion during the first trimester of pregnancy and of vertical transmission during the third trimester, as intrapartum maternal viremia can lead to severe neonatal infection associated with fever, poor feeding, pain, distal edema, and skin manifestations [23].

## Chronic stage

The chronic stage can include transient exacerbation within the first 3 months, long-lasting rheumatism and unexpected relapses. Early tenosynovitis is common on wrists and finger extensors and is sometimes responsible for distal dysesthesia when hypertrophic (carpal and/or

cubital tunnel syndromes). Transitory peripheral vascular disorders such as Raynaud's phenomenon or erythermalgia (red, hot, and painful extremities) have been reported during the second and third months after disease onset. Rheumatic disorders can begin during the first weeks after the acute stage and are dominated by persistent pain, inflammatory or sometimes mechanical, commonly involving previously injured joints and bones. Joint stiffness and morning pain usually improve partially with movement. Consequently, infected people often suffer from an important loss of quality of life, sometimes with depressive syndromes and/or suicide attempts (F. Simon, unpublished data). In early descriptions of CHIKV infection, pain and/or stiffness were more severe and more prolonged in older patients and patients with previous rheumatism. This was confirmed by the Reunion

**Table 11.2**  Epidemiological and clinical differences between chikungunya-infected natives and travelers.

|  | Native population [21] | Travelers [14] |
|---|---|---|
| **Recruitment of patients** | 157 cases in acute stage in Reunion Island | 47 cases imported from western Indian Ocean to mainland France |
| **Epidemiological data** | | |
| Mean/median age (years) | 57.9 | 45 (0.5–73) |
| Sex ratio M/F | 1.2 | 0.88 |
| Underlying disease | 71% | 64% |
| **Symptoms and signs** | | |
| Fever (duration) | 95.9% | 96% (3.7 days) |
| Headache | 47.1 | NR |
| Nausea, vomiting | ND | NR |
| Skin manifestations | 40.1% | 51% |
| Pruritis | 54% | 19% |
| Mucous bleeding | 2% | 4% |
| Arthralgia/arthritis | 96.1% | 100% |
| Symmetry of arthralgia | 73.2% | 64% |
| Periarticular edema | 31.8% | 41% |
| Spinal involvment | 34.4% | 47% |
| Peripheral lymphadenopathy | 8.9% | NR |
| Persistent arthralgia | NR | 48% after 6 months |
| Complications | Neurologic involvement: 12%; hematemesis/hemoptysia: 2% 3%, (mean age: 79.4 years) | 4% (acute myocarditis: 1, pancytopenia: 1) |
| Mortality | | 0 |

experience, where more than a half of CHIKV-infected patients reported persistent joint pain and/or stiffness after one year [24].

## Differences between travelers and natives

Clinical manifestations in travelers are quite different from those in autochthonous people in developing or developed countries (Table 11.2). Indeed, travelers are classically young and healthy, although there has been an obvious recent increase in the number of travelers with underlying diseases traveling throughout the world, including tropical countries. Data from the Indian Ocean outbreaks demonstrate that underlying disease and advanced age are the most important negative prognostic factors [21, 22]. Nevertheless, in the Reunion Island outbreak, most CHIK-related deaths were observed in patients more than 80 years of age. As far as we know, no death has been reported among the thousands of CHIKV-infected travelers, but acute complications such as myocarditis or pancytopenia have been reported in French travelers [14].

## Diagnosis

CHIKV infection must be considered in two situations when encountering a traveler after a stay in a possibly endemic or epidemic area (Figure 11.1): first, febrile polyarthritis, with or without rash, within 10 days after return, and second, persisting travel-acquired rheumatism. The choice of diagnostic tools is based on the time interval after disease onset, as is true for other arboviral infections. In the acute stage, viremia can be detected in uncoagulated blood sampled (in an EDTA-containing tube). Viral culture performed on mosquito cells, mammalian cells, or mice is the gold standard, but its sensitivity is low after 5 days of disease and its feasibility is limited [25]. Molecular detection with RT-PCR is faster, more feasible, and more sensitive than culture and is specific as well in determining the genotype. From the fifth day, anti-CHIKV IgM antibodies may be detected by direct ELISA and a few weeks later IgG may be detected by ELISA following immunocapture [26]. This indirect diagnosis has good sensitivity but renders false negative results (F. Simon,

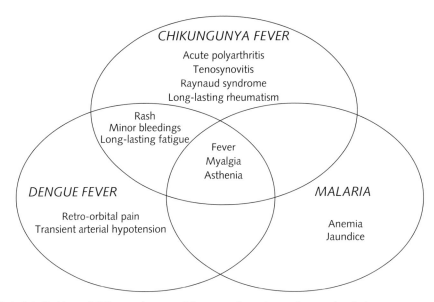

**Figure 11.4** Clinical similarities and differences between chikungunya fever, dengue fever, and malaria.

submitted for publication) and cross reactions with Ross River, O Nyong Nyong, and Mayaro may occur in non-epidemic settings [27].

The acute stage of CHIKV infection shares clinical signs and symptoms with various worldwide and tropical infections, notably malaria and dengue (Figure 11.4). Clinical analysis can identify the presence or absence of signs suggestive of chikungunya or other imported diseases. At this time, presence of painful wrist tenosynovitides is highly suggestive of CHIKV infection. However, the diagnosis of chikungunya fever should only be made after the more severe and treatable diseases, such as malaria or leptospirosis, have been ruled out. When acute or chronic

polyarthritis is the main symptom, physicians should consider other travel-acquired rheumatisms (Table 11.3). In addition to bacterial rheumatic infections, one should also think about other alphaviruses (O Nyong Nyong, Sindbis group, Ross River, Mayaro, Barmah Forest, Semliki) that induce similar polyarthritis and share antigenic similarities with CHIKV (cross-reactions). (See Chapter 40.)

## Treatment

To date, there is no specific antiviral treatment for CHIKV infection. Patients receive empirical and symptomatic

**Table 11.3** Etiologies of travel-acquired rheumatisms.

|  | Acute rheumatism | Chronic rheumatism |
| --- | --- | --- |
| Disseminated gonococcal infection | + |  |
| Reiter's syndrome<br>Sexually acquired: *Chlamydiae trachomatis*, HIV<br>Enterically acquired: *Yersinia, Shigella, Campylobacter,* etc. | + | + |
| Alphaviruses<br>Chikungunya, O Nyong Nyong, Sindbis group, Ross River, Mayaro,<br>   Barmah forest, Semliki | + | + |
| Helminth-related rheumatism<br>Taeniasis, hookworm, filariasis, strongyloidiasis, anisakiasis, etc. |  | + |

treatment such as paracetamol and nonsteroidal anti-inflammatory drugs (NSAIDs), which can induce iatrogenic complications (hepatotoxicity, digestive perforation). During the chronic stage, patients can be helped with painkillers, such as general NSAIDs and other analgesics (as strong as morphine). Local treatments such as physiotherapy are of great interest in refractory isolated arthritis. Short-term corticosteroid therapy can occasionally be used when NSAIDs are contraindicated or ineffective. Patients dramatically improve with this treatment, but relapses are not rare after steroid treatment discontinuation and multiple complications are possible after repeated use of steroids (hip necrosis, osteoporosis, etc.) [1]. Chloroquine sulfate has not demonstrated efficacy, either as a curative or as a preventive treatment [1].

## Prevention

The first approach to primary prevention consists of personal protection and antivector measures. Travelers should use personal protection to avoid mosquito bites. It should be remembered that *Aedes* spp. bite people during the daytime, which makes personal protection more difficult. Travelers should wear pretreated (permethrin, deltamethrin), clothing that covers the arms and legs, set the air conditioning to a low temperature in hotels, and apply repellent on exposed skin.

Measures to prevent breeding sites around properties are important, such as covering all water containers with lids, emptying water in old tires, and changing water daily in pets' water bowls [13].

The main public measures against vectors are educating the population, destroying water-containing receptacles, recycling tires, residual spraying, and dispersing insecticides. Internet surveillance networks give information on epidemics in real time [16]. Public health measures include mandatory reporting of CHIKV, education of general practitioners, research programs, and elimination of the nosocomial risk (altruistic use of bed netting for febrile patients, screening of blood units for transfusions).

While working on CHIKV as a potential threat, the US Army developed a live vaccine. Results from a phase II trial were consistent with safety, good tolerance, and high immunogenicity [28]. Unfortunately, funding for this project was discontinued and to date there is still no vaccine available. Since 2006 in France, research on this topic is once again becoming a priority (VacciChik project).

## Conclusions

Vector-transmitted infections are evolutionary threats in the modern world, even in temperate, industrialized countries. Travelers can be sentinels whose surveillance helps both to alert public health officials and to define clinical features of disease. (See Chapter 4.) More important, travelers are potent transporters and transmitters of the disease to naive populations in nonendemic areas, as demonstrated in the recent outbreak in Italy. The current large-scale CHIKV outbreak in the Indian Ocean, India, and eastern Asia has revealed the extraordinary adaptive capacity and clear potential for global extension of this previously neglected arbovirus. There is a new epidemiological profile of CHIK fever, that of global dissemination, in which travelers play a key role. CHIK fever should definitely be considered a threat to global public health. In addition to adequate international actions (research programs, surveillance, prompt local alerts, rapid confirmation of outbreaks), physicians in CHIKV-free areas should be prepared to suspect and confirm possible cases promptly [1].

## References

1 Simon F, Savini H, Parola P. Chikungunya: a paradigm of emergence and globalisation of vector-borne diseases. *Med Clin North Am* 2008;92:1323–43.

2 Charrel RN, de Lamballerie X, Raoult D. Chikungunya outbreaks—the globalization of vectorborne diseases. *N Engl J Med* 2007;356(8):769–71.

3 Parola P, de Lamballerie X, Jourdan J, Rovery C, Vaillant V, Minodier P, et al. Novel chikungunya virus variant in travelers returning from Indian Ocean islands. *Emerg Infect Dis* 2006;12(10):1493–9.

4 Rezza G, Nicoletti L, Angelini R, Romi R, Finarelli AC, Panning M, et al. Infection with chikungunya virus in Italy: an outbreak in a temperate region. *Lancet* 2007;370(9602):1840–46.

5 Powers AM, Logue CH. Changing patterns of chikungunya virus: re-emergence of a zoonotic arbovirus. *J Gen Virol* 2007;88(Pt 9):2363–77.

6 Chevillon C, Briant L, Renaud F, Devaux C. The Chikungunya threat: an ecological and evolutionary perspective. *Trends Microbiol* 2008;16(2):80–88.

7 Ledrans M, Quatresous I, Renault P, Pierre V. Outbreak of chikungunya in the French Territories, 2006: lessons learned. *Euro Surveill* 2007;12(9):E070906.

8 Chhabra M, Mittal V, Bhattacharya D, Rana U, Lal S. Chikungunya fever: a re-emerging viral infection. *Indian J Med Microbiol* 2008;26(1):5–12.

9 Schuffenecker I, Iteman I, Michault A, Murri S, Frangeul L, Vaney MC, et al. Genome microevolution of chikungunya viruses causing the Indian Ocean outbreak. *PLoS Med* 2006;3(7):e263.

10 De Lamballerie X, Leroy E, Charrel RN, Ttsetsarkin K, Higgs S, Gould EA. Chikungunya virus adapts to tiger mosquito via evolutionary convergence: a sign of things to come? *Virol J* 2008;5:33.

11 Vazeille M, Moutailler S, Coudrier D, Rousseaux C, Khun H, Huerre M, et al. Two Chikungunya isolates from the outbreak of La Reunion (Indian Ocean) exhibit different patterns of infection in the mosquito, *Aedes albopictus. PLoS ONE* 2007;2(11):e1168.

12 Vazeille M, Jeannin C, Martin E, Schaffner F, Failloux AB. Chikungunya: a risk for Mediterranean countries? *Acta Trop* 2008;105(2):200–202.

13 Straetemans M. Vector-related risk mapping of the introduction and establishment of *Aedes albopictus* in Europe. *Euro Surveill* 2008;13(7).

14 Simon F, Parola P, Grandadam M, Fourcade S, Oliver M, Brouqui P, et al. Chikungunya infection: an emerging rheumatism among travelers returned from Indian Ocean islands. Report of 47 cases. *Medicine (Baltimore)* 2007;86(3):123–37.

15 Lanciotti RS, Kosoy OL, Laven JJ, Panella AJ, Velez JO, Lambert AJ, et al. Chikungunya virus in US travelers returning from India, 2006. *Emerg Infect Dis* 2007;13(5):764–7.

16 Wilson ME, Freedman DO. Etiology of travel-related fever. *Curr Opin Infect Dis* 2007;20(5):449–53.

17 Reiskind MH, Pesko K, Westbrook CJ, Mores CN. Susceptibility of Florida mosquitoes to infection with chikungunya virus. *Am J Trop Med Hyg* 2008;78(3):422–5.

18 Simon F, Paule P, Oliver M. Chikungunya virus-induced myopericarditis: toward an increase of dilated cardiomyopathy in countries with epidemics? *Am J Trop Med Hyg* 2008;78(2):212–13.

19 Parola P, Simon F, Oliver M. Tenosynovitis and vascular disorders associated with Chikungunya virus-related rheumatism. *Clin Infect Dis* 2007;45(6):801–2.

20 Hochedez P, Hausfater P, Jaureguiberry S, Gay F, Datry A, Danis M, et al. Cases of chikungunya fever imported from the islands of the South West Indian Ocean to Paris, France. *Euro Surveill* 2007;12(1).

21 Borgherini G, Poubeau P, Staikowsky F, Lory M, Le MN, Becquart JP, et al. Outbreak of chikungunya on Reunion Island: early clinical and laboratory features in 157 adult patients. *Clin Infect Dis* 2007;44(11):1401–7.

22 Renault P, Solet JL, Sissoko D, Balleydier E, Larrieu S, Filleul L, et al. A major epidemic of chikungunya virus infection on Reunion Island, France, 2005–2006. *Am J Trop Med Hyg* 2007;77(4):727–31.

23 Gerardin P, Barau G, Michault A, Bintner M, Randrianaivo H, Choker G, et al. Multidisciplinary prospective study of mother-to-child chikungunya virus infections on the island of La Reunion. *PLoS Med* 2008;5(3):e60.

24 Borgherini G, Poubeau P, Jossaume A, Gouix A, Cotte L, Michault A, et al. Persistent arthralgia associated with chikungunya virus: a study of 88 adult patients on Reunion Island. *Clin Infect Dis* 2008;47(4):469–75.

25 Pialoux G, Gauzere BA, Jaureguiberry S, Strobel M. Chikungunya, an epidemic arbovirosis. *Lancet Infect Dis* 2007;7(5):319–27.

26 Grivard P, Le RK, Laurent P, Fianu A, Perrau J, Gigan J, et al. Molecular and serological diagnosis of chikungunya virus infection. *Pathol Biol (Paris)* 2007;55(10):490–94.

27 Calisher CH, el-Kafrawi AO, Al-Deen Mahmud MI, Travassos Da Rosa AP, Bartz CR, Brummer-Korvenkontio M, et al. Complex-specific immunoglobulin M antibody patterns in humans infected with alphaviruses.*J Clin Microbiol* 1986;23(1):155–9.

28 Edelman R, Tacket CO, Wasserman SS, Bodison SA, Perry JG, Mangiafico JA. Phase II safety and immunogenicity study of live chikungunya virus vaccine TSI-GSD-218. *Am J Trop Med Hyg* 2000;62(6):681–5.

# 12

# Ross River Virus

Joseph Torresi

Austin Hospital, University of Melbourne, Heidelberg, VC, Australia

## Introduction

Ross River virus (RRV) is a mosquito-transmitted alphavirus that is endemic and enzootic in Australia and Papua New Guinea [1–4]. RRV is an RNA virus belonging to the family Togaviridae, which contains the genera *Alphavirus* and *Rubivirus*. The virus was first isolated in 1959 from *Aedes vigilax* mosquitoes trapped beside the Ross River in Townsville, North Queensland. RRV is maintained in nature by infection of macropods (including wallabies and kangaroos), although urban epidemics may originate from infection of opossums, flying foxes (fruit bats), and birds. During epidemics, human–mosquito–human transmission also occurs. The major mosquito vectors of RRV infection in Australia are *A. vigilax*, *A. camptorhynchus*, and *Culex annulirostris* [5–7]. Other mosquito species, in particular *A. notoscriptus*, may also be involved in RRV transmission in Australia. In contrast, *A. polynesiensis* may be responsible for transmission of RRV in the South Pacific.

RRV is the most common arboviral disease in Australia and is characterized by fever, rash, and arthralgias and in some instances by disabling joint pains that may persist for several months [8, 9]. Absence of fever is not infrequent, and patients may present with rheumatological problems alone. Hence, this illness is more widely referred to as RRV disease than as Ross River fever. RRV has also been responsible for large epidemics in Fiji, New Caledonia, Samoa, and the Cook Islands [5, 10–13]. Although RRV has caused large epidemics in Oceania, the risk of this infection for travelers to these regions is less well established.

Barmah Forest virus (BFV) is a closely related arbovirus that is spread by the same mosquito vectors, and hence epidemics of mixed RRV and BFV have been reported.

RRV and BFV produce clinical illnesses that are essentially indistinguishable. As RRV is far more prevalent than BFV, this chapter will focus predominantly on the epidemiology and clinical features of RRV.

## Epidemiology of RRV

From the first reports of a syndrome consistent with RRV (epidemic polyarthritis) in 1928 in New South Wales [4, 14], RRV has spread to become established in most parts of Australia, resulting in several outbreaks in the Northern Territory, Queensland, Victoria, and New South Wales [4, 15–18]. RRV has also extended to Papua New Guinea and the South Pacific, causing large epidemics in Fiji, the Cook Islands, and Samoa [4, 5, 10–13]. RRV antibody prevalence among the Australian population increases with age and varies according to geographical area, ranging from 19% in southeast Queensland to 64% in the Cape York Peninsula of Queensland [19]. In New South Wales and Victoria, antibody prevalence ranges from 13% to 39%, whereas in South Australia, it is 8%. The overall incidence of RRV disease in Australia is approximately 22/100,000/year, although, like seroprevalence, this varies widely according to season and different geographical regions. The incidence of RRV disease in Queensland is 61/100,000/year, although this varies from 24 to 144/100,000 annually; in the Northern Territory, it varies from 32 to 203/100,000 annually (Table 12.1) [4, 20]. The number of cases reported in Australia between 1993 and 2007 averaged 4058 per year, peaking at 7823 in 1996 and 6686 in 1997. The number of annual notifications rises to a maximum between the months of February and April in each year [20] (Figure 12.1). Barmah Forest virus (BFV) is much less prevalent than RRV, with an annual notification rate of only 6/100,000/year. As with RRV, the notification rates for BFV are highest in the Northern Territory and Queensland (Table 12.1) and peak between the months of February and May (Figure 12.1B).

*Tropical Diseases in Travelers*, 1st edition. Edited by E. Schwartz.
© 2009 by Blackwell Publishing, ISBN: 978-1-4051-8441-0.

**Table 12.1** Notification rates (per 100,000 annually) for RRV and BFV averaged from 1993 to 2007.

| STATE | RRV notification rate (/100,000 annually) Mean (SEM) | RRV notification rate (/100,000 annually) Range (1993–2007) | RRV notification rate (/100,000 annually) Mean (SEM) | BFV notification rate (/100,000 annually) Range (1995–2007) |
|---|---|---|---|---|
| Australian Capital Territory | 1.9 (0.4) | 0.3–4.9 | 0.6 (0.2) | 0.0–1.8 |
| New South Wales | 12.9 (1.9) | 2.7–32.8 | 5.9 (0.6) | 3.0–9.4 |
| Northern Territory | 108.5 (12) | 31.8–202.9 | 18.9 (4.4) | 5.5–60.5 |
| Queensland | 60.5 (7.4) | 23.3–143.7 | 14.7 (7.4) | 8.7–22.9 |
| South Australia | 13.2 (4.1) | 1.4–52.7 | 1.6 (0.9) | 0.0–11.9 |
| Tasmania | 5.8 (1.8) | 1.0–24.5 | 0.08 (0.04) | 0.0–0.4 |
| Victoria | 5.8 (2.1) | 0.7–26.7 | 0.5 (0.09) | 0.2–1.2 |
| Western Australia | 29.8 (5.6) | 5.5–80.4 | 3.4 (0.6) | 1.1–10.2 |

*Source*: Adapted from Australian Government, Department of Health and Ageing, National Notifiable Diseases Surveillance System (http://www9.health.gov.au/cda/Source/Rpt_4_sel.cfm).
SEM: Standard error of the mean.

## Epidemiology in travelers

Reports of RRV disease in international travelers visiting Australia are infrequent [21–23]. In one report from New Zealand, 43% of patients suspected of having contracted RRV while traveling overseas were found to be antibody-positive. In addition, these patients had rising serum antibody titers indicating recent infection [21]. A report from Germany describes a traveler returning from the South Pacific with an acute febrile illness accompanied by generalized myalgia, arthralgia of the large joints, and positive serum IgG and IgM for RRV [22]. A more recent report of a Dutch traveler returning after a recent visit to the Northern Territory of Australia describes a febrile illness associated with arthralgia and a maculopapular rash on the trunk and limbs; a diagnosis of RRV disease was confirmed by positive serum IgM and IgG against RRV [23]. RRV disease can develop in travelers visiting endemic regions, but its true incidence in travelers is not known. Clinically apparent disease is likely to reflect the syndrome already well described in residents of endemic countries like Australia. The likelihood of a traveler becoming infected with RRV is also likely to reflect the local disease prevalence. It may, therefore, be expected that travel to destinations with the highest incidence and during seasons of peak disease transmission pose the highest risk for international travelers. However, the paucity of reports of symptomatic RRV infection in international travelers might also suggest that clinically significant disease is an infrequent problem for travelers; alternatively, it may reflect a lack of awareness of RRV disease among physicians practicing outside Australia and a general lack of availability of serological tests in many Western countries.

## Clinical aspects

RRV disease most commonly affects adults aged 25–39 years with a male-to-female ratio of approximately 1:1. The incubation period for RRV ranges from 7 to 9 days, although it may be as long as 21 days or as short as 3 days [4, 18, 24–28].

## Clinical manifestations

RRV disease causes a characteristic syndrome, including constitutional effects, rash, and rheumatic manifestations [4, 18, 29]. Rash, fever, and arthralgia may occur in any sequence. For the majority of patients, RRV disease will produce an illness of relatively short duration and will not significantly impact daily living. However, hospitalization for symptomatic relief may be required in 10–20% of patients.

### Constitutional manifestations

Fever in RRV disease affects between one-third and one-half of patients and is short-lived, lasting 1–3 days. Myalgia

(a)

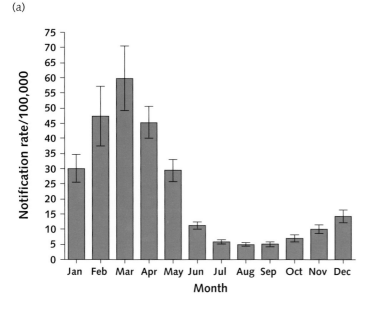

(b)

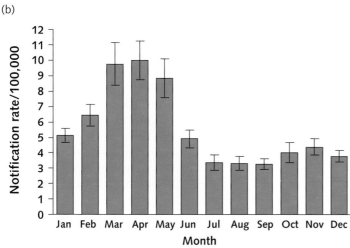

**Figure 12.1** (a) Notification rates (mean/SEM) for RRV according to month, for Australia between 1993 and 2007. (b) Notification rates (mean/SEM) for BFV according to month, for Australia between 1995 and 2007. (From Communicable Diseases Network, Australia New Zealand. URL: http://www.health.gov.au/pubhlth/cdi/nndss/.)

frequently accompanies arthralgia and is reported in over 50% of patients [25, 29]. Fatigue (affecting over 50% of patients), malaise, and lymphadenopathy are all common; sore throat and coryza are infrequent manifestations [29].

## Joint manifestations

Joint symptoms and signs are acute in onset and generally consist of arthralgia and joint effusions, usually symmetrical. They range from tenderness with minor restriction of movement to severe redness, joint swelling, and significant disability. The peripheral joints, particularly wrists, fingers (metacarpophalangeal joints), ankles, and knees,

are predominantly involved, although it is not unusual for patients to experience pain in proximal and axial joints (Figure 12.2) [4, 17, 29].

## Rash

Rash affects approximately 50% of people with RRV disease. The rash is most commonly maculopapular, but may also be vesicular or purpuric [4, 29]. It generally lasts 5–10 days, and in a small proportion of cases, it may be the sole manifestation of infection. The rash appears mainly on the limbs and trunk, but may also occur on the palms, soles, digits, face, and scalp.

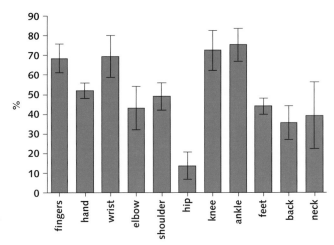

**Figure 12.2** Frequency of joint involvement in RRV disease. (Adapted from [4].)

## Rare presentations

Less common manifestations of RRV disease include splenomegaly, hematuria, glomerulonephritis, paresthesias, headache, neck stiffness, photophobia, and rarely meningitis and encephalitis [4, 29].

## Illness duration and prognosis

Initial reports of RRV disease suggested that the majority of patients experience a relatively short clinical course, with most recovering over a period of 1–4 weeks. Joint swelling generally persists for 4–7 days, and arthralgia tends to resolve a few days after the swelling subsides. More recent reports, however, suggest that long-term complications are not infrequent. In a small proportion of patients (3–10%), joint swelling and painful limitation of movement may persist for longer than 3 months [4, 15]. In a report by Fraser et al. [29], 50% of patients suffering from RRV disease had recovered after 6 months and 75% in just over 12 months. However, 5% of patients were still experiencing joint symptoms four years after infection, although progression to degenerative arthropathy was unusual. In a more recent review of cases of RRV disease acquired in far north Queensland, up to 27% of patients were found to have persisting joint abnormalities (based on tenderness, effusion, enthesopathy, swelling, heat, or other abnormal examination findings) up to 7 months after the onset of illness. However, the median number of painful joints decreased from 4 to 1 over the first 4 months, reaching 0 after 5–7 months (Figure 12.3) [4]. These investigators also assessed difficulties with activities of daily living, functional disability, and physical, psychological, and social function and found that patients had returned to normal function physically over 4–6 months and psychologically over 2–5 months.

## Laboratory diagnosis

The diagnosis of RRV disease essentially relies on serological testing. Isolation of RRV from humans is rarely successful because the virus does not persist in serum beyond the early stages of disease. Both IgG and IgM can be detected by enzyme-linked immunosorbent assay (ELISA). The detection of immunoglobulin M (IgM) in an acute-phase specimen provides a presumptive

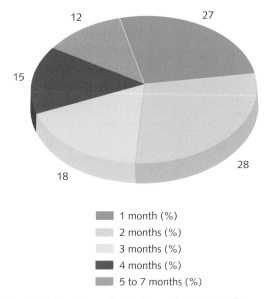

**Figure 12.3** Prevalence of joint abnormalities in RRV disease over time. Joint abnormalities were based on objective signs on joint examination and included tenderness, effusion, enthesopathy, swelling, heat, and other abnormal findings. (Adapted from [4].)

diagnosis of recent RRV infection; however, this is generally of low titer and does not persist for long periods in serum [4, 30]. A confirmed diagnosis requires a fourfold or greater increase in antibody titer in two sera obtained 10–14 days apart and tested in parallel. It is, therefore, important that the acute-phase serum be collected within 7 days of the onset of illness and that convalescent-phase serum be collected within 2–4 weeks of disease onset. The most commonly available assay is the indirect ELISA kit manufactured by PanBio. The sensitivity of the PanBio ELISA kit is 98.5% and 84.6% and the specificity is 96.5% and 97.6% for IgM and IgG, respectively [4]. However, false positive ELISA results may be caused by infection with the closely related Barmah Forest virus (BFV), which is also known to cause epidemic polyarthralgia. False positive results from rubella and Q fever infections and from noninfectious causes such as connective tissue disorders associated with the presence of rheumatoid factor in serum may also occur [4, 31].

Laboratory contacts for RRV and Barmah Forest virus serology include Victorian Infectious Diseases Reference Laboratory (available from http://www.vidrl.org.au/); Central Sydney Laboratory Service (available from http://www.cs.nsw.gov.au/csls/); and Queensland Medical Laboratory (available from http://www.qml.com.au/).

## Treatment

Treatment for RRV disease essentially consists of symptomatic and supportive management of joint pain and disability. The use of nonsteroidal anti-inflammatory drugs (NSAIDs) can produce a rapid improvement in joint symptoms. These drugs appear to be more effective than paracetamol, although the two have not been compared in clinical trials. For patients with more severe and disabling joint symptoms, rest also helps to provide symptomatic relief. For patients who have minimal disability and only mild joint symptoms, the use of NSAIDs may not be necessary; simple rest and physical therapy may be sufficient [4, 27].

## References

1 Scrimgeour EM, Aaskov JG, Matz LR. Ross River virus arthritis in Papua New Guinea. *Trans R Soc Trop Med Hyg* 1987;81:833–4.

2 Flexman JP, Smith DW, Mackenzie JS, et al. A comparison of the diseases caused by Ross River virus and Barmah Forest virus. *Med J Aust* 1998;169:159–63.

3 Hii J, Dyke T, Dagoro H, Sanders RC. Health impact assessments of malaria and Ross River virus infection in the Southern Highlands Province of Papua New Guinea. *P N G Med J* 1997;40:14–25.

4 Harley D, Sleigh A, Ritchie S. Ross River virus transmission, infection, and disease: a cross-disciplinary review. *Clin Microbiol Rev* 2001;14:909–32.

5 Mackenzie JS, Lindsay MD, Coelen RJ, Broom AK, Hall RA, Smith DW. Arboviruses causing human disease in the Australasian zoogeographic region. *Arch Virol* 1994;136:447–67.

6 Russell RC. Arboviruses and their vectors in Australia: an update on the ecology and epidemiology of some mosquito-borne arboviruses. *Rev Med Vet Entomol* 1995;83:141–58.

7 Russell RC. Vectors vs. humans in Australia: who is on top down under? An update on vector-borne disease and research on vectors in Australia. *J Vector Ecol* 1998;23:1–46.

8 Fraser JRE. Epidemic polyarthritis and Ross River virus disease. *Clin Rheum Dis* 1986;12:369–88.

9 Mackenzie JS, Broom AK, Hall RA, et al. Arboviruses in the Australian region, 1990 to 1998. *Commun Dis Intell* 1998;22:93–100.

10 Aaskov JG, Mataika JU, Lawrence GW, et al. An epidemic of Ross River virus infection in Fiji, 1979. *Am J Trop Med Hyg* 1981;30:1053–9.

11 Fauran P, Donaldson M, Harper JW, Oseni RA, Aaskov JG. Characterization of Ross River viruses isolated from patients with polyarthritis in New Caledonia and Wallis and Futuna Islands. *Am J Trop Med Hyg* 1984;33:1228–31.

12 Rosen L, Gubler DJ, Bennett PH. Epidemic polyarthritis (Ross River) virus infection in the Cook Islands. *Am J Trop Med Hyg* 1981;30:1294–1302.

13 Tesh RB, McLean RG, Shroyer DA, Calisher CH, Rosen L. Ross River virus (Togaviridae: *Alphavirus*) infection (epidemic polyarthrits) in American Samoa. *Trans R Soc Trop Med Hyg* 1981;75:426–31.

14 Nimmo JR. An unusual epidemic. *Med J Aust.* 1928;1:549–50.

15 Sibree EW. Acute polyarthritis in Queensland. *Med J Aust* 1944;2:565–7.

16 Fuller CO, Warner P. Some epidemiological and laboratory observations on an epidemic rash and polyarthritis occurring in the upper Murray region of South Australia. *Med J Aust* 1957;2:117–20.

17 Harley D, Bossingham B, Purdie DM, Nirmala Pandeya N, Sleigh AC. Ross River virus disease in tropical Queensland: evolution of rheumatic manifestations in an inception cohort followed for six months. *Med J Aust* 2002;177:352–5.

18 Jacups SP, Whelan PI, Currie BJ. Ross River virus and Barmah Forest virus infections: a review of history, ecology, and predictive models, with implications for tropical northern Australia. *Vector Borne Zoonotic Dis* 2008;8:283–98.

19 Doherty RL, Gorman BM, Whitehead RH, Carley JG. Studies of arthropod-borne virus infections in Queensland. V. Survey of antibodies to group A arboviruses in man and other animals. *Aust J Exp Biol Med Sci* 1966;44:365–78.

20 Owen R, Paul W Roche, Hope K, et al. Australia's notifiable diseases status, 2005: annual report of the National Notifiable

Diseases Surveillance System. *Commun Dis Intell* 2007;31:1–70.

21 Maguire T. Do Ross River and dengue viruses pose a threat to New Zealand? *The N Z Med J* 1994;107(989):448–50.

22 Proll S, Dobler G, Pfeffer M, Jelinek T, Nothdurft HD, Loscher T. [Persistent arthralgias in Ross-River-Virus disease after travel to the South Pacific]. *Dtsch Med Wochenschr* 1999;124(24):759–62.

23 Visser LG, Groen J. [Arthralgia and rash from Australia caused by Ross river virus]. *Ned Tijdschr Geneeskd* 2003; 147(6):254–7.

24 Fraser JRE, Cunningham AL. Incubation time of epidemic polyarthritis. *Med J Aust* 1980(1):550–51.

25 Mudge PR, Aaskov JG. Epidemic polyarthritis in Australia, 1980–1981. *Med J Aust* 1983;2:269–73.

26 Hawkes RA, Boughton CR, Naim HM, Stallman ND. A major outbreak of epidemic polyarthritis in New South Wales during the summer of 1983/1984. *Med J Aust* 1985;143: 330–33.

27 Condon RJ, Rouse IL. Acute symptoms and sequelae of Ross River virus infection in South-Western Australia: a follow-up study. *Clin Diagn Virol* 1995;3:273–84.

28 Westley-Wise VJ, Beard JR, Sladden TJ, Dunn TM, Simpson J. Ross River virus infection on the north coast of New South Wales. *Aust N Z J Public Health* 1996;20: 87–92.

29 Fraser JRE. Epidemic polyarthritis and Ross River virus disease. *Clin Rheum Dis* 1986;12:369–88.

30 Mackenzie JS, Broom AK, Calisher CH, et al. Diagnosis and reporting of arbovirus infections in Australia. *Arbovirus Res Aust* 1993;6:89–93.

31 Rich G, McKechnie J, McPhan I, Richards B. Laboratory diagnosis of Ross River virus infection. *Commun Dis Intell* 1993;17:208–9.

# 13 Viral Hemorrhagic Fevers

## Annelies Wilder-Smith

National University of Singapore, Singapore

## Introduction

Viral hemorrhagic fevers (VHF) are a group of febrile illnesses caused by several distinct families of viruses that share a number of properties, but differ in others. These groups include the arena-, bunya-, filo-, and flaviviruses (Table 13.1). Flaviviruses that cause diseases such as dengue and yellow fever also belong to the group of VHF, but differ in many aspects from the other viral hemorrhagic fevers. They are excluded from this chapter, as they are covered elsewhere (Chapters 7, 10). Ebola and Marburg, Lassa fever, Rift Valley fever (RVF), and Crimean–Congo hemorrhagic fever viruses, hantapulmonary syndrome, and hemorrhagic fever with pulmonary syndrome are the best-known diseases among the classical VHF.

Each virus is associated with one or more nonhuman host or vector species; however, the reservoir hosts for Ebola and Marburg viruses have not yet been identified. Some VHF have aerosol infectious properties and, therefore, could be used in bioterrorism. Spread can occur via aerosolization of rodent excreta or by mosquitoes or ticks.

Pathogenesis varies among the diseases, with direct viral damage, disseminated intravascular coagulation (DIC), hepatic damage, vascular damage, and cytokine release being implicated to varying degrees. Table 13.2 summarizes the clinical characteristics of VHF.

Taken together, the viruses that cause VHF are distributed over much of the globe. Table 13.3 summarizes the main reservoirs for the different VHF, as well as measures to prevent VHF. Travelers can be incidentally infected when their destination countries are experiencing outbreaks. However, the risk of VHF for travelers is overall very low [2, 3]. Travelers are also known to have introduced VHF into nonendemic countries, for example, by transmitting the diseases to health care workers [4].

Table 13.4 summarizes cases of VHF in travelers and mortality rates.

## Epidemiology

The various families of viruses that cause VHF are distributed widely. Each virus is associated with one or more nonhuman host or vector species, which determine the geographical distribution. Rodents are the main reservoir for hantavirus infections, hemorrhagic fever with renal syndrome, and Lassa fever. *Aedes* mosquitoes are the vectors for Rift Valley fever and ticks for Crimean–Congo hemorrhagic fever [5–7]. The viruses usually are transmitted to humans where the habitats of infected reservoir hosts or vectors and humans overlap. In general, travelers are rarely affected, and humans are incidental, dead-end hosts for these enzootic diseases.

## Arenaviruses

Each arenavirus is associated with one or more closely related rodent species that constitute its natural reservoir. Lassa fever, the South American hemorrhagic fevers, lymphocytic choriomeningitis, and several other African and South American viruses related to Lassa have been discovered [5]. Arenaviruses can be divided into two groups: the New World complex and the Old World or lymphocytic choriomeningitis virus (LCMV)/Lassa complex. Rodents are distributed across most of the globe, including Europe, Asia, Africa, and the Americas, although the individual viruses (with the exception of LCMV) are restricted to limited geographic areas. The following section describes Lassa fever.

### Lassa fever

#### Epidemiology
Lassa fever is limited to rural areas of West Africa. The main reservoir is *Mastomys* rodents. Lassa fever is different

*Tropical Diseases in Travelers*, 1st edition. Edited by E. Schwartz.
© 2009 by Blackwell Publishing, ISBN: 978-1-4051-8441-0.

**Table 13.1** Viral hemorrhagic fevers.

| Family | Disease (virus) | Main geographical distribution |
|---|---|---|
| Arenaviridae | Lassa fever | West Africa |
| | South American hemorrhagic fevers: | South America |
| | —Argentine HF* (Junin virus) | |
| | —Bolivian HF (Machupo virus) | |
| | —Brazilian HF (Sabia virus) | |
| | —Venezuelan HF (Guanarito virus) | |
| Bunyaviridae | Rift Valley fever | Africa, Middle East |
| | Crimean–Congo HF | Korea, Europe, Asia, |
| | HF with renal syndrome | Africa |
| | Hantavirus pulmonary syndrome (Sin Nombre, | Asia, Europe |
| | Andes, others) | North and South America |
| Filoviridae | Marburg HF | Africa (Marburg was first identified in Germany after |
| | Ebola HF | importation of green monkeys from West Africa) |
| Flaviviridae | Dengue | Subtropics and tropics, worldwide |
| | Japanese encephalitis | Large parts of Southeast Asia and South Asia |
| | Yellow fever | Large parts of South America and Africa, USA, |
| | West Nile fever | Middle East |

*HF: hemorrhagic fever.

from other arenaviral diseases in its ability to spread from person to person. Outbreaks typically include a few health care workers because of their close exposure to patients and infectious body fluids without barrier nursing precautions and because of their residence in the endemic area. Lassa fever was initially recognized in a Nigerian hospital, where three nurses became ill successively. Since then, extensive transmission with occasional nosocomial outbreaks has been reported from Nigeria, Sierra Leone, Guinea, and Liberia. Serologic studies and occasional cases have shown its presence in every country of West Africa between Nigeria and Senegal. Nosocomial outbreaks usually occur during the dry season (January to April), whereas endemic transmission occurs throughout the year. Endemic transmission takes place by aerosol and direct contact with infected rodents, and probably person to person in homes. Capture of rodents as a supplemental food source is another high risk factor for infection. *Mastomys* rodents are common in houses and in the nearby bush in West Africa. In some areas, they are found in virtually all homes, leading to high infection rates.

Peridomestic exposure to infected rodents is the most likely source of human infections for most of the arenaviruses. Rodent infestation facilitated by inappropriate food storage increases the risk of human infection. Person-to-person spread of Lassa viruses has also been described,

most notably by large droplet and contact transmission in health care settings.

### International travelers and Lassa fever
Since 1970, at least 25 cases have been reported in travelers [4]. All were acquired in West Africa; about one-third of those were reported in health care workers and aid workers. Lassa fever has also been reported in military personnel and professionals serving in Africa. About 10 cases have occurred in individual travelers, mainly to Sierra Leone. Fatal outcomes occurred in 7 cases. There were no secondary cases.

### Clinical manifestations
The incubation period varies from 3 to 16 days, usually lasting 7–12 days, when infection is transmitted from person to person. It is assumed to be similar in rodent-transmitted infections. All ages and both sexes are infected equally. Based on serologic data, there may be 20 mild or inapparent infections for each hospitalized case. In contrast, retrospective studies among white missionaries suggest, but do not yet prove, that moderately severe or even fatal illness usually follows infection. Severe multisystem disease occurs only in 5–10% of infections. Case fatality rates in hospitalized patients average from 1–25%. Clinical manifestations are nonspecific and include fever, chest pain, sore throat, cough, abdominal

**Table 13.2** Mode of transmission and clinical characteristics for the most important viral hemorrhagic fevers.

| Disease | Incubation time | Mode of transmission | Major clinical features | Treatment |
|---|---|---|---|---|
| Lassa fever | 5–6 days | Exposure to infected rodents, inhalation of aerosols from rodent urine, ingestion of rodent-contaminated food, direct contact of broken skin with rodent excreta. Nosocomial infection and laboratory transmission possible. | Mild to severe hemorrhagic febrile disease | Ribavirin |
| Rift Valley fever (RVF) | 2–5 days | Mosquitoes (*Aedes*), percutaneous inoculation, exposure to aerosols from contaminated blood or fluids of infected animals | Acute febrile illness with occasional retinietis, hemorrhagic fever, or encephalitis | Supportive |
| Crimean–Congo hemorrhagic fever (CCHF) | 3–12 days | Ticks | Severe hemorrhagic fever | Ribavirin |
| Hantavirus pulmonary syndrome (HPS) | 7–28 days | Aerosols from rodent excreta | Fever, shock, pulmonary edema | Ribavirin |
| Hemorrhagic fever with renal syndrome (HFRS) | 9–35 days | Aerosols from rodent excreta | Fever, shock, bleeding, renal failure | Ribavirin |
| Ebola | 3–16 days | Nosocomial and laboratory transmission | Fever, hemorrhage, multiorgan failure; mortality 80% | Supportive |
| Marburg | 3–16 days | Nosocomial transmissions; infection of gold miners from an unknown natural source | Hemorrhage, febrile illness; mortality around 20% | Supportive |

pain, and gastrointestinal symptoms. A combination of fever, pharyngitis, retrosternal pain, and proteinuria correctly predicted 70% of laboratory-confirmed Lassa fever cases. During the second week of illness, the patient may deteriorate and develop a capillary leak syndrome with reduced urinary output, facial edema, pleural effusions, and ascites, often accompanied by hemorrhages from mucosal surfaces.

## Diagnosis

Viruses can be isolated from blood during the first 7–10 days of illness by inoculating cell cultures. Serodiagnosis by detection of IgM antibodies by IFA or enzyme-linked immunosorbant assay (ELISA) is rapid and sensitive. A high degree of Lassa viremia is correlated with poor prognosis. The diagnosis of past infection is done by ELISA.

## Treatment

Intravenous administration of ribavirin reduced the mortality rate from 55% to 5% in Lassa patients if treatment was started before day 7 of the disease [5]. The loading dose is 30 mg/kg, followed by 15 mg/kg every 6 hours for 4 days and then 7.5 mg/kg three times daily for 6 additional days. Reversible anemia was the main side effect. Ribavirin is teratogenic. Volume replacement therapy with the judicious use of colloids should be started before the appearance of clinical shock, and electrolyte balance should be maintained.

## Prevention and control

Given the pervasive nature of *Mastomys*, control campaigns cannot be expected to prevent the disease, although model intensive efforts in a village in Sierra Leone resulted

**Table 13.3** Summary of important facts and prevention measures for viral hemorrhagic fevers for travelers.

| Viral hemorrhagic fever (VHF) | Reservoir | Prevention | Main areas of risk | Main travel populations at risk |
|---|---|---|---|---|
| Lassa fever | Rodents | Avoid direct contact with rodents, including inhalation of aerosols and contact/inhalation of rodent urine; infection control measures in hospitals. | West Africa | Missionaries, aid workers, health care workers, individual travelers, soldiers |
| Rift Valley fever (RVF) | Livestock (cattle, sheep, etc.) | Avoid mosquito bites. Avoid percutaneous inoculation. Avoid livestock, in particular, exposure to aerosols from contaminated blood or fluids of infected animals. | Sub-Saharan Africa, Middle East | Persons handling livestock; Hajj pilgrims |
| Crimean–Congo hemorrhagic fever (CCHF) | Livestock | Avoid ticks. Do not crush ticks. Avoid contact with blood or body fluids of domestic animals. In hospital: take infection control measures. | Africa, former Soviet Union, Middle East, Western China | Military populations |
| Hantavirus pulmonary syndrome (HPS) | Rodents (deer, mice) | Avoid contact with rodent urine, droppings, saliva, and nesting materials. | North and South America | Individual travelers |
| Hemorrhagic fever with renal syndrome (HFRS) | Rodents (striped field mice, yellow-necked mice, rats, or bank voles) | Avoid contact with rodent urine, droppings, saliva, and nesting materials. | Worldwide, but mainly in East Asia and Europe | Military populations |
| Ebola | Unknown | Avoid hospitals that do not practice standard infection control measures. | Africa | Health care workers; laboratory workers |
| Marburg | Unknown reservoir (African green monkeys from Uganda caused transmission to laboratory workers in Marburg in 1967) | Avoid mines, in particular, gold mines. Avoid fruit bats. Avoid hospitals without standard infection control. | Africa | Health care workers, laboratory workers, individual travelers |

**Table 13.4** Cases of viral hemorrhagic fever in travelers.

| Disease | Cases in travelers [4] | Reported mortality in nonendemic population | Case fatality in local population |
|---|---|---|---|
| Marburg | 31 cases in Germany (including 6 secondary cases), 1975–1990, 5 cases (including 1 secondary case) | 7/31 | 25% |
| Ebola | 1996, 1 secondary case | 1/1 | 30–90% |
| Lassa fever | Between 1969–2004, 23 cases were imported into Europe and North America, mainly medical staff; no secondary cases | 7/23 | 30% |
| Crimean–Congo hemorrhagic fever (CCHF) | 1997–2004, 2 travelers. | 1/2 | 10–50% |
| Rift Valley fever (RVF) | 1970s–8, Swedish soldiers in Egypt; 2002–2, French soldiers in Chad | 1/10 | 1% |
| Hanta pulmonary syndrome (HPS) | 1998–2006, 4 travelers | 2/4 | 30% |
| Hemorrhagic fever with renal syndrome (HFRS) | 1986–2008, 20 cases, all except 1, were soldiers either in Korea or in the Balkans | 2/20 | 5–15% |

*Source*: Adopted from GIDEON at http://web.gideononline.com/.

in a temporary fourfold reduction in transmission to humans. During nosocomial outbreaks, isolation of patients and barrier nursing are indicated. To prevent laboratory-acquired Lassa fever, only special laboratories with biological safety level 4 should be used.

### Prevention for travelers
Travelers should avoid rodents, and not stay in any local accommodation that is infested by rodents. Needlestick injury should be avoided. Universal precautions should be taken for any blood handling; reuse of needles or syringes is to be avoided.

## Bunyaviridae

Diseases caused by the family Bunyaviridae include Crimean–Congo hemorrhagic fever (CCHF), Rift Valley fever, hantavirus pulmonary syndrome, and hemorrhagic fever with renal syndrome [7–10]. They are zoonoses that are variously transmitted to humans by mosquitoes or direct/indirect transmission (Rift Valley fever), by ticks or direct handling of infected animals or carcasses (Crimean–Congo hemorrhagic fever), and through contact with urine, feces, or saliva of infected rodents (hantavirus pulmonary syndrome; hemorrhagic fever with renal syndrome).

## Crimean–Congo hemorrhagic fever
### Epidemiology
Crimean–Congo hemorrhagic fever was first described in the Crimea in 1944 and later equated with an illness that occurred in the Congo in 1956. Widely scattered cases were subsequently confirmed in Europe and Asia, most commonly among adult males (engaged in the livestock industry). The highest risk is reported among cattle owners, farmers, and shepherds. Sporadic cases are also encountered in soldiers, campers, veterinarians, forest workers, and health staff. Evidence for the virus has been found in ticks in Africa, Asia, the Middle East, and Eastern Europe. The virus is transmitted to man through the bites of ixodid ticks (*Hyalomma*) or contact with infected blood and tissues from livestock. As of 2000, the number of CCHF virus-transmitting ticks has been increasing worldwide,

which may be linked to global warming. The CCHF virus may infect a wide range of domestic and wild animals. The virus has been found in cattle, goats, sheep, hares, and hedgehogs. Tick vectors also lodge in small wild animals such as mice or rabbits and in wild birds. Many bird species are resistant to infection, but ostriches are susceptible and may show a high prevalence of infection in endemic areas. Human-to-human transmission has also been described. In rare instances, health care workers have been infected through patient contact and conjunctival exposure to blood.

### International travelers

Only two cases have been reported in international travelers (Table 13.4) [4]. In 1997, a fatal case of probable CCHF was reported in an English visitor to Zimbabwe. In 2004, a nonfatal case of imported CCHF (nonfatal) was reported in a traveler returning to France from Senegal.

### Clinical manifestations

Clinical manifestations include severe hemorrhagic fever with shock, disseminated intravascular coagulation, frequent extensive bleeding, and severe thrombocytopenia. Mortality ranges from 20–35%.

### Prevention and control

Because CCHF virus infects humans principally by the bite of adult *Hyalomma* ticks, avoidance of tick bites is important. Milkers and shepherds are frequent victims. It is also dangerous to crush infected ticks. Asymptomatically viremic sheep and cattle have been implicated in transmission to abattoir workers, even outside known endemic areas. Nosocomial transmission of CCHF has frequently been reported; therefore, universal precautions and hygiene are the mainstay of prevention.

### Prevention in travelers

Travelers should avoid tick bites and not crush ticks. Contact with livestock should be avoided. Hospitals with poor hygiene and infection control measures should be avoided.

## Rift Valley fever

### Epidemiology

Rift Valley fever (RVF) was first identified in Kenya in 1931 [8, 11]. RVF primarily affects livestock but may also infect humans. It is transmitted by several means, including the bites of mosquitoes, percutaneous inoculation, and exposure to aerosols from contaminated blood or fluids of infected animals. It is recognized as a disease of farm-

ers, veterinarians, and abattoir workers who have close contact with blood shed by sick domestic livestock or fresh carcasses containing a high concentration of virus. There is some evidence that humans may also become infected with RVF by ingesting the unpasteurized or uncooked milk of infected animals. RVF is maintained in Sub-Saharan Africa via transovarial transmission in *Aedes* mosquitoes, notably *A. mcintoshi*. In 1977, the virus was introduced to Egypt and resulted in widespread epidemic disease in humans and domestic animals; it reappeared in Egypt in 1992. After an extensive epidemic in Kenya in 1997–1998, RVF was introduced into the Arabian peninsula [12]. The annual influx of over 2 million pilgrims for the Hajj in Saudi Arabia, as well as the large migrant population in this region, generates high human and animal traffic that presents a risk of introducing both the vector and the livestock. In 2006–2007, an epidemic of RVF occurred in Ethiopia, Kenya, Somalia, and the United Republic of Tanzania following unusually heavy rainfall.

### International travelers

Eight Swedish soldiers serving in Egypt during the 1970s were found to be seropositive for RVF virus [4]. In 2002, two nonfatal cases of RVF were confirmed among French military personnel serving in Chad [11].

### Clinical manifestations

Although most human cases are relatively mild, a small percentage of patients develop a much more severe form of the disease. This usually appears as one or more of three distinct syndromes: ocular (eye) disease (0.5–2% of patients), meningoencephalitis (<1%), or hemorrhagic fever (<1%) [8].

In the *ocular form* of the disease, the usual symptoms associated with the mild form of the disease are accompanied by retinal lesions. The onset of the lesions in the eyes is usually 1–3 weeks after appearance of the first symptoms. Patients usually report blurred or decreased vision. The disease may resolve itself with no lasting effects within 10–12 weeks. However, when the lesions occur in the macula, 50% of patients will experience permanent loss of vision. Death is uncommon in patients with only the ocular form of the disease.

The onset of the *meningoencephalitis form* of the disease usually occurs 1–4 weeks after the first symptoms of RVF appear. Clinical features include intense headache, loss of memory, hallucinations, confusion, disorientation, vertigo, convulsions, lethargy, and coma. Neurological complications can appear later (>60 days). The death rate in patients who experience only this form of the disease is low, but residual neurological deficit, which may be severe, is common.

The symptoms of the *hemorrhagic fever form* of the disease appear 2–4 days after the onset of illness and begin with evidence of severe liver impairment, such as jaundice. Signs of hemorrhage appear subsequently, such as vomiting blood, passing blood in the feces, purpuric rash or ecchymoses (caused by bleeding in the skin), bleeding from the nose or gums, menorrhagia, and bleeding from venipuncture sites. The case fatality ratio for patients developing the hemorrhagic form of the disease is approximately 50%. The total case fatality rate has varied widely between different epidemics but, overall, has been less than 1% in those documented. Most fatalities occur in patients who develop the hemorrhagic icteric form.

## Diagnosis

Acute RVF can be diagnosed using several different methods. Serological tests such as enzyme-linked immunoassay may confirm the presence of specific IgM antibodies to the virus. The virus itself may be detected in blood during the early phase of illness, or in post-mortem tissue using a variety of techniques, including virus propagation (in cell cultures or inoculated animals), antigen detection tests, and real time polymerase chain reaction (RT-PCR).

## Treatment and vaccine

Most human cases of RVF are relatively mild and of short duration. No specific treatment is required for these patients. For the more severe cases, the predominant treatment is general supportive therapy.

An inactivated vaccine has been developed for human use. However, this vaccine is not licensed and is not commercially available. It has been used experimentally to protect veterinary and laboratory personnel at high risk of exposure to RVF. Other vaccines are under investigation.

## Prevention and control

Outbreaks of RVF in animals can be prevented by a sustained program of animal vaccination. Both modified live attenuated virus and inactivated virus vaccines have been developed for veterinary use. Only one dose of the live vaccine is required to provide long-term immunity, but the vaccine that is currently in use may result in spontaneous abortion if given to pregnant animals. The inactivated virus vaccine does not have this side effect, but multiple doses are needed to provide protection, which may prove problematic in endemic areas.

Animal immunization must be implemented before an outbreak if an epizootic is to be prevented. Once an outbreak has occurred, animal vaccination should not be implemented, because there is a high risk of its intensifying the outbreak. During mass animal vaccination campaigns, animal health workers may inadvertently transmit the virus through the use of multidose vials and the reuse of needles and syringes. If some animals in the herd are already infected and viremic (although not yet displaying obvious signs of illness), the virus will be transmitted among the herd, and the outbreak will be amplified. Restricting or banning the movement of livestock may be effective in slowing the expansion of the virus from infected to uninfected areas. Because outbreaks of RVF in animals precede human cases, the establishment of an active animal health surveillance system to detect new cases is essential for providing early warning to veterinary and human public health authorities.

During an outbreak of RVF, close contact with animals, particularly with their body fluids, either directly or via aerosols, has been identified as the most significant risk factor for RVF virus infection. In the absence of specific treatment and an effective human vaccine, raising awareness of the risk factors of RVF infection, as well as the protective measures individuals can take to prevent mosquito bites, is the only way to reduce human infection and deaths.

Public health messages for risk reduction should focus on reducing the risk of animal-to-human transmission as a result of unsafe animal husbandry and slaughtering practices. Gloves and other appropriate protective clothing should be worn and care taken when handling sick animals or their tissues and when slaughtering animals.

All animal products (blood, meat, and milk) should be thoroughly cooked before consumption.

The importance of personal and community protection against mosquito bites by using impregnated mosquito nets and personal insect repellent, if available; by wearing light-colored clothing (long-sleeved shirts and trousers); and by avoiding outdoor activity at peak biting times of the vector species should be emphasized in public health education. Vector control needs to be implemented. In hospitals, infection control measures should be practiced at all times.

## Prevention of RVF for travelers

Travelers should avoid direct contact with the blood and body fluids of sick or dead animals, particularly during the slaughter, manipulation, or burial of carcasses, fetuses, and the products of conception.

Frequent hand washing, in particular after contact with blood or body fluids from infected animals, is advised. Food safety is improved by cooking meat and avoiding the consumption of raw milk and blood. Personal and community protection should be used against mosquito bites, such as insecticide-impregnated mosquito bed nets and personal insect repellent (if available); and light-colored clothing should be worn (including long-sleeved shirts and trousers).

## Hantavirus infections

Hantaviruses are fundamentally parasites of wild rodents and perhaps insectivores. As such, hantaviruses are the exception to the general rule that Bunyaviridae are arthropod-borne viruses [7]. Hantaviruses that cause hanta virus pulmonary syndrome (HPS) are present in the Americas; those that cause hemorrhagic fever with renal syndrome (HFRS) occur worldwide.

## Hanta pulmonary syndrome

The number of cases and the geographical spread of HPS have increased in the Americas since the syndrome was first identified in 1993 in the USA. It has now been reported in Argentina, Bolivia, Brazil, Canada, Chile, Paraguay, Peru, and Uruguay. A total of 350–400 HPS cases have been confirmed in the Americas, most of them in Argentina and the USA [10]. HPS is caused by several distinct hantaviruses that are each associated with a specific rodent host. Once infected, rodents shed the virus throughout their lifetime. Humans are infected by inhaling aerosols of fresh or dried rodent excreta (feces, urine, and saliva). Investigation of an epidemic in Argentina in 1995 provided strong evidence for person-to-person transmission, not observed in studies in the USA.

### International travelers

There have been only a few reported cases in international travelers [4]. A patient in Chile died of HPS acquired in Bolivia in the late 1990s. In 2001, a French tourist acquired nonfatal HPS in Chile. In 2002, a nonfatal imported case of HPS (Andes virus) from Chile was reported in the United States. In 2006, a patient in Canada died of HPS acquired in Bolivia.

### Clinical manifestations

HPS begins with a febrile prodrome, followed by a severe increase in pulmonary vascular permeability and shock. If hypoxia is managed and shock is not fatal, the vascular leak reverses in a few days and recovery is apparently complete. About 45% of the reported cases were fatal.

The high fatality rate is associated with the sudden onset of pulmonary edema and respiratory distress.

### Diagnosis

HPS should be suspected when an otherwise healthy adult develops unexplained pulmonary edema or adult respiratory distress syndrome without one of the known causes being present. Thrombocytopenia is a particularly useful finding early in the course, associated with an elevated hematocrit, leukocytosis, left shift, and mildly elevated transaminases. Serological tests (IgM and IgG against hantaviruses) are useful. Hantaviruses can be recovered only with difficulty in cell culture or animal hosts, but the agent can be detected in blood or tissues by RT-PCR or in tissues by immunohistochemical staining.

### Treatment

There is no specific treatment for HPS, although prompt diagnosis is important for appropriate management of respiratory distress.

### Prevention and control

Control measures in endemic areas focus on rodent control, with particular emphasis on excluding rodents from buildings and reducing suitable habitats around inhabited dwellings. Many infections have resulted from cleaning rodent-infested areas. The use of readily available disinfectants such as chlorine bleach to decontaminate potentially infectious droppings and debris before cleaning is recommended. If available, respiratory protection should be used during this high-risk activity. Strict barrier nursing techniques are recommended for management of HPS.

### Prevention for travelers

Travelers should avoid contact with rodents.

## Hemorrhagic fever with renal syndrome

### Epidemiology

Hemorrhagic fever with renal syndrome (HFRS) is the most frequent hantavirus infection and viral hemorrhagic fever. HFRS occurs worldwide. Approximately 200,000 cases of HFRS occur annually, with a case fatality rate ranging from less than 1–10%. HFRS includes diseases such as Korean hemorrhagic fever, epidemic hemorrhagic fever, and nephropathy epidemica [13]. The viruses that cause HFRS include Hantaan, Dobrava-Belgrade, Seoul, and Puumala. Haantan virus is widely distributed in eastern Asia, particularly in China, Russia, and Korea. Puumala virus is found in Scandinavia, Western Europe, and Russia. Dobrava virus is found primarily in the Balkans, and Seoul virus is found worldwide. Rodents are the natural reservoir for hantaviruses. Known carriers include the striped field mouse (*Apodemus agrarius*), the reservoir for Hantaan virus; the brown or Norway rat (*Rattus norvegicus*), the reservoir for Seoul virus; the bank vole (*Clethrionomys glareolus*), the reservoir for Puumala virus; and the yellow-necked field mouse (*Ap. flavicollis*), which carries Dobrava virus.

People can become infected with these viruses and develop HFRS after exposure to aerosolized urine, droppings, or saliva of infected rodents or after exposure to dust from their nests. Transmission may also occur when infected urine or these other materials are directly introduced onto broken skin or onto the mucous membranes of the eyes, nose, or mouth. In addition, people who work with live rodents can be exposed to hantaviruses through bites from infected animals. Transmission from one human to another may occur, but is extremely rare.

### International travelers
Large numbers of military personnel have been affected by HFRS in the past decades, notably during the Korean War [4]. Since 1986, only 20 cases have been reported in travelers, 19 of whom were military personnel serving either in Korea (reported 1986) or in the last decade in the Balkans, in Bosnia-Herzegovina or Slovenia. Two fatal cases were reported among US soldiers in Korea. The only traveler who contracted the disease was a traveler from Taiwan who acquired hantavirus infection in China in 2008.

### Clinical manifestations
Symptoms of HFRS usually develop within 1–2 weeks after exposure to infectious material, but in rare cases, they may take up to 8 weeks to develop. Initial symptoms begin suddenly and include intense headaches, back and abdominal pain, fever, chills, nausea, and blurred vision. Individuals may have flushing of the face, inflammation or redness of the eyes, or a rash. Later symptoms can include shock, vascular leakage, and acute renal failure, which can cause severe fluid overload. The severity of the disease varies with the virus causing the infection. Hantaan and Dobrava virus infections usually cause severe symptoms, whereas Seoul and Puumala virus infections are usually moderate.

### Diagnosis
Positive IgM and IgG antibodies against hantaviruses are present. Hantavirus antigen can be found in tissue by immunohistochemical staining and microscope examination, or evidence of hantavirus RNA sequences in blood or tissue.

### Treatment
Ribavirin, a guanosine analogue, was effective in the treatment of HFRS in a double-blind placebo-controlled study in China using the intravenous dosing regimen established for Lassa fever. Effective supportive care is important. Early management of hantavirus patients should avoid excessive administration of fluids. Cardiotonic drugs should be used early because of the hemodynamic profile of decreased cardiac output and increased systemic vascular resistance. Some patients will need hemodialysis or peritoneal dialysis. Heparin is not recommended for the treatment of disseminated intravascular coagulation in HFRS.

### Prevention and control
Rodent control is the primary strategy for preventing hantavirus infections. Rodent populations near human communities should be controlled, and rodents should be excluded from homes. People should avoid contact with rodent urine, droppings, saliva, and nesting materials.

### Prevention for travelers
Travelers should avoid contact with rodents, rodent urine, droppings, saliva, and nesting materials.

## Filoviruses

### Ebola and Marburg Virus
Ebola and Marburg viruses belong to the family Filoviridae. They can cause severe hemorrhagic fever with high mortality in humans and nonhuman primates. The name of the viral family comes from their characteristic thread-like morphology, and this has made their recognition in tissues or clinical samples with electron microscopy unusually readily achieved. This viral family is characterized by a mysterious natural history. Primates are the only disease targets identified to date, but they are not thought to serve as reservoirs. In epidemics, it has usually been possible to trace the epidemic back to a human or nonhuman primate index case, but no further. Suspects have included spiders, soft ticks, bats, and monkeys, but there is no field evidence to incriminate any of these. Ebola hemorrhagic fever tends to appear in the humid rain forests of central and western Africa, and Marburg hemorrhagic fever in the drier and more open areas of central and eastern Africa. Filoviruses are prime examples of emerging

pathogens. Factors that may be involved in emergence are international commerce and travel, limited experience in diagnosis and case management, import of nonhuman primates, and the potential of filoviruses for rapid evolution [14].

## Ebola virus

### Epidemiology

Ebola virus was first recognized in 1976, when two unrelated epidemics occurred in northern Zaire and southern Sudan; 88% of the patients in 318 recognized cases died in the former, and 53% in 284 in the latter. Further outbreaks occurred in Sudan and Zaire again in the following year, but Ebola went into a silent mode for the following 2 decades. Then, in 1995–1996, an additional Ebola subtype (Cote d'Ivoire) was isolated from a human patient, and epidemics occurred in Gabon and Zaire [6]. Notably, one Gabon patient imported the disease to South Africa and transmitted the disease to a single nurse. More recently, smoldering outbreaks of the Sudan and Zaire virus subtypes have occurred in Uganda and Congo. The exact routes of transmission are not well known. Needlestick injury has been well documented, but mucous membrane contact with virus-laden material has probably been responsible from most recognized human infections. Blood and skin carry high titers of the virus. Almost all dermal structures are infected; this probably accounts for the additional risk to those participating in traditional burial preparation of cadavers and mourners touching cadavers. Filoviruses are also highly infective in small particle aerosols; nonetheless, airborne infection plays a minor role, if any, in interhuman spread [6].

### International travelers and Ebola

In 1996, a fatal case was reported in South Africa in a nurse involved in treating a patient transferred from Gabon [4].

## Marburg virus

### Epidemiology

Marburg virus was first identified in 1967. Transmission to humans occurred via African green monkeys that had been imported from Uganda to the city of Marburg (Germany) for use in vaccine production and biomedical research. Close contact with monkey blood or with cell cultures was present in all primary cases. Secondary cases were mainly among hospital staff and were associated with blood exposure. In total, there were 7 deaths among the 25 primary and 6 secondary human cases.

Marburg virus from an unknown natural source has repeatedly infected gold miners. The world's first extensive outbreak of Marburg virus infection occurred 1998–1999 in the Democratic Republic of Congo, involving 103 cases (69 fatal). An additional 16 cases were diagnosed at Durba-Watsa, Congo, during 2000 [6]. Follow-up antibody surveys in 2000 suggested that over 150 persons had been infected during the outbreak. Viral RNA was identified in insectivorous and fruit bats inhabiting a cave associated with the outbreak. In 2004 to 2005, a large outbreak (374 cases, 329 fatal) was reported in Angola. In 2007, an outbreak (5 cases suspected, 4 confirmed, 1 fatal) was reported among gold miners in Uganda.

### International travelers and Marburg viral hemorrhagic fever

Several cases have occurred in travelers since 1975. In 1975, a young hitchhiking Australian man was admitted to a Johannesburg hospital in South Africa after having toured Rhodesia (now Zimbabwe). Two secondary cases occurred, one being in the first patient's travel companion, and the other in a South African nurse [15]. In 1980, a French engineer working in Kenya developed Marburg virus disease and infected his physician. In 1987, a Danish tourist was infected in Kenya. In 1990, a tourist returning to Sweden from Kenya was found to have Marburg disease (diagnosis speculative). In 1994, a case of laboratory infection with Marburg virus was identified in Russia. In July 2008, a Dutch tourist visited a cave in Western Uganda and later died of Marburg hemorrhagic fever. A US citizen contracted Marburg disease while visiting the same cave in Uganda.

### Clinical manifestations of Ebola and Marburg virus infections

The incubation time is 3–16 days (5–10 days typical range). There is abrupt onset of fever, accompanied by myalgia and headache, followed by vomiting, abdominal pain, diarrhea, chest pain, cough, and pharyngitis. Thrombocytopenia and leucopenia with elevated transaminase levels are characteristic. As the disease progresses, wasting becomes evident and bleeding manifestations occur. Bleeding is often from multiple sites, most commonly from the gastrointestinal tract, lungs, and gingivae. In the second week, the patient either improves or progresses to multiorgan dysfunction accompanied by disseminated intravascular coagulation, anuria, and liver failure. Hemorrhage and oropharyngeal lesions carry a particularly poor prognosis. The mortality of Marburg is around 25%, whereas it is around 80% for Ebola. Studies during epidemics show that subclinical infections are uncommon.

## Diagnosis

Culture is positive during the acute stage. IgM antibodies detected in capture ELISA are also useful. IgG serologic testing has not been reliable. False positive or irreproducible results are common with the indirect fluorescent antibody test. Confirmation should be done with seroconversion. Seroconversion occurs around days 8–12. Antigen detection or PCR amplification of reverse transcription products provides a practical and sensitive method of diagnosis. Virus isolation should be the gold standard. In convalescence, virus has been isolated from semen for several weeks and from anterior chamber fluid in a case of late uveitis. Fatal cases can be diagnosed by immunohistochemical staining of postmortem skin samples.

## Treatment

In the absence of specific antiviral therapy, management is supportive. Hydration is the mainstay, with replacement of coagulation factors and platelets if indicated. Heparin may be indicated in cases of disseminated intravascular coagulation. Convalescent plasma, interferon, and ribavirin have not proven useful. Nematode anticoagulant protein c2 is undergoing investigation as a potential treatment for Ebola.

## Prevention and control

Prevention of epidemics rests on early recognition of initial cases and prompt institution of barrier nursing. At the community level, properly sterilized injection equipment, protection from body fluids and skin contact during preparation of the dead, and routine barrier nursing precautions are indicated. Extensive quarantine precautions are now in place to prevent the movement of infected monkeys.

## Prevention for travelers

Travelers should not enter or approach mines. They should avoid needlestick injuries, hospitalization at times of Ebola or Marburg virus outbreaks, and avoid hospitals with poor standards of hygiene and infection control.

## Conclusion

Risk of VHF is associated with human encroachment into areas where the reservoir hosts or vectors exist. Travelers are rarely affected by VHF. However, numerous cases of Lassa fever have been confirmed in international travelers who were living or staying in traditional dwellings in the countryside or in small villages. HFRS has been described frequently in military populations. The VHF most commonly associated with nosocomial disease are CCHF and Ebola, and spread is usually associated with extensive exposure to blood in a setting of poor hospital hygiene.

The fatality rate reported in travelers seems to be of the same order of magnitude (although numbers are relatively low) as reported among local populations, despite the fact that the vast majority of them were treated in developed countries.

Travelers should not visit locations where an outbreak is occurring. However, surprises can also occur in one's home country, as the outbreak of Marburg fever in Germany has shown. A high index of suspicion, detailed investigation of the travel and exposure history of the patient, and a basic understanding of the incubation periods and distributions of the various reservoirs of HFV are imperative, as are prompt notification and laboratory confirmation. Clinical management is largely supportive, with special emphasis on safe nursing practices to prevent nosocomial transmission [16].

## References

1 Khan A KT, Peters CJ. Viral hemorrhagic fevers. *Semin Pediatr Infect Dis* 1997;8:64–73.
2 Isaacson M. Viral hemorrhagic fever hazards for travelers in Africa. *Clin Infect Dis* 2001;33:1707–12.
3 Gear JH. Hemorrhagic fevers, with special reference to recent outbreaks in southern Africa. *Rev Infect Dis* 1979;1: 571–91.
4 Gideon Informatics [Online]. Available from URL: http://web.gideononline.com/∞.
5 Peters C. Lymphocytic choriomeningitis virus, Lassa virus, and the South American hemorrhagic fevers. In: Mandell GLBJ, Dolin R, editors. *Principles and Practice of Infectious Diseases.* 6th ed. Philadelphia: Elsevier; 2005. vol. 2, p. 2090–98.
6 Peters C. Marburg and Ebola virus hemorrhagic fevers. In: Peters CS, Simpson GL, Levy, H, eds. *Principles and Practice of Infectious Diseases.* Philadelphia: Elsevier; 2005. vol. 2, p. 2057–9.
7 Mandell GL, Bennett SE, Dolin R., eds. Spectrum of hantavirus infection: hemorrhagic fever with renal syndrome and hantavirus pulmonary syndrome. *Annu Rev Med* 1999;50:531–45.
8 World Health Organization. *Rift Valley Fever.* Available from URL: http://www.who.int/mediacentre/factsheets/fs207/en/.

9 Jaureguiberry S, Tattevin P, Tarantola A, et al. Imported Crimean–Congo hemorrhagic Fever. *J Clin Microbiol* 2005; 43:4905–7.

10 World Health Organization. *Hantavirus Pulmonary Syndrome in the Americas.* Available from URL: http://www .who.int/csr/don/1997_10_02b/en/.

11 Durand JP, Bouloy M, Richecoeur L, Peyrefitte CN, Tolou H. Rift Valley fever virus infection among French troops in Chad. *Emerg Infect Dis* 2003;9:751–2.

12 Fagbo SF. The evolving transmission pattern of Rift Valley fever in the Arabian Peninsula. *Ann N Y Acad Sci* 2002; 969:201–4.

13 Centers for Disease Control. *Hemorrhagic Fever with Renal Syndrome.* 2008. Available from URL: http://www .cdc.gov/ncidod/dvrd/spb/mnpages/dispages/hfrs.htm.

14 Feldmann H, Slenczka W, Klenk HD. Emerging and reemerging of filoviruses. *Arch Virol Suppl* 1996;11:77–100.

15 Gear JS, Cassel GA, Gear AJ, et al. Outbreak of Marburg virus disease in Johannesburg. *Br Med J* 1975;4:489–93.

16 Bausch DG, Ksiazek TG. Viral hemorrhagic fevers including hantavirus pulmonary syndrome in the Americas. *Clin Lab Med* 2002;22:981–1020, viii.

# 14 Rabies and the Traveler

Henry Wilde and Thiravat Hemachudha

Faculty of Medicine, Chulalongkorn University, Bangkok, Thailand

## Introduction

Rabies is again expanding to regions where it had been controlled or was never present. Travelers may be exposed to it in a foreign environment under conditions that are unfamiliar and at locations that are unable to provide adequate care [1]. Rabies is most commonly transmitted by bites from infected mammals. The rabies virus can infect any mammal. In human beings, it is a fatal disease, but some mammals are known to recover from it. The rabies virus can be found on all land areas except Greenland, Antarctica, and some isolated islands. In Australia, previously considered rabies-free, fruit as well as insect-eating bats harbor Australian bat lyssavirus, which has caused a fatal rabies-like illness in two humans [2]. Regions harboring stray unvaccinated dogs present the greatest risk to human beings, and dogs are the principal vectors worldwide. Raccoons, skunks, foxes, wolves, and other wild carnivores are threats in some parts of the world, but account for few human deaths. Bats are the principal transmitting vector to humans among wildlife, particularly in the Americas. Fifty-six nontransplant-associated cases of bat rabies were identified from 1950 to 2007 in bats within the United States and Canada [3]. Monkey bites are not uncommon in tourists. If they occur in a canine rabies-endemic region, this should be considered a rabies exposure and dealt with in the same manner as a dog or cat bite. Asian rats can be large and live in close proximity to dogs and cats. Rabies in rats is extremely rare but has been reported. A local expert should be consulted in the event of a severe rat bite.

Rabies reporting is unreliable in many endemic countries. The number of human deaths annually from rabies is unknown but thought to be well over 55,000. Nearly half of these are in children. Small children are less able to defend themselves against biting animals and are more likely to be bitten severely in high-risk body regions such as the face, head, and hands. Rabies is responsible for more deaths than polio, yellow fever, Japanese encephalitis, SARS, or meningococcal meningitis. India alone has over 20,000 estimated annual human rabies deaths and Pakistan approximately 5000 [4]. The disease is not reportable in these countries and the numbers are estimates. Rabies is emerging again in China, which was virtually rabies-free under the rule of Mao Zedong. There were over 3000 reported annual human cases in China between 1991 and 2005 and, in contrast to the rest of Asia, most appeared to have been from domestic dogs [5]. Japan, Taiwan, Malaysia, Singapore, and South Korea eliminated canine rabies decades ago, but bat rabies may still be a hidden danger. Disease control can only be effective by strict enforcement of canine and feline vaccination rules and elimination of unsupervised dogs. This is not yet a universal practice in canine rabies-endemic countries [6].

Rabies can be transmitted by bites from virtually any mammal, through the inhalation of bat secretions, and through the transplantation of infected tissues [7,8]. Bats do not often interact with human beings, but transmission to humans and pets has been documented in the Americas, Europe, and Australia. Indigenous bat lyssaviruses have now been identified in the Philippines, Thailand, Siberia, Central Asia, and Cambodia, as well as in Europe, Australia, and Africa. It is likely that there are still undetected bat lyssaviruses in many parts of the world, and one must assume that any bat contact anywhere in the world may present a rabies exposure [9]. Britain, previously considered rabies-free, recently experienced a human death from a European bat lyssavirus. Bat bites are often virtually painless and the rabies virus variants that infect bats have an increased ability to infect skin cells. Bats have been shown to harbor several other viruses potentially dangerous to human beings, such as Nipah and Hendra viruses in Australia and in South and Southeast Asia [10]. Most bats are migratory and are able to fly long distances. Dogs, cats, and other vector animals are

*Tropical Diseases in Travelers*, 1st edition. Edited by E. Schwartz.
© 2009 by Blackwell Publishing, ISBN: 978-1-4051-8441-0.

occasionally transported from rabies-endemic regions to rabies-free ones. The introduction of rabies to rabies-free Flores Island by Indonesian fishermen from Sulawesi resulted in an ongoing rabies outbreak with over 100 human deaths [11].

Rabies may present special problems to the international traveler. Modern vaccines or immunoglobulins or the staff to administer them may not be readily available [1]. Animal contacts such as exposure to bites, licks, or saliva of potentially rabid mammals are not uncommon in travelers. Potential rabies exposures are now being increasingly reported.

Recent reports from the GeoSentinel database showed that 1.4% of all post-travel visits were due to animal bites. These were more frequent in travelers returning from South and Southeast Asia. The main contacts were with dogs in 51% and monkeys in 21% of cases. The GeoSentinel database did not report human rabies in travelers, but several other reports have documented cases in travelers and immigrants, notably GIDEON, the Global Infectious Disease Database [available from http://www.gideononline.com]. Even though travel clinics in developed countries are usually able to provide advice on pre-exposure immunization as well as the vaccines to administer it, not all have up-to-date information about the actual risk in the area that is to be visited. When a traveler has experienced a potential rabies exposure, this is usually accompanied by severe anxiety and often doubts that locally obtained advice and services offered are adequate or trustworthy. A call to the travel clinic or family doctor back home often follows and often fails to provide the correct advice, due to lack of local knowledge. We have also encountered cases in which the wrong advice was given, for instance, that a patient bitten by a potentially rabid animal should immediately return to Europe, Australia, or America rather than proceed to the nearest facility with adequate care, which is often nearby.

## Clinical diagnosis of rabies

Rabies presents in two forms, furious and paralytic, but atypical presentations are also seen. Diagnosis of canine and feline rabies is not difficult when it is of the furious form. Irritability, aggression, increased salivation, and indiscriminate biting with damaged and inflamed oral structures suggest rabies. The dumb or paralytic form of rabies (approximately 30% in dogs) is usually associated with paralysis of the hind limbs initially and with minimal or no aggression. It is difficult to diagnose because the clinical picture is similar to that of other canine infections, such as distemper [12]. Given the similarity to other illnesses, euthanasia and brain examination using the direct fluorescent antibody test must be considered whenever possible in rabies-endemic regions. However, this may not always be available and it is, therefore, safest to start postexposure prophylaxis (PEP) immediately in a possibly exposed human. A free interactive computer program (available from http://www.soonak.com/ rabies in English and Thai versions) can aid in the clinical diagnosis of canine and human rabies.

The furious human form is characterized by vague, often flu-like prodromal symptoms, fever, headache, myalgia, and even diarrhea. Pain or abnormal sensation in or near the bite site is seen in 30% of cases associated with dog variants but is more common with bat variants. This is followed by the neurological phase, consisting of alternating intervals of severe anxiety, agitation, aggression, and coherent calmness. Hydrophobic and aerophobic spasms of the neck and diaphragm may occur intermittently; they may not appear together or be present in every case. Autonomic dysfunctions may start early but usually become prominent in the neurological phase. They consist of excessive salivation, fluctuating blood pressure, urinary incontinence, cardiac arrhythmias, pupillary dysfunctions, and neurogenic pulmonary edema. Hallucinations and seizures are rare in dog-related cases but can often be seen in bat-related cases. Coma soon ensues with respiratory failure, leading to rapid demise unless life is prolonged by cardiopulmonary support. One-third of human cases present as the paralytic form, resembling the Guillain–Barré syndrome, which is difficult to diagnose without experience and sophisticated laboratory help. Phobic spasms can be seen in only half of paralytic cases. Survival time is longer than in the furious form (11 vs 5 days) [13]. The paralytic form of rabies in humans is not due to different virus characteristics. We have found that the same dog can cause the furious form in one victim and the paralytic form in another. The clinical signs and symptoms appear to be due to different host responses and are caused largely by immune dysfunction of peripheral nerves and an earlier brain immune response with a delay in neuroinvasiveness [14].

Rabies must be considered in any patient presenting with an unclear encephalopathy. An acute psychosis or use of illicit drugs, medications, or alcohol may mislead clinicians. A history of recent animal encounters (which may be absent in cryptic bat-related cases or unsupervised small children), fever, muscular paralysis with preserved consciousness and intact sensory function, urinary incontinence, percussion myoedema, inspiratory spasms, and rapid progression to respiratory failure suggest paralytic rabies. Rabies awareness is inadequate worldwide. This became tragically evident in recent transplantation-related disasters in Germany and the United States [8].

## Laboratory diagnosis of rabies

Postmortem brain examination for rabies antigen by the direct fluorescent antibody test (DFA) or for rabies RNA using molecular techniques is the gold standard for diagnosing rabies. Antemortem laboratory diagnosis of rabies in animals is not recommended because the distribution of virus in organs may vary and viral shedding in saliva, urine, and spinal fluid is intermittent [15]. Several saliva-based rapid tests have been proposed, but they have never been adequately field-tested. They should be considered unreliable, if for no other reason than that virus excretion in saliva is intermittent.

There were no false negative results in a prospective study of 8987 brain impression smears using the DFA test carried out by an experienced laboratory [16]. Brain tissue, dried on filter paper, can be kept at room temperature for many days for rabies virus RNA detection [17]. To be of clinical value, results must be rapidly available, sensitive, and specific, because they will contribute to evidence-based postexposure management decisions [7]. In contrast to the above-mentioned methods, detection of classical Negri bodies (by Sellers stain) in histopathological specimens is neither sensitive nor specific. The genetic sequence of rabies virus is useful for epidemiological surveillance and the study of transmission dynamics and should be obtained wherever possible [18]. New and simplified tests that may one day replace the DFA test, which requires an expensive fluorescent microscope and conjugate reagents, are also emerging [19, 20].

Real time-polymerase chain reaction (RT-PCR) and other molecular techniques can be performed, with results known within a day or less. Saliva, cerebrospinal fluid, urine, hair follicles, and tears should be tested simultaneously and repeatedly when results are negative, owing to the varied distribution of the virus and to the intermittency of virus secretion. Negative results require repeated testing when there is clinical suspicion of rabies [21]. CT is of virtually no diagnostic value in rabies other than to exclude other diseases. Carefully carried out MRI can be helpful and is the subject of several recent studies that also analyzed viral and cytokine distribution in relation to MRI abnormalities [22]. However, results are variable and closely related to the time when the MRI is performed. MRI performed early in the clinical course may show only trivial changes. Significant findings appear late (Figure 14.1) [13, 23]. In the recent transplant-related rabies cases, MRI abnormalities were extensive. Brain biopsy is now rarely done in rabies patients, but can demonstrate the virus using DFA or molecular techniques. The authors do not recommend using tissue donors who have unclear neurological disease. We know of one case where a homeless street person was fatally struck by a truck and used as a corneal donor. Two recipients died of rabies [unpublished data]. If, however, such a donor is still considered, multiple brain samples should be examined before any tissue is used for transplants [8]. A limited brain necropsy can be done via the superior orbital fissure using a kidney or liver biopsy needle. This is invaluable for confirming the diagnosis and obtaining tissue for sequencing the virus when a complete necropsy cannot be performed. A VDO demonstration of this procedure can be seen at www.soonak.com and at www.cueid.org.

## Management of human rabies patients

Treatment of human rabies was the subject of a 2002 Canadian- and US Centers for Disease Control and Prevention (CDC)-sponsored conference in Toronto. The convened experts agreed that supportive and comfort care is the first goal. There have been many past efforts to cure rabies using antiviral agents, such as ribavirin, interferons, and intrathecal immunoglobulin [24]. The authors treated one patient with 900 mL of intravenous (IV) human rabies immunoglobulin to no avail. The dosage (amount of IgG used) was equivalent to the IV immunoglobulin treatment in immune-mediated diseases such as the Guillain-Barré syndrome. This patient did not show detectable antibodies in the cerebrospinal fluid (CSF), presenting convincing evidence that the blood–brain barrier remained intact [25]. Intensive curative efforts should be reserved for a time when promising new drugs become available and have been shown to be effective in animal studies. There are as yet no proven antiviral agents against lyssaviruses. However, the survival of a 15-year-old girl bitten by a bat in the USA, who had not received PEP, created hope and much media interest. Treatment consisted of intensive care and induced coma with periodic burst suppression using ketamine and benzodiazepine to lessen excitotoxicity mechanisms in the brain, as well as ribavarin and amantadine [26]. This patient was unusual in that she had neutralizing antibodies on admission in both serum and spinal fluid but no demonstrable viable virus. No viral RNA or antigen could be identified throughout her hospital course. Her case was similar to that of the 6-year-old survivor, who also had a

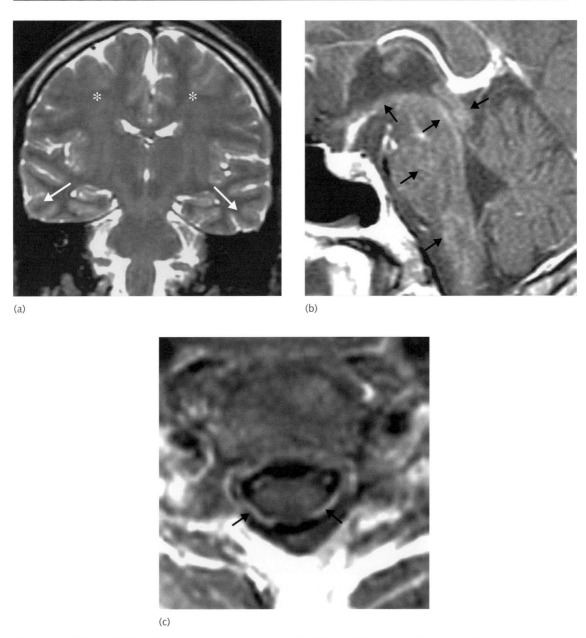

(a)

(b)

(c)

**Figure 14.1** (a) Coronal T2W of the brain reveals only nonspecific ill-defined mild hypersignal T2 change of the cortical grey matter (small white arrows) and subcortical white matter (white asterisks) seen in both paralytic and furious forms. (b) Post gadolinium midline sagittal T1W of the brain reveals enhancement along the hypothalamus, midbrain, tectal plate, pons, and medulla, which can be seen in comatose furious and paralytic cases (small black arrows). (c) Post gadolinium axial T1W of the cervical spine reveals vivid enhancing spinal nerve roots, especially the dorsal nerve roots that is clearly seen in paralytic case (small black arrows). (Photos courtesy of Jiraporn Laothamatas, MD.)

bat bite and early antibodies in serum and spinal fluid. He received PEP but still developed rabies. He was treated with supportive care only and made a full recovery [27]. His virus, or its antigen, could not be identified and he was found to have antibody in the CSF. We suggest that these bat-derived agents could have been of less virulence or that the two young patients were able to mount more rapid cellular and humoral immune responses that contained the disease. There have now been six documented survivors of rabies. With the exception of the two cases discussed above, all had severe neurological sequelae, and antibodies were found in serum and CSF early in the course of their illness. No virus could be recovered from any of them [28]. We treated one rabies patient with the coma induction regimen with ketamine and ribavarin. He never developed neutralizing antibodies and died on the eighth day of hospitalization for multisystem failure. Ample viral RNA was identified throughout his hospital course [29]. Approximately 25% of our dog-related human patients developed serum neutralizing antibodies regardless of the form of rabies. However, none had significant titer in the CSF. Similar coma induction regimens have now been applied to 10 other patients in the USA, Canada, Mexico, Europe, and India, all without success.

## Postexposure prophylaxis

PEP requires immediate vigorous cleansing of bite wounds with flowing water and soap, preferably under pressure. This is followed by application of a viricidal agent—iodophore, benzalkonium chloride, or Dakins solution (diluted household bleach). Alcohol is not recommended because it causes tissue irritation and disturbs healing. Washing with water may decrease the size of the virus inoculum; soap and antiseptic agents denature the virus and may prevent invasion. This is followed by risk evaluation. Even though modern PEP carries few risks of serious adverse reactions, it can be painful and is expensive (approximately $2500–$3000 in the USA). In countries with a well-developed public health care system and few if any rabies risk factors, it is often decided to observe the dog or to euthanize it and have it examined by a competent laboratory. This takes time and can result in delayed PEP, which may come too late. In a canine rabies-endemic country with a large stray dog population, it is a different story. The risk is high and the threshold for PEP is and should be much lower. To play Russian roulette in such a setting is not wise. Monkeys, cats, other domestic and

**Table 14.1** Tissue culture and avian culture vaccines.

| Vaccine | Country | Manufacturer | Diluent |
|---|---|---|---|
| **HDCV 1.0** | **France** | **Sonofi-Pasteur** | **lyophylized** |
| **HDCV 1.0** | **Germany** | **Chiron** | **lyophylized** |
| **PCEC 1.0** | **Germany** | **Chiron** | **lyophylized** |
| *PCEC 1.0* | *India* | *Chiron* | *lyophylized* |
| *PCEC 1.0* | *Japan* | *Kaketsuken* | *lyophylized* |
| *PDEV 1.0* | *India* | *Cadila* | *lyophylized* |
| *PVRV 0.5* | *France* | *Sonofi-Pasteur* | *lyophylized* |
| *PVRV 0.5* | *Colombia* | *VECOL* | *lyophylized* |
| PVRV 0.5 | India | Immunologicals | lyophylized |
| PVRV 0.5 | India | Conoor | lyophylized |
| PVRV 0.5 | India | Barat Biotech | lyophylized |
| PVRV 1.0 | China | Wuhan | lyophylized |
| PVRV 1.0 | China | Hainan | lyophylized |
| PHK 1.0 | China | Wuhan | lyophylized |
| PHK 1.0 | China | Lanzhou | liquid form |
| PHK 1.0 | China | Changchun | liquid form |
| PHK 1.0 | China | Shanghai | liquid form |
| PHKC 1.0 | Russia | Poliom Moscow | liquid form |
| PHKC 3.0 | Russia | Ufa | liquid form |

*Italic:* WHO recommended
**Bold:** US-CDC and WHO recommended
Black: recommended in country of origin and others

agricultural mammals, and even rodents are potential accidental hosts, as they live in close proximity to dogs and bats. However, rodents and rats usually are not capable of transmitting disease among themselves and are considered rare accidental vectors. After careful wound care, PEP follows by administration of a course of tissue culture vaccine (Table 14.1). It is important to understand that it takes 7–10 days for a significant level of vaccine-induced natural antibody to develop. This may leave time for the virus to invade peripheral nerves. Once inside a peripheral nerve, the virus can be reached by rabies antibody and other immune mechanisms, but may not be inactivated and may advance to the central nervous system (CNS). One of our studies suggests that this may be the mechanism for the syndrome of paralytic rather than encephalitic rabies [13, 30]. Passive immunity must therefore be provided as soon as possible after the bite to prevent invasion of peripheral nerves. This is done by aggressively injecting antirabies immunoglobulin (RIG) into and around the bite wounds to neutralize the virus at the inoculation site [31, 32]. Immunoglobulin, if injected intramuscularly (IM) at a site distant from the wound, may be useless. However, the ancient recommendation to inject any RIG left over after

**Table 14.2** Guide for postexposure rabies prophylaxis.

| Category | Contact | Treatment |
|---|---|---|
| I | Touching, feeding animal | None if history reliable[a] |
| | Licking over intact skin | None |
| II | Licks over broken skin, minor bites or scratches without bleeding | Start vaccine and stop treatment if animal is well after 10 days or FAT negative |
| III | Single or multiple transdermal bites at any site or licks over mucous membranes | Inject RIG into and around bite sites. Rest (if any) IM, followed by vaccine series. Stop vaccine if animal well 10 days later or FAT is negative |

*Source*: Adopted and modified from the WHO and US CDC recommendations by the Rabies Advisory Committee of the Thai Red Cross Society.

The US Centers for Diseases Control and Advisory Committee on Immunization Practices recognize only one category of possible rabies exposure from a bite. "Any penetration of the skin by teeth constitutes a bite exposure and requires the use of immunoglobulin injected into and around bite wounds followed by vaccine." Their recommendations regarding non-bite and bat exposures are essentially the same as those of WHO [51].

Rabies vaccination of the responsible animal in a canine rabies endemic region does not exclude rabies. This is particularly true if only one vaccination had been given. Canine and feline vaccine failures and short duration of immunity are common in endemic countries.

Whether an attack is provoked or unprovoked is often difficult to evaluate. Unprovoked attacks are more likely to come from a rabid dog or cat.

In a low-rabies or rabies-free region, observing a biting dog for 10 days before starting rabies prophylaxis may be considered. However, doing this in a canine rabies-endemic country could place patients at grave risk.

[a]Children may present an unreliable history. This is a good time to start pre-exposure vaccination in rabies endemic countries.

adequate wound injection IM elsewhere is still the World Health Organization (WHO) and US CDC party line and must be followed [13, 33]. Following application of immunoglobulin, a WHO- or US CDC-approved vaccine series is started to induce active immunity by endogenous antibody production.

Consultation with an infectious disease expert is advised when unusual problems are encountered. Unusual cases of potential rabies exposure and management problems are not infrequently encountered. To discuss them all here is not possible. Common ones are delay in seeking treatment (which should be started anyway) and the patient being started on a vaccine or regimen that is either not available or not used in his or her home country (treatment should proceed using the Essen IM regimen for whatever injections are still needed). Many other dilemmas often seen have been discussed by Sriaroon [34]. Not all problems have been defined in WHO and US CDC publications or textbooks. A common sense approach and/or consultation with an expert are clearly indicated when an unusual problem is encountered.

Pre- and postexposure rabies prophylaxis is expensive and often not properly performed. Delay in starting PEP must be avoided at all cost. Rabies incubation periods may be as short as a few days, or as long as years. It remains unknown which mechanisms are responsible for this extreme variation in the incubation period. PEP is therefore mandatory irrespective of delay in presentation. This is recommended even if weeks or months have gone by, and the virus may be in the silent phase (in which PEP may or may not help).

Table 14.2 summarizes the approach to rabies-exposed patients. It is best to initiate PEP unless immediate necropsy of the animal excludes rabies. There are no reliable *in vivo* tests on animals that would eliminate rabies. If the animal (this applies only for dogs and cats) is observed and later found free of the virus, the vaccine series can be discontinued. There are no contraindications to rabies PEP. Postexposure rabies vaccination with modern tissue culture vaccines and immunoglobulins has been used safely with pregnant mothers and their fetuses [35]. An infected bite wound can be injected safely with RIG as long as good wound care and antibiotics are applied [36]. A history of vaccination for the dog is not an absolute justification for not providing PEP to a bite victim. It might be considered if the vaccination has been thoroughly documented and reliably administered [37]. The observation that a dog bite was provoked has limited value in excluding rabies [38].

WHO recognized the following postexposure treatment regimens, of which only the first is also approved by the US CDC:

**1** The *gold standard Essen regimen* consists of IM full dose (1 ampoule) injections using a WHO recognized tissue or avian culture vaccine on days 0, 3, 7, 14, and 28 (5 clinic visits).

**2** The *Zagreb or 2–1–1 regimen* consists of 2 full-dose IM injections at different sites on day 0 and 1 each on days 7 and 21 (3 clinic visits).

**3** The *Thai Red Cross intradermal regimen* consists of 2 injections of 0.1 mL of any WHO recognized potent tissue culture vaccine at 2 different lymphatic drainage sites on days 0, 3, 7, and 28 (4 clinic visits).

**4** The *Oxford intradermal or 8-site regimen* consists of 1 injection of 0.1 mL at 8 different body sites on day 0, at 4 sites on day 7, and at 1 site on days 28 and 90 (4 clinic visits).

Intramuscular injections of vaccine must be administered in the deltoid or lateral thigh regions, avoiding fat. Intradermal vaccines are injected into arms or legs at different lymphatic drainage sites. In the Oxford Regimen, injections are also made into the abdominal and intrascapular regions [31]. Just as with BCG vaccination and tuberculin testing, the appearance of a bubble at the injection site demonstrates successful intradermal and not subdermal administration. If the bubble has not appeared (the dose went subdermal), simply repeat the injection nearby. Reduced-dose intradermal PEP (schedules 3 and 4) significantly decreases the cost of vaccine and have been used at rabies control clinics in several countries for nearly two decades. Many studies have shown equivalent immunogenicity and efficacy of the four regimens. There is even some experimental evidence that intradermal rabies vaccination induces an earlier cellular immune response than the IM schedules, which might be clinically significant [39].

WHO recognized tissue culture rabies vaccines have excellent safety records. Adverse reactions are minor and equivalent to those seen with vaccines against polio, mumps, and measles. These vaccines are far less reactogenic than tetanus toxoid.

Transient erythema, discomfort, and itching at injection sites, as well as mild regional lymphadenopathy (particularly with ID regimens), are reported with rabies vaccine injections. Mild transient fever, headache, and malaise are rare. Human diploid cell rabies vaccine (HDCV), and rarely other tissue culture vaccines, may cause reactions similar to serum sickness in individuals who had a prior series and are later given frequent boosters. These are not from the rabies antigen but from immune complexes, usually between serum albumin and propiolactone. Vaccines alone will protect the vast majority of rabies-exposed patients, but it is not possible to predict who will die if not also given passive immunization using immunoglobulin injected into and around the bite wounds. Patients with facial, head, and hand bites are at the highest risk of death, and they represent a priority group if immunoglobulin is in short supply. Patients often present to a clinic after having received vaccine without immunoglobulin. It has been shown that RIG can be administered without significant suppression of the immune response up to 7 days after the first vaccine dose was given [40].

Human rabies immunoglobulin (HRIG) is the first choice for provision of passive immunity. It has a low rate of adverse reactions but is in very short supply, very expensive, and usually not available where it is needed the most (in poor developing canine rabies-endemic countries). See Table 14.3.

The original equine or sheep serum-derived antisera had a deserved bad reputation for serum sickness and anaphylaxis. Second generation highly purified equine anti-rabies immunoglobulins (ERIG) have an acceptable safety margin, causing only 1–7% serum sickness reactions depending on the product, equine protein content, and batch [41]. These systemic reactions almost always appear after approximately 1 week. An effort was later made to reduce serum sickness and the local reaction rate by heat treatment and chromatography purification and by splitting the IgG antibody using pepsin digestion. Whether splitting the IgG by pepsin digestion and other purification steps reduces efficacy remains to be determined, because treated products have a shorter half-life than whole IgG immunoglobulins [42]. Several new manufacturers of ERIG have emerged in Thailand, India, the Russian Federation, South America, and China. Some are currently undergoing WHO preapproval studies and may soon appear on the international market. Unfortunately, all are pepsin-digested split IgG products. However, they are the only RIG products currently available in most of the canine rabies-endemic world and thus must remain an essential biological that is used when RIG is indicated and HRIG is not available. Serum sickness can be

**Table 14.3** Manufacturers of immunoglobulins.

| Human origin (HRIG) (dose is 20 IU/kg) | Equine origin (ERIG)[a] (dose is 40 IU/kg) |
|---|---|
| Sonofi- Pasteur, France | Butantan, Brazil |
| Chiron Corporation, Germany | Laboratorios Biologicas de Mexico (Birmax), Mexico |
| Bayer Corporation, USA | Institut Pasteur de Tunis, Tunisia |
| Razi Vaccine and Serum Institute, Iran | Biorarma, Indonesia |
| Berna, Swtzerland | Central Research Institute Kasauli, India |
| | Sonofi-Pasteur, France |

This listing is based on information available at the time of printing, and may be incomplete. The authors regret any unintentional omissions.

[a]Several commercial firms discontinued production of equine rabies immunoglobulin (ERIG) in 2001. Some of these international firms may be reconsidering their positions regarding ERIG production under WHO pressure.

managed using analgesics, antihistamines, and good communication with the patient. Steroids are contraindicated, as they will suppress the immune response to the vaccine. Using purified ERIG products (of the whole IgG molecule) in Bangkok, we encountered only two cases of anaphylaxis among more than 150,000 ERIG recipients. Both occurred within 30 minutes of the ERIG treatment, and recipients could be managed as outpatients. Transient local injection site reactions are common with ERIG, usually appear within hours, and are best managed by antihistamines and reassurance of the patient. However, facilities that use equine serum products, antibiotics, and other parenteral medications likely to cause rare anaphylaxis must have a protocol and regularly update their emergency procedures. A very promising monoclonal rabies antibody technology has emerged and was found safe and effective in animal experiments. At least two products are currently undergoing human studies, but it will take time for them to become commercially available worldwide [43].

Because brain-tissue-derived Semple (SV) and suckling mouse brain (SMB) vaccines are still being used in some countries, one can expect to encounter patients who have rabies exposure but had prior vaccination with SV or SMB. How should such a patient be handled? A study has shown that antibody responses in such patients are unpredictable. The vaccine batch may have been of high or even no antigenicity [1]. At least one vaccine manufacturer in Asia has consistently made a Semple vaccine with little or no potency. WHO and the Thai Red Cross, therefore, recommend that patients treated previously with nerve-tissue-derived vaccine be dealt with as if they have never been vaccinated, unless an immediate serum antibody titer is obtained from the victim [31].

Lack of funding for PEP is a major problem for physicians and nurses in developing countries. Even when the least expensive reduced-dose intradermal regimen with equine rabies immunoglobulin is used, it amounts to approximately 10 days' wages for a laborer in most developing countries. This is even worse for those working outside large cities and in village health centers, which often have to manage canine bites in patients who do not have the funds to travel to a nearby medical center where they can receive inexpensive intradermal vaccination. The Thai Red Cross intradermal schedule has reduced the cost of a PEP treatment by up to 70% from the standard IM regimens. However, use of the intradermal regimen, where one new bite victim or less is seen daily, makes splitting a vaccine ampoule between more than one patient impossible unless the lyophilized vaccine is stored after reconstitution. Several studies have demonstrated that tissue culture vaccine can be reconstituted and used on the same patient for the day 0, 3, and 7 injections as long as it is held under sterile conditions in a refrigerator. The loss of potency over this 1 week is negligible. This method has been successfully applied in the field but is not WHO approved [44].

## Postexposure treatment failures

Failures of PEP have been reported. Most are due to omissions of or deviations from WHO recommendations. However, there are documented cases where all appear to have been followed correctly in a normal host, including proper wound care, timely start of PEP, use of potent WHO recognized vaccine, and HRIG or ERIG injected into and around bite wounds. A recent paper collected seven such cases [45]. We recently found one more case in the older literature. An 8-year-old American military dependent was treated with daily duck embryo rabies vaccine and whole IgG antirabies serum that was injected into and around the wound. He developed furious rabies 3 months later and died. Autopsy confirmed the diagnosis by mouse brain inoculation test [46]. It is likely that an overwhelming viral load may have been injected into a peripheral nerve or close to its endings in these eight cases. Virus then propagated and advanced toward the CNS within a relatively short time. It is not surprising that severely immune-compromised subjects, particularly those with full-blown AIDS and very low CD4 counts, do not develop antibodies to rabies vaccine PREP or PEP [47]. The best possible wound care and diligent injection of immunoglobulin into and around the wounds may be life-saving in such a rabies-exposed subject. A regular WHO approved PEP vaccine schedule using a WHO-approved regimen must still be administered. There have been no reported treatment failures in subjects who had received PREP or PEP previously and had the WHO and US CDC recommended postexposure boosters.

In addition to immediate and vigorous wound cleansing, antibiotic treatment should be considered in most cases. Even relatively minor cat bites are notorious for causing rapid and often very progressive cellulitis, usually due to *Pasteurella multocida*. Of importance is the fact that *Macaca* monkeys such as *M. resus*, *M. cyanomogulus*, and pigtail macaques in Africa and Asia often carry the simian herpesvirus (Virus-B) that causes encephalitis in humans. The responsible monkeys are usually asymptomatic carriers but may have oral ulcers. This virus responds to acyclovir or valacyclovir. Patients with severe bites require careful wound cleansing, as in the case of rabies prophylaxis. A 2-week course of acyclovir or valacyclovir should be considered.

## Pre-exposure vaccination

Human and equine rabies immunoglobulins are not available in many rabies-endemic regions, and PEP is often not carried out to WHO standards [1,45]. Pre-exposure prophylaxis (PREP) is therefore recommended for travelers to endemic countries, certain occupations that are likely to come in contact with infected animals, and laboratory workers regularly exposed to lyssaviruses. One study from Thailand showed that 9% of tourists had canine contacts

that could have resulted in rabies exposure. This suggests that PREP for tourists to high-risk regions should be encouraged.

Recent studies have demonstrated that immunity following WHO recommended tissue culture vaccine injections is very long-lasting. Neutralizing antibodies can be detected as long as 2 decades after a PREP or PEP series. Booster injections then result in an accelerated antibody response [48]. WHO recommends one IM or intradermal booster injection on each of days 0 and 3 in an individual who experiences a possible rabies exposure after having had reliable PREP or PEP with a WHO recognized tissue culture vaccine at any time in the past. An alternate method is to administer intradermal injections of 0.1 mL of vaccine at four sites (deltoid and lateral thigh) at one setting. This saves clinic costs and travel time and actually results in higher antibody titers than the conventional injections on days 0 and 3 [49]. Persons who are continuously exposed and for whom specific exposures are likely to go unrecognized, such as researchers working with potentially rabid animals or with live virus at high concentrations, are still advised to have periodic antibody titer determinations every 6 months and receive booster only when neutralizing antibody level is below 0.5 IU/Ml to avoid unnecessary immunization. Some diplomatic missions, nongovernmental organizations, and military and United Nations (UN) teams recommend PREP for their staff when they are transferred to canine rabies-endemic countries. Most tourists or business travelers visit rabies-endemic countries for less than 2 months. They are also reluctant to pay the US $300–$400 usually charged for a full three-injection series of PREP by travel clinics in Western countries. Often, there is not enough time before departure to complete such a series. Recent promising preliminary studies have shown that one IM injection of rabies vaccine is sufficient to generate memory cells that respond well to subsequent boosters within 6 months [50]. This discovery may be of interest to military personnel or UN staff who may have to be dispatched on very short notice to high-risk regions, however, this study must to be repeated using a larger population.

Many countries are failing to control canine rabies, yet harbor large stray and uncontrolled dog populations. Cultural and religious barriers, as well as lack of motivation by governments, are mostly responsible for this sad state. Children represent half the world's rabies deaths. This has led to suggestions to include rabies vaccine as part of routine childhood immunizations for high-risk populations. Cost–benefit considerations and priority of funding for other vaccinations have, however, prevented implementation so far. It is gratifying to note that the Gates Foundation is now taking an interest in this.

## References

1 Parviz S, Luby S, Wilde H, et al. Post-exposure treatment of rabies in Pakistan. *Clin Infect Dis* 1998;27:751–6.

2 Delmas O, Holmes EC, Talbi C, Larrous F, Dacheux L, Bouchier C, et al. Genomic diversity and evolution of the lyssaviruses. *PLoS ONE* 2008;3:e2057.

3 De Serres G, Dallaire F, Côte M, Skowronski DM. Bat rabies in the United States and Canada from 1950 through 2007: human cases with and without bat contact. *Clin Infect Dis* 2008;46:1329–37.

4 World Health Organization. *World Survey of Rabies* No. 34. Geneva: WHO; 1998.

5 Zhang YZ, Xiong CL, Xiao DL, Jiang RJ, Wang ZX, Zhang LZ, et al. Human rabies in China. *Emerg Infect Dis* 2005;11: 1983–4.

6 Wyatt J. Rabies—update on a global disease. *Pediatr Infect Dis J* 2007;4:351–2.

7 Hemachudha T, Wacharapluesadee S, Laothamatas J, Wilde H. Rabies. *Curr Neurol Neurosci Rep* 2006;6:460–68.

8 Bronnert J, Wilde H, Tepsumethanon V, Lumlertdacha B, Hemachudha T. Organ transplantations and rabies transmission. *J Travel Med* 2007;14:177–80.

9 Nel LH, Rupprecht CE. Emergence of lyssaviruses in the Old World: the case of Africa. *Curr Top Microbiol Immunol* 2007;315:161–93.

10 Wacharapluesadee S, Lumlertdacha B, Boongird K, Wanghongsa S, Chanhome L, Rollin P, et al. Bat Nipah virus, Thailand. *Emerg Infect Dis* 2005;11:1949–51.

11 Windiyaningsih C, Wilde H, Meslin FX, et al. The rabies epidemic on Flores Island, Indonesia (1998-2003). *J Med Assoc Thai* 2004;87:1389–93.

12 Tepsumethanon V, Wilde H, Meslin FX. Six criteria for rabies diagnosis in living dogs. *J Med Assoc Thai* 2005;88: 419–22.

13 Hemachudha T, Wacharapluesadee S, Mitrabhakdi E, Wilde H, Morimoto K, Lewis RA. Pathophysiology of human paralytic rabies. *J Neurovirol* 2005;11:93–100.

14 Laothamatas J, Wacharapluesadee S, Lumlertdacha B, Ampawong S, Tepsumethanon V, Shuangshoti S, et al. Furious and paralytic rabies of canine origin: neuroimaging with virological and cytokine studies. *J Neurovirol* 2008;14: 119–29.

15 Hemachudha T, Laothamatas J, Rupprecht CE. Human rabies, a disease of complex neuropathogenic mechanisms and diagnostic challenges. *Lancet – Neurol* 2002;2:217–19.

16 Tepsumethanon V, Lumlertdacha B, Mitmoonpitak C, Fagen R, Wilde H. Fluorescent antibody test for rabies: prospective study of 8,987 brains. *Clin Infect Dis* 1997 Dec;25:1459–61.

17 Wacharapluesadee S, Phumesin P, Lumlertdaecha B, Hemachudha T. Diagnosis of rabies by use of brain tissue dried on filter paper. *Clin Infect Dis* 2003;36:674–5.

18 Denduangboripant J, Wacharapluesadee S, Lumlertdacha B, Ruankaew N, Hoonsuwan W, Puanghat A, et al. Transmission dynamics of rabies virus in Thailand: Implications for disease control. *BMC Infect Dis* 2005;5:52.

19 Khawplod P, Inoue K, Shoji Y, Wilde H, Ubol S, Nishizono A, et al. A novel rapid fluorescent focus inhibition test for rabies virus using a recombinant rabies virus visualizing a green fluorescent protein. *J Virol Methods* 2005;125:35–40.

20 Durr S, Naissengar S, Mindekem R, Diguimbye C, Niezgoda M, Kuzmin I, et al. Rabies diagnosis for developing countries. *PLoS Negl Trop Dis.* 2008;3:e206.

21 Hemachudha T, Wacharapluesadee S. Antemortem diagnosis of human rabies. *Clin Infect Dis* 2004;39;1085–6.

22 Laothamatas J, Wacharapluesadee S, Lumlertdacha B, Ampawong S, Tepsumethanon V, Shuangshoti S, et al. Furious and paralytic rabies of canine origin: neuroimaging with virological and cytokine studies. *J Neurovirol* 2008;14: 119–29.

23 Laothamatas J, Hemachudha T, Mitrabhakdi E, Wannakrairot P, Tulayadaechanont S. MR imaging in human rabies. *AJNR Am J Neuroradiol.* 2003;24:1102–9.

24 Jackson AC, Warrell MJ, Rupprecht CE, et al. Management of rabies in humans. *Clin Infect Dis* 2003;36:60–63.

25 Hemachudha T, Sunsaneewitayakul B, Mitrabhakdi E, Suankratay C, Laothamathas J, Wacharapluesadee S, et al. Paralytic complications following intravenous rabies immune globulin treatment in a patient with furious rabies. *Int J Infect Dis* 2003;7:76–7.

26 Wiloughby RE Jr, Tieves KS, Hoffman GM, et al. Survival after treatment for rabies with induction of coma. *N Engl J Med* 2005;352:2508–14.

27 Hattwick MA, Weis TT, Stechschulte CJ, Baer GM, Gregg MB. Recovery from rabies. A case report. *Ann Intern Med* 1972;76:931–42.

28 Wilde H, Hemachudha T, Jackson AC. Management of human rabies. *Trans R Soc Trop Med Hyg*, in press.

29 Hemachudha T, Sunsaneewitayakul B, Desudchit T, Suankratay C, Sittipunt C, Wacharapluesadee S, et al. Failure of therapeutic coma and ketamine for therapy of human rabies. *J Neurovirol* 2006;12:407–9

30 Mitrabhakdi E, Shuangshoti S, Wannakrairot P, Lewis RA, Susuki K, Laothamatas J, et al. Difference in neuropathogenetic mechanisms in human furious and paralytic rabies. *J Neurol Sci* 2005;238:3–10.

31 World Health Organization. *Recommendations on Rabies Post-exposure Treatment and the Correct Technique of Intradermal Immunization against Rabies.* Geneva: WHO; 1996.

32 Briggs DJ. Public health management of human rabies. In: Jackson AC and Wunner WH, editors. Rabies. Amsterdam: Academic Press; 2002. p. 401–28.

33 Anderson DC. WHO guidelines dealing with immunoglobulin use impede rabies prevention. *Asian Biomed* 2007;1: 103–7.

34 Sriaroon C, Jaijaroensup W, Tantavichien T, et al. Common dilemmas in managing rabies exposed subjects. *Travel Med Infect Dis* 2005;3:1–7.

35 Chutivongse S, Wilde H, Benjavogkulchai M, Chomchey P, et al. Postexposure rabies vccination during pregnancy; effect on 102 woman and their infants. *Clin Infect Dis* 1995;20: 818–20.

36 Wilde H, Bhanganada K, Chutivongse S, Siakasem A, Boonchai W, Supich C. Is injection of contaminated animal bite wounds with rabies immune globulin a safe practice? *Trans R Soc Trop Med Hyg* 1992;86:86–8.

37 Sage G, Khawplod P, Wilde H, Lobaugh C, Hemachudha T, Tepsumethanon W, et al. Immune response to rabies vaccine in Alaskan dogs: failure to achieve a consistently protective antibody response. *Trans R Soc Trop Med Hyg* 1993;87: 593–5.

38 Siwasontiwat D, Lumlertdacha B, Polsuwan C, Hemachudha T, Chutvongse S, Wilde H. Rabies: is provocation of the biting dog relevant for risk assessment? *Trans R Soc Trop Med Hyg* 1992;86:443.

39 Phanuphak P, Khawplod P, Sirivichayakul S, Siriprasomsub W, Ubol S, Thaweepathomwat M. Humoral and cell-mediated immune responses to various economical regimens of purified Vero cell rabies vaccine. *Asian Pac J Allergy Immunol* 1987;5:3–7.

40 Khawplod P, Wilde H, Yenmuang W, Benjavongkulchai M, Chomchey P. Immune response to tissue culture rabies vaccine in subjects who had previous postexposure treatment with Semple or suckling mouse brain vaccine. *Vaccine* 1996;14:1549–52.

41 World Health Organization. Rabies vaccines. *Weekly Epidemiol Rec* 2002;14:109–19.

42 Hanlon CA, Niezgoda M, Morrill PA, et al. The incurable wound revisited, progress in human rabies prevention. *Vaccine* 2001;19:2273–9.

43 Nagarajan T, Rupprecht CE, Dessain SK, Rangarajan PN, Thiagarajan D, Srinivasan VA. Human monoclonal antibody and vaccine approaches to prevent human rabies. *Curr Top Microbiol Immunol* 2008;317:67–101.

44 Khawplod P, Tantawichien T, Wilde H, Limusanno S, Tantawichien T, Saikasem A, et al. Use of rabies vaccines after reconstitution and storage. *Clin Infect Dis* 2002;34:404–6.

45 Wilde H. Failures of post-exposure rabies prophylaxis. *Vaccine* 2007;25:7605–9.

46 Anderson JA, Daly FT, Kidd JC. Human rabies after antiserum and vaccine postexposure treatment. *Ann Intern Med* 1966;64:1297–1302.

47 Pancharoen C, Thisyakorn U, Tantawichien T, Jaijaroensup W, Khawplod P, Wilde H. Failure of pre- and postexposure rabies vaccinations in a child infected with HIV. *Scand J Infect Dis* 2001;33:390–91.

48 Suwansrinon K, Wilde H, Benjavongkulchai M, Banjongkasaena U, Lertjarutorn S, Boonchang S, et al. Survival of neutralizing antibody in previously rabies vaccinated subjects: a prospective study showing long lasting immunity. *Vaccine* 2006;24:3878–80.

49 Khawplod P, Benjavongkulchai M, Limusanno S, Chareonwai S, Kaewchompoo W, Tantawichien T, et al. Four-site intradermal postexposure boosters in previously rabies vaccinated subjects. *J Travel Med* 2002;9:153–5.

50 Suandork P, Pancharoen C, Kumperasart S, et al. Accellerated antibody response to rabies vaccination six month after a single intramuscular pre-exposure dose. *Asian Biomed* 2007;1:211–12.

# 15 Enterically Transmitted Hepatitis: Hepatitis A and E

Nancy Piper Jenks[1] and Eli Schwartz[2]

[1] Hudson River Healthcare, Peekskill, NY, USA
[2] Chaim Sheba Medical Center, Tel Hashomer, Israel and Sackler School of Medicine, Tel Aviv University, Tel Aviv, Israel

## Introduction

Enteric infection and diarrheal diseases are the most common medical problems among travelers to tropical and semitropical areas. The risk for diarrhea is largely determined by hygienic conditions in particular areas of the world and the immune status of the traveler. The incidence of travelers' diarrhea among persons from low-risk areas visiting high-risk areas can be as high as 90%. Rates of travelers' diarrhea can serve as a surrogate marker not just for poor sanitation in an area but also for the likelihood of contracting other gastrointestinal infections.

Travelers to the Indian subcontinent are perhaps at the highest risk for enteric infections [1]. These infections include two known enterically transmitted hepatitis viruses, hepatitis A (HAV) and hepatitis E (HEV). Although the two viruses are distinctly different infectious agents (HAV, a picornavirus, and HEV, a hepevirus), they have similar clinical pictures. Their incubation periods are comparable and except for a high mortality rate during the third trimester of pregnancy with HEV, the clinical courses are similar. Both HAV and HEV are considered acute diseases without chronic infection (although there are some recent data regarding possible chronic infection with HEV, as discussed below).

Despite their similarities, HAV is regarded as the most common vaccine-preventable disease in travelers; HEV remains rare in this population. The reason for this difference in incidence among travelers is not yet fully understood.

*Tropical Diseases in Travelers*, 1st edition. Edited by E. Schwartz.
© 2009 by Blackwell Publishing, ISBN: 978-1-4051-8441-0.

For clinicians who see returning travelers, enterically transmitted hepatitis will be the dominant condition. In fact, in two travel medicine clinics, one in Nepal where travelers are seen during travel and one in Israel where they are seen post-travel, about 90% of cases with a known diagnosis were either hepatitis A or E. Interestingly, with the increased use of hepatitis A vaccine, hepatitis E, despite its low incidence, has become an important pathogen. In Nepal, about 40% of the cases were due to hepatitis E, and of the Israeli cases, 52% were hepatitis E (unpublished data).

## Hepatitis A

HAV infection is the leading cause of viral hepatitis throughout the world, responsible for about 1.4 million new infections worldwide each year [2]. The virus is predominantly transmitted by a person-to-person fecal–oral route among close contacts. HAV can, however, remain infectious in the environment, allowing waterborne and foodborne outbreaks and sporadic cases to occur. The virus is extremely resistant to degradation by the environment and can persist as long as 6 months in contaminated ground water. In contrast, HEV is less stable under difficult environmental conditions such as high salt concentration or repeated freeze–thawing. It is also more susceptible to heat than HAV is [3].

HAV is a member of the family Picornaviridae. Because of its unique features, HAV has been put into its own genus, *Hepatavirus* [4]. HAV is a nonenveloped spherical virus, 27–28 nm in diameter, containing single-stranded RNA. The genomic RNA has positive polarity. There are four recognized human and three simian genotypes of HAV.

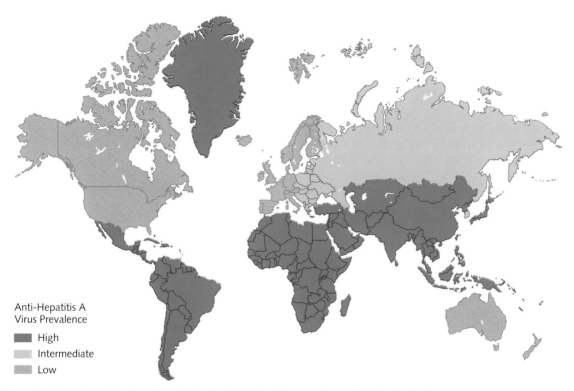

Anti-Hepatitis A
Virus Prevalence

■ High
▨ Intermediate
▨ Low

**Figure 15.1** Global distribution of hepatitis A virus (HAV; based on prevalence of HAV antibodies).

There appears to be only one HAV serotype throughout the world [5]. Thus, persons infected in one part of the world are immune to HAV if exposed in another area of the world.

## Epidemiology

Hepatitis A occurs throughout the world, although there are significant variations in endemicity in different geographic areas, affecting the epidemiologic features (Figure 15.1). Highly endemic countries are typically less developed, lacking public health infrastructure, and have lower standards of hygiene and worse sanitary conditions. With limited access to clean water and inadequate disposal of human feces, HAV in highly endemic areas affects most residents early in life. Often these infections are subclinical and entire populations are immune before reaching adolescence, as demonstrated by age-specific anti-HAV antibody surveillance. Nonimmune adults living in these areas are at high risk of infection and disease, but outbreaks are rare, due to the high level of immunity within the population.

Countries where public health infrastructure has been improving are often moderately endemic for HAV. In these areas of the world, there is a shift to a greater average age of HAV infection than in highly endemic countries. Ironically, the overall incidence of clinical disease is thus higher because there are more susceptible older individuals. An example of a large outbreak of HAV occurred in Shanghai in 1988, with over 300,000 cases after exposure to harvested clams infected with human sewage. Most of those admitted to the hospital were between the ages of 20 and 40. The mortality from fulminant hepatitis increased with the increase of age and in those with chronic hepatitis B [6]. As economic conditions continue to improve in the historically highly endemic HAV countries, early childhood infection and universal immunity will no longer be apparent. The transition to moderate endemicity will likely mean that a substantial proportion of the population will remain susceptible to disease at a greater age. This of course puts these individuals at risk for hepatitis A-related morbidity and mortality. A recent study from Delhi, India, reported that the incidence of clinical HAV disease has increased from 3.4% to 12.3% in adults over a period of 5 years [7]. Data suggest that throughout India there has been a shift in the epidemiology of HAV [8].

Universal vaccination in developing countries, particularly those that are highly endemic for HAV, is not yet indicated, simply because early childhood infection is nearly universal and disease is uncommon. However, in the countries of transition, implementing vaccine programs may become cost-effective. For example, in Israel, which was the first country to implement hepatitis A vaccine as a universal vaccine, there was a dramatic decline in hepatitis A, not only among children but, due to marked herd protection, also in the general population [9].

Ironically, as standards of living and public health infrastructure improve, in the immediate future the global burden of hepatitis A may well increase, as a larger proportion of populations will be susceptible to HAV infection in their adolescent and adult years.

In countries of low endemicity, outbreaks of hepatitis A infection have occurred, for example, secondary to food importation from an HAV-endemic region, as shown with a significant HAV outbreak in the USA as a result of green onions imported from Mexico [10].

## Epidemiology in travelers

Hepatitis A is considered the most common vaccine-preventable disease in travelers to endemic regions of the world. In the 1980s and 1990s, prospective studies of European and American travelers who had not received immune globulin showed a risk of infection of 3–5/1000 per month of stay. Travelers eating and drinking under poor hygienic conditions were estimated to have a rate of 20/1000 per month [11, 12]. More recent epidemiological data have been analyzed looking at the risk of HAV in non-immune travelers to destinations with high or intermediate risk of transmission. These estimates are significantly less than previously thought, with a risk of 6–11/100,000 per month in all travelers to high or intermediate endemic areas and 6–30/100,000 per month in those presumed to be nonimmune [13]. This occurrence seems to reflect the improvement of hygiene in many endemic countries, and travelers are sentinels for this shift.

In the USA, although the absolute number of cases of hepatitis A associated with international travel has stayed about the same, the proportion of cases attributable to travel exposure has increased, accounting for 14.7% of all US cases in 2006. About 70% of these travel-related cases were the result of travel to Mexico or Central or South America [14]. In Sweden, between 1999 and 2004, 35% of all HAV cases were from travel abroad [15].

The use of hepatitis A vaccine in place of immune globulin will continue to dramatically decrease the number of cases of hepatitis A among international travelers. This is of particular significance in long-term travelers, who in the past may not have sought out or had access to repeated doses of immune globulin. In countries such as the USA where hepatitis A vaccine has been adopted as part of a routine childhood vaccination schedule, there should eventually be a sustained reduction in disease incidence. In industrialized countries, childhood vaccine recommendations to include hepatitis A vaccine may have particular impact on children from immigrant communities who are visiting friends and relatives in their parents' countries of origin. If they are vaccinated, this important source of cases of hepatitis A will also be eliminated.

The expectation that hepatitis A vaccine will confer lifelong protection gives successive cohorts of children who have been vaccinated the opportunity to travel internationally as adults without the risk of hepatitis A being associated with their travels.

On the other hand, adult and elderly travelers to endemic areas may prove to be at greater risk for HAV. Their risk stems from two factors: a lack of awareness that they are susceptible to hepatitis A due to the changing pattern of native immunity in their homeland, and a lack of awareness that hepatitis A is not a mild disease but a potentially severe disease among older adults. They, therefore, may not seek immunization before travel.

## Clinical course

The incubation period of HAV ranges from 2 to 6 weeks, with a mean incubation period of 28 days [16]. Shorter incubation periods are seen in those infected parenterally than in those infected through the more common fecal–oral transmission [17]. The spectrum of clinical disease is wide. There are infected persons, as demonstrated by the detection of HAV immunoglobulin M (IgM) antibody in serum, who never develop symptoms and have no elevation of serum aminotransferase levels. In contrast, there are asymptomatic individuals with detected IgM with elevated serum aminotransferase levels. In addition, there are infected individuals who are symptomatic, and the course of the disease can be complicated, including the possibility of fulminant hepatitis and death.

The frequency and severity of symptoms with HAV is highly associated with the age of those infected. Studies demonstrate that 50–90% of children under the age of 5 have asymptomatic disease [18]. In contrast, 70–90% of adults with HAV are likely to have symptoms.

Hospitalization rates of those with clinical hepatitis were reported among cases in the US from 2001 to 2005. Among children under the age of 5, 13.4% were hospitalized in contrast to 42.1% of those ages 60 and above.

Case fatality rates in the United States from 2001 to 2005, as reported through this same national surveillance, ranged from 0% among children less than 5 years to 1.5% in those over 60 [19]. Fulminant hepatitis and death due to hepatitis A occur almost exclusively in individuals infected after age 50. The age distribution of reported deaths over 8 years in the USA demonstrated a mortality rate of over 2.5% in those over age 50 with hepatitis A. In addition to advanced age, those patients with underlying liver disease, such as alcoholic liver disease or chronic hepatitis from other viral agents, are at much greater risk for severe manifestations and fulminant hepatitis [20]. The mortality rate for those with fulminant hepatitis A is 60% [21].

The entire acute illness may last from one to several weeks. Prodromal symptoms include malaise, fever, headache, fatigue, myalgias, abdominal pain, nausea, and vomiting. Among smokers, a loss of desire to smoke can be an early sign of disease (and this reverses itself at the beginning of recovery). Dark urine, light-colored stools, and jaundice may follow. There may also be hepatomegaly and liver tenderness. The fever in the prodromal stage is usually accompanied by significant headaches and cannot be distinguished from the clinical presentation of other classical tropical diseases such as malaria, dengue fever, or typhoid fever. Usually after 3–5 days, fever subsides and jaundice appears, and at this stage the diagnosis becomes more obvious.

Elevated levels of serum bilirubin and serum alanine aminotransferase (ALT), aspartate aminotransferase (AST), alkaline phosphatase, and gamma-glutamyltranspeptidase occur and are much higher than in the other tropical diseases. AST and ALT may precede the onset of symptoms by 1 week or more and usually return to normal within 2–3 months after the onset of illness [22] (Figure 15.2).

The duration of illness is variable, but most individuals begin to feel better within several weeks. In an epidemic of Hepatitis A in Shanghai in 1988, 90% of 1 group of 8647 hospitalized patients recovered completely in 4 months and all recovered after 1 year [6]. There is no carrier state associated with HAV.

Because HAV has the same mode of fecal–oral transmission as several other diseases in endemic areas, it is not surprising that there have been reported concomitant infections with other enteric diseases. Reports include cases of co-infection with HAV and typhoid fever, HAV and amebic liver abscess, and HAV and HEV [23–25]. An

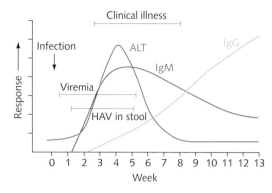

**Figure 15.2**  Events in hepatitis A virus (HAV) infection.

important clue to dual infection in patients is the presentation of an unusual course of HAV disease, such as prolonged fever after the appearance of jaundice.

## Diagnosis

On clinical grounds, hepatitis A cannot be distinguished from other forms of viral hepatitis; therefore, acute disease must be proven with the detection of HAV-specific IgM antibody in serum. HAV-specific IgM antibody is present early in the course of the disease and declines to undetectable levels after 6–12 months [26]. Because wild-type HAV is very difficult to isolate in cell culture, viral detection assays have not been useful. The viral shedding in stool peaks before the onset of clinical illness, and therefore antigen detection is generally not sufficiently sensitive to detect HAV in stool samples. PCR is difficult to conduct and is expensive, and therefore is not used commercially [27, 28]. However, the IgM serology is a highly sensitive and specific test and is readily available. Serological tests that measure total anti-HAV are also readily available but not applicable to diagnosing acute disease, because those with past HAV infection or past active vaccination maintain lifelong antibodies.

## Treatment

There is no specific treatment for hepatitis A outside of supportive therapy. Studies have not demonstrated benefits of activity restriction. Medications that are metabolized by the liver should be used sparingly. Those who are hospitalized are often dehydrated from vomiting and need intravenous hydration. Some patients with fulminant hepatitis are candidates for liver transplantation, although criteria to make that decision are not established.

## Prevention

Immune globulin is 80–90% effective in preventing hepatitis A if given before exposure or within 2 weeks after exposure [29]. Until the development of hepatitis A vaccine, this approach was the only available and effective preventive measure. Studies showed that the rate of HAV infection among Peace Corps volunteers went from 1.6 to 2.1 cases per 100 per year to 0.1 to 0.3 cases per 100 per year after the Peace Corps mandated that volunteers receive immune globulin every 4 months while living overseas [30].

In the 1990s, two inactivated hepatitis A vaccines were developed and licensed worldwide, Havrix (Glaxo-SmithKline Biologicals, Rixensart, Belgium) and VAQTA (Merck & Co, Inc., West Point, PA). These vaccines are available in both pediatric and adult formulations. Studies have shown that the inactivated hepatitis A vaccines are highly immunogenic. In general, 1 month after one dose of vaccine, 90–100% of children 1 year of age or older and adults respond with protective antibodies. The second dose, given 6–12 months subsequently, boosts antibody concentration to what is considered long-term protection. In vaccinated adults, antibodies to HAV have been shown to persist at least 10–12 years after vaccination [31]. The anamnestic responses after the second vaccine have therefore proven to be robust and rapid. With the average incubation period for hepatitis A being 4 weeks, it is likely that those who have seroconverted by vaccine will be protected even if their antibody levels drop below what are considered protective levels. A recent study from Kazakhstan demonstrated that active vaccine given as prevention postexposure is not inferior to immune globulin [32]. It is, therefore, clear that immune globulin is becoming obsolete for the prevention of hepatitis A, in that the vaccine grants specific protection for longer duration. Moreover, it has been shown that for travelers, the hepatitis vaccine can be given even shortly before departure.

## Hepatitis E

HEV is the single most important cause of *acute clinical* hepatitis among adults in many areas of the developing world, specifically the Indian subcontinent and Southeast Asia [33].

HEV is a spherical, nonenveloped virus that is approximately 30–32 nm in diameter and contains a single-stranded, positive sense RNA genome 7.2 Kb in length [34]. HEV is the only member of a new genus, *Hepevirus*, in a new virus family, Hepeviridae. There are five genotypes, each with a unique geographic distribution. Genotypes 1 and 2 have been isolated only from humans; 3 and 4 from humans and swine; 5 is an avian virus that may only infect chickens and other birds. HEV has been recovered from other animals, such as rats, cattle, and sheep, but the impact of these strains on human disease is unclear. There are four genotypes of human HEV and only one recognized serotype [33, 35].

The existence of HEV was suspected for many years on epidemiological grounds. A large outbreak of waterborne hepatitis during the winter of 1955–1956 in New Delhi led researchers, two decades later, to consider the existence of a new virus. The significant monsoon flooding in New Delhi caused the Jamuna River to change direction. The waters ran through the city sewage and then into uptake pipes feeding a treatment plant that supplied water to most of New Delhi. The treatment facility broke down and contaminated water ran through the city's water supply. Subsequently, the hospitals in New Delhi were overwhelmed with hepatitis cases. There were reported to be over 30,000 cases of hepatitis. It was assumed that the etiology of this outbreak was hepatitis A. It was considered unusual at the time to have such a large number of cases when most people were presumably immune to hepatitis A. It was speculated that the contamination of the water supply was so great that it overwhelmed any previous immunity individuals had to hepatitis A. At the time of the epidemic, it was noted that women with hepatitis in the third trimester of pregnancy had a high mortality rate, something not seen in the past with hepatitis A. In spite of these inconsistencies, the belief that this hepatitis outbreak was due to hepatitis A continued for many years.

In 1973, with electron microscopy, Drs. Robert Purcell and Stephen Feinstone identified the hepatitis A virus. During this same time period, the hepatitis B virus was also identified using electron microscopy [36]. This led to the discovery of the serological tests for hepatitis A and B. It was fortunate that during the hepatitis outbreak in New Delhi, sample sera from those with hepatitis had been collected and stored. With the availability of serological tests for hepatitis A and B, it was proven by the late 1970s that the outbreak victims from New Delhi had not been infected with hepatitis A or B. Clearly, a new virus was responsible for the outbreak. The name "enterically-transmitted non-A, non-B hepatitis virus" was coined for this virus [37]. The virus was finally isolated in 1990 and named hepatitis E virus (HEV) [38].

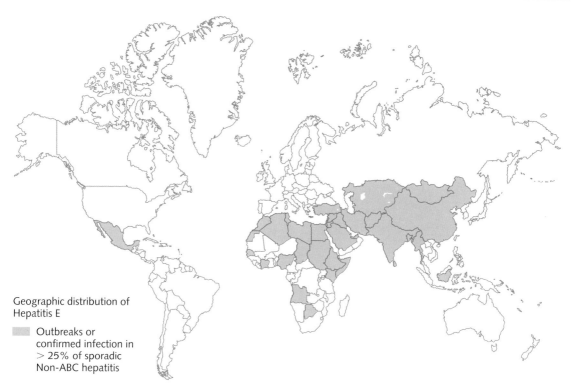

Geographic distribution of
Hepatitis E

Outbreaks or
confirmed infection in
> 25% of sporadic
Non-ABC hepatitis

**Figure 15.3** Global distribution of hepatitis E virus (HEV). Regions of the world where outbreaks or >25% of sporadic non-ABC hepatitis are due to hepatitis E virus (HEV) are in a darker shade.

## Epidemiology

Hepatitis E virus infection is a major cause of both epidemic and acute sporadic hepatitis in much of the developing world (Figure 15.3). Because it is most often a self-limited hepatitis (with the exception of high case-fatality rates in pregnant women) and occurs in areas of the world where serological testing is not readily available, the true burden of the disease is unknown. It has been estimated, however, based on seroprevalence studies, that one-third of the world's population has been infected with HEV [39]. Outbreaks, including massive waterborne epidemics, commonly occur in Asia, Africa, Central and South America, and the Middle East. More than 100,000 cases of HEV were reported in the Xinjiang region of China between 1986 and 1988 [40]. The Kanpur outbreak in India in 1991 recorded over 79,000 cases [41]. More recent outbreaks have been reported in refugee camps in Darfur, Sudan and in Chad [42]. The lifetime risk of infection in countries such as India is as high as 60%, corresponding to hundreds of thousands of cases annually [43].

The peak incidence of clinical disease and seroprevalence occur among older children and young adults. This is in sharp contrast to hepatitis A in developing countries, where virtually all children have antibodies to hepatitis A by the age of 10, often in the absence of clinical disease. The reason for this later onset is not understood.

Seroprevalence studies conducted in various HEV-endemic countries have demonstrated higher seropositivity with increasing age (Figure 15.4) [44–47]. The seroprevalence of HEV seldom exceeds 40%, although some countries, such as India, Egypt, and some parts of China, have a higher prevalence of anti-HEV [44]. A recent seroprevalence study in rural areas of southern China demonstrated a prevalence of anti-HEV that ranged from 25% to 63%, with higher rates in males and those between the ages of 25 and 29 [48]. In Bali, 20% (52/276) of serum samples demonstrated positive HEV IgG antibodies. This contrasted with Lombok and Surabaya, with 4% and 0.05%, respectively. From these same three areas, Bali, Lombok, and Surabaya, seroprevalence studies demonstrated positive hepatitis A antibodies in 95%, 90%, and 89% of the population [49]. Persons from Bali are mostly Hindu and often consume pork, whereas Lombok and Suraby, both Muslim areas, do not. This difference may highlight

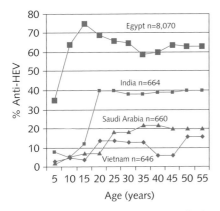

**Figure 15.4** Age-specific prevalence of serum antibody to hepatitis E virus ( HEV) in endemic countries.

the role of zoonotic transmission of the disease from swine.

## Epidemiology in industrialized countries

Clinical HEV has rarely been reported in industrialized countries in North America and Europe. However, seroprevalence studies among healthy blood donors without antecedent travel have demonstrated rates of 0.4–3.9% (Figure 15.5) [50–55]. It is unclear if this level of seropositivity without evidence of clinical disease reflects false positive results or real, subclinical infection.

Seroprevalence studies have also demonstrated that within a number of industrialized countries there are variations of rates of seropositivity. In southwest France, for example, one study demonstrated rates of seroprevalence to be 19.1%, differing from the results of other seroprevalence studies within France [56]. In southwest England, in a study among blood donors, there was a similar finding of

a seroprevalence rate of 16% [57]. There have been seroprevalence studies showing rates of anti-HEV to exceed 20% among US veterinarians who treat swine [58].

During the last decade, more reports of acute HEV infection in industrialized countries have appeared. Many of these cases are among people returning from endemic areas (see below), but clearly there are also a number of reports of autochthonous disease without any recorded travel history [57, 59, 60]. In southwest England, there was a recent report of acute HEV in 21 patients. The genotype matched that of the swine in the geographic area. All of the patients were adults or elderly, and they included more men than women. The cases all occurred during the spring, summer, and autumn months. All of the patients recovered fully [61].

Recently, when the different genotypes of HEV were discovered, it was shown that HEV strains associated with sporadic acute hepatitis isolated from serum samples in North America [62] and Europe (Italy, Greece, Spain, and the United Kingdom) [63, 64] are genetically divergent from strains from HEV-endemic countries [65]. The autochthonous disease in industrialized countries is thought to be spread zoonotically, principally from swine. Thus, the level of seroprevalence of HEV in industrialized countries may truly reflect the existence of the infection. These recent reports underscore the importance of HEV testing in all patients with hepatitis, regardless of their travel history.

## Epidemiology in travelers

The incidence of HEV in travelers is not well defined, but appears to be very low, on the order of 1 case per 1 million travelers [66]. This is a striking phenomenon taking into account that the disease has a fecal–oral route of transmission and is highly endemic in many countries, especially the Indian subcontinent, which is a popular travel destination (the World Tourism Organization reports over 4 million travelers annually to India). Moreover, travelers are not immune to the disease. In a national survey in Israel, only 5 cases of HEV were identified from 1992–1998; all five were in travelers who had gone to the Indian subcontinent [67].

A thorough review of the literature from 1989 to 1999 identified 161 reported cases of acute HEV in travelers and military personnel. The areas of acquisition of the disease were mainly the Indian subcontinent and Southeast Asia [66]. Recent GeoSentinel surveillance data from returning travelers during the period from 1999 to 2005 report 33 cases of acute HEV. The majority of these cases were in travelers visiting the Indian subcontinent [68].

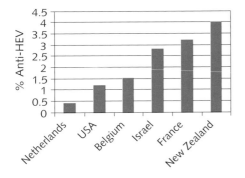

**Figure 15.5** Seroprevalence of antibody to hepatitis E virus (HEV) among healthy blood donors in industrialized countries.

From 1994 to 2003, there were 30 cases of documented Hepatitis E among travelers, expatriates, and Peace Corps volunteers in Nepal who presented for care at three local clinics in Kathmandu (unpublished data). In 2004, in Australia, there were seven reported cases of travelers with acute HEV infection. Five of the seven had traveled to India, the remaining two to Thailand and Vietnam [69]. During a world cruise in 2008, seven UK citizens contracted acute HEV infection during their 12-week voyage, which included visiting several port cities [70]. There have been additional sporadic reports of travelers from industrialized countries contracting HEV.

The total number of reported HEV cases in travelers is in fact very low. However, it is not possible to determine how many cases of HEV in travelers go undocumented. The reason for this is threefold. First, there is a lack of awareness of HEV infection among physicians in industrialized countries, and the diagnosis of HEV may not be included in their differential diagnosis. Second, there is a lack of commercial diagnostic tools in many industrialized countries, preventing confirmation of the diagnosis. Finally, not every proven case is published. Therefore, there is a real likelihood of underreporting,

Seroconversion studies among travelers could prove helpful in the determination of HEV risk to travelers from a low to a highly endemic region of the world. A small number of published HEV antibody seroconversion studies in travelers have been performed to date, as summarized in Table 15.1. A prospective seroconversion study was conducted in 1993 among 356 American short-term business or vacation travelers to developing countries. Of the 236 initially seronegative patients for whom post-travel sera samples were available at 6 months, 4 (1.7%) seroconverted to HEV IgG positive. All four were asymptomatic. The median age was 47.5 years (range 41–55) and the median travel time was 2 weeks (range 8–21 days) [71]. A 1995 retrospective study of 328 North American missionaries serving in various locations in Africa, Asia,

and Central and South America between 1967 and 1984 demonstrated no seroconversion [72]. Two more recent studies show similar results. Among 84 Israeli travelers to Asia (including the Indian subcontinent) and South America, none seroconverted during a mean travel period of 6.1 months [73]. Another large seroconversion study took place in Nepal from June 1997 to December 1998. This study was conducted to determine the seroprevalence of anti-HEV among foreigners living in Nepal and to determine seroconversion rates over a 12-month period. Among the 373 who were negative for IgG antibodies against HEV, there was one case of acute HEV infection, for a seroconversion rate of 0.3%. There were no cases of asymptomatic seroconversion [74]. These seroconversion studies support the impression that HEV is uncommon in travelers (Table 15.1).

Characteristics of the reported cases of acute HEV infection associated with travel are mean age 30 (range 6–65) and 48% male. Seventy-seven percent (53/69) of these individuals had traveled to the Indian subcontinent (India, Nepal, Pakistan, and Sri Lanka). The mean duration of travel was about 3 months, but there was a report of disease acquisition after only 1 day in an endemic area (range 1 day to 12 months) [69].

## Mode of transmission

Transmission of HEV occurs predominantly by the fecal–oral route, although parenteral routes and vertical transmission occur. In endemic countries, contaminated water, resulting in waterborne epidemics, is commonly the source of infection. Less usual are foodborne transmission and person-to-person infection. In regions of the world where HEV is not endemic, the mode of transmission is not well understood. In contrast to other hepatitis viruses, HEV has animal reservoirs. Transmission of HEV from swine and deer has been reported, both epidemiologically and through direct evidence [75, 76].

**Table 15.1** Hepatitis E seroconversion rate in travelers.

| Year of study [ref] | Group | Number in study | Seroconversion rate |
| --- | --- | --- | --- |
| 1967–1984 [72] | US missionaries | 328 | 0% |
| 1993 [71] | US travelers (<3 months) | 236 | 1.7% |
| 1998 [73] | Israeli travelers (6 months) | 84 | 0% |
| 1997–1998 [74] | Nepal expatriates (12 months) | 373 | 0.3% |

## Clinical course

Clinically hepatitis E cannot be differentiated from other types of viral hepatitis. The incubation period is from 15 to 60 days, with an average incubation period of 40 days. Hepatitis E is typically a self-limited illness, lasting 1–4 weeks. Clinical signs and symptoms may include malaise, anorexia, abdominal pain, nausea, vomiting, fever, and jaundice. Serum levels of liver enzymes can be elevated and there can be bilirubinemia. These markers usually return to normal within 6 weeks of onset.

Most patients recover completely within a few months. Long-term postinfection immunity against subsequent HEV infection has been suggested, but lifelong immunity has not been confirmed.

The severity of infections can range from subclinical disease to fulminant hepatitis. There is overall mortality ranging from 0.1% to 4%. The mortality rate among pregnant women infected with HEV during their third trimester is as high as 25% [77]. Fulminant hepatitis is also associated with patients with chronic liver disease [78]. Some patients, however, progress to fulminant hepatitis without any apparent precipitating factors. In 2004, 23 patients presented with fulminant hepatitis at a tertiary hospital in Dhaka. More than half (13/23) of those with fulminant hepatitis were HEV IgM positive. The mortality rate was 87% in this study [79].

## Clinical course in travelers and in industrialized countries

The incubation period and typical clinical course in travelers are identical to what has been noted in HEV-endemic areas for acute HEV. The reported outcomes in one review of travelers with HEV showed that 96% (155/161) completely recovered with no sequelae [66]. Among these travelers, 2.5% (4/161) were reported to have developed fulminant hepatitis. Of those with fulminant hepatitis, two died. One of these was a 65-year-old man with chronic hepatitis C and the other was a woman with no reported underlying liver disease. The case fatality in this review was 1.2% (2/161). The mortality rate of indigenous persons with acute HEV infection in endemic countries is reported to be 0.5–4%, with a significantly higher mortality rate among women in later pregnancy, as discussed earlier.

The very high fatality rate among pregnant women in endemic areas cannot be evaluated in the traveler population or in industrialized countries because cases are very rare. Reports of "severe hepatitis" in two pregnant women from the UK in their third trimesters were noted [66]. Another case of liver transplantation due to fulmi-

nant HEV occurred in an Israeli woman a few days after an uneventful delivery, and she had no history of travel (E. Schwartz, unpublished data).

Hepatitis E seems to be a disregarded disease in Western countries, and many physicians do not consider the diagnosis when there is no history of travel to endemic areas. In a study done in Japan, 18 cases of non-A, non-B, non-C fulminant hepatitis were evaluated. Three of the 18 cases (17%) were diagnosed having acute HEV without a travel history or a history of contact with pigs or rats. The patients were all male, were all over 60, and all had a fatal course [80].

There have been recent reports of chronic HEV infection in organ-transplant recipients. These were cases of HEV acquired in France in patients without travel history. The patients had persistent elevated liver-enzyme levels, viral RNA in blood and stool, which continued for over 6 months, and liver biopsies showing patterns of chronicity [81]. HEV infection in these cases led to both chronic hepatitis and cirrhosis in these patients. This phenomenon is unique in enterically transmitted hepatitis.

## Diagnosis

The diagnosis of hepatitis E is made by detecting viral RNA (RT-PCR) in the serum and/or feces during the incubation phase or in the early acute phase of the disease. HEV can also be diagnosed by demonstration of anti-HEV IgM or a rising titer of anti-HEV IgG in the serum during the late acute or convalescent phase of the illness (Figure 15.6). Commercial ELISA tests for antibody detection are available in Europe, Canada, and parts of Asia. In the USA, however, these tests are not commercially available. In research settings, there are tests for detecting hepatitis E virus antigen (HEVAg) in the serum. Rapid

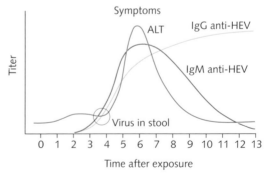

**Figure 15.6** Events in hepatitis E virus (HEV) infection.

**Table 15.2** Comparison of hepatitis A virus (HAV) and hepatitis E virus (HEV).

|  | Hepatitis A | Hepatitis E |
|---|---|---|
| Family | Picornaviridae | Hepaeviridae |
| Size | 27–28 nm | 30–32 nm |
| Structure | +(sense) ssRNA, 7.8 kb | +(sense) ssRNA, 7.2 kb |
| Stability | Extremely resistant to degradation by the environment, can persist for at least 6 months in the environment, can be concentrated by shellfish | Susceptible virus, sensitive to high salt concentration, degraded when freeze-thawed, more susceptible to heat |
| **Diagnosis** |  |  |
| Serology IgM | Up to 6 months, commercially available | Up to 3 months, not easily available, sensitivity and specificity not clear |
| Serology IgG | Lifelong, serology commercially available | Longevity not clear; serology not easily available, sensitivity and specificity not clear |
| PCR blood | Not useful | During incubation period or early acute stage |
| PCR stool | Not useful | Same as above |
| **Clinical aspects** |  |  |
| Incubation time | 2–6 weeks | 2–9 weeks |
| Common age of infection in endemic regions | First decade | Second decade |
| Risk for nonimmune travelers | High | Low |
| High-risk group for severe disease | Adults over age 50 | Pregnant women in second and third trimesters |
| Chronicity | None | Rare; reported in immuno-compromised patients |
| Prevention | Active vaccine, highly efficient HAV vaccine; passive immunization, immune globulin | Active vaccine under investigation (phase 3); passsive immunization not available |
| Mode of transmission | Fecal–oral, person-to-person, or contaminated food or water | Fecal–oral, contaminated water supplies, person-to-person uncommon |
| Reservoir | Humans (rare in nonhuman primates) | Humans, zoonosis (pigs, cattle, chicken, deer) |

immunochromatographic assays for serologic diagnosis are under development [82].

Diagnosing HEV remains a challenge given the lack of available diagnostic methods. PCR is not available in many areas of the world and serology cannot be relied upon.

## Prevention

Individuals with prior exposure to HEV, demonstrated by pre-existing anti-HEV, appear to be protected when subsequently exposed to the virus [83]. The use of immune globulin prepared in HEV-endemic regions of the world does not appear to provide significant protection. This may be because there are relatively low titers of anti-HEV in the general population. There have, however, been studies of the protective efficacy of anti-HEV when immune globulin from patients in the convalescent period of natural infection is pooled [84].

A recombinant HEV vaccine has been developed and a phase II/phase III trial of the vaccine was carried out in seronegative members in the Nepalese military. The three-part vaccine (doses at 0, 1, and 6 months) was proven highly efficacious, with protective rates of 95.5% in subjects who received all three doses. The duration of protection is not known, but the vaccine appeared to render significant protection for at least 2 years after vaccination [85]. The studied vaccine regimen of three doses over a period of 6 months is impractical for travelers. It is also unclear if the vaccine's use can prevent asymptomatic HEV infection, which may be important in terms of transmission through viral shedding and maintaining a reservoir of HEV.

Current preventive strategies lie solely in food and water precautions.

The need for HEV vaccine remains uncertain in that the attack rate is travelers remains low. On the other hand, with excellent vaccines now available for both hepatitis A and hepatitis B virus, the prevalence of these viruses may decline significantly and HEV may become the dominant hepatitis among travelers. In addition, due to the zoonotic factor in transmission, there may be an overall increase in HEV infection worldwide.

## Conclusions

HEV and HAV have a number of similarities, including mode of transmission, incubation time, clinical symptoms, and outcome of infection. However, there are several important differences in the modes of transmission as well as the reservoirs of the viruses (Table 15.2). The two viruses are endemic in many areas of the developing world. For the nonimmune traveler, there is a greater risk of acquiring HAV than HEV. It is clear, however, with a greater uptake of HAV vaccine among nonimmune travelers, more attention may be focused on HEV.

Clinicians who see returning travelers should bear in mind that acute hepatitis after travel in travelers immune to hepatitis A and B is very likely to be hepatitis E.

Through nonimmune travelers who contract HEV, a clearer picture of the pathophysiology of HEV infection may emerge.

## References

1 Greenwood Z, Black J, Weld L, O'Brien D, Leder K, Von Sonnernberg F, et al. Regional relative risks of gastrointestinal infection among international travelers globally. *J Trav Med* 2008;15(4):221–8.

2 World Health Organization. Hepatitis A vaccines. *Wkly Epidemiol Rec* 2000;75:38–44.

3 Emerson SU, Arankalle VA, Purcell RH. Thermal stability of hepatitis E virus. *J Infect Dis* 2005;192(5):930–33.

4 Melnick JL. Properties and classification of hepatitis A virus. *Vaccine* 1992; 10 Suppl 1:S24–S26.

5 Lemon SM, Jansen RW, Brown EA. Genetic, antigenic and biological differences between strains of hepatitis A virus. *Vaccine* 1992;10 Suppl 1:S40–S44.

6 Halliday ML, Kang LY, Zhou TK, Hu MD, Pan QC, Fu TY, et al. An epidemic of hepatitis A attributable to the ingestion of raw clams in Shanghai, China. *J Infect Dis* 1991;164 (5):852–9.

7 Hussain Z, Das BC, Husain SA, Murthy NS, Kar P. Increasing trend of acute hepatitis A in north India: need for identification of high-risk population for vaccination. *J Gastroenterol Hepatol* 2006;21:689–93.

8 Kar P. Viral hepatitis—is it still a challenge in the Indian subcontinent? *Indian J Med Res* 2007;125:608–11. [Erratum in *Indian J Med Res* 2007;126(1):88.]

9 Dagan R, Leventhal A, Anis E, Slater P,Ashur Y, Shouval D. Incidence of hepatitis A in Israel following universal immunization of toddlers. *JAMA* 2005;294(2):202–10.

10 Wheeler C, Vogt TM, Armstrong GL, Vaughan G, Weltman A, Nainan OV, et al. An outbreak of hepatitis A associated with green onions. *N Engl J Med* 2005;353(9):890–7.

11 Steffen R, Kane MA, Shapiro CN, Billo N, Schoellhorn KJ, Van Damme P. Epidemiology and prevention of hepatitis A in travelers. *JAMA* 1994;272:885–9.

12 Steffen R. Hepatitis A in travelers: the European experience. *J Infect Dis* 1995;171(suppl 1):S24–S28.

13 Mutsch M, Spicher VM, Gut C, Steffen R. Hepatitis A virus infections in travelers, 1988–2004. *Clin Infect Dis* 2006;42(4):490–97.

14 Wasley A, Grytdal S, Gallagher K. Surveillance for acute viral hepatitis—United States, 2006. *MMWR Morb Mortal Wkly Rep* 2008;57(SS02):1–24.

15 Swedish Institute for Infective Disease Control [Online]. 2008 [cited 2008 Apr 19]. Available from: URL:http://www .smittskyddsinstitutet.se/in-english/.

16 Neefe JR, Gellis SS, Stokes J Jr. Homologous serum hepatitis and infectious (epidemic) hepatitis: studies in volunteers bearing on immunological and other characteristics of the etiological agents. *Am J Med* 1946;1:9.

17 Purcell RH, Wong DC, Shapiro M. Relative infectivity of hepatitis A virus by the oral and intravenous routes in 2 species of nonhuman primates. *J Infect Dis* 2002;185:1668–1771.

18 Hadler SC, Webster HM, Erben JJ, Swanson JE, Maynard JE. Hepatitis A in day-care centers; a community-wide assessment. *N Engl J Med* 1980;302:1222–7.

19 Centers for Disease Control and Prevention. Surveillance for acute viral hepatitis—United States 2005. *MMWR Morb Mortal Wkly Rep* 2007;56(SS-3):1–24.

20 Lemon S. Type A viral hepatitis: epidemiology, diagnosis, and prevention. *Clin Chem* 1997;43:1494–9.

21 Ciocca M. Clinical course and consequences of hepatitis A infection. *Vaccine* 2000;18:S71–S74.

22 Koff RS. Clinical manifestations and diagnosis of hepatitis A virus infection. *Vaccine* 1992;10(suppl 1):S15–S17.

23 Schwartz E, Jenks NP, Shlim DR. 'Typhoid hepatitis' or typhoid fever and acute viral hepatitis. *Trans R Soc Trop Med Hyg* 1994;88(4):437–8.

24 Schwartz E, Piper-Jenks N. Simultaneous amoebic liver abscess and hepatitis A infection. *J Travel Med* 1998;5(2):95–6.

25 Rodriguez L, Quintana A, Villaba MC, Lemos G, Corredor MB, Moreno AG, et al. Dual infection with hepatitis A and E viruses in outbreaks and in sporadic clinical cases: Cuba 1998–2003. *J Med Virol* 2008;80(5):798–802.

26 Kao HW, Ashcavai M, Redeker AG. The persistence of hepatitis A IgM antibody after acute clinical hepatitis A. *Hepatology* 1984;4:933–936.

27 Jansen RW, Siegl G, Lemon SM. Molecular epidemiology of human hepatitis A virus defined by an antigen-capture polymerase chain reaction method. *Proc Natl Acad Sci USA* 1990;87:2867–71.

28 Hutin YJ, Pool V, Cramer EH, Nainan OV, Weth J, Williams IT, et al. A multistate, foodborne outbreak of hepatitis A. *N Engl J Med* 1999;340:595–602.

29 Winokur PL, Stapleton JT. Immunoglobulin prophylaxis for hepatitis A. *Clin Infect Dis* 1992;14:580–86.

30 Pierce PF, Cappello M, Bernard KW. Subclinical infection with hepatitis A in Peace Corps volunteers following immune globulin prophylaxis. *Am J Trop Med Hyg* 1990;42:465–9.

31 Van Damme P, Banatvala J, Fay O, Iwarson S, McMahon B, Van Herck K, et al. Hepatitis A booster vaccination: is there a need? *Lancet* 2003; 362:1065–71.

32 Victor J, Monto A, Surdina TY, Suleimenova SZ, Vaughan G, Nainan OV, et al. Hepatitis A vaccine versus immune globulin for post exposure prophylaxis. *N Engl J Med* 2007;357:1685–94.

33 Purcell RH, Emerson SU. Hepatitis E virus. In: Mandell GL, Bennett JE, Dolin R, editors. *Mandell, Douglas, and Bennet's Principles and Practice of Infectious Diseases*, 6th ed. Philadelphia: Elsevier; 2005, p. 2204–17.

34 Emerson SU, Anderson D, Arankalle A, et al. Virus taxonomy. In: Fauquet CM, Mayo MA, Maniloff J, et al., editors. VIIIth Report of the International Committee of the Taxonomy of Viruses. London: Elsevier/Academic Press; 2004. p. 279–96.

35 Purcell RH, Emerson SU. Animal models of hepatitis A and E [Review]. *ILAR J* 2001;42(2):161–77.

36 Dane DS, Cameron CH, Briggs NM. Virus-like particles in serum of patients with Australia antigen-associated hepatitis. *Lancet* 1970;1:695–98.

37 Wong DC, Purcell RH, Sreenivasan MA, Prasad SR, Pavri KM. Epidemic and endemic hepatitis in India: evidence for a non-A, non-B hepatitis virus aetiology. *Lancet* 1980;2(8200):876–9.

38 Reyes GR, Purdy MA, Kim J, Luk KC, Young LM, Fry KE, Bradley DW. Isolation of cDNA from the virus responsible of enterically-transmitted non-A, non-B hepatitis. *Science* 1990;247:1335–9.

39 Purcell RH, Emerson SU, Prevention. In : Thomas HC, Lemon S, Zuckerman AJ, editors. *Viral Hepatitis*. Malder, MA: Blackwell Publishing; 2005, p. 635–45.

40 Zhuang H. Hepatitis E and strategies for its control. Viral hepatitis in China: problems and control strategies. *Monogr Virol* 1992;19:126.

41 Ray R, Aggarwal R, Salunke PN, Mehrotra NN, Talwar GP, Naik SR. Hepatitis E virus genome in stools of hepatitis patients during large epidemic in North India. *Lancet* 1991;338:783–4.

42 Nicand E, Armstrong GL, Enouf V, Guthmann JP, Guerin JP, Caron M, et al. Genetic heterogeneity of hepatitis E virus in Darfur, Sudan and neighboring Chad. *J Med Virol* 2005;77:519.

43 Worm HC, Wirnsberger G. Hepatitis E vaccines: progress and prospects. *Drugs* 2004;64:1517–31.

44 Fix AD, Abdel-Hamid M, Purcell RH, Shehata MH, Abdel-Aziz F, Mikhail N, et al. Prevalence of antibodies to hepatitis E in two rural Egyptian communities. *Am J Trop Med Hyg* 2000;62:519–23.

45 Arankalle VA, Tsarev SA, Chadha MS, Alling DW, Emerson SU, Banerjee K, Purcell RH. Age-specific prevalence of antibodies to hepatitis A and E viruses in Pune, India, 1982 and 1992. *J Infect Dis* 1995;171(2):447–50.

46 Arif M. Enterically transmitted hepatitis in Saudi Arabia: an epidemiological study. *Ann Trop Med Parisitol* 1996;90(2):197–201.

47 Hau CH, Hien TT, Tien NT, Khiem HB, Sac PK, Nhung VT, et al. Prevalence of enteric hepatitis A and E viruses in the

Mekong River Delta region of Vietnam. *Am J Trop Med Hyg* 1999;60(2):277–80.

48 Li RC, Ge SX, Li YP, Zheng YJ, Nong Y, Guo QS, et al. Seroprevalence of hepatitis E virus infectrion, rural southern People's Republic of China. *Emerg Infect Dis* 2006;12(11):1682–8.

49 Wibawa ID, Muljono DH, Mulyanto, Suryadarma IG, Tsuda F, Takahashi M, et al. Prevalence of antibodies to hepatitis E virus among apparently healthy humans and pigs in Bali, Indonesia: identification of a pig infected with a genotype 4 hepatitis E virus. *J Med Virol* 2004;73(1):38–44.

50 Zaaijer HL, Kok M, Lelie PN, Timmerman RJ, Chau K, van der Pal HJ. Hepatitis E in the Netherlands: imported and endemic [Letter]. *Lancet* 1993:341:826.

51 Mast EE, Kuramoto IK, Favorov MO, Schoening VR, Burkholder BT, Shapiro CN, et al. Prevalence of and risk factors for antibody to hepatitis E Virus seroreactivity among blood donors in northern California. *J Infect Dis* 1997;176: 34–40.

52 Vranckx R, Van Damme P, Coenjaerts A. HEV infections in selected Belgium populations. In: Buisson Y, Coursaget P, Kane M, editors. *Enterically Transmitted Hepatitis Viruses, Proceedings of the International Symposium on Enterically Transmitted Hepatitis Viruses.* Joue-les-Tours (France): La Simarre; 1996, p. 225–7.

53 Karetnyi YV, Favorov MO, Khudyakova NS, Weiss P, Bar-Shani S, Handsher R, et al. Serological evidence for hepatitis E virus infection in Israel. *J Med Virol* 1995;45(3):316–20.

54 Boutrouille A, Bakkali-Kassimi L, Cruciere C, Pavio N. Prevalence of anti-hepatitis E virus antibodies in French blood donors. *J Clin Microbiol* 2007;45(6):2009–10.

55 Dalton HR, Fellows HJ, Gane EJ, Wong P, Gerred S Schroeder B, et al. Hepatitis E in new Zealand. *J Gastroenterol Hepatol* 2007;22(8):1236–40.

56 Mansuy JM, Legrand-Abravanel F, Calot JP, Peron JM, Alric L, Agudo S, et al. High prevalence of anti-hepatitis E virus antibodies in blood donors from Southwest France. *J Med Virol* 2008;80(2):289–93.

57 Dalton HR, Stableforth W, Hazeldine S, Thurairajah P, Ramnarace R, Warshow U, et al Autochthonous hepatitis E in Southwest England: a comparison with hepatitis A. *Eur J Clin Microbiol Infec Dis* 2008;27(7):579–85.

58 Meng XJ, Wiseman B, Elvinger F,Guenette DK, Toth TE, Engle RE, et al. Prevalence of antibodies to hepatitis E virus in veterinarians working with swine and in normal blood donors in the United States and other countries. *J Clin Microbiol* 2002;40:117–122.

59 De Silva AN, Muddu AK, Iredale JP, Sheron N, Khakoo SI, Pelosi E. Unexpectedly high incidence of indigenous acute hepatitis E within South Hampshire: time for routine testing? *J Med Virol* 2008;80(2):283–8.

60 Renou C, Moreau X, Pariente A, Cadranel JF, Maringe E, Morin T, et al. A national survey of acute hepatitis E in France. *Aliment Pharmacol Ther* 2008;27(11):1086–93.

61 Dalton HR, Thurairajah PH, Fellows HJ, Hussaini HS, Mitchell J, Bendall R et al. Autochthonous hepatitis E in southwest England. *J Viral Hep* 2007;14(5):304–9.

62 Kwo PY, Schlauder GG, Carpenter HA, Murphy PJ, Rosenblatt JE, Dawson GJ, et al. Acute hepatitis E by a new isolate acquired in the United States. *Mayo Clin Proc* 1997;72:1133–6.

63 Pina S, Buti M, Cotrina M, Piella J, Girones R. HEV identified in serum from humans with acute hepatitis and in sewage of animal origin in Spain. *J Hepatol* 2000;33:826–33.

64 Zanetti AR, Schlauder GG, Romano L, Tanzi E, Fabris P, Dawson GJ, et al. Identification of a novel variant of hepatitis E virus in Italy. *J Med Virol* 1999;57:356–60.

65 Schlauder GG, Mushaahwar IK. Genetic heterogeneity of hepatitis E virus. *J Med Virol* 2001;65:282–92.

66 Piper Jenks N, Horowitz H, Schwartz E. The risk of hepatitis E infection to travelers. *J Travel Med* 2000;7:194–9.

67 Schwartz E, Piper Jenks N, Van Damme P, Galun E. Hepatitis E virus infection in travelers. *Clin Infect Dis* 1999;29;1312–14.

68 Reed C, Freedman DO, Castelli F,Chen L, Pandy P, Parola P et al. Increase in hepatitis E among travelers reported to the GeoSentinel surveillance system [Abstract]. 43rd Annual Meeting of the Infectious Diseases Society of America. San Francisco; October 2005.

69 Cowie B, Adamopoulos J, Carter K, Kellly H. Hepatitis E infections, Victoria Australia. *Emerg Infect Dis* 2005;11(3): 482–4.

70 Promed. *Hepatitis E, world cruise.* 2008 May 1. Available from URL: http://www.promedmail.org, archive number: 20080501.1503.

71 Ooi W, Gawoki J, Yarbough P, Pankey G. Hepatitis E Seroconversion in United States travelers abroad. *Am J Trop Med Hyg* 1999;61(5):822–24.

72 Smalligan R, Lange W, Frame J, et al. The rik of viral hepatitis A,B, C and E among North American missionaries. *Am J Trop Med Hyg* 1995;53:233–6.

73 Potasman I, Koren L, Peterman M, Srugo I. Lack of hepatitis E infection among backpackers to tropical countries. *J Travel Med* 2000;7:208–10.

74 Shlim DR, Pandey P, Scott R, Vaughn DW. Risk of Hepatitis E infection among foreigners living in Nepal [Abstract FC 1.4]. In: *Proceedings of the 6th Conference of the International Society of Travel Medicine*, Montreal; 1999.

75 Masuda J, Yano K, Tamada Y, Takii Y, Ito M, Omagari K, Kohno S. Acute hepatitis E of a man who consumed wild boar meat prior to the onset of illness in Nagasaki, Japan. *Hepatol Res* 2005;31:178–83.

76 Tei S, Kitjima N Takahashi K, Mishiro S. Zoonotic transmission of hepatitis E virus from deer to human beings. *Lancet* 2003;362:371–3.

77 Khuroo MS, Teli MR, Skidmore S, Sofi MA, Khuroo MI. Incidence and severity of viral hepatitis in pregnancy. *Am J Med* 1981;70:252–5.

78 Ramachandran J, Eapen C, Kang G, Abraham P, Hubert DD, Kurian G, et al. Hepatitis E superinfection produces severe

decompensation in patients with chronic liver disease. *J Gastroenterol Hep* 2004;19:134–8.

79 Mantab MA, Rahman S, Khan M, Marmum AA, Afroz S. Etiology of fulminant hepatic failure: experience from a tertiary hospital in Bangladesh. *Hepatobilary Pancreat Dis Int* 2008;7(2):161–2.

80 Suzuki K, Aikawa T, Okamoto H. Fulminant Hepatitis E in Japan. *N Engl J Med* 2002;347:1456.

81 Kamar N, Selves J, Mansuy JM, Ouezzani L, Peron JM, Gutard J, et al. Hepatitis E virus and chronic hepatitis in organ-transplant recipients. *N Engl J Med* 2008;358:811–17.

82 Myint KS, Guan M, Chen HY, Lu Y, Anderson D, Howard T, et al. Evaluation of a new rapid immunochromatographic assay for serodiagnosis of acute hepatitis E infection. *Am J Trop Med Hyg* 2005;73:942.

83 Bryan JP, Tsarev SA, Iqbal M, Ticehurst J, Emerson S, Ahmed A, et al. Epidemic hepatitis E in Pakistan: patterns of serologic response and evidence that antibody to hepatitis E virus protects against disease. *J Infect Dis* 1994;170:517–21.

84 Pillot J, Turkoglu S, Dubreuil P, Cosson A, Lemaigre G, Meng J, et al. Cross-reactive immunity against different strains of the hepatitis E virus transferable by simian and human sera. *C R Acad Sci III* 1995;318:1059–64.

85 Shresta MP, Scott RM, Joshi DM, Mammen MP Jr, Thapa GB, Thapa N, et al. Safety and efficacy of a recombinant hepatitis E vaccine. *N Engl J Med* 2007;365:895–903.

# 16 Typhoid and Paratyphoid Fever

Eli Schwartz

Chaim Sheba Medical Center, Tel Hashomer, Israel and Sackler School of Medicine, Tel Aviv University, Tel Aviv, Israel

## Introduction

Enteric fever is the inclusive term for the systemic infections that are caused by the bacterium *Salmonella enterica*, serotype *S. typhi*, and by *S. enterica*, serotype *S. paratyphi*. Because *S. typhi* is the predominant pathogen, the term *typhoid fever* is often used for both typhoid and paratyphoid fever.

Typhoid fever (TF) is a fecal–oral transmissible disease, and therefore it is primarily found where overcrowding, poor sanitation, and untreated water are the norm. It used to have a worldwide distribution, including the Western world (the USA and Europe), until early in the twentieth century. Sanitation and hygiene have been largely responsible for the dramatic decrease witnessed through the last century. Today, most typhoid infections occur in less developed countries, where sanitary conditions remain poor and water supplies are not treated. Cases in industrialized countries are imported by travelers or migrants. Humans are the only known reservoir, and transmission occurs through food and water contaminated by acutely ill or chronic carriers of the organism.

## Epidemiology

According to WHO data, there are 16–33 million cases of typhoid fever annually, with a yearly death toll of approximately 500,000 [1]. However, it is difficult to obtain accurate data on disease burden in developing countries because the diagnosis of typhoid fever is often a clinical one, without blood culture confirmation, and most patients are treated as outpatients [2]. Public health figures may, therefore, underestimate typhoid incidence compared to community-based studies. The greatest burden of disease

*Tropical Diseases in Travelers*, 1st edition. Edited by E. Schwartz.
© 2009 by Blackwell Publishing, ISBN: 978-1-4051-8441-0.

is in Asia, where there are an estimated 13 million cases, with 400,000 deaths annually [3] (Figure 16.1). There has been a rise in cases since the 1990s [4].

Annual incidence rates of up to 198 per 100,000 in the Mekong Delta region in Vietnam [5] and 980 per 100,000 in Delhi, India [6] have recently been reported. In these places, the highest incidence of the disease is found among schoolchildren age 5–15, although high rates are also found among children aged less than 5 years. The incidence may vary considerably, even within a country, or within a city where it predominantly affects the urban slums [1].

### Epidemiology of typhoid fever in developed countries

In developed countries where typhoid fever used to be endemic, there have been two major changes in the pattern of disease. One is a marked decline in incidence in the past half century, and the other is that the disease has become predominantly travel-associated (Figure 16.2). In the United States, the number of typhoid cases fell from 35,994 in 1920 to an average of 500 cases annually (mostly imported) in the 1990s, which can be translated to an annual incidence that has dropped from 7.5 per 100,000 in 1940 to 0.2 per 100,000 in the 1990s. Correspondingly, the proportion of cases related to foreign travel increased from 33% in 1967–1972 to 81% in 1996–1997 [7–9]. In Israel, the change was even more marked, with an annual incidence of 90/100,000 in the early 1950s that dropped to 0.23/100,000 in 2003, of which 57% were acquired abroad [10]. Altogether, the range of reported annual incidence in industrialized countries in the last decade is from 0.13 to 1.2 cases per 100,000 population, with the overwhelming majority being imported [9, 11, 12].

### Epidemiology of typhoid fever in travelers

The risk for travelers appears to vary with geographic region visited and with the economic development of the country (Table 16.1). Several reports indicate that travel

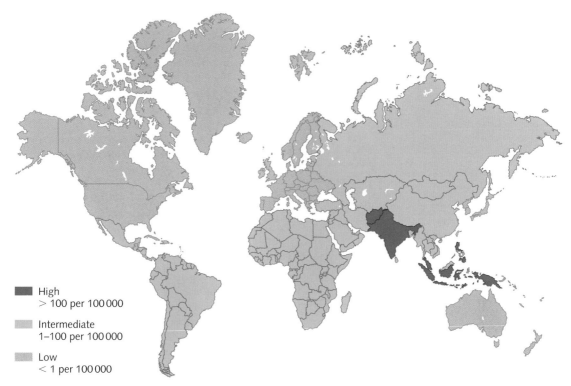

**Figure 16.1** Annual incidence of typhoid fever worldwide. (Reprinted from Connor BA, Schwartz E. Typhoid and paratyphoid fever in travelers. *Lancet Infect Dis* 2005;5:623–8, with permission from Elsevier.)

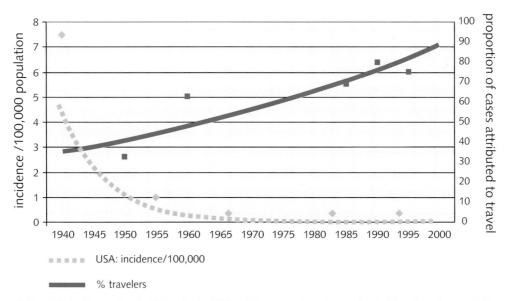

**Figure 16.2** Trends in incidence of typhoid fever in the USA and the proportion of cases of typhoid attributed to travel. (Reprinted from Connor BA, Schwartz E. Typhoid and paratyphoid fever in travelers. *Lancet Infect Dis* 2005;5:623–8, with permission from Elsevier.)

**Table 16.1** Incidence of typhoid fever in Israeli and American travelers to selected destinations vs local incidence.

| Country | World Bank income group[a] | Cases/100,000 travelers | Cases/100,000 local residents |
|---|---|---|---|
| Mexico | Upper middle | 0.13 | Not available |
| Jordan | Middle | 0.3 | 2.3 |
| Egypt | Middle | 0.3 | 13 |
| Thailand | Middle | 0.4 | 53.8 |
| Morocco | Middle | 0.7 | 8.2 |
| Turkey | Middle | 1.0 | 3.8 |
| Nepal | Low | 7.9 | 162 |
| India | Low | 27–81 | 980 |

*Source*: From [16].

[a] Low income, $765 or less; middle income, $766–$3,035; upper middle income, $3,036–$9,368 (annual per capita income).

to the Indian subcontinent carries the highest risk of acquiring TF.

For example, among travelers from the United States, the overall risk of travel to the Indian subcontinent was 18 times higher than for travel to any other geographic region. In addition, whereas the incidence of typhoid fever among US travelers to Mexico decreased from 0.19 to 0.13 per 100,000 during the 10-year period 1985–1994, the incidence amongst travelers to the Indian subcontinent increased from 23.4 to 81.2 per 100,000 [9]. British data show a similar trend. In a review of cases in northwest England from 1996 to 1998, 85% of the imported cases related to travel to India or Pakistan [13], and in another review of 200 cases in England and Wales, 80% of cases acquired abroad were related to travel to the Indian subcontinent [14]. In another British report, 75% of cases of typhoid fever were in travelers, and their global risk of ty-

phoid fever was 1 per 100,000 visits, as compared to 30 per 100,000 visits for travel to the Indian subcontinent [15]. In Israel, 74% of imported typhoid fever cases were acquired in India, and the calculated attack rate was 24/100,000 travelers, 100 times higher than for travelers to Thailand or to Middle Eastern countries [16]. Reports from France and Germany also indicate the Indian subcontinent as the main geographic source [17, 18].

As expected, travel to rural areas with poor sanitation is associated with higher risk. Not following food and water precautions and not receiving pretravel consultation increased the risk tenfold [19].

The length of stay is another factor. An analysis of typhoid cases among US travelers demonstrated that 60% of cases were in those staying up to 6 weeks, but it is important to note that 5% of cases had visits of 1 week or less [20].

A special group with increased risk is travelers visiting friends and relatives (VFRs), that is, immigrants who return to visit their homelands. In addition to engaging in more travel to rural areas, VFR travelers are less likely to have received pretravel advice, are less likely to follow food and water precautions, and do not receive typhoid vaccine prior to travel [21].

## Microbiology of enteric fever

Enteric fever (EF) is caused by several members of the species *Salmonella enterica*, which are rod-shaped, gram-negative bacteria. They are all restricted human pathogens, which unlike many other salmonellae do not readily infect poultry, reptiles, or mammalian livestock. The main causative agent of EF is *S. enterica* serovar Typhi, which accounts for 60–80% of cases [4, 22]. The other *S. enterica* serovars are *paratyphi* species A, B, and C, which differ in geographical distribution (Table 16.2).

**Table 16.2** Geographical distribution of *S. paratyphi* species A, B, and C.

| Bacteria | Group | Geographic distribution |
|---|---|---|
| *S. paratyphi A* | *S. enterica* Group A | Indian subcontinent |
| *S. paratyphi B* | *S. enterica* Group B | Indonesia, Malaysia, the Mediterranean region, and South America |
| *S. paratyphi C* | *S. enterica* Group C | Africa |
| *S. typhi* | *S. enterica* Group D | Developing countries, mainly the Indian subcontinent and Southeast Asia |

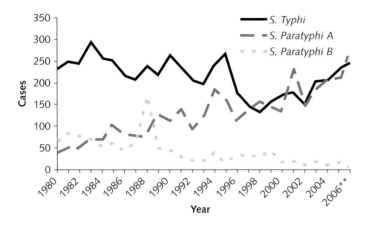

**Figure 16.3** Annual cases of *S. typhi* and *S. paratyphi* in the UK. (Courtesy of the Health Protection Agency, http://www.hpa.org.uk/webw/ HPAweb&HPAwebStandard/HPAweb _C/1195733753804?p=1191942172078.)

The newly emerging pathogen is *S. paratyphi* A, which was considered to be of minor epidemiological importance. However, among travelers, the incidence of disease caused by *S. paratyphi* A was found to be significant. In reports from Nepal, more than a decade ago, the proportions of *S. paratyphi* A and *S. typhi* were 70% versus 30% among travelers, whereas this ratio was reversed, as expected, in the local population [23]. The same holds true in the UK, where the number of cases of *S. paratyphi* A, mostly acquired in the Indian subcontinent, exceeded the number of cases of *S. typhi* infection (Figure 16.3).

Several recent reports from Southeast Asia and the Indian subcontinent have shown a similar trend. For example, *S. paratyphi* A was found in 64% of culture-positive cases in Hechi (China) and in 15–25% of cases in Kolkata (India) and Karachi (Pakistan) [24].

The disproportionate number of cases of *S. paratyphi* in travelers may be the effect of the vaccine, which gives protection only for *S. typhi*. This was clearly shown among Israeli travelers, where among vaccinated patients 29% had *S. paratyphi* A, whereas among nonimmunized patients only 4% had *S. paratyphi* A ( $p = 0.016$ ) [16]. It is interesting to examine whether a similar trend follows mass typhoid vaccination campaigns in endemic countries (e.g., in Hechi, China, where 64% of positive cultures were caused by paratyphi A, typhoid vaccination is part of routine immunization).

## Clinical features

The incubation time from ingestion of S. *enterica* serotype Typhi or Paratyphi to the onset of fever is usually 2–3 weeks (range 3–60 days).

At this early stage of the infection and until the establishment of bacteremia, there are usually no symptoms or clinical signs. However, gastrointestinal symptoms may exist as a result of co-infection with other fecal–oral pathogens, which are common in travelers to these areas.

The hallmark of EF is fever. Classically, the temperature rises steadily for the first few days, and then a persistent fever is established. The three main symptoms at presentation are usually high fever, dull frontal headache, and prostration. This typical persistent fever is often not noted, probably because of the widespread use of antipyretics.

Patients typically present after the onset of fever with influenza-like symptoms, including chills (although rigors are rare), a dull frontal headache, malaise, anorexia, and nausea, but with few physical signs. Cough is a common symptom, but secondary pneumonia is a rare occurrence. In the majority of cases, abdominal signs and symptoms eventually appear. These include abdominal pain, constipation, diarrhea, nausea, and vomiting. Again, the exact percentage of patients with diarrhea caused by EF is hard to establish, because other gastrointestinal co-infections may exist.

On physical examination, hepatomegaly and splenomegaly may exist. Relative bradycardia is considered common in typhoid, although it is not specific for it. Rose spots, which are blanching erythematous maculopapular lesions normally 2–4 mm in diameter, are reported in 5–30% of cases. They usually occur on the abdomen and chest and are easily missed in dark-skinned patients. In one study, which compared S. *typhi* to S. *paratyphi* in travelers, rose spots were not found in those with paratyphi infection [25]. Fever often occurs in a stepwise fashion, with 5–7 days of daily increments in maximal temperature of 0.5–1 °C and the peak of fever usually occurring in the afternoon. This is followed by a period of 10–14 days of sustained fever of 39–41 °C, and then the fever slowly decreases. Travelers usually seek medical attention early in the clinical course, and therefore the stepwise fever curve and sustained fevers are usually not seen in this population.

Without treatment, fever and ancillary signs of EF may continue for many weeks, leaving the patient very weak and debilitated and prone to other infections. Even with antimicrobial treatment, the temperature drops, not immediately, but after a median of 5–7 days. However, the persistence of fever for a week or more on antimicrobial therapy should prompt a search for metastatic spread with abscess formation or antimicrobial resistance. A sudden worsening of abdominal pain should suggest bowel perforation. This complication of EF is probably associated with the majority of fatal cases.

## Complications

Case fatality rates as high as 30% have been reported in endemic countries [26]. However, in travelers, this rate appears to be significantly lower. The serious complications, such as gastrointestinal bleeding, intestinal perforation, and typhoid encephalopathy, which may occur in 10–15% of patients in endemic countries, are rarely seen in travelers, most likely because of early access to medical care.

Secondary metastatic foci may occur in many organs and may lead to splenic abscesses, endocarditis, osteomyelitis, arthritis, and acute cholecystitis.

Relapse may occur, even with appropriate antimicrobial therapy, in both S. typhi and S. paratyphi [16]. This reflects the difficulty of eradicating the organism.

Chronic biliary carriage may occur in 2–5% of cases, even after treatment. Biliary carriage is defined as continuous shedding of the organism for more than a year. Carriers can present a public health risk, especially if working in the food service industry. This complication is now hardly ever seen in travelers.

## Death

A review of CDC surveillance data from 1985 to 1994 included 2445 cases of typhoid with 0.4% mortality. Fatal cases occurred exclusively in immigrants, not short-term travelers [9]. In a study of 45 travelers with enteric fever in Nepal, no death was reported [25]. In addition, accounts of typhoid fever in hospitalized returning travelers in France, Germany, and Israel reported no deaths [16–18].

Paratyphi infection is perceived as less severe than typhi infection. Similarly, cases of vaccine failure (those who contract S. typhi despite having been vaccinated) are thought to be less severe. Few data exist on these issues in general, and particularly in travelers. A study among Israeli travelers has shown that the clinical outcome in cases of vaccine failure and that associated with S. paratyphi A is indistinguishable from that of S. typhi, with complications occurring in about the same percentage of patients [16, 25].

## Diagnosis and laboratory findings

Physical examination does little to aid the clinician in establishing the diagnosis. All patients are febrile, and the temperature pattern is rarely diagnostic. The examination occasionally reveals relative bradycardia, but this sign is neither universal nor diagnostic. Rose spots are a more specific sign, but identifying them requires vigilance and experience, and their incidence varies markedly between series. In addition, they are even rarer in S. paratyphi A infection.

Laboratory tests are nonspecific as well. Mild liver function abnormalities are common (2–3 times the upper limit of normal) with a hepatocellular pattern more frequently seen. Leukopenia, thrombocytopenia, and mild anemia occur, but are neither universal nor diagnostic; they may occur in other tropical diseases, such as dengue and malaria.

Typically, the eosinophil count is very low, as well as the sedimentation rate. A high sedimentation rate may be associated with abscess formation or osteomyelitis, and eosinophilia, if present, should prompt an investigation for concomitant parasitic infections acquired during travel.

Typhoid hepatitis has been described in patients in endemic countries [27] and is characterized by significant liver damage. Study of this phenomena in travelers revealed that this syndrome was in fact related to co-infection with either hepatitis A or E, which are also fecal–oral transmissible pathogens [28].

### Serological tests

The well-established test is the *Widal test*. This test measures agglutinating antibody levels against O and H antigens. Usually, O antibodies appear on days 6–8 and H antibodies on days 10–12 after the onset of the disease. Thus, the ideal is to have paired tests. The first test is performed on an acute serum (at the time of first contact with the patient), and a convalescent serum should ideally also be collected, so that paired titrations can be performed. In practice, however, this is often difficult.

Moreover, the test has only moderate sensitivity and specificity. It can be negative in up to 30% of culture-proven cases of typhoid fever. This may be because of prior antibiotic therapy that has blunted the antibody response. Further, *S. typhi* shares O and H antigens with other *Salmonella* serotypes and has cross-reacting epitopes with other Enterobacteriacae, and this can lead to false positive results. Such results may also occur under other clinical conditions, such as malaria, typhus, bacteremia caused by other organisms, and cirrhosis. In areas of endemicity, there is often a low background level of antibodies in the normal population. In travelers who were vaccinated for typhoid, the vaccine itself may cause positive results [29].

Travel medicine practitioners should be aware that in many developing countries the Widal test is readily available and is performed frequently on ill travelers. Positive findings can lead to a diagnosis of typhoid fever without these limitations being taken into account. Thus, many travelers without any clinical picture of typhoid are given this diagnosis.

In response to the need for a quick and reliable diagnostic test to replace the Widal test, several new rapid tests have been developed. The IDL Tubex test detects IgM O9 antibodies (specific for *S. typhi*). Another rapid serological test, Typhidot, was developed in Malaysia and detects specific IgM and IgG antibodies against a 50-kD antigen of *S. typhi*. A newer version of the test, Typhidot-M, was recently developed in the Netherlands to detect specific IgM antibodies only [30]. These tests are targeted only for *S. typhi* infection. They normally have better sensitivity and specificity than the Widal test, but there has not been much experience with them in travelers, and in many industrialized countries they are still not available.

The optimal serological test should approach 100% sensitivity, specificity, and positive and negative predictive values and require only a single acute sample. In addition, it should have the capacity to diagnose both *S. typhi* and *S. paratyphi*.

## Cultures

The diagnosis, therefore, should be based on recovery of the pathogen in blood or stool cultures. Although historically reported as only 50–70% positive, updated culture systems will detect bacteremia in 80–100% of patients [31].

There is a decline in the diagnostic sensitivity of blood cultures with increasing duration of illness. A review of the literature reported that 89% of blood cultures were positive during the first week of typhoid fever, 73% in the second, 60% in the third, and only 26% in the fourth and subsequent weeks. Updated blood culture media may be better at growing smaller numbers of bacteria than those used previously, but the trend is the same. The declining number of bacteria in blood coincides with their accumulation in Peyer's patches and is associated with severe necrosis of the gut wall [32].

Many patients may have started antibiotics, and in these instances, blood cultures may be negative. Bone marrow culture in this circumstance can still provide a better chance of recovery of the organism, up to 90% [33]. However, in practice, physicians usually give empirical antibiotic treatment rather than doing bone marrow culture.

The organism may also be cultured from the rose spots.

Stool culture may occasionally be positive even when blood culture is negative, especially if it is taken more than a week after the onset of fever. Because prolonged stool carriage of *S. typhi* occurs, the interpretation of a positive stool culture merits caution in local populations. However, in travelers from industrialized countries, where carriage is very uncommon, a typical clinical setting combined with positive stool for *S. typhi* or *paratyphi* is strongly suggestive of the diagnosis.

Molecular methods for detecting *S. typhi* exist. Detection by PCR in blood and stool samples has a sensitivity and specificity of nearly 100% when compared to culture [31], but this is not commercially available.

## Treatment and drug resistance

The outcome of typhoid fever is usually good when effective antimicrobial therapy is provided in a timely manner, with a fatality rate of less than 1%, and a low rate of serious complications. However, even with proper antimicrobial treatment, the temperature does not drop immediately but only after a median of 5–7 days. This probably reflects the relative difficulty of eradicating intracellular organisms.

Historically, typhoid fever was treated with chloramphenicol, ampicillin, or trimethoprim/sulfamethoxazole, but starting in the 1950s there were initial reports of resistance to one or two of these. By 1972, chloramphenicol resistance became widespread and, since 1989, resistance to all three has occurred, first noted in strains in India, Pakistan, China, and the Arabian Gulf. Resistance appears to be plasmid-mediated, allowing the simultaneous acquisition of resistance to multiple drugs and the emergence of multidrug-resistant strains. A decade ago, 50–80% of isolates from China and the Indian subcontinent were multidrug-resistant [34] and 93% were reported in an outbreak in Tajikistan [35].

A major advance in therapy was the introduction of fluoroquinolones, which were found to be highly effective and well tolerated and could be administered orally. Ciprofloxacin 500 mg b.i.d. quickly became a first-line agent. Treatment was also reduced from 14 days to as short as 5 days duration [36]. Unfortunately, within the last decade, multidrug-resistant strains, now including quinolone-resistant strains, have become prevalent in the Indian subcontinent and have also been reported in other countries, such as Tajikistan and Vietnam. In some areas, approximately 80% of cases display quinolone resistance [35, 37, 38].

Drug resistance increases the magnitude of the problem of typhoid fever in the endemic areas. Multi-drug-resistant strains require expensive therapies, which may be less effective and in many cases are not available for the local population.

### Drug therapy in travelers

In industrialized countries, where most cases are imported, the problem of resistance reflects the same situation as seen in endemic countries. In the United States, multidrug-resistant strains of S. typhi have increased dramatically over two decades. From 1975 to 1984, only 5% of isolates were resistant to any of the commonly used drugs and 0.1% were resistant to all [8]. From 1990 to 1994, 30% were resistant to at least one and 12% were resistant to the three first-line agents [9]. The same pattern of resistance is now being seen in S. paratyphi A infection [22].

Because most imported cases are acquired in the Indian subcontinent, quinolones are no longer recommended as the drug of first choice. Laboratory proof of quinolone sensitivity must rely on MIC or on performing disk diffusion tests on quinolones and nalidixic acid. Strains that are apparently sensitive to fluoroquinolones but resistant to nalidixic acid should not be considered quinolone-sensitive, as clinical failure is expected [39].

The drugs of choice for people acquiring the disease in areas endemic to quinolone- or nalidixic acid-resistant strains are third-generation cephalosporins such as ceftriaxone, 2 g daily [40]. Where isolates have been found to be fluoroquinolone-sensitive, standard doses of a fluoroquinolone, such as ciprofloxacin 500 mg b.i.d, may be used.

Clinical experience in endemic areas shows a slower response to treatment in recent years, even when the pathogen is sensitive in vitro to quinolones or ceftriaxone [41]. Similar phenomena have been reported in returned travelers from the India subcontinent infected with S. paratyphi A [42]. Our experience with travelers in recent years has also shown that those who were treated for typhoid and paratyphoid with ceftriaxone alone tended to respond slowly to therapy, even though the infecting strains were sensitive in vitro, and complications such as abscesses and endocarditis were excluded.

Another promising option that has been tested in the last few years is azithromycin. This agent shows results similar to those for ciprofloxacin and ofloxacin [43, 44]. Oral azithromycin was comparable to intravenous ceftriaxone in uncomplicated typhoid fever in children and adolescents [40].

Thus, our recent policy has been to use a combination therapy, with azithromicin and cephalosporin. Combined therapy of ceftriaxone, 2 gr daily for 14 days, along with azithromycin, 500 mg daily for 5–7 days, seems to be highly effective, with a shorter defervescent time (3–4 days) and without relapses (E. Schwartz, unpublished data).

In conclusion, travelers who are suspected to have typhoid or paratyphoid fever and who acquired the disease outside the Indian subcontinent can still be treated empirically with oral quinolones until sensitivity results are completed. In those who have returned from the Indian subcontinent, the drug of choice should be intravenous ceftriaxone, preferably with azithromycin.

### Prevention of typhoid fever

The basic rule for typhoid fever prevention is improved sanitation. In industrialized countries, the disease was effectively controlled through improvement of water and food sanitation. However, in developing countries, a new and effective infrastructure is unlikely in the near future, particularly in slum areas, where the highest disease burden occurs. Among travelers, strict observance of hygiene rules to avoid contaminated food and water has always been stressed. However, the efficacy of these precautions is known to be poor, if judged by their failure in preventing traveler's diarrhea.

Vaccine can play a major role in prevention. To date, three types of typhoid vaccines exist: live attenuated oral vaccine, with the Ty21a strain (Vivotif, Berna), Vi capsular polysaccharide vaccine (Typhim Vi—Aventis Pasteur and Typherix—GlaxoSmithKline), and a new protein-conjugated capsular vaccine.

The live oral vaccine is an attenuated *S. typhi* strain, Ty21a, which is a mutant of Ty2 with a uridine diphospho-galactose 4-epimerase defect. It is avirulent (lacking the Vi antigen) but contains immunogenic cell wall polysaccharides. Primary vaccination consists of one enterically coated capsule or lyophilized sachet on alternate days for 3–4 doses. It causes a vigorous secretory IgA and cell-mediated response. Its efficacy is about 50–78% and the duration of protection is 3–4 years [45]. The disadvantage of the vaccine is that concurrent use of antibiotics or antimalarials may interfere with the antibody response. This vaccine also needs to be refrigerated, cannot be given to children under 6, and relies on the traveler's adherence (and memory) to complete the 3–4 required doses [46, 47]. In addition, this vaccine is contraindicated in pregnancy and in those with cell-mediated immunosuppression.

The Vi vaccine is the purified capsular polysaccharide antigen. The Vi antigen is the virulence antigen that allows *S. typhi* to survive in blood, leading to septicemia. The Vi vaccine contains only the Vi component of *S. typhi* and gives rapid seroconversion after one dose. It is safe to co-administer with other travel vaccines, as well as antimalarials, with no diminution in antibody response. It can be administered from the age of 2 onward. However, as a polysaccharide vaccine, it gives no boosting effect from revaccination, and the duration of protection appears to be between 2 and 3 years, with an efficacy of 50–67% [45].

In recent years, this vaccine became available in combination with hepatitis A vaccine (Hepatirix—Glaxo-SmithKline, Viatim—Sanofi Pasteur).

A new *S. typhi* conjugating Vi to a carrier protein (similarly to the conjugated pneumococcal and meningococcal vaccines) has also been developed and has the advantage of increasing immunogenicity, giving a higher efficacy of about 90% and a prolonged protection time [48].

An important caveat is that all estimates of vaccine efficacy are derived from studies on local populations, which might be different from travelers. On one hand, local populations may have a degree of pre-existing immunity, and are likely to have more repeated exposure than travelers, with immune enhancement and, therefore, vaccine efficacy is expected to be less in travelers. On the other hand, typhoid vaccine is unique because its protection is influenced by the dose of inoculum. A higher inoculum of infection may overcome the vaccine protection. Thus, among travelers who live and eat in a more sanitary environment than local populations, vaccine efficacy might be even higher. Indeed, in a retrospective analysis of vaccine

efficacy in travelers in Nepal, vaccine efficacy was found to be about 90% [23].

A major disadvantage of the vaccine is its lack of protection against *S. paratyphi* infection. The purified Vi vaccine protects by eliciting serum antibodies against Vi, an antigen that does not exists in *S. paratyphi*. Thus, even the new conjugate vaccine does not add to protection against *S. paratyphi*.

The attenuated *S. typhi* Ty21a, which does not express Vi, but rather mediates protection by eliciting serum and mucosal antibodies to *S. typhi* O and H and other antigens and by stimulating an array of cell-mediated immune responses (including cytotoxic T cells) may give some protection against paratyphi infection. In fact, an Israeli study demonstrated that Vi vaccine gave better protection against *S. typhi* among travelers to India, whereas Ty21a gave better protection against *S. paratyphi* A [16].

A recent retrospective analysis of pooled data of Ty21a vaccine studies, which was done in Chile, showed some protection of this vaccine against paratyphoid B fever only (efficacy of 49%) [49].

## Conclusions

Typhoid fever is still a major health problem in many developing countries and is far from being eradicated. Although it is no longer endemic in most developed countries, it is seen in travelers returning from endemic countries, especially from the Indian subcontinent. With the continued increase in worldwide travel and of migration from endemic regions, physicians should be well acquainted with the disease. Unfortunately, the current vaccines available offer only moderate protection against *S. typhi* and almost no protection against *S. paratyphi*, which has become a more dominant pathogen. Taken together with the increase in multi-drug-resistant strains, cases are expected to continue to increase and to become even more of a challenge to treat.

## References

1  DeRoeck D, Jodar L, Clemens J. Putting typhoid vaccination on the global health agenda. *N Engl J Med* 2007;357:1069–71.
2  Parry CM, Hien TT, Dougan G, et al. Typhoid fever. *N Engl J Med* 2002;347:1770–82.
3  Ivanoff B. Typhoid fever: global situation and WHO recommendations. *Southeast Asian J Trop Med Public Health* 1995;26(suppl 2):1–6.

4 Crump JA, Luby SP, Mintz ED. The global burden of typhoid fever. *Bull World Health Organ* 2004;82:346–53.

5 Lin FY, Ho VA Bay PV, et al. The epidemiology of typhoid fever in the Dong Thap Province, Mekong Delta region of Vietnam. *Am J Trop Med Hyg* 2000;62:644–8.

6 Sinha A, Sazawal S, Kumar R, et al. Typhoid fever in children less than 5 years. *Lancet* 1999;354:734–7.

7 Taylor DN, Pollard RA, Blake PA. Typhoid in the United States and the risk to the international traveler. *J Infect Dis* 1983;148:599–602.

8 Ryan CA, Hargrett-Bean NT, Blake PA. *Salmonella typhi* infections in the United States, 1975–1984: increasing role of foreign travel. *Rev Infect Dis* 1988;2:1–8.

9 Mermin JH, Townes JM, Gerber M, et al. Typhoid fever in the United States, 1985–1994. *Arch Intern Med* 1998;158:633–8.

10 Meltzer E. Yosipovitch O., Sadik C., Dan M, Schwartz E. Epidemiology and clinical aspects of typhoid fever in Israel. *Am J Trop Med Hyg* 2006;74:540–45

11 Lester A, Mygind O, Jensen KT, Jarlov JO, Schonheyder HC. Typhoid and paratyphoid fever in Denmark 1986–1990. Epidemiologic aspects and the extent of bacteriological follow-up of patients. *Ugeskr Laeger* 1994;156:3770–5.

12 Yew FS, Goh KT, Lim YS. Epidemiology of typhoid fever in Singapore. *Epidemiol Infect* 1993 Feb; 110: 63–70.

13 Lighton LL. Follow up in north west England of cases of enteric fever acquired abroad, April 1996 to March 1998. *Commun Dis Public Health* 1999;2:145–6.

14 UK Department of Health. Typhoid. In: Salisbury DM, Begg NT, editors. *Immunisation against Infectious Disease.* London: UK Department of Health; 1996. p. 243–9.

15 Behrens R, Carroll B. The 10 year trend of travel associated infections imported into the U.K. In: *Proceedings of the 7th Conference of the International Society of Travel Medicine (CISTM7),* Innsbruck 2001; p. 86.

16 Meltzer E, Sadik C, Schwartz E. Enteric fever in Israeli travelers: a nation-wide study. *J. Travel Med.* 2005;12:275–81.

17 Caumes E, Ehya N, Nguyen J, et. al. Typhoid and paratyphoid fever: a 10-year retrospective study of 41 cases in a Parisian hospital. *J Travel Med* 2001;8:293–7.

18 Jelinek T, Nothfurft HD, Sonnenburg FV, et al. Risk factors for typhoid fever in travelers. *J Travel Med* 1996;3:200–203.

19 O'Brien D, Tobin S, Brown GV, et al. Fever in returned travelers: review of hospital admissions for a 3-year period. *Clin Infect Dis* 2001;33:603–9.

20 Steinberg EB, Bishop R, Haber P, Dempsey AF, Hoekstra RM, Nelson JM, Ackers M, Calugar A, Mintz ED. Typhoid fever in travelers: who should be targeted for prevention? *Clin Infect Dis* 2004;39:186–91.

21 Leder K, Tong S, Weld L, et al. GeoSentinel Surveillance Network. Illness in travelers visiting friends and relatives: a review of the GeoSentinel surveillance network. *Clin Infect Dis* 2006 1;43:1185–93.

22 Safdar A, Kaur H, Elting L, Rolston KV. Antimicrobial susceptibility of 128 *Salmonella enterica* serovar typhi and paraty-

phi A isolates from northern India. *Chemotherapy* 2004;50: 88–91.

23 Schwartz E, Shlim DR, Eaton M, et al. The effect of oral and parenteral typhoid vaccination on the rate of infection with *Salmonella typhi* and *Salmonella paratyphi* A among foreigners in Nepal. *Arch Intern Med* 1990;150:349–51.

24 Ochiai RL, Wang X, von Seidlein L, et al. *Salmonella paratyphi* A rates, Asia. *Emerg Infect Dis* 2005;11:1764–6.

25 Shlim DR, Schwartz E, Eaton M. Clinical importance of *Salmonella paratyphi* A infection to enteric fever in Nepal. *J Travel Med* 1995;2:165–8.

26 Edelman R, Levine MM. Summary of an international workshop on typhoid fever. *Rev Infect Dis* 1986;8:329–49.

27 Khosla SN. Typhoid hepatitis. *Postgrad Med J* 1990;66:923–5.

28 Schwartz E, Jenks NP, Shlim DR. 'Typhoid hepatitis' or typhoid fever and acute viral hepatitis. *Trans R Soc Trop Med Hyg* 1994;88:437–8.

29 Olopoenia LA, King AL. Widal agglutination test—100 years later: still plagued by controversy. *Postgrad Med J* 2000;76: 80–84.

30 World Health Organization. *The Diagnosis, Treatment and Prevention of Typhoid Fever.* World Health Organization; May 2003.

31 Sanchez-Jimenez MM, Cardona-Castro N. Validation of a PCR for diagnosis of typhoid fever and salmonellosis by amplification of the hilA gene in clinical samples from Colombian patients. *J Med Microbiol* 2004;53:875–8.

32 Wain J, Diep TS, Ho VA, et al. Quantitation of bacteria in blood of typhoid fever patients and relationship between counts and clinical features, transmissibility, and antibiotic resistance. *J Clin Microbiol* 1998;36:1683–7.

33 Gilman RH, Terminel M, Levine MM, et al. Relative efficacy of blood, urine, rectal swab, bone-marrow, and rose-spot cultures for recovery of *Salmonella typhi* in typhoid fever. *Lancet* 1975;1(7918):1211–13.

34 Gupta A. Multidrug-resistant typhoid fever in children: epidemiology and therapeutic approach. *Pediatr Infect Dis J* 1994;13:134–40.

35 Mermin JH, Villar R, Carpenter J, et al. A massive epidemic of multi-drug resistant typhoid fever in Tajikistan associated with consumption of municipal water. *J Infect Dis* 1999;17:1416–22.

36 Alam MN, Haq SA, Das KK, et al. Efficacy of ciprofloxacin in enteric fever: comparison of treatment duration in sensitive and multidrug-resistant *Salmonella. Am J Trop Med Hyg* 1995;53: 306–11.

37 Murdoch DA, Banatvala NA, Bone A, et. al. Epidemic ciprofloxacin-resistant *Salmonella typhi* in Tajikistan. *Lancet* 1998;351:339.

38 Parry C, Wain J, Chinh NT, e al. Quinolone resistant *Salmonella typhi* in Vietnam. *Lancet* 1998;351:3.

39 Parry CM. The treatment of multidrug-resistant and nalidixic acid-resistant typhoid fever in Viet Nam. *Trans R Soc Trop Med Hyg* 2004;98:413–22.

40 Frenck RW, Nakhla I, Sultan Y, et al. Azithromycin versus ceftriaxone for the treatment of uncomplicated typhoid fever in children. *Clin Infect Dis* 2000;31:1134–8.

41 Slinger R, Desjardins M, McCarthy AE, et al. Suboptimal clinical response to ciprofloxacin in patients with enteric fever due to *Salmonella* spp. with reduced fluoroquinolone susceptibility: a case series. *BMC Infect Dis.* 2004;20(4)(1):36.

42 Piersma D, Overbosch D, Petit P, van Genderen PJ. Protracted fever after a journey to India and Nepal: a case of persistent *Salmonella paratyphi* infection. *J Travel Med* 2004;11:257–9.

43 Girgis NI, Butler T, Frenck RW, Sultan Y, et al. Azithromycin versus ciprofloxacin for treatment of uncomplicated typhoid fever in a randomized trial in Egypt that included patients with multidrug resistance. *Antimicrob Agents Chemother* 1999;43:1441–4.

44 Chinh NT, Parry CM, Ly NT, et al. A randomized controlled comparison of azithromycin and ofloxacin for treatment of multidrug-resistant or nalidixic acid-resistant enteric fever. *Antimicrob Agents Chemother* 2000;44:1855–9.

45 Engels EA, Falagas ME, Lau J, et al. Typhoid fever vaccines: a meta-analysis of studies on efficacy and toxicity. *BMJ* 1998;316:110–16.

46 Stubi CL, Landry PR, Petignat C, et al. Compliance to live oral Ty21a typhoid vaccine and its effect on viability. *J Travel Med* 2000;7:133–7.

47 Cryz SJ. Patient compliance in the use of Vivotif Berna® vaccine, typhoid vaccine, live oral Ty21a. *J Travel Med* 1998;5:14–17.

48 Lanh, MN, Lin FYC, Bay PV, et al. Persistence of antibodies and efficacy against typhoid fever 28–46 months following Vi conjugate vaccine (Vi-*r*EPA) in 2 to 5 years-old children. *N Engl J Med* 2003 349:1390–91.

49 Levine MM, Ferreccio C, Black RE, Lagos R, San Martin O, Blackwelder WC. Ty21a live oral typhoid vaccine and prevention of paratyphoid fever caused by *Salmonella enterica* Serovar Paratyphi B. *Clin Infect Dis* 2007;45 Suppl 1:S24–S28.

50 Connor BA, Schwartz E. Typhoid and paratyphoid fever in travelers. *Lancet Infect Dis* 2005;5:623–8.

# 17 Bacterial Diarrhea

## Herbert L. DuPont

The University of Texas–Houston School of Public Health and Medical School, Baylor College of Medicine, and St. Luke's Episcopal Hospital, Houston, TX, USA

## Introduction

In this review, we deal with the bacterial causes of travelers' diarrhea (TD) and consider bacterial agents as causes of endemic diarrhea (ED) in the developing world. Bacterial enteropathogens explain more than 60% of travelers' diarrhea (TD) and cause a similar rate of ED in young children living in the same areas. In contrast, the bacterial agents can be shown to cause 10–20% of diarrhea in older children and adults living in developing regions where TD is seen. This chapter is organized into epidemiology, clinical syndromes, diagnosis, treatment, and prevention of bacterial diarrhea of travelers.

## Epidemiology of travelers' diarrhea and endemic diarrhea

In this chapter, we deal with TD and ED occurring in developing tropical and semitropical regions of Latin America, Africa, and southern Asia. TD and ED are more common in warmer summer months, particularly when summer and rainy seasons coincide. The illnesses produced by bacterial enteropathogens or their toxins often produce characteristic syndromes that may allow a tentative etiologic diagnosis. Each will be discussed below.

### Etiologic classifications

Table 17.1 lists the important bacterial enteropathogens causing acute diarrhea along with comments about their importance as causes of TD and ED. The bacterial enteropathogens cause two general types of enteric disease in both travelers and the locals living in tropical and semitropical areas: (1) enteric infection with an incuba-

tion period of 14 hours to 9 days and (2) intoxication, or ingestion of preformed bacterial toxins, with an incubation period of 2–7 hours.

## Enteric infection and intoxications in travelers

Most cases of TD are caused by bacterial enteropathogens. Although research groups can identify a bacterial pathogen in approximately 60% of TD cases, bacteria actually explain a higher percentage of the cases. Strong indirect evidence suggests that bacterial pathogens may explain up to 80% of TD cases in which antibacterial drugs shorten bacterial diarrhea and the illness is not associated with a detectable pathogen [1]. Use of PCR methods has enhanced the detection of bacterial enteropathogens, particularly enterotoxigenic *Escherichia coli* (ETEC) and other diarrheagenic *E. coli*, helping to reduce the percentage of cases without a detectable agent.

Although ETEC is the principal cause of TD worldwide, it is more important as a cause of TD in Latin America and the Caribbean and in Africa, explaining from one-third to 40% of illness. In Asia, it is the most common pathogen of TD, but it is less important, causing approximately 20% of illness. There are other regional differences in frequency of bacterial enteropathogens in TD. *Campylobacter jejuni*, *Aeromonas* spp., and *Salmonella* strains appear to be more common as causes of TD in those visiting countries of southern Asia, compared with other developing regions. Noncholera vibrios such as *Vibrio parahaemolyticus* are an important cause of TD in people traveling to coastal areas of Southern Asia. An occasional cause of recurrent illness complicating fluoroquinolone therapy of TD is *Clostridium difficile* diarrhea [2].

## Enteric infection and intoxications in endemic diarrhea in children and adults

Children who live in developing regions frequently experience bacterial infection with the same pathogens seen

*Tropical Diseases in Travelers*, 1st edition. Edited by E. Schwartz.
© 2009 by Blackwell Publishing, ISBN: 978-1-4051-8441-0.

**Table 17.1** Etiologic agents in travelers' diarrhea (TD) and endemic diarrhea (ED) in developing regions: enteric infections and intoxications (ingestion of preformed toxins).

| Etiologic agent | Characteristic syndrome |
| --- | --- |
| *Shigella* spp. | Important reservoir—infected persons; dysentery (passage of bloody stools) is seen in half of affected patients; the organism causes 6–10% of TD and ED |
| Nontyphoid *Salmonella* spp. | Poultry and hens' eggs are the important reservoir; causes acute diarrhea and fever, complicated by bacteremia in 6–8% of healthy people and up to 50% of those who have underlying illness; the organism causes 6–10% of TD and ED |
| *Campylobacter jejuni* | Poultry reservoir; dysentery is seen in half the affected patients; major definable cause of Guillain–Barré syndrome; the organism causes ~10% of TD in Asia and in ED ~5% of TD in Latin America and Africa |
| *Clostridium difficile* | Major cause of antibiotic-associated colitis in hospitalized patients; currently there is a widespread epidemic of a hypervirulent strain with more serious outcomes being seen in Europe, Canada, and the USA; *C. difficile* is a more important cause of ED in developing regions |
| Enterotoxigenic *Escherichia coli* (ETEC) | The major cause of TD and of diarrhea involving children living in developing tropical and semitropical regions; the organism is a less common cause of ED in adults in developing regions, and causes occasional foodborne outbreaks in industrialized regions |
| Enteropathogenic *E. coli* (EPEC) | Typical EPEC strains characteristically cause nursery outbreaks; atypical strains are important causes of TD and ED in adults and children in many settings |
| Enteroinvasive *E. coli* (EIEC) | Occasional cause of TD and large foodborne outbreaks of dysentery throughout the world |
| Enterohemorrhagic or Shiga toxin-producing *E. coli* (EHEC or STEC) | Important reservoir is cattle; the early outbreaks were associated with ground beef; now produce growing in fields contaminated with cattle manure is the most important vehicle of transmission; the organism also causes hemolytic uremic syndrome in a substantial percentage (~10%) of children and is less common in the elderly; rare cause of TD |
| *Aeromonas* spp. | Common cause of TD and ED in Asia |
| *Plesiomonas* spp. | An important cause of seafood-associated TD and ED |
| *Vibrio*, cholera and noncholera | Cholera is a rare cause of TD; noncholera vibrios are important causes of diarrhea in coastal areas of southern Asia |
| Intoxication with preformed toxin of *Staphylococcus aureus* (SA), *Bacillus cereus* (BC), and *Clostridium perfringens* (CP) | After ingestion of heat-stable SA enterotoxin, vomiting occurs with an incubation period (i.p.) of 2–7 hours; with ingestion of CP organisms and toxin, watery diarrhea without vomiting occurs after an i.p. of 12–16 hours; with BC toxin ingestion two syndromes are seen: (1) vomiting with an i.p. of 2–7 hours (like SA) and (2) watery diarrhea after 12–16 hours (like CP). |

in international travelers to their country. ETEC is common in this population, as it is in visitors to these areas. We have shown that although ETEC infection is less common in local adults in the developing region of Mexico than in international travelers from industrialized regions [3], ETEC diarrhea can occur in Mexican adults with diarrhea [4], providing evidence that ETEC immunity in endemic areas is short-term. The frequency of finding a bacterial enteropathogen when older children and adults with endemic diarrhea are studied is no more than 10%–15% in all countries of the world. In addition, antibiotics are not effective in treating the 85–90% of cases of ED in these age groups that are without a definable bacterial pathogen. An unappreciated bacterial cause of ED in developing countries is *C. difficile* [5]. It is not considered an important pathogen in these settings, because it is not generally sought by local investigators.

## Regional occurrence of TD

The average rate of TD is 40% for persons from industrialized countries traveling to high-risk countries of Latin America, Africa, and southern Asia. These rates of TD have not changed in the more than 50 years that they have been studied. The rates of TD during travel from low-risk areas to the intermediate-risk regions of the Middle East, the Caribbean, Thailand, China, and Russia appears to be less than half the rate for travel to high-risk regions (<20%).

## Source of TD

The important sources of TD due to bacterial enteropathogens are contaminated foods and occasionally beverages, the result of reduced hygiene in developing regions. The foods and beverages served in developing tropical and semitropical regions can be classified as often safe and recommended or often contaminated and unsafe based on known principles. Heating food or beverages to 60°C will inactivate all enteric bacterial pathogens [6], explaining the safety of steaming hot food items. Bacteria need moisture for propagation, so dry foods such as bread are generally safe to eat. Fruits that have been peeled or can be peeled by the traveler, including citrus and bananas, are usually safe. Finally, foods with very high sugar content, such as syrups, honey, jams, and jellies, are safe from bacterial contamination.

Any food items that are served moist at room temperature should be considered a potential source of enteric bacterial pathogens. Berries, grapes, and tomatoes that have not been carefully washed by the traveler also should be considered unsafe.

## Clinical aspects of enteric bacterial infection

Five syndromes are seen in international travelers with enteric bacterial disease. The first is acute gastroenteritis, in which the subjects experience vomiting with little or no diarrhea. The preformed toxin of *Staphylococcus aureus*, showing an incubation period of 2–7 hours, is the common cause of this syndrome. This intoxication is not an enteric infection and the illness is short-lasting, with recovery occurring within 12–18 hours or less. A second intoxication is seen with *C. perfringens*. In *C. perfringens*,

enteric infection and free toxin appear to be important. The incubation period for *C. perfringens* foodborne disease is 8–14 hours, and watery diarrhea without vomiting is the clinical illness typically produced. *Bacillus cereus* produces two different toxins that explain the two syndromes produced by this form of intoxication: either a *S. aureus*-type disease with vomiting with an incubation period of 2–7 hours or a *C. perfringens*-type illness with watery diarrhea without vomiting, with an incubation period of 8–14 hours.

The second syndrome of TD is dysentery, where subjects pass grossly bloody stools, generally with measurable fever. The major causes of dysenteric TD are *Campylobacter* and *Shigella* spp. Rarely, Shiga toxin-producing *E. coli* (including *E. coli* O157:H7) can cause this syndrome in international travelers. Noncholera *Vibrio* and *Aeromonas* spp. also cause bloody diarrhea.

The third syndrome of bacterial TD is acute watery diarrhea with or without low-grade fever. All of the bacterial enteropathogens listed in Table 17.1 can cause this syndrome, which lasts approximately five days if untreated. For the vast majority of cases of TD, it is not possible to determine the bacterial cause of the illness on clinical grounds.

The fourth syndrome is febrile illness with systemic toxicity, fitting the pattern of enteric or typhoid fever. A person with enteric fever may or may not have diarrhea.

The fifth syndrome is persistent diarrhea, where illness lasts 14 days or longer. The bacterial agents known to cause persistent diarrhea in travelers and in children living in developing regions are *Shigella* spp., enteroaggregative *E. coli*, *Aeromonas* spp., *Plesiomonas* spp., *Campylobacter*, and *Salmonella* spp.

## Diagnosis of travelers' diarrhea

Because TD is a syndrome, it can be diagnosed without laboratory studies. In fact, the laboratory is not useful in making an etiologic diagnosis of the major bacterial causes, because nearly half of the illness is due to diarrhea-producing *E. coli* that cannot be detected by routine diagnostic methods.

The diagnosis of TD is made whenever a person from an industrialized country develops diarrhea (passage of three or more unformed stools in 24 hours plus another sign or symptom of enteric infection, such as abdominal pain or cramps, nausea, vomiting, tenesmus, dysentery, or fecal urgency) while traveling in a developing region of Latin America, Africa, or southern Asia. The illness

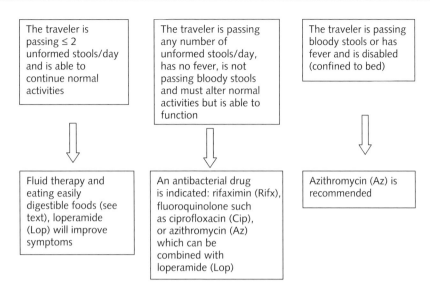

**Figure 17.1** Algorithm for the treatment of travelers' diarrhea caused by bacterial enteropathogens. Lop—loperamide dose: 4 mg initially followed by 2 mg after each unformed stool, not to exceed 8 mg/day; can take up to 48 hours. Rifx—rifaximin dose: 200 mg three times a day for 3 days. Cip—ciprofloxacin dose: 750 mg once a day for 1–3 days. Az—azithromycin dose, 1 g in a single dose.

may also develop shortly after returning home because of infection late in the trip and a prolonged incubation period that may be as long as 9 days after ingestion. It is important to ask people with acute diarrhea if they have recently traveled to a developing region.

Patients with TD that persists more than 14 days should have a workup for protracted illness. The workup for bacterial enteropathogens should include a stool culture looking for *Shigella*, *Salmonella*, *Campylobacter*, *Aeromonas*, and *Plesiomonas*. If the diarrhea occurred during travel to a coastal area of southern Asia, the laboratory should also be asked to look for vibrios, including *V. parahaemolyticus*. This will require culturing the stool on special media.

The common diarrheagenic *E. coli* can be sought only by working with research laboratories. In the case of persistent illness with fever, blood cultures should be obtained. Nontyphoid *Salmonella* and *S. typhi* may be responsible for this enteric fever syndrome. Diagnostic testing is generally not indicated for the short-lasting gastroenteritis associated with preformed toxins.

## Treatment of travelers' diarrhea due to bacterial causes

The treatment of TD caused by bacterial diarrhea consists of attention to diet, fluid and salt replacement, treatment to improve symptoms, and antibacterial drugs. Each has an important place in the treatment of bacterial TD. See Figure 17.1 for principles of therapy of TD due to bacterial enteropathogens.

## Diet alteration

It is a mistake to withhold food from people with TD. They should be given easily digestible foods such as steamed or baked fish, chicken, and vegetables, as well as toast, bananas, and applesauce. Fried and spicy foods should not be consumed, and milk should be withheld from the diet of adults with TD for approximately 2 days. Bacterial enteropathogens cause damage to the intestinal lining, and calories are needed for enterocyte renewal, recovery from injury, and rapid recovery from diarrhea.

## Fluid and electrolytes

Bacterial TD can lead to dehydration. Those with illness must pay attention to fluid and salt intake. Soups and broths are ideal to provide calories and to replace both fluid and electrolytes. In addition to soups, soft drinks, dilute fruit juice, saltine crackers, and bananas can keep up with important fluid and salt losses. If travelers experience any degree of dehydration with their diarrhea and cannot keep up with fluid losses, they should seek medical attention and may need intravenous fluid therapy.

## Symptomatic therapy

The primary mechanism of diarrhea in bacterial TD is mucosal secretion, or transport of fluid and electrolytes from the vascular serosal surface of the gut across the mucosa to the lumen, resulting in passage of unformed stools. Loperamide is considered the most effective symptomatic treatment for acute diarrhea, whether it is TD or ED. Loperamide works by causing segmental intestinal contractions, slowing the transit of the luminal fluid, which causes increased fluid and electrolyte absorption. The drug also has weak anti-calmodulin effects and blocks secretion in that way. Clays that bind to water will make stools more formed but have little effect in improving diarrhea. Bismuth subsalicylate (BSS) is an antisecretory drug that works through salicylate mechanisms. Where loperamide reduces diarrhea (number of stools passed during illness) by approximately 60%, BSS will reduce the number of stools passed in bacterial diarrhea by approximately 40%.

## Antimicrobial therapy

The mainstay of treatment of TD due to bacterial enteropathogens is one of several antibiotics with predictable activity against prevalent etiologic organisms. The drugs with significant activity against the diarrhea-producing *E. coli* are rifaximin, given in a dose of 200 mg three times a day for 3 days, ciprofloxacin, in a dose of 750 mg once a day for 1–3 days, and azithromycin, in a single 1-g dose. For febrile dysentery, the drug of choice is azithromycin [7], because rifaximin is not useful in enteric disease, due to invasive bacterial enteropathogens and ciprofloxacin-resistant *Campylobacter* strains that are found worldwide.

For nonfebrile and nondysenteric TD due to bacterial enteropathogens, the combination of antibacterial therapy and loperamide (given in the doses provided in Figure 17.1) will provide the most rapid relief from diarrhea [8]. For typhoid fever or systemic nontyphoid *Salmonella* disease, a fluoroquinolone is given to adults and a third generation cephalosporin to children.

## Prevention of bacterial TD

### Diet and beverage selection

The source of TD due to bacterial enteropathogens is reduced hygiene, seen at all levels in developing regions. The food served in hotels and restaurants is characteristically contaminated with bacterial enteropathogens. Figure 17.2 offers an approach to preventing TD due to bacterial enteropathogens, focusing on ingestion of usually safe food and beverages and targeted use of chemoprophylaxis with rifaximin or bismuth subsalicylate. In the single prospective study looking at the value of exercising care in food/beverage selection during international travel, the number of errors made in selecting items to consume is directly related to the rate of TD [9], offering hope of preventing a large proportion of TD by attention to diet.

In some parts of the world, rifaximin or bismuth subsalicylate is not available. In Europe, there is general concern about bismuth toxicity from using BSS for prophylaxis. Most authorities in the US believe this nonsoluble form of bismuth can be safely given to healthy persons, provided it is not given in excessive doses or to persons with intestinal absorptive capacity, as may be seen with advanced AIDS or inflammatory bowel disease.

## Chemoprophylaxis

Chemoprophylaxis was first successfully used more than 50 years ago. At the 1968 international Olympics in Mexico City, many competing teams from industrialized countries such as the UK, the USA, and Australia took preventive antibiotics. The effectiveness of antibiotics in preventing the disease in the 1950s and 1960s was the first evidence available that bacterial enteropathogens were responsible for TD [10]. This approach was largely discounted in the mid-1980s, when a Consensus Development Conference expressed concern about the development of resistance among extra-intestinal bacterial flora and development of adverse reactions to the agents when absorbed drugs were employed [11]. With the availability of nonabsorbed (<0.4%) rifaximin, the concept is being reconsidered [12, 13]. Chemoprophylaxis can be considered for people who have an underlying disease that could suffer complications as a result of TD (e.g., insulin-dependent diabetes mellitus, cancer, or congestive heart disease), when the trip is vital and an 8–10 hour illness cannot be tolerated (e.g., politician, athlete, musician, lecturer), when people have been affected by TD in a previous trip or are taking proton pump inhibitors regularly, suggesting increased susceptibility, and when travelers request chemoprophylaxis [12]. If available to travel medicine specialists and future travelers, the ideal drug for TD prevention is rifaximin.

## Immunoprophylaxis

One vaccine for prevention of the principal cause of TD, ETEC, is currently licensed in 50 countries. The vaccine, Dukoral, is a combination of whole cell *V. cholerae* strains plus the recombinant binding subunit of cholera toxin, which is closely related to the binding subunit of the

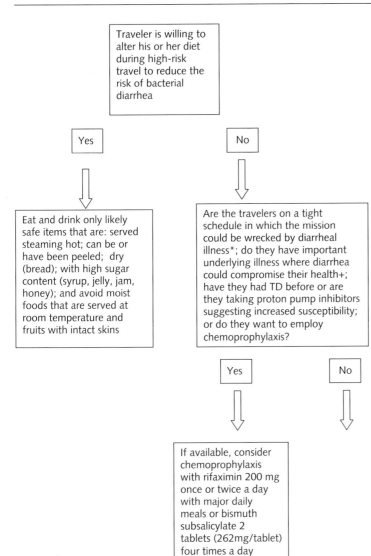

**Figure 17.2** Prevention of travelers' diarrhea due to bacterial enteropathogens.
\*: Politician, musician, athlete, lecturer.
+: Insulin-dependent diabetics, cancer patients, and persons with congestive heart failure.

heat-labile enterotoxin of ETEC. This ETEC vaccine is given in two oral doses and provides short-term protection against ETEC diarrhea [14]. A second vaccine, which is being developed and is not currently licensed, is purified heat-labile enterotoxin (LT) of ETEC, given transcutaneously as a skin patch. The vaccine is given twice before travel and provides high-level protection against severe forms of TD [15]. Vaccines against ETEC look promising as a means of preventing the most important pathogen causing TD [12].

## References

1 DuPont HL, Haake R, Taylor DN, Ericsson CD, Jiang ZD, Okhuysen PC, et al. Rifaximin treatment of pathogen-negative travelers' diarrhea. *J Travel Med* 2007;14(1): 16–19.

2 Norman F, Perez-Molina J, de Ayala P, Jimenez B, Navarro M, Lopez-Velez R. *Clostridium difficile*-associated diarrhea after antibiotic treatment for traveler's diarrhea. *Clin Infect Dis* 2008;46:1060–63.

3 DuPont HL, Olarte J, Evans DG, Pickering LK, Galindo E, Evans DJ. Comparative susceptibility of Latin American and United States students to enteric pathogens. *N Engl J Med* 1976;295(27):1520–21.

4 Bouckenooghe AR, Jiang ZD, De La Cabada FJ, Ericsson CD, DuPont HL. Enterotoxigenic *Escherichia coli* as cause of diarrhea among Mexican adults and US travelers in Mexico. *J Travel Med* 2002;9(3):137–40.

5 Garcia C, Samalvides F, Vidal M, Gotuzzo E, Dupont HL. Epidemiology of *Clostridium difficile* associated diarrhea in a Peruvian tertiary care hospital. *Am J Trop Med Hyg* 2007;77(5):802–5.

6 Bandres JC, Mathewson JJ, DuPont HL. Heat susceptibility of bacterial enteropathogens. Implications for the prevention of travelers' diarrhea. *Arch Intern Med* 1988;148(10): 2261–3.

7 Tribble DR, Sanders JW, Pang LW, Mason C, Pitarangsi C, Baqar S, et al. Traveler's diarrhea in Thailand: randomized, double-blind trial comparing single-dose and 3-day azithromycin-based regimens with a 3-day levofloxacin regimen. *Clin Infect Dis* 2007;44(3):338–46.

8 Dupont HL, Jiang ZD, Belkind-Gerson J, Okhuysen PC, Ericsson CD, Ke S, et al. Treatment of travelers' diarrhea: randomized trial comparing rifaximin, rifaximin plus loperamide, and loperamide alone. *Clin Gastroenterol Hepatol* 2007;5(4):451–6.

9 Kozicki M, Steffen R, Schar M. 'Boil it, cook it, peel it or forget it': does this rule prevent travellers' diarrhoea? *Int J Epidemiol* 1985;14(1):169–72.

10 Kean BH. The diarrhea of travelers to Mexico. Summary of five-year study. *Ann Intern Med* 1963;59:605–14.

11 Gorbach S, Edelman, R. Travelers' diarrhea: National Institutes of Health Consensus Development Conference. 1986;8(Suppl 2):S109–S233.

12 DuPont HL. Systematic review: prevention of travellers' diarrhoea. *Aliment Pharmacol Ther* 2008;27(9):741–51.

13 DuPont HL, Jiang ZD, Okhuysen PC, Ericsson CD, de la Cabada FJ, Ke S, et al. A randomized, double-blind, placebo-controlled trial of rifaximin to prevent travelers' diarrhea. *Ann Intern Med* 2005;142(10):805–12.

14 Peltola H, Siitonen A, Kyronseppa H, Simula I, Mattila L, Oksanen P, et al. Prevention of travellers' diarrhoea by oral B-subunit/whole-cell cholera vaccine. *Lancet* 1991;338(8778):1285–9.

15 Frech SA, DuPont HL, Bourgeois AL, et al. Protection against travelers' diarrhea in a randomized, double-blind, placebo-controlled field trial of a patch containing heat-labile toxin from *Escherichia coli. Lancet*, in press.

# 18 Rickettsial Diseases

Mogens Jensenius[1] and Philippe Parola[2]

[1] Ullevål University Hospital, Oslo, Norway
[2] Institut de Médicine Tropicale du Service de Santé des Armées, Le Pharo, Université de la Méditerranée and Hôpital Nord, AP-HM, Marseille, France

## Introduction

Rickettsial diseases are caused by obligate intracellular, gram-negative bacteria belonging to the order Rickettsiales. The taxonomy of Rickettsiales is complex and continues to be modified as new data become available, but currently the order contains four distinct genera that include recognized human pathogens: *Rickettsia, Orientia, Ehrlichia,* and *Anaplasma.* However, it was just recently that *Coxiella burnetii* (the causative agent of Q fever) and *Bartonella* spp. (the causative agents of the bartonelloses) were removed from the order, and for historical reasons they are included in this overview. Diseases caused by *Rickettsia* and *Orientia* species are often collectively referred to as "rickettsioses" (see below) [1].

During the past few decades, several hundred travelers infected with rickettsial diseases in tropical and subtropical areas have been reported in the literature, the majority of cases being African tick bite fever, Mediterranean spotted fever, murine typhus, scrub typhus, and Q fever. Many rickettsial diseases are transmitted by arthropods that favor particular environmental biotopes and are restricted to remote areas or niches beyond the tourist mainstream. Importantly, because ecotourism and adventure travel are increasingly popular worldwide, the incidence of imported cases is likely to escalate in the years to come. Here, we summarize current knowledge of the epidemiology, clinical presentation, diagnosis, and treatment of rickettsial diseases in international travelers to the tropics.

## Rickettsioses

Rickettsioses are febrile diseases caused by members of the genera *Rickettsia* and *Orientia* that invade endothelial cells and induce the formation of vasculitis. They are transmitted by various arthropods, such as ticks, mites, fleas, and lice, and involve arthropod and mammal reservoirs. The 16 currently recognized rickettsioses are divided into three groups: the spotted fever group, the typhus group, and the scrub typhus group (Table 18.1). Until the mid-1980s, travel-associated rickettsioses were considered rarities, but since then, several hundred cases have been reported in the literature, in particular in returnees from Sub-Saharan Africa and Southeast Asia [2]. In a recent GeoSentinel study of 17,353 ill travelers presenting at centers in North America, Europe, and Oceania, spotted fever group rickettsiosis was found to be the second most commonly diagnosed disease in returnees from Sub-Saharan Africa with systemic febrile illness, only surpassed by malaria [3]. A GeoSentinel study specifically focusing on fevers in returned travelers suggests that up to 2% of cases may be caused by rickettsioses and that 20% of these are hospitalized [2].

## African tick bite fever

African tick bite fever is caused by *R. africae*, a spotted fever group rickettsia transmitted by *Amblyomma* ticks (Figure 18.1). The disease is ubiquitous in Sub-Saharan Africa and the Eastern Caribbean in grassy woodlands, including savannahs. Its incubation period is typically one week (range 5–10 days). The clinical presentation is characterized by acute fever, headache, nuchal myalgia, and one or several eschars, that is, painless, centimeter-sized erythemas with central necrotic lesions at the sites of the preceding tick bites (Figures 18.2 and 18.3). Lesser frequent signs include regional lymphadenitis, draining lymphangitis (Figure 18.3), aphthous stomatitis, and a vesicular rash (Figure 18.4). Most cases are mild and self-limited and so far no fatalities have been reported in the literature [4].

From being virtually unknown in travel medicine only two decades ago, African tick bite fever has emerged as an

*Tropical Diseases in Travelers*, 1st edition. Edited by E. Schwartz.
© 2009 by Blackwell Publishing, ISBN: 978-1-4051-8441-0.

**Table 18.1** Features of the common rickettsioses in travelers to the tropics.

| Disease | Pathogen | Vector | Distribution | High-risk activities | Common presentation | Outcome |
|---|---|---|---|---|---|---|
| African tick bite fever | *R. africae* | Cattle ticks | Sub-Saharan Africa (mainly southern Africa) | Safari, game park walk | Fever, myalgia + multiple eschars | Benign |
| Mediterranean spotted fever | *R. conorii* | Dog ticks | Mediterranean rim and focally in Sub-Saharan Africa | Contact with local dogs | Fever, myalgia, rash + single eschar | Multiorgan failure may occur |
| Murine typhus | *R. typhi* | Rodent fleas | Worldwide in rodent-infested areas | Visit to harbor areas and beach resorts | Fever, myalgia, rash | Multiorgan failure may occur |
| Scrub typhus | *O. tsutsugamushi* | Mites | South and Southeast Asia | Trekking, rafting, camping | Fever, myalgia, rash + single eschar | Multiorgan failure may occur |

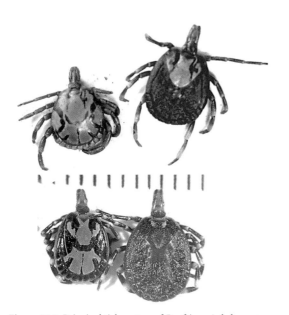

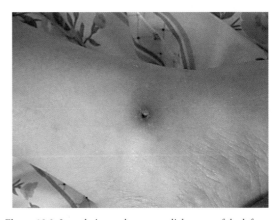

**Figure 18.2** Inoculation eschar on medial aspect of the left ankle in a Norwegian traveler with African tick bite fever.

**Figure 18.1** Principal tick vectors of *R. africae*: *A. hebraeum*, male and female (upper panel), and *A. variegatum*, male and female (lower panel). Scale is millimetric.

important cause of acute febrile illness in travelers to Sub-Saharan Africa, in particular to South Africa and neighboring countries. It is overwhelmingly the most common tick-borne rickettsiosis diagnosed in visitors to the region. In a retrospective series of 119 cases of tick-borne rickettsioses diagnosed in returnees from Sub-Saharan Africa, 118 (99%) were caused by *R. africae* and only one (1%) by *R. conorii*, the agent of Mediterranean spotted fever (see below) [5]. In the only prospective study so far of any rickettsial disease in travelers, the incidence of African tick bite fever among 940 mostly short-term Norwegian safari travelers to Sub-Equatorial Africa was 4%, ranging from

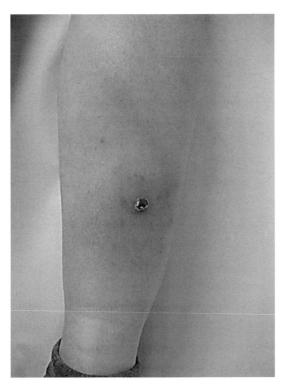

**Figure 18.3** Inoculation eschar with draining lymphangitis on shin of a Norwegian traveler with African tick bite fever.

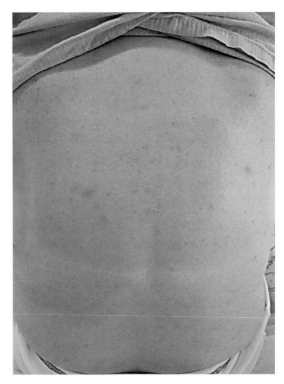

**Figure 18.4** Vesicular rash on the back of a Norwegian traveler with African tick bite fever.

2% in leisure safari tourists to an impressive 25% in game hunters [6]. *Amblyomma* ticks are highly aggressive and can attack humans in great numbers; this is especially true for the minute larval and nymph forms that may swarm over clothes and exposed skin within a few minutes after exposure. The ticks usually bite where the skin is soft and humid, typically behind the knees and in the perianal area, the groin, and the axillae. Tourists are often infected during bush walks, camping, or hunting, and the disease sometimes occurs in spectacular clusters that may affect up to 100% of a group of travelers. Cases of African tick bite fever may occur 12 months a year, although the risk is highest during the rainy season from January to April [6]. Most travel-associated cases resolve uneventfully, but complications such as myocarditis, prolonged fever, reactive arthritis (Figure 18.5), subacute neuropathy, and neuropsychiatric manifestations are occasionally reported [4].

## Mediterranean spotted fever

Mediterranean spotted fever is caused by *R. conorii*, a spotted fever group rickettsia closely related to *R. africae*. The disease is transmitted by the brown dog tick, *Rhipi-*

*cephalus sanguines*, and occurs primarily in urban areas with canines in the Mediterranean basin and in parts of Africa. Mediterranean spotted fever usually presents 6–10 days after the infective tick bite with a maculopapular rash that may involve the palms and soles, a high fever, and an

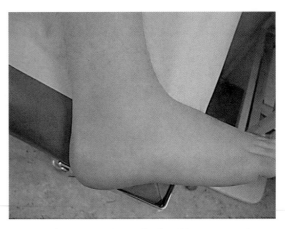

**Figure 18.5** Reactive arthritis of right ankle in a Norwegian traveler with African tick bite fever.

inoculation eschar at the tick bite site. The disease is potentially more severe than African tick bite fever and may, if left untreated, result in neurological involvement, gangrene, respiratory distress syndrome, multiorgan failure, and death [7].

Mediterranean spotted fever is occasionally reported in travelers to the tropics, including Sub-Saharan Africa. Most patients can recall direct physical contact, such as patting or playing with local dogs. The clinical course of Mediterranean spotted fever in travelers is usually benign, but cases complicated by neurological deficits or multiorgan failure and death have been reported in visitors to Africa [8].

### Murine typhus

Murine typhus is caused by *R. typhi*, a typhus group rickettsia transmitted by rat fleas. The disease is ubiquitous in tropical areas, particularly in rodent-infested areas, such as harbors, garbage dumps, and food deposits. It is generally accepted that most people become infected when flea feces contaminated with *R. typhi* contaminate disrupted skin or are inhaled into the respiratory tract. Rarely, the infection may result from the fleabite itself. As for other rickettsioses, the incubation period for murine typhus is about 7 days. The clinical presentation is nonspecific, with fever, constitutional symptoms, and an often poorly visible maculopapular exanthema on the trunk as its main features. Importantly, patients with murine typhus never develop inoculation eschars. Most cases are mild, although the fatality rate may be up to 4%.

Murine typhus is sometimes diagnosed in travelers returning from Asia, including Indonesian islands, such as Bali, and Africa [2, 9]. Typical itineraries include travel to port cities or beach resorts, and some patients can recall direct contact with dead or living rodents. Usually, murine typhus is a mild disease in travelers, but aseptic meningitis, deafness, deep venous thrombosis, and even fatalities have been reported [2].

### Scrub typhus

Scrub typhus is one of a few mite-borne rickettsioses in humans. It is common in South and Southeast Asia and the Pacific, where an estimated one million cases occur each year, mainly among persons engaged in outdoors occupational activities. The disease is caused by *O. tsutsugamushi* (formerly *R. tsutsugamushi*), which is transmitted by the bites of larval trombiculid mites, also called chiggers. These mites occur year-round on grassy vegetation, although their prevalence fluctuates with temperature and rainfall. Humans are usually bitten on the lower extrem-

ities or in the genital region. The time from mite bite to symptom onset (incubation period) is usually 7–10 days. Most patients present with fever, constitutional symptoms, and a generalized lymphadenitis, and up to 90% have visible inoculation eschars at the sites of the mite bites. About 50% of patients develop nonpruritic macular or maculopapular rashes that begin on the abdomen and spread to the extremities and face. Cases are usually mild, but respiratory distress, meningoencephalitis, disseminated intravascular coagulation, and renal failure are commonly seen. The fatality rate of scrub typhus may be up to 35%, depending on bacterial virulence, host factors, and delay in treatment [10].

Scrub typhus is occasionally reported in international travelers to endemic areas. Most patients are infected in Thailand and neighboring countries, but some cases are acquired in Sri Lanka and India [11]. Typical case histories include camping, trekking, or rafting and may occur after visits to coral atolls, rice paddies, canals, or palm oil plantations. The clinical course in travelers is usually benign, although devastating complications have been reported in misdiagnosed returnees from Thailand and Burma [2].

### Other rickettsioses

Tick-borne rickettsioses that have occasionally been reported in travelers to the tropics include Astrakhan fever and Indian tick typhus, caused by two distinct subspecies of *R. conorii*, and *R. aeschlimannii* infection [2]. Basically, however, tick-borne rickettsioses are prevalent throughout the world, and many areas can be considered potentially risky to travelers [12].

Recently, a spotted fever group rickettsiosis caused by *R. felis* and associated with several flea species throughout the world was described, but no cases have yet been reported in travelers [13]. Specific travelers, such as health workers or military personnel, may occasionally be exposed to epidemic typhus caused by *R. prowazekii*, a typhus group rickettsia transmitted by human body lice in crowded settings, including refugee camps and prisons [2].

### Q fever

Q fever is a zoonosis of worldwide distribution caused by *C. burnetii*, which is transmitted from infected mammals (usually sheep, goats, cattle, cats, and dogs) to humans by contaminated aerosols or ingestion of unpasteurized diary products. *C. burnetii* exists in two antigenic phases, called phase I and phase II. This antigenic difference is important in diagnosis and in distinguishing between acute and chronic Q fever (see below). Sporulated bacteria may be spread from infected animals by the wind over large distances, a few kilometers or more. Human-to-human transmission is probably very rare [14].

The disease is divided into two clinical forms: acute Q fever and chronic Q fever. The incubation period of acute Q fever ranges from 2 to 6 weeks but is usually around 20 days. Acute Q fever typically presents as a nonspecific flulike illness with high fever, chills, headache, and myalgia. In a minority of cases, atypical pneumonia or granulomatous hepatitis may develop. Chronic Q fever, which is defined as an infection lasting for more than 6 months, typically manifests as endocarditis or vasculitis. It occurs in 1–5% of patients infected with *C. burnetii*, but virtually only in those with certain predisposing conditions, including cardiac valvular disease, vascular aneurysms, immunodeficiency, or pregnancy. The prognosis of chronic Q fever is dire; as many as 65% of patients may die of the disease.

Q fever is sometimes diagnosed in travelers to the tropics. In a Spanish retrospective study of 708 febrile travelers evaluated at a university clinic, 5 (0.7%) were diagnosed with acute Q fever acquired in Africa (3 cases), Asia, and South America [15]. In Sweden and Norway, 32 cases of imported Q fever were diagnosed from 2000 to 2007, of which approximately 50% were acquired in tropical areas, with the Canary Islands being the most common destination (Sirkka Vene, personal communication). In a series of 10 cases of acute Q fever imported to France, 3 were acquired in Sub-Saharan Africa (Mali, Chad, and Congo), one in the Indian Ocean (Reunion), and one in South America (Guyana) [16]. Outbreaks of Q fever among travelers are rare but were reported in a group of Israeli visitors to rural Kenya [17]. Many infected travelers can recall visits to local farmlands and direct physical contact with domestic animals [15]. Others, however, have only stayed in typical hotel or resort areas and are likely to have been infected by windborne *Coxiella* spores from nearby animal farms or roaming mammals [18].

Most infected travelers develop benign acute Q fever, although fatalities have been reported [19]. Chronic Q fever is seemingly rare in travelers. Occasionally travelers with Q fever may be co-infected with other tropical diseases, including falciparum malaria and African tick bite fever, which may preclude correct diagnosis and treatment [20, 21].

## Bartonelloses

Three bartonella species are responsible for most cases of human bartonellosis: *B. bacilliformis*, transmitted by sandflies in the Andean region of South America and the agent of Carrion's disease, a biphasic illness with an acute, life-threatening febrile stage (Oroya fever) and a chronic, benign cutaneous stage (verruga peruana); *B. quintana*, transmitted by body lice worldwide and the cause of trench fever, endocarditis, bacillary angiomatosis, and chronic bacteremia; and *B. henselae*, transmitted by felines and their fleas and the causative agent of cat scratch disease, endocarditis, and bacillary angiomatosis.

Bartonelloses appear to be extremely rare in travelers to the tropics. In the GeoSentinel surveillance network database, which currently contains information on >90,000 ill travelers and immigrants evaluated since 1996, only five cases of bartonellosis are reported (David Freedman, personal communication). In the literature, just a handful of cases have been published, including an Italian tourist to Peru and an Equadorian expatriate who were both diagnosed with Carrion's disease [22, 23]. A third case of imported bartenollosis was recently seen in a US returnee from Peru who developed a febrile illness with splenomegaly and bacteremia caused by a new flea-associated species, *B. rochalimae* [24].

## Diagnosis

Routine blood tests in patients with rickettsioses and Q fever usually show nonspecific and modest aberrations only. Mild leukopenia, lymphopenia, and thrombocytopenia are common, as are elevated serum C-reactive protein and liver transaminases [10, 14, 25].

The microbiological diagnosis of rickettsioses and Q fever relies in most cases on serology performed on acute and convalescent phase sera. Immunofluorescence assay (IFA) is the reference serological method, although other less sensitive and specific tests, such as the archaic Weil–Felix test and novel dipstick slide tests, are in use at many laboratories worldwide [26]. Sophisticated serological analyses for rickettsial diseases, including multiantigen IFA (where reactions to several rickettsial antigens may be compared directly) and Western blot, are available at reference centers to which serum samples may be shipped at ambient temperature.

Currently, there are commercial IFA kits based on several rickettsial antigens: some of the spotted fever group rickettsiae (e.g., *R. conorii* and *R. rickettsii*, the agent of Rocky Mountain spotted fever in America), the typhus group rickettsiae, *O. tsutsugamushi*, and *C. burnetii*. It should be noted that an IFA specifically based on *R. africae* is not commercially available; however, most patients with African tick bite fever will test positive in assays based on *R. conorii* and *R. rickettsii* antigens because of cross reactions. Most patients with rickettsial diseases will seroconvert by IFA within 10–14 days after symptom onset. The major exception to this rule is African tick bite fever, where seroconversion usually occurs beyond three weeks after symptom onset [27], or not at all in mild cases or in those treated early with doxycycline [28].

*C. burnetii* exists in two antigenic phases called phase I and phase II. In acute Q fever, the antibody level against phase II is usually higher than that against phase I, often by several orders of magnitude, whereas the reverse is true in chronic Q fever. Due to the serious prognosis of chronic Q fever, patients diagnosed with acute Q fever and at risk for chronic disease should be followed with monthly IFA for at least six months to detect any rising IgG antibody titers against *C. burnetii* phase I antigens.

With the exception of the bartonellae, which may grow (if very slowly) in standard blood culture bottles, bacteria discussed in this chapter cannot be isolated in cell-free media. Isolation attempts on cell cultures can be performed on buffy coat and tissue samples, including eschar biopsies. Cell culture, however, is technically cumbersome, is usually negative in patients pretreated with antibiotics, and is potentially hazardous and should only be performed at laboratories with biosafety level 3 facilities [26].

Blood and tissue samples may also be submitted for PCR, a sensitive, specific, and rapid diagnostic test. In contrast to cell culture, PCR is usually positive irrespective of any prior antibiotic treatment. Primer sets targeting various rickettsial genes, including those encoding 16S DNA, have been described and can be used in any laboratory with suitable facilities. If PCR-based testing is delayed for more than 24 hours, samples should be stored at $-20°C$ [26].

## Treatment

Importantly, drugs against rickettsial diseases must be active intracellularly. Chloramphenicol was the first antibiotic shown to be effective but has since been largely been replaced by doxycycline and other tetracyclines. Institution of treatment is usually followed by rapid resolution of symptoms, including fever, and a delayed response beyond 48 hours should call the diagnosis in question. The standard dose of doxycycline is 100 mg twice daily given for 3–5 days in African tick bite fever and mild cases of scrub typhus, and for 2 weeks in patients with Q fever. Alternative drugs include the new macrolides (e.g., azithromycin) and fluoroquinolones [2]. The treatment of the bartonelloses is more complex and should be based on combinations of doxycycline, rifampicin, aminoglycosides, and fluoroquinolones [29]. Patients with chronic Q fever endocarditis should be treated with a combination of doxycycline and hydroxychloroquine for a minimum of 18 months [18].

## Prevention

The best preventive measure against rickettsial diseases is to avoid typical risk settings when traveling in endemic areas. This is particularly important for immunocompromised individuals, for whom some of the diseases can have a devastating course. Dogs, cats, rodents, and domestic livestock (dead or alive) should not be touched, and bush vegetation likely to be infested with ticks or mites should not be entered. If this course cannot be followed, measures aimed at minimizing the risk of arthropod bites should be implemented. Travelers to regions highly endemic for African tick bite fever in Africa or for scrub typhus in Asia should walk wide trails and wear protective clothing with long sleeves and long trousers impregnated with permethrin, an acaricide derivate of the chrysanthemum family. Repellents containing dimethylmetatoluamide (DEET) should be applied to exposed skin every 1–2 hours [30]. Daily tick checks are recommended during stays in tick-infested areas, and any attached tick should be swiftly removed. To avoid Q fever, travelers should not visit animal farms or ingest unpasteurized diary products. A weekly 200-mg dose of doxycycline prevents scrub typhus in military personnel deployed to endemic areas [31]. The efficacy against scrub typhus and other rickettsioses of the daily 100-mg doxycycline regimen used for malaria chemoprophylaxis is untested and unknown. No vaccines against rickettsial diseases are readily available for travelers.

## Concluding comments

Ecotourism and adventure travel are increasingly popular and now constitute the fastest-growing segment of the leisure travel industry. Numerous visitors travel off the beaten track and participate in trekking, rafting, bush walks, safaris, camping, and other outdoor recreational activities. To this, add aid workers and military personnel deployed to remote areas, where they may live in close proximity to local populations and their animals. Because some of these new destinations are important biotopes for rickettsioses, Q fever, and bartonelloses, a continuing increase of travel-associated cases should be anticipated in the years to come.

Despite these current trends, rickettsial diseases are still surprisingly rarely reported in travelers to the tropics. The reason for this is probably complex, although under-diagnosis and underreporting are likely to be common. Most diseases in question have a nonspecific presentation and may easily confuse the less experienced physician but should always, in the absence of other plausible explanations, be considered in a febrile returnee from the tropics, irrespective of the season. In severely ill cases, empirical treatment with doxycycline is vindicated. Importantly, microbiological tests can only provide a retrospective diagnosis, and a negative result in the acute phase can therefore never rule out the presence a rickettsial disease. Travelers to endemic areas should be informed about the importance of avoiding bites by arachnids and insects by not entering heavily infested biotopes and of refraining from physical contact with local animals, both domesticated and wild.

## References

1 Rolain JM, Jensenius M, Raoult D. Rickettsial infections in travelers. *Curr Opin Infect Dis* 2004;17:433–7.

2 Jensenius M, Fournier PE, Raoult D. Rickettsioses and the international traveler. *Clin Infect Dis* 2004; 39: 1493–9.

3 Freedman DO, Weld LH, Kozarsky PE, et al. Spectrum of disease and relation to place of exposure among ill returned travelers. *N Engl J Med* 2006;354:119.

4 Jensenius M, Fournier PE, Kelly P, Myrvang B, Raoult D. African tick bite fever. *Lancet Infect Dis* 2003;3:557–64.

5 Raoult D, Fournier PE, Fenollar F, et al. *Rickettsia africae*, a tick-borne pathogen in travelers to Sub-Saharan Africa. *N Engl J Med* 2001;344:1504–10.

6 Jensenius M, Fournier PE, Vene S, et al. African tick bite fever in travelers to rural Sub-Equatorial Africa. *Clin Infect Dis* 2003;36:1411–17.

7 Raoult D, Weiller PJ, Chagnon A, Chaudet H, Gallais H, Casanova P. Mediterranean spotted fever: clinical, laboratory and epidemiological features of 199 cases. *Am J Trop Med Hyg* 1986;35:845–50.

8 Rutherford JS. Fatal spotted fever rickettsiosis, Kenya. *Emerg Infect Dis* 2004;10:910–13.

9 Azuma M, Nishioka Y, Ogawa M, Takasaki T, Sone S, Uchiyama T. Murine typhus from Vietnam, imported into Japan. *Emerg Infect Dis* 2006;12:1466–8.

10 Watt G, Parola P. Scrub typhus and tropical rickettsioses. *Curr Opin Infect Dis* 2003;16: 429–36.

11 Jensenius M, Montelius R, Berild D, Vene S. Scrub typhus imported to Scandinavia. *Scand J Infect Dis* 2006;38: 200–202.

12 Parola P, Paddock CD, Raoult D. Tick-borne rickettsioses around the world: emerging diseases challenging old concepts. *Clin Microbiol Rev* 2005;18:719–56.

13 Labruna MB, Ogrzewalska M, Moraes-Filho J, Lepe P, Gallegos JL, López J. *Rickettsia fells* in Chile. *Emerg Infect Dis* 2007;13:1794–5.

14 Raoult D, Tissot-Dupont H, Foucault C, et al. Q fever 1985-1998. Clinical and epidemiologic features of 1,383 infections. *Medicine (Baltimore)* 2000;79:109–23.

15 Ta TH, Jiménez B, Navarro M, Meije Y, González FJ, Lopez-Velez R.Q Fever in returned febrile travelers. *J Travel Med* 2008;15:126–9.

16 Imbert P, Rapp C, Jagou M, Saillol A, Debord T. Q fever in travelers: 10 cases. *J Travel Med* 2004;11:383–5.

17 Potasman I, Rzotkiewicz S, Pick N, Keysary A. Outbreak of Q fever following a safari trip. *Clin Infect Dis* 2000;30: 214–15.

18 Cohen NJ, Papernik M, Singleton J, Segreti J, Eremeeva ME. Q fever in an American tourist returned from Australia. *Travel Med Infect Dis* 2007;5:194–5.

19 Isaksson HJ, Hrafnkelsson J, Hilmarsdóttir I. Acute Q fever: a cause of fatal hepatitis in an Icelandic traveler. *Scand J Infect Dis* 2001;33:314–15.

20 Rolain JM, Gouriet F, Brouqui P, et al. Concomitant or consecutive infection with Coxiella burnetii and tickborne diseases. *Clin Infect Dis* 2005;40:82–8.

21 Brouqui P, Rolain JM, Foucault C, Raoult D. Short report: Q fever and Plasmodium falciparum malaria co-infection in a patient returning from the Comoros archipelago. *Am J Trop Med Hyg* 2005;73:1028–30.

22 Matteelli A, Castelli F, Spinetti A, Bonetti F, Graifenberghi S, Carosi G. Short report: verruga peruana in an Italian traveler from Peru. *Am J Trop Med Hyg* 1994;50:143–4.

23 Lydy SL, Eremeeva ME, Asnis D, et al. Isolation and characterization of Bartonella bacilliformis from an expatriate Ecuadorian. *J Clin Microbiol* 2008;46:627–37.

24 Eremeeva ME, Gerns HL, Lydy SL, et al. Bacteremia, fever, and splenomegaly caused by a newly recognized bartonella species. *N Engl J Med* 2007;356:2381–7.

25 Jensenius M, Fournier PE, Hellum KB, et al. Sequential changes of hematological and biochemical parameters in African tick bite fever. *Clin Microbiol Infect* 2003;9:678–83.

26 La Scola B, Raoult D. Laboratory diagnosis of rickettsioses: current approaches to diagnosis of old and new rickettsial diseases. *J Clin Microbiol* 1997;35:2715–27.

27 Fournier PE, Jensenius M, Laferl H, Vene S, Raoult D. Kinetics of antibody responses in *Rickettsia africae* and *Rickettsia conorii* infections. *Clin Diagn Lab Immunol* 2002;9: 324–8.

28 Jensenius M, Fournier PE, Vene S, Ringertz SH, Myrvang B, Raoult D. Immunofluorescence assay, Western blotting and cross-adsorption for the diagnosis of African tick bite fever. *Clin Diagn Lab Immunol* 2004;11:768–8.

29 Rolain JM, Brouqui P, Koehler JE, Maguina C, Dolan MJ, Raoult D. Recommendations for treatment of human infections caused by *Bartonella* species. *Antimicrob Agents Chemother* 2004;48:1921–33.

30 Jensenius M, Pretorius AM, Clarke F, Myrvang B. Efficacy of four commercial DEET repellents against *Amblyomma hebraeum* (Acari: Ixodidae), the principal vector of *Rickettsia africae* in southern Africa. *Trans R Soc Trop Med Hyg* 2005;99:708–11.

31 Olson JG, Bourgeois AL, Fang RC, Coolbaugh JC, Dennis DT. Prevention of scrub typhus. Prophylactic administration of doxycycline in a randomized double blind trial. *Am J Trop Med Hyg* 1980;29:989–97.

# 19 Relapsing Fever

## Gil Sidi[1] and Eli Schwartz[2]

[1]Memorial Sloan Kettering Cancer Center, New York, USA
[2]Chaim Sheba Medical Center, Tel Hashomer, Israel and Sackler School of Medicine, Tel Aviv University, Tel Aviv, Israel

## Introduction

Relapsing fever has been known since ancient times and was recognized to be a tick-transmitted disease in 1905, when Dutton and Todd demonstrated spirochetes in *O. moubata* ticks in West Africa [1, 2]. The disease has since been reported in North and South America, Africa, Asia, and Europe. It is caused by *Borrelia* species, which infect humans through tick or louse bites.

Although relapsing fever is still endemic in many regions of the world, it has attracted little attention in recent years and is likely being underdiagnosed. With the increase in worldwide travel, more cases are being diagnosed in travelers to endemic areas, increasing the need for physicians in nonendemic countries to be aware of this disease.

## Epidemiology

*Borrelia* are helical, 8–30 μm long, and 0.2–0.5 μm wide, have 3–10 loose spirals, are actively motile, and divide by transverse fission [3]. There are two types of relapsing fever *Borrelia*, each with distinct epidemiological and clinical features: louse-borne relapsing fever (LBRF) and tick-borne relapsing fever (TBRF) [3, 4].

LBRF is transmitted by the human body louse, *Pediculus humanus*, infected with *B. recurrentis*. The louse causes infection when it is crushed, causing its fluids to contaminate mucous membranes or breaks in the skin. LBRF, also termed epidemic relapsing fever, is found in areas of crowding and poor sanitation and was associated with vast outbreaks in soldiers and civilians during World War I and after World War II. LBRF is currently an important

disease only in northeastern Africa, especially the highlands of Ethiopia. Humans are the only known reservoir of infection [4].

The TBRF *Borrelia* is the more important disease, as it still endemic in many Western countries and is more relevant to travelers as well. TBRF is transmitted to humans by the bite of an infected *Ornithodoros* tick. The *Ornithodoros* species of ticks belong to the family Argasidae (soft ticks), which have nocturnal feeding habits and painless bites (Figure 19.1). They are long-lived, often surviving many years without food. The primary reservoirs of *Borrelia* in the USA are rodents, such as deer mice, chipmunks, squirrels, and rats, and lagomorphs, such as rabbits and hares [4]. In East Africa, chickens and pigs are suspected to act as reservoirs [5]. An article by Schwan et al. suggested that birds may have a role as reservoirs of *Borrelia* and in dispersing it in the natural environment [6]. Tick-borne *Borrelia* can remain viable in their natural tick vectors for up to 12 years [7].

The *Borrelia* species have the genetic ability to vary their surface antigens extensively, leading to repeated stimulation of the immune system by new antigens and causing the typical recurrent attacks. This pattern, in animals, allows the bacteremia to persist long enough to permit transmission to feeding ticks, thereby completing the life cycle [8].

Acquisition of human TBRF is generally restricted to the geographical range of the tick vectors. A number of *Ornithodoros* species have been described worldwide, each with its characteristic *Borrelia* types. Each *Borrelia* species that causes relapsing fever appears to be specific to its tick vector. *Ornithodoros* species endemic to the United States include *O. hermsi*, which harbors *B. hermsii* [3], *O. turicata*, which harbors *B. turicatae* [9], and *O. parkeri*, which harbors *B. parkeri* [10]. Species described in other parts of the world include *O. moubata*, which harbors *B. duttoni* (Africa), *O. erraticus*, which harbors *B. hispanica*

*Tropical Diseases in Travelers*, 1st edition. Edited by E. Schwartz.
© 2009 by Blackwell Publishing, ISBN: 978-1-4051-8441-0.

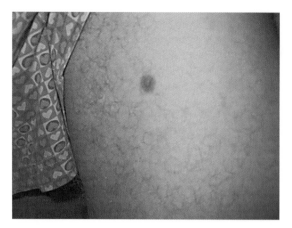

**Figure 19.1** Typical tick bite of *Ornithodoros*.

Exposure to the ticks occurs in their natural places of habitat. In the western USA, *O. hermsi*, which harbors *B. hermsii*, has most commonly been described as infecting persons sleeping in tick-infested cabins. The nocturnal ticks seek their hosts and feed within 15–90 minutes, after which they return to their refuge in the walls, floor, or attic [6]. In Texas, *O. turicata*, which harbors *B. turicatae*, has been described as infecting persons visiting caves [9] Similarly, *O. tholozany*, in the Middle East and Central Asia, is primarily found in dark moist areas, such as caves and abandoned buildings. In an Israeli study, 64% of TBRF cases were associated with exposure to caves [12]. Due to this correlation, TBRF in Israel has traditionally been called "cave fever."

## Epidemiology in travelers

and *B. crocidurae* (Spain, Portugal, North Africa), and *O. verrucosus*, which harbors *B. caucasica* (Central Asia) [4]. *Borrelia persica*, whose host is *O. tholozany*, is thought to be the cause of most cases of TBRF in Israel and is prevalent in other Middle Eastern countries such as Jordan and in Central Asian countries, such as Russia, China, and Iran [11] (Figure 19.2).

LBRF is limited to its endemic areas in Ethiopia; short-term visitors to these areas are at almost no risk of acquiring it. It can be acquired by persons who have long-term close contact with the LBRF population, such as health relief workers. It has historically spread out of its endemic areas during periods of war and famine [4]. The detection of high seroprevalence for *B. recurrentis* among homeless

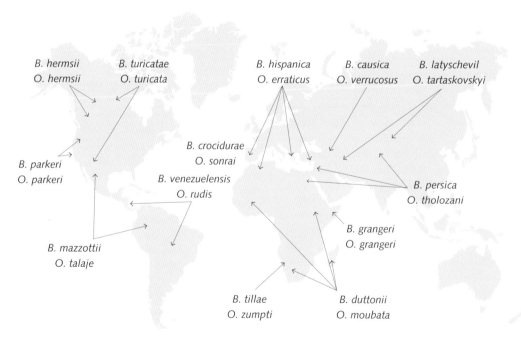

**Figure 19.2** Geographical distribution of common species of *Borrelia* and *Ornithodoros*.

people in Marseilles suggests that this disease may play an important role in future epidemics [13].

TBRF, on the other hand, despite becoming less common in developed countries, where the population is increasingly urbanized [12], is emerging as a disease of travelers to rural areas. In recent years, rural areas have become more popular as travel destinations for tourists from developed countries. Several studies have described TBRF in travelers to endemic countries.

Several features of TBRF make it hazardous for travelers. *Ornithodoros* ticks are long-lived and can remain in the environment for prolonged periods without feeding. The ticks feed for a short period, and their bite is painless, reducing their chance of being detected. Because TBRF is not well known to physicians in nonendemic areas, and because the symptoms are nonspecific and could be confused with those of another disease such as malaria, travelers who acquire the disease may be incorrectly diagnosed or may be diagnosed late in the course of the disease.

This disease also exists in rural areas of industrialized countries. There are reports of importation of the disease from Israel [14] and from Spain[15 ], in addition to importation from developing countries in Africa [15, 16] and Central America [17]. In an epidemiological study of relapsing fever in Israel in 1971–2003, three cases were described in travelers returning from Africa and four cases were described in soldiers who were on military duty in Lebanon and acquired the disease there [12].

Residents of endemic countries who are normally not at risk for the disease may become exposed as a result of engaging in high-risk activities. An article describing TBRF cases in the United States and British Columbia found that 40% of cases occurred in persons traveling out of their states of residence, with exposures to TBRF through cave exploration, rustic cabin dwelling and hiking [18]. In Israel, exposure most commonly occurs in persons engaging in outdoor activities, including travelers to rural areas and soldiers involved in activities that require lying on the ground for prolonged periods [12].

## Clinical aspects

TBRF and LBRF have similar clinical manifestations (Table 19.1). The incubation period lasts an average of 7 days (range 2–18 days), after which the illness characteristically begins abruptly with high fever (usually reaching 40°C), chills, headache, myalgia, arthralgia, abdominal pain, and malaise. Other symptoms can include diarrhea, dry cough, photophobia, rash, neck pain, eye pain, dysuria, and confusion. A small subset of patients develop symptoms and signs of meningitis. The disease is characterized by intensification of the symptoms for several days, ending in a crisis, after which the fever ceases. This is followed by a quiescent period lasting on average 9 days in LBRF and 7 days in TBRF, after which a relapse can occur. Untreated patients with TBRF can have up to 13 relapses, which tend to be milder and farther apart as the disease runs its course [19]. Patients with LBRF characteristically have only one or two relapses [4]. The spikes of high temperature are associated with bacteremia, in which the number of *Borrelia* in the blood can reach $10^8$ ml$^{-1}$ [8]. The febrile attack in each cycle cannot be differentiated from other febrile diseases of travelers, but the history of recurrent attacks makes this disease unique and can give a clue to the diagnosis.

The most common findings on physical examination are fever and tachycardia. There can be significant arthralgia but not arthritis. Some patients have meningismus. A pleural rub may be auscultated, and the liver and spleen may be enlarged and tender to palpation. Some patients have rashes, which can be petechial, maculopapular, or papulovesicular [4].

Death in TBRF is rare and limited mainly to infants and the elderly [7]. Death in LBRF is more common, but this may be due to the presence of malnutrition and co-infections in the population it commonly affects.

## Laboratory findings

Common nonspecific laboratory findings include thrombocytopenia, hematuria, and proteinuria [20]. Other common laboratory findings that were noted in a review of cases of TBRF in Israel between 1975 and 2003 included anemia (78% of cases), leukopenia (14%), leukocytosis (14%), and thrombocytopenia (33%). The blood chemistry panels were normal in most of the cases (72%). Common abnormalities included elevated lactate dehydrogenase levels, elevated indirect bilirubin levels, elevated fibrinogen levels, and mildly elevated transaminase levels. The ESR was elevated, in the range of 50–120 mm/hour, in 95% [the authors, unpublished data].

## Diagnosis

Relapsing fever should be suspected in a person who inhabits or has traveled to an endemic area and has engaged in high-risk behavior (living in tick-infested cabins,

**Table 19.1** Symptoms, signs, and laboratory findings.

| | Tick-borne | | | Louse-borne |
|---|---|---|---|---|
| | Sidi, Schwartz Unpublished data | Lerman et al. [26] | Dworkin et al. [20] | Ramos et al. [27] |
| Number of patients | 97 | 83 | 182 | 170 |
| Percent male | 74% | 99% (soldiers) | 57% | 59% |
| Location | Israel | Israel | North America | Ethiopia |
| Prevalent *Borrelia* spec. | *B. persica* | *B. persica* | *B. hermsii* | *B. recurrentis* |
| | | Symptoms | | |
| Headache | **42%** | **70%** | 94% | 54% |
| Nausea/vomiting | 23% | 28% | **76%** | 23% |
| Myalgia | 17% | **34%** | 92% | NA |
| Abdominal pain | 11% | **18%** | **44%** | 18% |
| Arthralgia | 7% | **8%** | 73% | NA |
| Dry cough | NA | **12%** | 27% | 24% |
| Eye pain | NA | NA | **26%** | NA |
| Diarrhea | 2% | **18%** | 25% | NA |
| Weight loss | 2% | **4%** | NA | NA |
| Dysuria | 1% | **7%** | 13% | NA |
| Syncope | 1% | NA | NA | NA |
| | | Signs | | |
| Fever | NA | NA | 100% | 100% |
| Confusion | NA | NA | **38%** | NA |
| Icterus | NA | 10% | NA | 2% |
| Rash | **9%** | **12%** | **18%** | 2% |
| Splenomegaly | NA | 47% | NA | 5% |
| Hepatomegaly | NA | 29% | NA | NA |
| Lymphadenopathy | NA | 40% | NA | NA |
| Nuchal rigidity | NA | 5% | NA | 2% |
| | | Lab results | | |
| Leukocytosis | NA | 44% | NA | NA |
| Leukopenia | NA | 3% | NA | NA |
| Anemia | NA | NA | NA | NA |
| Elevated bilirubin | NA | 25% | NA | NA |
| Elevated transaminase | NA | 8% | NA | NA |
| Proteinuria | NA | 27% | 46% | NA |
| Hematuria | NA | 39% | 30% | NA |
| Pyuria | NA | 50% | NA | NA |
| Death | 0% | NA | NA | 6% |
| J–H reaction | NA | NA | 54% | NA |

visiting caves), who presents with the typical clinical picture of recurring febrile attacks with a few afebrile days between them. It may be more difficult to identify the disease within the first febrile attack.

Diseases that should be considered in the differential diagnosis include typhus, typhoid fever, malaria, dengue, leptospirosis, viral hemorrhagic fevers, and, in the United States, Colorado tick fever [4].

Laboratory confirmation is made by observing spirochetes on a Wright's or Giemsa-stained smear of peripheral blood (Figure 19.3). Smears obtained during a febrile period have a sensitivity of nearly 70% when performed

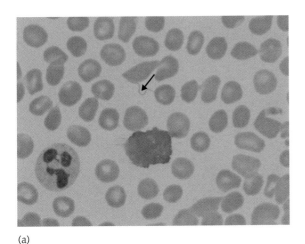

(a)

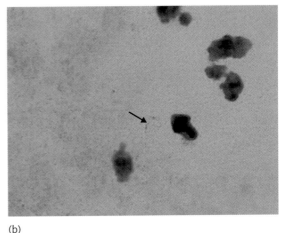

(b)

**Figure 19.3** Spirochetes on a Wright–Giemsa-stained smear of peripheral blood showing the spiral shape of the borrelia. (a) In a thin blood smear (see arrow). (b) In a thick blood smear (see arrow). (Courtesy of Dr. G. Smollen, Department of Clinical Microbiology. Sheba Medical Center, Israel.)

by an experienced observer. Enzyme immunoassays or immunofluorescent assays for antibodies to the *Borrelia* species that cause TBRF are available, but have not been standardized, and may not be positive in the early stages of the disease. The most specific diagnostic test is culture of *Borrelia* from blood, but this procedure is neither rapid nor widely performed [21].

Another test that has recently become available is PCR, which has been evaluated in several trials. An Israeli trial evaluated PCR targeting the glycerophosphodiester phosphodiesterase (GlpQ) gene and found it to be highly sensitive and specific for the detection of *B. persica* during febrile periods [22]. PCR was also found to be useful in a trial in Senegal [23].

## Treatment

Doxycycline (or another tetracycline) is the drug of choice, based on clinical experience. Erythromycin and chloramphenicol are also effective. Penicillin therapy appears to be associated with an increased rate of relapse, and rare failures have been reported with doxycycline. The typical dose of doxycycline is 100 mg q12 given for 7 days. In LBRF a single dose of 100 mg of doxycycline has been shown to be highly effective [4].

The *Jarisch–Herxheimer reaction*, which consists of chills, fever, tachycardia, and hypotension, is a serious consequence of antimicrobial therapy for relapsing fever. This reaction occurs in up to half of patients and typi-

cally begins within 1–4 hours after the administration of antimicrobial agents. The severity of the reaction is positively correlated with the density of spirochetes in the blood at the time of treatment [4, 20, 21].

Because this reaction is quite common, our recommendation is starting antibiotic treatment under medical observation. In our experience, some patients even needed ICU observation. Because this reaction only occurs after the first dose of the treatment, continuation of treatment can be given out of the hospital.

## Prevention

Environmental measures can be used to attempt to control tick infestation in endemic areas. Spraying of tick-infested sites with insecticides has been evaluated, and was shown to be effective in reducing the number of cases of TBRF [24]. Another environmental method that may be effective is rodent proofing of homes and vacation cabins. Of 15 cases of TBRF acquired in the Grand Canyon, 14 occurred after overnight stays in cabins that had not been rodent-proofed [16]. Environmental control may be difficult to achieve for several reasons. The ticks causing relapsing fever belong to the family Argasidae, which spend most of their lives in cracks in the ground or below ground in their habitats. The ticks are very hardy and can survive for many years without feeding. These characteristics make it difficult to eradicate the ticks from their natural habitats.

For travelers, more effective prevention would be based on personal protection. Measures that can be taken include avoidance of rodent- and tick-infested sites and, during visits to at-risk sites, use of protective clothing as well as application of repellents to exposed skin and clothing [4].

Another way of preventing the disease is through postexposure prophylaxis. In a study conducted in the Israeli army, a 5-day course of doxycycline was shown to be effective in preventing TBRF in soldiers who had been bitten by ticks. No side effects were recorded and no occurrence of the Jarisch–Herxheimer reaction was documented [25].

## References

1  Dutton JE, Todd JL. The nature of tick fever in the eastern part of the Congo Free State, with notes on the distribution and bionomics of the tick. *Br Med J* 1905;2:1259–60.

2  Raoult D, Roux V. The body louse as a vector of reemerging human diseases. *Clin Infect Dis* 1999;29:888–911.

3  Goubau PF. Relapsing fevers. A review. *Ann Soc Belge Med Trop* 1984;64:335–64.

4  Dennis DT, Campbell GI. Relapsing fever. In: Braunwald E, Hauser SL, Fauci AS, Longo DL, Kasper DI, Jameson JL, editors. *Harrison's Principles of Internal Medicine.* New York: McGraw-Hill; 2005.

5  McCall PJ, Hume JC, Motshegwa K, Pignatelli P, Talbert A, Kisinza W. Does tick-borne relapsing fever have an animal reservoir in East Africa? *Vector Borne Zoonotic Dis* 2007;7(4):659–66.

6  Schwan TG, Raffel SJ, Schrumpf ME, Porcella SF. Diversity and distribution of *Borrelia hermsii. Emerg Infect Dis* 2007 Mar;13(3):436–42.

7  Johnson DW, Golightly LM. Borrelia species (relapsing fever). In: Mandell GL, Bennett JE, Dolin R, editors. *Mandell, Douglas, and Bennett's Principles and Practice of Infectious Diseases*, 5th ed. Philadelphia: Churchill Livingstone; 2000: 2502–4.

8  Norris SJ. Antigenic variation with a twist—the *Borrelia* story. *Mol Microbiol* 2006;60(6):1319–22.

9  Rawlings JA. An overview of tick-borne relapsing fever with emphasis on outbreaks in Texas. *Tex Med* 1995;91: 56–9.

10  Thompson RS, Burgdorfer W, Russel R, Francis BJ. Outbreak of tick-borne relapsing fever in Spokane County, Washington. *JAMA* 1969;210:1045–50.

11  Megido D. A case survey of acute relapsing fever in Israel. *Harefuah* 1984;107:142–5.

12  Sidi G, Davidovitch N, Balicer RD, Anis E, Grotto I, Schwartz E. Tickborne relapsing fever in Israel. *Emerg Infect Dis* 2005;11(11):1784–6.

13  Brouqui P, Stein A, Dupont HT, et al. Ectoparasitism and vector-borne diseases in 930 homeless people from Marseilles. *Medicine (Baltimore)* 2005;84(1):6–8.

14  McNamara JJ, Kay HH. Relapsing fever (*Borrelia*) in an adolescent tourist in Israel. *J Adolesc Health Care* 1988;9(5): 421–3.

15  Wyplosz B, Mihaila-Amrouche L, Baixench MT, et al. Imported tickborne relapsing fever, France. *Emerg Infect Dis* 2005;11(11):1801–3.

16  Colebunders R, De Serrano P, Van Gompel A, et al. Imported relapsing fever in European tourists. *Scand J Infect Dis* 1993;25(4):533–6.

17  Heerdink G, Petit PL, Hofwegen H, van Genderen PJ. A patient with fever following a visit to the tropics: tick-borne relapsing fever discovered in a thick blood smear preparation. *Ned Tijdschr Geneeskd* 2006;150(43):2386–9.

18  Paul WS, Maupin G, Scott-Wright AO, Craven RB, Dennis DT. Outbreak of tick-borne relapsing fever at the north rim of the Grand Canyon: evidence for effectiveness of preventive measures. *Am J Trop Med Hyg* 2002;66(1):71–5.

19  Southern PM Jr, Sanford JP. Relapsing fever: a clinical and microbiological review. *Medicine* 1969;48:129–49.

20  Dworkin MS, Anderson DE Jr, Schwan TG, et al. Tick-borne relapsing fever in the northwestern United States and southwestern Canada. *Clin Infect Dis* 1998;26:122–31.

21  Spach DH, Liles WC, Campbell GL, Quick RE, Anderson DE Jr, Fritsche TR. Tick-borne diseases in the United States. *N Engl J Med* 1993;329:936–47.

22  Halperin T, Orr N, Cohen R, et al. Detection of relapsing fever in human blood samples from Israel using PCR targeting the glycerophosphodiester phosphodiesterase (GlpQ) gene. *Acta Trop* 2006;98(2):189–95.

23  Brahim H, Perrier-Gros-Claude JD, Postic D, Baranton G, Jambou R. Identifying relapsing fever *Borrelia*, Senegal. *Emerg Infect Dis* 2005;11(3):474–5.

24  Talbert A, Nyange A, Molteni F. Spraying tick-infested houses with lambda-cyhalothrin reduces the incidence of tick-borne relapsing fever in children under five years old. *Trans R Soc Trop Med Hyg* 1998; 92(3):251–3.

25  Hasin T, Davidovitch N, Cohen R, et al. Postexposure treatment with doxycycline for the prevention of tick-borne relapsing fever. *N Engl J Med* 2006;13;355(2):148–155.

26  Lerman Y, Koufman Z, Egoz N. The clinical picture of relapsing fever in the Israel Defense Forces, 1966–1976. *Harefuah* 1978;95:365–7.

27  Ramos JM, Malmierca E, Reyes F, et al. Characteristics of louse-borne relapsing fever in Ethiopian children and adults. *Ann Trop Med Parasitol* 2004;98:191–6.

# 20 Leptospirosis

## Eyal Leshem and Eli Schwartz

Chaim Sheba Medical Center, Tel Hashomer, Israel and Sackler School of Medicine, Tel Aviv University, Tel Aviv, Israel

## Introduction

Leptospirosis is a zoonosis caused by infection with pathogenic *Leptospira* species. The disease occurs worldwide and is regarded as a re-emerging infection. Leptospirosis has a wide spectrum of clinical manifestations, ranging from subclinical infection through mild self-limited febrile illness to severe multiorgan failure with high mortality rates. Because of the nonspecific presentation of many patients, leptospirosis is often overlooked by caregivers, and a high level of suspicion is needed to accurately diagnose and treat it.

Historically, Adolf Weil described a clinical syndrome of fever, jaundice, and nephritis in 1886, now referred to as Weil's disease [1]. Nearly 30 years later, Inada and Ido were the first to report a spirochete as the cause of infectious jaundice in Japanese miners [2]. They further demonstrated *Leptospira*-specific antibodies in their patients. Leptospirosis was simultaneously described by two German groups studying the "French disease" affecting German soldiers stationed in the trenches of northeast France.

*Leptospira* are thin, coiled, motile spirochetes 6–20 $\mu$m in length and 0.1–0.2 $\mu$m in diameter (see Figure 20.1), sharing features of both gram-positive and gram-negative bacteria. They are obligate aerobes with unique nutritional requirements for long-chain fatty acids. At least eight genomically identifiable *Leptospira* species are pathogenic to humans. Pathogenic *Leptospira* are serologically classified into 24 serogroups further divided into over 230 serovars.

*Leptospira* infect a variety of wild and domestic animals. Infected animals chronically excrete the spirochete in their urine, contaminating the environment. *Leptospira* proliferate in fresh water, damp soil, vegetation, and mud. The microorganism can survive weeks to months in environmental temperatures from 28°C to 32°C.

*Tropical Diseases in Travelers*, 1st edition. Edited by E. Schwartz.
© 2009 by Blackwell Publishing, ISBN: 978-1-4051-8441-0.

Transmission of the infection to humans occurs by direct contact with infected animal urine or tissues or indirectly by contact with contaminated water or damp soil. Spirochetes may enter through broken skin, mucous membranes, or conjunctiva. Other modes of transmission include infection via intact skin following prolonged immersion, drinking contaminated water, inhalation of aerosols, and even sexual intercourse [2].

Leptospirosis was traditionally considered to be an occupational risk in industrialized countries and endemic in rural tropical areas. Today, the disease is re-emerging as a travel-related infection, both sporadic cases and outbreaks following water-related sports events [3–6]. Each year, millions of travelers visit tropical countries and adventure tourism expands, with water recreational activities becoming more popular. Thus, the risk of water exposure-related infections in travelers is increasing.

Clinicians must be aware of the risks related to water exposure, and leptospirosis must be considered in the differential diagnosis of any febrile illness in returning travelers, especially those reporting fresh water contact during their travels [5].

## Epidemiology—general

Leptospirosis is thought to be the most common zoonosis globally [7]. Due to its ubiquitous distribution, leptospirosis is said to be found wherever it is sought. The disease is considered a significant health problem in many parts of the world, but there is no precise estimate of the global burden. Although the distribution of leptospirosis is worldwide, the incidence of the infection is significantly higher in tropical regions [8].

The epidemiology of leptospirosis varies with local geographic and demographic features and with the activity engaged in by the infected individual (Table 20.1, Figure 20.2).

**175**

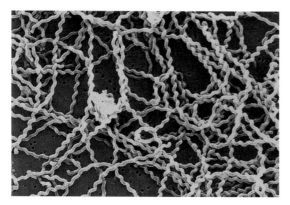

**Figure 20.1** *Leptospira*. (From Centers for Disease Control and Prevention. Content provider: CDC/NCID/Rob Weyant. Photo Credit: Janice Haney Carr.)

In tropical areas, the disease has higher incidence and seroprevalence rates, with increased mortality compared to industrialized countries. Sporadic infection is common, mainly during the rainy season, when environmental conditions favor both increased pathogen–human contact and survival of the spirochete [9–11]. *Leptospira* exposure during daily activities, such as laundering, bathing, and walking barefoot in damp soil is common. Living in close proximity to animals may further expose vast populations in developing countries. In densely inhabited areas, mainly in urban slums, sewage overflow during heavy rainfall periods may expose large populations, causing outbreaks [12]. The importance of leptospirosis as a cause of acute febrile illness in Southeast (SE) Asia was assessed by Laras and colleagues [10]. In this study, evidence

of a recent *Leptospira* infection was detected in 17% of patients with jaundice (after hepatitis A through E were ruled out), in 13% of patients with nonmalarial fever, and in 3% of patients with hemorrhagic fever not related to dengue.

In Latin America, leptospirosis is more common in rural than in urban populations, occurring more frequently in men than in women [13]. In the Iquitos area of Peru, as many as 30% of patients who presented to local health posts with undifferentiated fever suffered from leptospirosis [9]. Large epidemics were described in urban settings in several reports from Brazil, Ecuador, and Nicaragua [12]. In Salvador, Brazil, during the rainy season of 1996, the calculated incidence of severe leptospirosis was 12.5 cases per 100,000 inner city inhabitants, and the authors estimated that the actual incidence was 10 times higher [12]. The reasons for this outbreak were related to the rapid increase in urban population combined with the creation of urban slums, inadequate sanitation, and climatic changes related to the El Niño phenomenon. The actual risk to exposed populations in endemic regions of Latin America of acquiring leptospirosis was estimated to be as high as 0.41 infections per person-year [13]. *Leptospira* IgG antibody, signifying past exposure, was detected in 37% of human sera collected from a cross-sectional community-based study in Lao [10]. Other seroprevalence studies in Asia and Latin America reported a seroprevalence ranging from 17% to 52% [13–15].

In industrialized countries, infection may occur as an occupational risk, or may be related to water sports or to travel [2] (see Table 20.1). Leptospirosis was traditionally considered an occupational disease affecting workers with direct contact with infected animals (cattle ranchers,

**Table 20.1** Epidemiologic differences between travel-related and locally acquired leptospirosis in industrialized and developing countries.

|  | Travelers | Industrialized countries | Developing countries |
|---|---|---|---|
| Estimated annual incidence per 100,000 population | NA | 0.009–0.8 [8, 20, 37, 51] New Zealand 2.6 [8] | 0.4–43.2 [8, 52–54] |
| Seroprevalence | NA | Rural Italy 10–12% [55] | 17–52% [10, 13–15] |
| Incidence in febrile patients | 0.3%–1.2% [28–30] | NA | SE Asia 13–17% [10] Nicaragua 6% [11] |
| Estimated mortality | None reported [3–5, 24, 56, 57] | 1.4%–7% [20, 37] | 2%–15% [12, 14] |
| Exposure | Water-related adventure activities, sporadic | Occupational, inner city dwellers, water-related activities, sporadic | Occupational, flooding-related epidemics, sporadic |

*Note.* NA: not available.

Water-related activities (water sports and adventure travel):

- Rafting

- Caving

- Swimming

- Jungle walking

- Fishing

Environmental risk:

- Heavy precipitation

- Muddy terrain

- Jungle

- Flooding

- Inner city

Daily activities:

- Occupational (farming, animal related work, water related work)

- Walking barefoot or with sandals

- Laundry and dishwashing

- Bathing in contaminated water sources

General:

- Skin lacerations or abrasions

- Drinking contaminated water

**Figure 20.2** Risk exposures associated with leptospirosis.

abattoir workers, veterinarians) and others exposed to contaminated water and soil (sewage workers, miners, garbage collectors, soldiers, and farmers, especially rice farmers working barefoot, and fish farmers) [16]. There seems to have been a decrease in the incidence of occupational leptospirosis reported from industrialized countries in recent years, because of several factors: increased disease awareness leading to glove use during occupational animal contact and mechanization of field cultivation and irrigation techniques [17]. However, the disease has been described in inner city dwellers exposed to rodents [18]. In developed countries, the incidence varies greatly, with a trend toward an increase in travel- and water sports-related cases [8, 17, 19, 20]. A study summarizing the epidemiology of leptospirosis in Israel showed a decline in annual incidence from 3.6/100,000 population in the 1960s to 0.05/100,000 population in the study period (1985–1999) [17]. In Germany, a steady decrease in incidence was shown from a mean annual of 0.11/100,000 population in 1962–1967 to 0.06 per 100,000 population in 1998–2003 [21]. In this study, 16% of the cases were travel-related, and 30% reported recreational exposure. A considerable number of outbreaks have been associated with group adventure water sports events and military activities in both tropical and temperate areas [5, 6, 22–26].

In both industrialized and developing countries, leptospirosis appears as a pathogen of increasing importance in the urban environment. This trend is partially explained by accelerated urbanization with inadequate infrastructure [12, 18].

Environmental conditions have a major influence on the prevalence of leptospirosis. Favorable conditions commonly found in the tropics are warm, humid climate, abundant rainfall and water sources, and nonacidic soil. During heavy rainfall, water saturates the soil and human contact with *Leptospira* present in mud and surface water is increased.

Some leptospiral serogroups are commonly associated with particular animal reservoirs. For example, the serogroup Icterohaemorrhagiae is transmitted by rats and commonly infects sewage water in cities [18, 27]. The serogroup Canicola infects dogs, and the serogroup Hardjo infects cattle and sheep (Table 20.2).

## Epidemiology in travelers

There is scarce information regarding the prevalence of leptospirosis in travelers (see Table 20.1). In a recent article describing the causes of fever in ill returned travelers presenting at specialized tropical medicine clinics around the world, only 25 (0.3%) of 6957 febrile patients were diagnosed with leptospirosis [28]. A similar rate was shown in another large series of febrile returned travelers from Antwerp, Belgium, where 6/1842 (0.3%) patients were

Table 20.2 Animal reservoirs of *Leptospira* serovars.

| Serogroup | Main reservoir |
| --- | --- |
| Icterohaemorrhagiae | Rats |
| Canicola | Dogs |
| Hardjo | Cattle, sheep |
| Ballum | Rats, mice |
| Bataviae | Rodents |
| Sejroe | House mice |
| Bim | House mice |
| Grypotyphosa | Cattle |
| Australis | Cattle |

diagnosed with leptospirosis [29]. In a series of hospitalized returned Israeli travelers, 2/163 (1.2%) patients suffered from leptospirosis [30]. These data probably represent underdiagnosis of leptospirosis as a cause of fever in returned travelers. No serologic data exist regarding leptospirosis seroconversion in returned travelers.

Most cases of leptospirosis in travelers are reported in outbreaks (Table 20.3), mainly occurring in settings of group water-related sports events, rafting, or military training. From these outbreak investigations, two statistically significant risk factors have been identified: ingesting contaminated water and prolonged immersion or submersion. There are several reports of leptospirosis outbreaks following ingestion of contaminated water [2]. Based on these reports, enteric transmission of leptospirosis should be considered as a common route of infection. Evidence supporting this observation derives from the identification of *Leptospira* in the mesenteric lymph nodes of infected patients [19]. Another important lesson from these reports is that rapid epidemiological investigation allows the identification of affected cases and prevents unnecessary diagnostic procedures. In one report, seven patients underwent lumbar punctures, two underwent cholecystectomy, and one had a renal biopsy before the correct diagnosis was established [19].

There is little data regarding the epidemiology of sporadic leptospirosis in travelers. Only two reports summarize the characteristics of sporadic leptospirosis in returned travelers (Table 20.4). Although these data probably represent only a minority of travel-related *Leptospira* cases, several conclusions can be drawn:

1 Most patients acquired the infection in SE Asia. (Among Israeli travelers, recreational activities in the Mekong river in Laos were the most common exposure.)

2 The majority of patients were male.

3 Most patients participated in water-related activities, but 9% did not participate in such activities. Thus, leptospirosis must not be ruled out in the absence of a history of water exposure.

4 There were no deaths associated with leptospirosis in either the outbreak reports or the sporadic travel-related cases.

Case reports of leptospirosis in travelers may present a biased clinical picture, because they focus on patients with severe or unusual presentations. Most cases are probably not reported even when a diagnosis is made [31, 32].

## Clinical aspects

Leptospirosis has a broad spectrum of clinical manifestations. Most symptomatic patients develop a mild febrile illness and do not come to clinical attention [2]. Some infected individuals may undergo asymptomatic seroconversion [19, 24].

Classically, leptospirosis is described as a biphasic disease. The incubation period is 1–21 days with a median of 8 days [20]. The first stage is the spirochetemic phase, which lasts for a week. This is followed by an immune stage, during which spirochetes cannot be cultured from the blood but are excreted in the urine. A short period (3–4 days) of relative improvement may separate the two stages, but the biphasic course is rarely seen in travelers and the fever is often continuous.

The clinical presentation and severity of leptospirosis depend on both host- and pathogen-related factors. Most of the case series do not correlate the clinical presentation of cases with the infecting serogroup. However, from analyzing case series with known clinical–serogroup correlation, it appears that the disease caused by *Leptospira* of the serogroup Icterohaemorrhagiae follows a severe course more frequently than other serogroups (Table 20.5).

Leptospirosis may be manifest in several clinical syndromes. The individual patient may present with a combination of symptoms, signs, and a clinical course that are not always typical of any of the syndromes.

### Anicteric leptospirosis

Anicteric leptospirosis presents as an acute onset febrile illness accompanied by chills, headache, myalgia, anorexia, nausea, vomiting, and diarrhea. Less often, conjunctival suffusion and a transient (<24 hours) maculopapular rash may be seen. Fever is present in virtually all clinical cases. Fever usually lasts up to 1 week but may follow a longer

**Table 20.3** Outbreaks of leptospirosis in water-related group events (travel-related, military training, and locally occurring in industrialized countries).

| | Panama 1961 [57] | Okinawa, Japan 1987 [24] | Costa Rica 1996 [6] | Malaysian Borneo 2000 [5] | Ireland 2001 [26] | Illinois 1998 [19] | Israel 2002 [23] |
|---|---|---|---|---|---|---|---|
| Number of patients/total participants | 9/365 (2%) | Combat skills 7/15 (47%); swimming 15/82 (18%) | 9/26 (34%) | 80/189 (42%) | 6/65 (9%) | 52/474 (11%) | 7/27 (26%) |
| Exposure | Military exercise: overnight jungle walk | Military: combat skills training or recreational swimming | White-water rafting | Multisport endurance event: swimming, kayaking, caving, mountain biking | Canoeing | Triathlon: swimming | Military combat skills training |
| Hospitalization | 9/9 (100%) | 9/9 (100%) | 2/9 (22%) | 29/80 (36%) | 5/6 (83%) | 21/52 (40%) | 1/7 (14%) |
| Deaths | 0 | 0 | 0 | 0 | 0 | 0 | 0 |
| Asymptomatic seroconversion | 8/167 (4%) | 2/86 (2%) | NA | NA | NA | 4/197 (2%) | 0/27 (0) |
| RR by ingesting water (95% CI) | NA | 78 (17–345) | 8.7 (1.5–∞) | 1.8 (1.2–2.9) | 17 (2.4–127) | 3.8 (1.8–7.9) | 1.43 (1.1–1.9) |
| RR due to characteristics of the immersion (95% CI) | NA | NA | 6 (1.1–∞)[a] | 2 (1.3–3.1) | 1.8 (1–3.5)[b] | 1.43 (1.1–1.9)[c] | 0 |

*Notes.* RR: relative risk; CI: confidence interval; NA: data not available.
[a]Being submerged underwater.
[b]Swim time >42 minutes.
[c]Exposure >20 hours.

**Table 20.4** Epidemiology of sporadic leptospirosis cases among travelers.

| | Van Crevel et al. [4] | Leshem et al. [3] | Total |
|---|---|---|---|
| Number | 32 | 16 | 48 |
| Nationality | Dutch | Israeli | |
| Acquired in SE Asia | 28 (87%) | 12 (71%) | 40 (83%) |
| Latin America and the Caribbean | 3 (9%) | 0 | 3 (6%) |
| Africa | 1 (3%) | 2 (14%) | 3(6%) |
| Oceania | 0 | 2 (14%) | 2 (4%) |
| Male sex | 26 (81%) | 16 (100%) | 42 (87%) |
| Mean age | 31 | 29 | 30 |
| Water-related activity | 31 (96%) | 11/14 (78%) | 42/46 (91%) |
| Hospitalized | 25 (78%) | 16 (100%) | 41 (85%) |
| Antibiotic treatment | 14 (44%) | 13/14 (93%) | 27/46 (58%) |
| Serogroup | | | |
| Icterohaemorrhagiae | 4 | 5 | 9/30 (30%) |
| Australias/autumnalis | 6 | 1 | 7/30 (23%) |
| Sejroe | 5 | 2 | 7/30 (23%) |
| Bataviae | 2 | 1 | 3/30 (10%) |
| Pyrogenes | 1 | 3 | 4/30 (13%) |

**Table 20.5** Clinical features of infection with serogroup Icterohaemorrhagiae versus non-Icterohaemorrhagiae.

| | Total number of cases described in series | Icterohaemorrhagiae (%) | Non-Icterohaemorrhagiae (%) | OR (95 % CI |
|---|---|---|---|---|
| Jaundice | 281 [3, 23, 26, 27, 53, 58, 59] | 76/111 (68%) | 20/111 (18%) | 9.8 (5.2–18) |
| Elevated bilirubin (>100 mg/L) | 469 [3, 20, 23, 27] | 84/101 (83%) | 81/165 (49%) | 5.1 (2.8–9.3) |
| Elevated LFT | 139 [3, 23, 37] | 42/49 (85%) | 34/31 (77%) | 1.7 (0.5–5.5) |
| Renal failure | 199 [3, 23 37, 59, 60] | 46/61 (75%) | 16/79 (20%) | 12 (5.4–26) |
| Dialysis | 374 [3, 20 ,23] | 10/113 (9%) | 1/128 (1%) | 12.3 (1.5–97) |
| Elevated BUN (>200 mg/L) | 469 [3, 20, 23, 27] | 92/143 (64%) | 53/191 (27%) | 4.6 (2.9–7.4) |
| Elevated creatinine (>15 mg/L) | 374 [3, 20, 23] | 51/76 (67%) | 26/74 (35%) | 3.7 (1.9–7.4) |
| Oliguria/anuria | 360 [20, 23] | 50/125 (40%) | 16/126 (12%) | 4.5 (1.9–7.4) |
| Thrombocytopenia | 35 [3, 23, 60] | 3/3 (100%) | 3/25 (12%) | NA |
| Severe disease (multiorgan failure) | 95 [23, 26, 59, 61] | 42/54 (77%) | 3/41 (7%) | 44 (11–169) |
| Death | 1545 [3, 20, 23, 27, 37, 51, 54, 58–60] | 47/591 (8%) | 46/922 (5%) | 1.6 (1.08–2.5) |

*Notes.* OR: odds ratio; LFT: liver function tests; BUN: blood urea nitrogen.

continuous or biphasic course. Headache is often severe, is retro-orbital, and may be accompanied by photophobia and meningeal irritation in up to 25% of patients. Myalgia may be severe and usually affects the calf and lumbar areas. Differentiating anicteric leptospirosis from other febrile illnesses may be difficult, and conjunctival suffusion and muscle tenderness are often suggested as distinguishing clinical findings [2].

## Icteric leptospirosis

The severe condition of icteric leptospirosis is present in approximately 5–10% of patients [33]. Mortality ranges between 5% and 15% of patients [33]. The syndrome may follow a fulminant, rapidly progressive course or appear during the second "immune" phase of the illness following a short period of relative remission. The disease is characterized by a combination of jaundice, renal failure, diffuse tissue hemorrhages, and refractory shock. Acute renal failure may present in oliguric or nonoliguric forms. Oliguric renal failure accompanied by hyperkalemia is an ominous prognostic sign and requires close follow-up and rapid intervention if the condition worsens.

Infection with different serogroups exerts a variable risk of developing icteric leptospirosis. Disease caused by serogroup Icterohaemorrhagiae probably poses the highest risk for severe disease, with a 10–12 odds ratio of developing jaundice and renal failure and death compared with other serogroups (Table 20.5).

Predictors of death from severe leptospirosis include altered mental status, oliguric renal failure, older age, respiratory insufficiency, and cardiac arrhythmia [12, 34].

## Severe pulmonary hemorrhagic leptospirosis

The clinical presentation of severe pulmonary hemorrhagic leptospirosis may range from mild fever, cough, dyspnea, and hemoptysis through intra-alveolar hemorrhage to fulminant acute respiratory distress syndrome (ARDS) and respiratory failure requiring mechanical ventilation [14]. Chest X rays usually disclose patchy alveolar infiltrates. Larger consolidations may indicate intra-alveolar hemorrhage.

In an urban outbreak of severe leptospirosis in Brazil, 90% of patients had serologic evidence of infection with serogroup Icterohaemorrhagiae [12]. In this outbreak, 19% suffered from respiratory insufficiency, 18% suffered from hemoptysis, 23% required peritoneal dialysis, and 16% suffered bleeding diasthesis. The syndrome of leptospirosis-associated pulmonary hemorrhage first came to international attention following a large epidemic

of leptospirosis in Nicaragua, resulting in high morbidity and mortality, mainly from pulmonary hemorrhage [11]. In this report, serologic evidence of infection with serogroup Canicola was detected in 54% of patients, and serogroup Icterohaemorrhagiae (serovars *icterohaemorrhagiae* and *copenhageni*) was detected in 40%. The severity of the pulmonary syndrome was unrelated to the presence of jaundice or renal dysfunction.

## Other clinical manifestations

Several other manifestations of leptospirosis are described in the literature. Cardiac involvement is common in leptospirosis. Cardiac disease may present as myocarditis accompanied by arrhythmias (atrial fibrillation and variable conduction blocks). In a series of severe leptospirosis patients from the Philippines, 39% had electrocardiographic anomalies [35]. Ocular involvement may progress to anterior uveitis in 2–3% of patients. Uveitis may present weeks, months, or even years following acute infection [2]. Aseptic meningitis may present in up to 25% of *Leptospira* patients. Cerebrospinal fluid examination may disclose increased opening pressure, elevated protein, normal glucose, and lymphocytic pleocytosis.

## Asymptomatic seroconversion

There are conflicting data regarding the prevalence of asymptomatic infection with *Leptospira*. Asymptomatic seroconversion is frequently reported in tropical areas, it is rarely found in studies of outbreaks among travelers and in industrialized countries (Table 20.3). The rate of asymptomatic infection in the tropics is derived from outbreak investigations such as that in Nicaragua, which showed that, among seropositive inhabitants, only 29% had a recent history of febrile disease [36]. Conversely, when outbreaks in industrialized countries and among travelers, where all participants in the same activity were checked for leptospirosis antibodies, were investigated, only 0–4% were found to have asymptomatic seroconversion (see Table 20.3). A possible explanation of the high rates of seropositivity in series from tropical countries may be that patients remain seropositive for many years (low titer) following *Leptospira* infection, and seropositive individuals in these series might have had past infections rather than recent asymptomatic infections. Thus, based on reports from industrialized countries and traveler outbreaks, which seem to be more reliable, it appears that asymptomatic infection with *Leptospira* is uncommon.

**Table 20.6** Clinical and laboratory features of sporadic leptospirosis in travelers.

| | Van Creval et al. [4] | Leshem et al. [3] | Grobusch et al. [62] | Sejvar et al. [5] | Total |
|---|---|---|---|---|---|
| Number of patients | 32 | 14 | 4 | 80 | 130 |
| Fever | 32 (100%) | 14 (100%) | 4 (100%) | 80 (100%) | 130 (100%) |
| Chills | 21 (65%) | 4 (28%) | 3 (75%) | 80 (100%) | 108 (84%) |
| Headache | 27/30 (90%) | 12 (85(%) | 2 (50%) | 80 (100%) | 121/128 (94%) |
| Myalgia | 24/31 (77%) | 10 (71%) | 4 (100%) | 80 (100%) | 118/129 (91%) |
| Nausea and vomiting | 14/28 (50%) | 9 (64%) | 2 (50%) | NA | 25/46 (54%) |
| Diarrhea | 16/30 (53%) | 9 (64%) | 2 (50%) | 62 (77%) | 89/128 (69%) |
| Conjuctival suffusion | 11/28 (39%) | 4 (28%) | 0 | 11 (13%) | 26/126 (20%) |
| Acute renal failure/oliguria | 10 (31%) | 5/12 (41%) | 1 (25%) | 0 | 16/126 (12%) |
| Jaundice | 8 (25%) | 5/11 (45%) | 2 (50%) | 0 | 15/127 (12%) |
| Thrombocytophenia | 5/24 (20%) | 5/13 (38%) | 0 | NA | 10/37 (27%) |
| Death | 0 | 0 | 0 | 0 | 0 |

*Note.* NA: not available.

## Clinical features in travelers

Leptospirosis may present as an undifferentiated febrile disease in the returned traveler. Additional nonspecific common complaints include headache, myalgia, nausea, vomiting, and diarrhea. Conjunctivitis is often regarded as a hallmark of leptospirosis, but it was present in a minority of cases in our experience, and is not a specific sign, because it may be present in other common causes of travel-related febrile illness, such as dengue fever. Some cases of travel-related leptospirosis present as severe disease with jaundice, renal failure, and respiratory failure. Severe cases in travelers are often associated with infection due to serogroup Icterohaemorrhagiae. This serogroup was the most prevalent cause of *Leptospira* infection among travelers in two published case series, presenting in 9/30 (30%) of the cases where microscopic agglutination test (MAT) determination of serogroup was performed (see Table 20.4). Thus, severe infection may be a common phenomenon among travelers diagnosed with leptospirosis. However, as previously noted, there were no reports of deaths associated with travel-related leptospirosis (see Tables 20.3 and 20.4). This is contrary to the mortality rate of 1.4% (5/353) reported in leptospirosis patients in Hawaii [20] and 7% reported from Denmark [37]. The difference in traveler mortality compared with the mortality rate in the general populations of industrialized countries may represent different epidemiologic features characterized by the healthier status of travelers engaging in adventure travel or underdiagnosis of leptospirosis as a cause of death in travelers.

Table 20.6 summarizes the clinical and laboratory features of leptospirosis in travelers. It is notable that a significant number of patients suffered from renal failure, jaundice, or thrombocytopenia, representing severe forms of leptospirosis. Over half the travelers suffered from diarrhea, suggesting the inclusion of leptospirosis in the differential diagnosis of fever and diarrhea in travelers [31]. Only 32% suffered conjunctival suffusion. Thus, one must consider leptospirosis in febrile travelers even in the absence of specific signs (conjuctival suffusion) or with atypical presentations (diarrhea).

## Differential diagnosis

Leptospirosis must be considered in the differential diagnosis of every febrile traveler. However, several other common infections must be ruled out before leptospirosis is diagnosed. Malaria, dengue fever, enteric fever, and rickettsiosis are all common causes of febrile travel-related illnesses and may present with similar manifestations. In a report of leptospirosis cases identified during a large urban dengue epidemic in Salvador, Brazil, as many as 61% of leptospirosis patients seeking medical aid for a febrile illness were wrongly diagnosed as suffering from dengue, thus delaying medical attention and treatment [38]. Atypical presentations of leptospirosis, such as infectious enteritis, have also been described [31]. It is important to rule out co-infections in febrile returned travelers. Co-infection with common causes of fever in the tropics, such as malaria [39] and scrub typhus [40], has been described in leptospirosis patients.

## Laboratory features

Tropical diseases common in travelers often cause leukopenia. However, in leptospirosis, the blood count often discloses leukocytosis with left shift, differentiating it from malaria, dengue, and other common causes of fever among travelers. Blood count may also disclose thrombocytopenia.

Liver function tests are often significant for hyperbilirubinemia, with moderate elevation of the aminotransferase levels and mild cholestasis. The discrepancy between high bilirubinemia and other liver function tests near normal is considered a unique characteristic of leptospirosis, especially caused by serogroup Icterohaemorrhagiae. Urinalysis shows leukocyturia, microscopic hematuria, proteinuria, hyaline casts, and granular casts. Oliguric renal failure may be accompanied by hyperkalemia or hypokalemia.

## Diagnosis

There are several tools to aid the clinician in the diagnosis of leptospirosis, but most methods are available only in reference or research laboratories, and usually results confirming infection are available only weeks after the acute infection. Thus, the initiation of treatment is often guided by clinical diagnosis rather than based on laboratory confirmation. A simple sensitive diagnostic test during the acute phase of leptospirosis is the focus of intensive research [41].

To understand the diagnostic methods used in leptospirosis, the taxonomy of *Leptospira* must be elucidated first. *Leptospira* are classified by two major classifications.

## Serological classification

Serological classification classifies a serovar based on antibodies directed against its lipopolysaccharid antigen. Antigenically related serovars are traditionally grouped into serogroups. By this method, there are two serological species. *L. interrogans*, comprising all *Leptospira* pathogenic to humans, is further divided into 24 sero-

groups and over 230 serovars. *L. biflexa* comprises over 60 nonpathogenic *Leptospira* serovars.

## Genetic classification

Genetic classification classifies *Leptospira* based on DNA relatedness. By this classification, the genus is divided into 17 species, of which 8 are pathogenic to humans. It is important to mention that one serovar may belong to more then one species and members of the same species may belong to different serogroups.

## Diagnostic methods

The main reason for missing leptospirosis as the cause of fever in returned travelers is that most cases present as a nonspecific febrile illness. Diagnosis requires awareness of the disease manifestations, a high level of suspicion, and repeated serology during convalescence.

## Serology

Serology is the most common method for diagnosis of *Leptospira*. Several serological methods are widely used and reported, but the MAT is regarded as the gold standard for the diagnosis of *Leptospira*. MAT uses *in vitro* cultivated live *Leptospira* of multiple serovars incubated with patient serum. After incubation, the serum–antigen mixture is tested for agglutination. Seroconversion, or a fourfold rise between acute and convalescent sera, or a single high titer (usually $\geq 1:200$ in areas of low endemicity) is often regarded as a positive test. MAT is serogroup specific and must be interpreted cautiously [2]. The two major limitations of this method are its availability only in reference laboratories and its low sensitivity during the acute phase of the disease.

Serology is usually negative in the first 5 days of the disease. Seroconversion occurs during the second week, and by the end of the second week, most patients have positive serology (high titer). Seronegative results during the acute illness mandate sending convalescent serum; however, at this stage, the test results may not alter the approach to the patient. Positive serology (albeit in low titer) may persist for years following infection and, in the absence of clinical symptoms suggesting *Leptospira* infection, the value of a positive serologic study in the diagnosis of a recent infection is questionable.

ELISA and lateral flow assays reach sensitivity and specificity of 70–80% when acute and convalescent sera are tested. Indirect hemagglutination is regarded as less sensitive. The development of these assays is intended to aid in "point of care" diagnosis. However, the problem of low sensitivity during the acute phase remains unresolved.

## Antigen detection

Several methods of *Leptospira* antigen detection have been evaluated in the past. These include radioimmunoassay, ELISA, and immunomagnetic antigen capture combined with fluoroimmunoassay, which recently showed increased sensitivity. However, none of these methods is widely used in the routine diagnosis of leptospirosis.

## Polymerase chain reaction

PCR is regarded as a sensitive and specific method and can differentiate between *Leptospira* species, but is performed only in reference laboratories. A study of 60 leptospirosis patients in Brazil found that PCR was 65% sensitive and 100% specific [42]. In this study, PCR samples of patient blood and urine were sent. PCR sensitivity was highest during days 9–14 of the disease (72%). Performing PCR may have clinical implications, as a definitive diagnosis can be achieved during the acute illness and can alter treatment decisions. Moreover, the quantity of *Leptospira* has been shown to correlate with disease severity [43].

## Direct visualization

It is possible to demonstrate *Leptospira* in blood, urine, and CSF using dark field microscopy. Microscopy may reveal *Leptospira* in blood during the first few days of the illness, but microscopy of the CSF is probably of little value at this time. Direct visualization is rarely used in clinical practice, because of its very low sensitivity. Staining methods, including immunohistochemical techniques, may increase the usefulness of direct visualization.

## Culture

*Leptospira* requires special media for isolation. During the septicemic phase (first 7–10 days of the disease), *Leptospira* may be isolated from blood, CSF, and peritoneal dialysate of patients. After the first week, only urine samples may yield positive cultures. Cultures are kept for a minimum of 16 weeks and are examined weekly by dark field microscopy before a negative result is reported. In practice, *Leptospira* cultures do not aid in treatment decisions and are mainly of academic value.

## Treatment

The evidence supporting antibiotic treatment in leptospirosis was reviewed in 2000 by Guidugli and colleagues [44]. In their review, the authors included only three randomized controlled trials (RCTs) comparing an-

tibiotic therapy to placebo and concluded that there was evidence that penicillin and doxycycline reduce the duration of fever, the length of hospital stay, and spirochetal urine isolation.

Since the publication of this review in 2000, several new studies have compared the efficacy of various antibiotic regimens in the treatment of leptospirosis. Ceftriaxone was compared with penicillin G in a prospective, open-label, randomized trial of 173 patients with severe leptospirosis in Thailand. There were no significant differences in the duration of fever, organ dysfunction, adverse events, or mortality [45]. In another prospective, open-label, randomized trial in Thailand, cefotaxime, penicillin G, and doxycycline were compared in 540 patients with suspected severe leptospirosis, of whom 264 had confirmed leptospirosis. In this trial, death rate, duration of fever, organ dysfunction, and failure rates were similar in the three antibiotic regimens [46]. In a recent trial in 296 febrile adults in Thailand, doxycycline was compared to azithromycin for the treatment of leptospirosis and scrub typhus. Sixty-nine patients had a final diagnosis of leptospirosis. The cure rate and defervescence with the two drugs were similar, and there were no deaths. The authors concluded that both drugs were effective [40]. In a large retrospective series of patients diagnosed in Hawaii, early initiation of treatment was associated with shortened illness duration [20]. However, one RCT showed that treatment with intravenous penicillin improved the outcome in patients with severe advanced leptospirosis, even when therapy was initiated late in the course of the disease [47].

In summary, there are no RCTs of antibiotic treatment for leptospirosis in travelers. However, based on trials in the tropics, several antibiotic options yielded similar results. This includes penicillin G (intravenous 1.5 million units every 6 hours for 7 days) or ampicillin (intravenous 1000 mg every 6 hours for 7 days) for severe cases, and doxycycline (oral 100 mg twice daily for 7 days) for mild or moderate disease. Modern studies confirm the efficacy of cephalosporins (intravenous ceftriaxone 1000 mg once daily for 7 days) and macrolides (azithromycin 1000 mg followed by 500 mg daily for 3 days) as treatment options for leptospirosis.

## Prevention

Preventive measures must be taken during pretravel consultation, especially for adventure travelers. Traveler education regarding the associated risks of fresh water exposure in endemic areas (leptospirosis, schistosomiasis) even for minor exposures such as walking barefoot or wearing sandals is highly important.

In the analyses of the leptospirosis outbreak among Eco-Challenge participants in Malaysian Borneo, doxycycline usage was protective, although not statistically significant (RR = 0.4, 95% CI 0.1–1.1) [5]. At least two RCTs confirmed the efficacy of doxycycline (200 mg once weekly) in preventing leptospirosis in heavily exposed groups [48, 49]. Therefore, doxycycline chemoprophylaxis is an attractive option for travelers planning to participate in water-related activities, especially in malaria risk areas [50].

There are no widely approved human vaccines for leptospirosis at the present time.

## References

1 Weil A. Uber eine eigentumliche, mit Milztumor, Icterus und Nephritis einhergehende akute Infektionskrankheit. *Dtsch Arch Klin Med* 1886;39:209–32.

2 Levett PN. Leptospirosis. *Clin Microbiol Rev* 2001;14(2):296–326.

3 Leshem E, Ostfeld I, Barnea A, Schwartz E. *Leptospirosis in Israeli Travelers*. Presented at the Annual Meeting of the Israel Society for Parasitology, Protozoology and Topical Diseases. Tel Aviv, Israel; Dec 17–18, 2008.

4 Van Crevel R, Speelman P, Gravekamp C, Terpstra WJ. Leptospirosis in travelers. *Clin Infect Dis* 1994;19(1):132–4.

5 Sejvar J, Bancroft E, Winthrop K, et al. Leptospirosis in "Eco-Challenge" athletes, Malaysian Borneo, 2000. *Emerg Infect Dis* 2003;9(6):702–7.

6 Centers for Disease Control and Prevention. Outbreak of leptospirosis among white-water rafters—Costa Rica, 1996. *JAMA* 1997;278(10):808–9.

7 Leptospirosis worldwide, 1999. *Wkly Epidemiol Rec* 1999;74(29):237–42.

8 Pappas G, Papadimitriou P, Siozopoulou V, Christou L, Akritidis N. The globalization ofleptospirosis: worldwide incidence trends. *Int J Infect Dis* 2007;12(4):351-7.

9 Bharti AR, Nally JE, Ricaldi JN, et al. Leptospirosis: a zoonotic disease of global importance. *Lancet Infect Dis* 2003;3(12):757–71.

10 Laras K, Cao BV, Bounlu K, et al. The importance of leptospirosis in Southeast Asia. *Am J Trop Med Hyg* 2002; 67(3):278–86.

11 Trevejo RT, Rigau-Perez JG, Ashford DA, et al. Epidemic leptospirosis associated with pulmonary hemorrhage—Nicaragua, 1995. *J Infect Dis* 1998;178(5):1457–63.

12 Ko AI, Galvao Reis M, Ribeiro Dourado CM, Johnson WD Jr, Riley LW. Urban epidemic of severe leptospirosis in Brazil. Salvador Leptospirosis Study Group. *Lancet* 1999;354(9181):820–25.

13 Lomar AV, Diament D, Torres JR. Leptospirosis in Latin America. *Infect Dis Clin North Am* 2000;14(1):23–39, vii–viii.

14 Segura ER, Ganoza CA, Campos K, et al. Clinical spectrum of pulmonary involvement in leptospirosis in a region of endemicity, with quantification of leptospiral burden. *Clin Infect Dis* 2005;40(3):343–51.

15 Sharma S, Vijayachari P, Sugunan AP, Natarajaseenivasan K, Sehgal SC. Seroprevalence of leptospirosis among high-risk population of Andaman Islands, India. *Am J Trop Med Hyg* 2006;74(2):278–83.

16 Tangkanakul W, Siriarayaporn P, Pool T, Ungchusak K, Chunsuttiwat S. Environmental and travel factors related to leptospirosis in Thailand. *J Med Assoc Thai* 2001;84(12): 1674–80.

17 Kariv R, Klempfner R, Barnea A, Sidi Y, Schwartz E. The changing epidemiology of leptospirosis in Israel. *Emerg Infect Dis* 2001;7(6):990–92.

18 Vinetz JM, Glass GE, Flexner CE, Mueller P, Kaslow DC. Sporadic urban leptospirosis. *Ann Intern Med* 1996;125(10): 794–8.

19 Morgan J, Bornstein SL, Karpati AM, et al. Outbreak of leptospirosis among triathlon participants and community residents in Springfield, Illinois, 1998. *Clin Infect Dis* 2002;34(12): 1593–9.

20 Katz AR, Ansdell VE, Effler PV, Middleton CR, Sasaki DM. Assessment of the clinical presentation and treatment of 353 cases of laboratory-confirmed leptospirosis in Hawaii, 1974–1998. *Clin Infect Dis* 2001;33(11):1834–41.

21 Jansen A, Schoneberg I, Frank C, Alpers K, Schneider T, Stark K. Leptospirosis in Germany, 1962–2003. *Emerg Infect Dis* 2005;11(7):1048–54.

22 Ricaldi JN, Vinetz JM. Leptospirosis in the tropics and in travelers. *Curr Infect Dis Rep* 2006;8(1):51–8.

23 Hadad E, Pirogovsky A, Bartal C, et al. An outbreak of leptospirosis among Israeli troops near the Jordan River. *Am J Trop Med Hyg* 2006;74(1):127–31.

24 Corwin A, Ryan A, Bloys W, Thomas R, Deniega B, Watts D. A waterborne outbreak of leptospirosis among United States military personnel in Okinawa, Japan. *Int J Epidemiol* 1990;19(3):743–8.

25 Russell KL, Montiel Gonzalez MA, Watts DM, et al. An outbreak of leptospirosis among Peruvian military recruits. *Am J Trop Med Hyg* 2003;69(1):53–7.

26 Boland M, Sayers G, Coleman T, et al. A cluster of leptospirosis cases in canoeists following a competition on the River Liffey. *Epidemiol Infect* 2004;132(2):195–200.

27 Lindenbaum I, Eylan E, Shenberg E. Leptospirosis in Israel: a report of 14 cases caused by icterohaemorrhagiae serogroup (1968-82). *Isr J Med Sci* 1984;20(2):123–9.

28 Wilson ME, Weld LH, Boggild A, et al. Fever in returned travelers: results from the GeoSentinel Surveillance Network. *Clin Infect Dis* 2007;44(12):1560–68.

29 Bottieau E, Clerinx J, Schrooten W, et al. Etiology and outcome of fever after a stay in the tropics. *Arch Intern Med* 2006;166(15):1642–8.

30 Stienlauf S, Segal G, Sidi Y, Schwartz E. Epidemiology of travel-related hospitalization. *J Travel Med* 2005;12(3): 136–41.

31 Paz A, Krimerman S, Potasman I. Leptospirosis masquerading as infectious enteritis. *Travel Med Infect Dis* 2004;2(2):89–91.

32 Gelman SS, Gundlapalli AV, Hale D, Croft A, Hindiyeh M, Carroll KC. Spotting the spirochete: rapid diagnosis of leptospirosis in two returned travelers. *J Travel Med* 2002;9(3):165–7.

33 Heath CW, Jr., Alexander AD, Galton MM. Leptospirosis in the United States. Analysis of 483 cases in man, 1949, 1961. *N Engl J Med* 1965;273(17):915–22.

34 Daher E, Zanetta DM, Cavalcante MB, Abdulkader RC. Risk factors for death and changing patterns in leptospirosis acute renal failure. *Am J Trop Med Hyg* 1999;61(4):630–34.

35 Watt G, Padre LP, Tuazon M, Calubaquib C. Skeletal and cardiac muscle involvement in severe, late leptospirosis. *J Infect Dis* 1990;162(1):266–9.

36 Ashford DA, Kaiser RM, Spiegel RA, et al. Asymptomatic infection and risk factors for leptospirosis in Nicaragua. *Am J Trop Med Hyg* 2000;63(5–6):249–54.

37 Holk K, Nielsen SV, Ronne T. Human leptospirosis in Denmark 1970–1996: an epidemiological and clinical study. *Scand J Infect Dis* 2000;32(5):533–8.

38 Flannery B, Pereira MM, Velloso LdF, et al. Referral pattern of leptospirosis cases during a large urban epidemic of dengue. *Am J Trop Med Hyg* 2001;65(5):657–63.

39 Wongsrichanalai C, Murray CK, Gray M, et al. Co-infection with malaria and leptospirosis. *Am J Trop Med Hyg* 2003; 68(5):583–5.

40 Phimda K, Hoontrakul S, Suttinont C, et al. Doxycycline versus azithromycin for treatment of leptospirosis and scrub typhus. *Antimicrob Agents Chemother* 2007;51(9):3259–63.

41 McBride AJ, Athanazio DA, Reis MG, Ko AI. Leptospirosis. *Curr Opin Infect Dis* 2005;18(5):376–86.

42 de Abreu Fonseca C, Teixeira de Freitas VL, Calo Romero E, et al. Polymerase chain reaction in comparison with serological tests for early diagnosis of human leptospirosis. *Trop Med Int Health* 2006;11(11):1699–1707.

43 Truccolo J, Serais O, Merien F, Perolat P. Following the course of human leptospirosis: evidence of a critical threshold for the vital prognosis using a quantitative PCR assay. *FEMS Microbiol Lett* 2001;204(2):317–21.

44 Guidugli F, Castro AA, Atallah AN. Antibiotics for treating leptospirosis. *Cochrane Database Syst Rev* 2000(2): CD001306.

45 Panaphut T, Domrongkitchaiporn S, Vibhagool A, Thinkamrop B, Susaengrat W. Ceftriaxone compared with sodium penicillin g for treatment of severe leptospirosis. *Clin Infect Dis* 2003;36(12):1507–13.

46 Suputtamongkol Y, Niwattayakul K, Suttinont C, et al. An open, randomized, controlled trial of penicillin, doxycycline, and cefotaxime for patients with severe leptospirosis. *Clin Infect Dis* 2004;39(10):1417–24.

47 Watt G, Padre LP, Tuazon ML, et al. Placebo-controlled trial of intravenous penicillin for severe and late leptospirosis. *Lancet* 1988;1(8583):433–5.

48 Takafuji ET, Kirkpatrick JW, Miller RN, et al. An efficacy trial of doxycycline chemoprophylaxis against leptospirosis. *N Engl J Med* 1984;310(8):497–500.

49 Gonsalez CR, Casseb J, Monteiro FG, et al. Use of doxycycline for leptospirosis after high-risk exposure in Sao Paulo, Brazil. *Rev Inst Med Trop Sao Paulo* 1998;40(1):59–61.

50 Guidugli F, Castro AA, Atallah AN. Antibiotics for preventing leptospirosis. *Cochrane Database Syst Rev* 2000(4): CD001305.

51 Christova I, Tasseva E, Manev H. Human leptospirosis in Bulgaria, 1989-2001: epidemiological, clinical, and serological features. *Scand J Infect Dis* 2003;35(11–12):869–72.

52 Merien F, Perolat P. Public health importance of human leptospirosis in the South Pacific: a five-year study in New Caledonia. *Am J Trop Med Hyg* 1996;55(2):174–8.

53 Vado-Solis I, Cardenas-Marrufo MF, Jimenez-Delgadillo B, et al. Clinical-epidemiological study of leptospirosis in humans and reservoirs in Yucatan, Mexico. *Rev Inst Med Trop Sao Paulo* 2002;44(6):335–40.

54 Everard CO, Edwards CN, Everard JD, Carrington DG. A twelve-year study of leptospirosis on Barbados. *Eur J Epidemiol* 1995;11(3):311–20.

55 Nuti M, Amaddeo D, Crovatto M, et al. Infections in an Alpine environment: antibodies to hantaviruses, leptospira, rickettsiae, and *Borrelia burgdorferi* in defined Italian populations. *Am J Trop Med Hyg* 1993;48(1):20–25.

56 Outbreak of leptospirosis among white-water rafters—Costa Rica, 1996. *MMWR Morb Mortal Wkly Rep* 1997;46(25): 577–9.

57 Mackenzie RB, Reiley CG, Alexander AD, Bruckner EA, Diercks FH, Beye HK. An outbreak of leptospirosis among U.S. army troops in the Canal Zone. *Am J Trop Med Hyg* 1966; 15(1):57–63.

58 Lecour H, Miranda M, Magro C, Rocha A, Goncalves V. Human leptospirosis—a review of 50 cases. *Infection* 1989;17(1):8–12.

59 Bishara J, Amitay E, Barnea A, Yitzhaki S, Pitlik S. Epidemiological and clinical features of leptospirosis in Israel. *Eur J Clin Microbiol Infect Dis* 2002;21(1):50–52.

60 Narita M, Fujitani S, Haake DA, Paterson DL. Leptospirosis after recreational exposure to water in the Yaeyama islands, Japan. *Am J Trop Med Hyg* 2005;73(4):652–6.

61 Ciceroni L, Stepan E, Pinto A, et al. Epidemiological trend of human leptospirosis in Italy between 1994 and 1996. *Eur J Epidemiol* 2000;16(1):79–86.

62 Grobusch MP, Bollmann R, Schonberg A, et al. Leptospirosis in travelers returning from the Dominican Republic. *J Travel Med* 2003;10(1):55–8.

# 21 Malaria in Travelers: Epidemiology, Clinical Aspects, and Treatment

## Eli Schwartz

Chaim Sheba Medical Center, Tel Hashomer, Israel and Sackler School of Medicine, Tel Aviv University, Tel Aviv, Israel

## Introduction

Despite the long and earnest efforts of many national and international agencies to combat malaria, it remains a major threat in many parts of the globe, with 2.5 billion people living under the threat of malaria, and an estimated 380–570 million infections annually. Malaria continues to be a major cause of mortality worldwide, and together with HIV and tuberculosis has been targeted by the World Health Organization (WHO) for control and eradication.

Malaria is caused by the protozoan *Plasmodium*, which is an intra-erythrocytic parasite. Four species are responsible for human diseases: *P. falciparum*, *P. vivax*, *P. ovale*, and *P. malariae*. These species are hosted in humans and transmitted from person to person by anopheline mosquitoes. Because the only reservoir for the parasite is humans, there was a theoretical hope that by mass treatment of human carriers of the disease, combined with mass anti-mosquito campaigns, malaria eradication could be achieved, a goal that thus far has been unattainable.

Recently, a parasite that usually causes malaria in monkeys, *P. knowlesi*, has established itself as the fifth species that can cause human malaria [1].

The mosquito vector responsible for transmitting malaria is a female mosquito of the anopheline genus. It is only the female that sucks blood because it needs protein to produce eggs. The anopheline species are active from sunset to sunrise, which necessitates protection for humans during nighttime hours. There are differences between the anopheline species in lifespan, seeking meals indoors or outdoors, etc. These entomological parameters are important in planning antimalarial campaigns.

In rare cases, malaria can be transmitted without the anopheline vector via blood transfusions, organ transplants, needlesticks, sharing needles and syringes, or vertical transmission from mother to newborn (congenital malaria). During the twentieth century, there have been a number of attempts to treat infectious diseases associated with neurological conditions such as neurosyphilis, and, more recently, Lyme disease [neuroborreliosis] and HIV infection, with malariotherapy, where malaria (usually *P. vivax*) was injected directly into the blood of the patient [2].

## Malaria life cycle within humans

During a blood meal of a female *Anopheles* mosquito, sporozoites are inoculated from the salivary glands of the mosquito into the bloodstream of the victim. The number of sporozoites varies from one or two to several hundred. The parasite hence begins its life cycle within the human body. The stages of development can be divided as follows (Figure 21.1).

**A** The *sporozoites*, which are small motile forms, enter the liver cells to begin their asexual reproduction period. This stage takes a few minutes.

**B** The *hepatic stage* (also called the pre-erythrocytic stage), when the sporozoite begins its asexual multiplication process, gives rise to thousands of daughter *merozoites*. The swollen hepatocytes will eventually burst and release thousands of merozoites into the blood stream (Table 21.1)); in this form, these are capable of invading

*Tropical Diseases in Travelers*, 1st edition. Edited by E. Schwartz.
© 2009 by Blackwell Publishing, ISBN: 978-1-4051-8441-0.

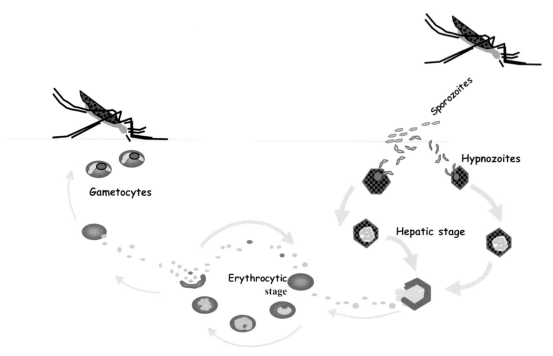

**Figure 21.1** Malaria life cycle.

the erythrocytes. This stage takes about 1 week; however, it varies between malaria species (Table 21.1).

**B1** In *P. vivax* and *P. ovale* infection a unique process occurs where part of the sporozoites that entered the liver cells, instead of developing into merozoites as described above, develop into smaller "sleeping" cells, appropriately referred to as *hypnozoites*. Not much is known about their development, but they are probably preprogrammed to develop into the hypnozoite form immediately upon entering the liver [3]. The hypnozoites have an intrinsic "clock" that wakes them up after several months (in

tropical areas, it normally happens after a short interval; in subtropical areas, it may take 9–12 months) [4]. After they awake, they turn into merozoites and burst into the bloodstream and the process continues as described below. This unique form of the malaria parasite is the cause for relapses, which characterize vivax and ovale infections.

**C** The *blood stage* (erythrocytic stage) occurs when the merozoites, which were released into the bloodstream, invade the erythrocytes. The entry occurs rapidly and is mediated via a specific receptor on the erythrocytes (e.g., *P. vivax* enters via a Duffy receptor, and therefore in West

**Table 21.1** Characteristics of human plasmodium.

|  | *P. falciparum* | *P. vivax* | *P. ovale* | *P. malariae* |
|---|---|---|---|---|
| Intrahepatic (days) | 5–7 | 7–8 | 9 | 14–16 |
| Incubation period [From mosquito bite to clinical symptoms], days (average) | 8–25 (12) | 8–27 (14) | 9–17 (14) | 16–59 (32) |
| Erythrocytic cycle (days) | 2 | 2 | 2 | 3 |
| Hypnozoites formation (relapse) | No | Yes | Yes | No |
| Number merozoites/hepatic schizont | 30,000 | 10,000 | 15,000 | 2000 |
| RBC preference | All RBC | Reticulocytes | Reticulocytes | Old RBC |

*Note:* RBC = Red blood cells.

Africa, where people are genetically lacking this receptor, vivax infection is uncommon).

Within the erythrocyte, the ring form matures and starts an asexual multiplication again, which causes the erythrocyte to burst open after about 48 hours (in *P malariae* 72 hours), releasing 6–32 merozoites, each capable of invading new erythrocytes.

The clinical symptoms of the infected patient start at this stage. These symptoms are attributed to the destruction of the red blood cells and the host's response to this destruction. The onset of symptoms typically occurs 12–14 days after the mosquito bite (Table 21.1).

**D** After a period of asexual reproduction, a proportion of the merozoites develop into a distinct sexual form, called *gametocytes*. This process usually takes at least 2 weeks. The mechanism that drives part of the cells to become gametes is still unknown. They are long-lived and are not associated with clinical illness, but they are crucial in continuing the life-cycle of malaria because it is only when they are ingested by the female mosquito that they can multiply within the mosquito gut and subsequently (at least 10 days later) be inoculated into human beings.

The different plasmodial forms in the various stages have distinctive antigenic profile expressions and differ-ent sensitivities to antimalarial drugs. Thus, in choosing antimalaria drugs, it is important to understand that no one drug can cover all stages of the parasite. For the hypnozoite and gametocyte stages, only one drug exists, primaquine (its hypnozoiticidal effect is discussed further in this chapter and in Chapter 23).

In cases of transfusion malaria (or any other non-mosquito route of infection) merozoites are injected directly into the bloodstream and, therefore, the incubation time will be 1–2 days (there is no hepatic stage development). In these cases, even in vivax infection, there will not be a need for primaquine treatment because hypnozoites were never inoculated.

## Epidemiology

Figure 21.2 shows the current malaria-endemic areas. The transmission of malaria occurs in more than 100 countries in Sub-Saharan Africa, Asia, Latin America, and Oceania. Diagnosis of malaria and survey data in the endemic areas are often unreliable; thus, the global malaria burden is an estimate extrapolating survey or prospective data to wider

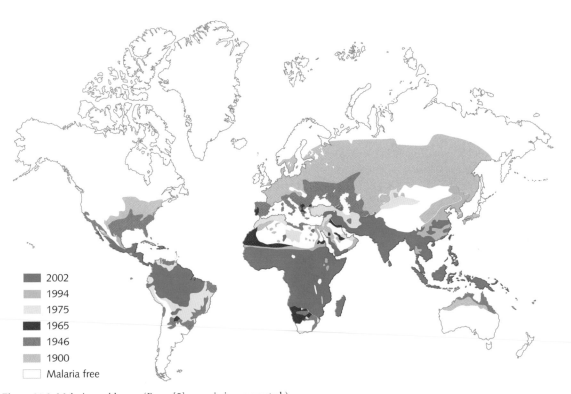

2002
1994
1975
1965
1946
1900
Malaria free

**Figure 21.2** Malaria world map. (From [5], permission requested.)

areas. The estimated number is 380–570 million, but this remains a best guess [5].

Similar problems are encountered with estimation of the death toll for malaria. The widely quoted estimate is about 1 million per year. Virtually all malaria deaths are due to *P. falciparum* infection and mostly occur in Sub-Saharan Africa among children under 5 years.

## Epidemiology in travelers

Until the middle of the twentieth century, malaria was also a disease of the currently industrialized countries. Several regions within North America, Europe, Australia, New Zealand, and Japan were infected (Figure 21.2). After continuous control programs, malaria was finally eradicated. Europe, for example, was declared malaria-free by the WHO in 1975. However, cases due to disease importation either by immigrants or by travelers are still diagnosed. With the increase of global mobility, including immigration from endemic countries, and with increased travel from nonendemic countries to the highly endemic malaria regions, a flow of malaria-infected persons will undoubtedly continue.

An estimated 30,000 cases of travel-associated malaria occur annually, even after short trips [6]. In a review of returned travelers within the GeoSentinel Surveillance Network from 1997–2006, 28% of the 24,920 visits were for febrile illnesses. Malaria was the most common etiology of fever in all returned travelers, comprising 21% of those with fever (14% *P. falciparum* and 6% *P. vivax*), and 33% of the deaths in travelers were attributed to malaria.

The risk for travelers varied significantly between different regions in the endemic areas. Among visitors to Sub-Saharan Africa and Oceania, the percentage of febrile illness due to malaria exceeded 40% [7]. An approximate relative risk (RR) of malaria acquisition by region (where very low-risk areas such as Europe and North America were taken as one) was determined in the GeoSentinel study. Sub-Saharan Africa had the highest RR of 208, followed by Oceania with a RR of 77. Lower risk areas were South Asia (RR 54), Central America (RR 38), Southeast Asia (RR 11.5), and South America (RR 8).

In the same study, it was shown that the risk also varied according to the reason for travel. Those who originally came from endemic countries and travel back to visit their friends and relatives (VFRs) are at higher risk for malaria. This group accounted for 35% of malaria cases, followed by those who traveled for tourism (26%) and for business (14%) [6].

Similar results were reported from Europe, where approximately 11,000 cases of malaria are estimated to occur annually, with 44% of these cases attributable to persons visiting friends and relatives (VFRs), 35% attributable to tourism, and 11% to business [8].

The USA has reported between 1000 and 1500 cases annually over the past 20 years; among them about 75% were US citizens. Based on purpose of travel, VFRs comprised 56% of these cases, whereas tourism accounted for 7 %, and business travel for 6% [9]. *P. falciparum* accounted for about 50% of the cases.

### *P. vivax*

Among the four human plasmodium species, *P. vivax and P. falciparum* are predominant, accounting for 95% of cases worldwide (see Figure 23.4). Whereas *P. falciparum* is the predominant species in Sub-Saharan Africa, *P. vivax* is predominant outside Sub-Saharan Africa. *P. falciparum* receives much more attention due to its severe and fatal consequences, but it should be noted that severe and fatal cases are well documented in *P. vivax* infection as well [10]. *P. vivax* is the predominant species among returning travelers in many Western countries [11].

*P. vivax* has a more complicated life cycle than *P. falciparum* because of the formation of liver hypnozoites, which can result in clinical relapse several months after the primary infection. Complete prevention of this infection is much more difficult (see Chapter 23).

Vivax malaria remains a major global public health problem. About 80,000,000 new cases are estimated to occur every year, and it is the most prevalent cause of malaria outside Africa [12]. *P. vivax* merozoites penetrate the red blood cells (RBC) via Duffy receptors, and because in Sub-Saharan African populations this receptor is frequently lacking, this type of malaria is less common. This is apparent in West Africa, where less than 1% of infection is due to *P. vivax* , whereas in East Africa it is more common, and in other areas, such as Ethiopia, up to 40% of cases reported are *P. vivax* [12].

Vivax malaria is also highly prevalent among returning travelers. Case series of travelers (excluding immigrants) show that vivax malaria accounts for 27–63% of all malaria cases (Table 21.2). This wide range may reflect the variation in favorite travel destinations among different groups of travelers.

The two large multinational databases on travelers' imported infections are GeoSentinel (an international reporting system) and TropNet (multiple European

**Table 21.2** Rate of *P. vivax* in returning travelers [44].

| Country | Years | Total cases | % vivax |
|---------|-------|-------------|---------|
| Israel | 1995–1999 | 300 | 52% |
| USA | 1992–1998 | 2822 | 47% |
| Australia | 1997–2001 | 100 | 63% |
| UK | 1969–1988 | 229 | 48% |
| Japan | 1990–2000 | 1253 | 49% |
| GeoSentinel | 1997–2006 | 1484 | 27% |

countries reporting system). Their data concerning imported vivax malaria mark the destinations where the disease was acquired [11, 13]. Remarkably, their data are very similar and Africa is surprisingly a major region contributing to vivax cases (Table 21.3). This could be explained by the high popularity of East Africa (compared to West Africa) among travelers, or the lack of efficient prophylaxis for vivax infection, or perhaps these data uncover an unexpected higher prevalence of vivax infection in Sub-Saharan Africa.

### *P. ovale* and *P. malariae*

Less than 5% of all malaria cases are caused by *P. ovale* and *P. malariae*. The distribution of *P. ovale* is mainly in Sub-Saharan Africa, but several foci exist in Asia, including India and Papua New Guinea.

The distribution of *P. malariae* coincides with that of *P. falciparum*. It is widespread throughout Sub-Saharan Africa and much of Southeast Asia, into Indonesia, and on many of the islands of the western Pacific. It is also reported in areas of the Amazon Basin of South America, along with *P. brasilianum*, a parasite commonly found in New World monkeys. This parasite is apparently the same species as *P. malariae* and has naturally adapted to grow in monkeys.

**Table 21.3** Area of acquisition of vivax malaria in returning travelers.

| Continent | GeoSentinel [11] | TropNet [13] |
|-----------|------------------|--------------|
| Africa | 29% | 33% |
| Asia | 27% | 28% |
| Pacific | 19% | 20% |
| Latin America | 16% | 17% |

Recently, in Southeast Asia, it has been shown that infections in humans with the monkey malaria parasite *P. knowlesi* have been misdiagnosed as being infections with *P. malariae*.

In many cases, the correct diagnosis of *P. malariae* infection is uncertain unless PCR techniques are used [14].

In the past, *P. malariae* was prevalent in Europe and in the United States. Because the blood stage of the parasites may persist for extremely long periods (reported even after 50 years), there have been reports of people who had never been in the currently known endemic areas, but who lived in the previously endemic areas of Europe or the USA, and whose infections recrudesced after many years of dormancy.

## Clinical aspects

Sir Patrick Manson, in a lecture given 100 years ago, enumerated the major findings seen in patients with malaria to facilitate making the diagnosis (see Chapter 2). He mentioned periodicity of the fever, splenomegaly, and anemia. The absence of leukocytosis was another helpful sign. Out of these findings, only the relative leukopenia remains a valid finding among travelers, with the others rarely seen in this population.

The clinical features seen in uncomplicated cases are similar in all human malaria species.

Headache, nausea, and vomiting, accompanied by a low-grade fever, mark the onset of malaria. Within a few hours, there is often a high fever with profuse sweating that resolves within a few more hours, but is then followed by severe shaking chills. The cycles of drenching sweats, fever, and "bed-shaking" chills called paroxysms tend to be more severe with vivax than with falciparum malaria. The relatively higher levels of inflammatory cytokines excreted during a vivax infection may account for this difference [15]. When all parasites are at the same stage of development, they are called synchronous. In a synchronous infection, both *P. vivax* and *P. falciparum* have an approximately 48-hour life cycle in the erythrocyte and the paroxysms occur every 48 hours or every third day. Thus, they were formerly referred to as "tertian" malarias. Vivax malaria was referred to as "benign tertian" malaria and falciparum malaria as "malignant tertian" malaria, because falciparum malaria was associated with significant risk of more severe disease and death. This synchronous pattern of the disease is uncommon in travelers, especially in falciparum malaria, where patients have continuous or almost

**Table 21.4** Prevalence of symptoms in imported malaria patients. (Adapted from [16].)

| Symptom | Total patients assessed | % of patients affected (95% CI) |
|---|---|---|
| Fever | 1104 | 97 (96–98) |
| Chills | 1315 | 78 (75–80) |
| Headache | 1669 | 74 (72–76) |
| Sweating | 801 | 64 (60–67) |
| Myalgia | 898 | 34 (31–37) |
| Nausea | 777 | 27 (24–30) |
| Vomiting | 678 | 27 (23–30) |
| Cough | 681 | 20 (17–23) |
| Diarrhea | 1741 | 18 (17–20) |
| Abdominal pain | 1192 | 13 (11–15) |

continuous fevers with some spikes. When a traveler has a synchronous infection, it is usually with vivax malaria. The *P. malariae* infection, which may be associated with a cycle of 72 hours, or every fourth day, is called "quartan malaria." This pattern is also rarely seen in travelers. When the synchronous attacks do occur, the patient may feel well between attacks.

The nonspecific nature of the initial malaria symptoms, which may those of resemble influenza, often leads to mistakes and delay in diagnosis. If the disease occurs during the influenza season, the chance for error is even higher.

The common symptoms are listed in Table 21.4 [16].

## Physical examination

The physical examination in patients with uncomplicated malaria is usually unremarkable. Splenomegaly, which is one of the hallmarks of malaria among the endemic population, is hardly ever seen in travelers. It should be remembered that in those with splenomegaly, this is a nonspecific finding that can occur with many other infections, such as dengue, which is often an important consideration in the differential diagnosis of the febrile patient. Mild jaundice may occur due to hyperbilirubinemia (usually indirect bilirubinemia, seldom due to direct bilirubinemia—see *Laboratory findings* below).

Because anemia typically does not occur in travelers, pallor is not seen.

The presence of certain physical findings may serve as evidence against malaria, such as rash or lymphadenopathy, which are not seen in malaria, unless there is a co-infection.

## Laboratory findings

The laboratory findings in uncomplicated malaria are similar in all malaria species.

The most common laboratory abnormality is thrombocytopenia (platelet count $<150 \times 10^9$/L), which is found in about 80% of cases. Typically, the blood count reveals a normal to low white cell count with a normal differential count. There is an absence of eosinophils in the peripheral blood (similar to the effect of corticosteroids). The presence of a high eosinophil count during the acute febrile illness should alert the clinician to the possibility of acute schistosomiasis (in cases where appropriate exposure has taken place) because both diseases are highly prevalent in Sub-Saharan Africa. Leukocytosis may be seen in complicated malaria or in co-infections with other bacterial infections. Anemia, which is the hallmark of malaria in endemic countries, is rarely seen in travelers, because they typically present within the first week of the febrile illness, before significant hemolysis and anemia develop. C-reactive protein and sedimentation rate are usually mildly elevated.

The coagulation factors are usually normal in uncomplicated cases, although D-dimer is elevated, mostly in *P. falciparum* infection, as a marker of endothelial damage.

Biochemistry can remain normal. Indirect bilirubinemia and elevated lactic dehydrogenase (LDH) may present as a consequence of the hemolysis process. Mild elevation of transaminases is not uncommon. In more severe cases with direct hepatic damage (mostly due to *P. falciparum*), direct bilirubinemia may present, along with significant elevations of the transaminases.

One of the most sensitive changes that occur during the acute attack is hypocholestrolemia. One study suggests that this is the strongest positive predictive value among the laboratory tests [17]. One of the early signs of recovery is the return of normal cholesterol levels.

## Severe malaria

*Severe malaria* is defined by the WHO as infection caused by *P. falciparum*, accompanied by end organ damage such as cerebral malaria, pulmonary edema, renal failure, or by metabolic or hematological manifestations, such as acidosis, hypoglycemia, coagulopathy, or circulatory collapse (Figure 21.3).

The pathophysiology of severe falciparum infection is considered to be *cytoadherence*, where infected red cells bind to venular and capillary endothelium. This process is attributed to adhesion proteins that develop on the surfaces of infected red cells ("knobs"), which leads

---

**Common in travelers:**

- **Cerebral Malaria:** Impaired consciousness, seizures, or coma

- **Acute renal failure:** Renal impairment (oliguria < 400ml/day + Creatinine > 3mg/dl or creatinine > 265μmol/l)

- **Respiratory failure:** Pulmonary edema *or* acute respiratory distress syndrome (ARDS)

**Less common in travelers:**

- Acidosis (pH < 7.3)

- Shock (algid malaria – BP < 90/60 mmHg)

- Anemia-Hemoglobin ≤ 8 g/dL

- Hypoglycaemia (< 2.2 mmol/l)

- DIC-Spontaneous bleeding/disseminated intravascular coagulation

- Hemoglobinuria (without G6PD deficiency)

**The following are not defined under "severe and complicated" but indicate severe disease:**

–Hyperparasitaemia (>2% in non-immunes, >10% in semi-immunes)

–Hyperpyrexia > 41C

–Jaundice (bilirubin > 3mg/dl)

–Hyponatraemia

–Prostration

**Figure 21.3** Major features of severe or complicated falciparum malaria in adults. (Adapted from [22].)

to adherence of infected erythrocytes to normal erythrocytes, forming *rosettes*. These cell aggregates are *sequestered* in the small vasculature of the vital organs, causing capillary blockage and release of cytokines, which are responsible for the clinical manifestations. This pathway is encoded by a gene family termed *var*, which is unique to the falciparum species [18].

Risk factors for acquiring severe malaria in endemic countries are youth and pregnancy, especially first pregnancy.

*Young children* are victims of severe malaria due to their lack of immunity to malaria, which is only acquired after several attacks. At infancy they are still protected by their mothers' antibodies, transmitted transplacentally, and usually those over the age of 5 years have acquired immunity from repeated attacks.

*Pregnancy* can be considered a temporarily acquired immune deficiency state in pregnant women. It is not clear

why mainly primigravidae are affected. The susceptibility of pregnant women to malaria is usually seen during the second and third trimesters and continues through the early postpartum period [19].

There is no clear evidence of whether the immune deficiency state of *HIV patients* in Africa increases their risk of acquiring severe malaria.

### Risk factors among travelers

In contrast to the situation in endemic countries, among travelers, older age appears to be a risk factor. In a nationwide Israeli study of 135 patients, all nonimmune travelers with falciparum malaria, 84 (62%) were <40 years old, and only 5% of the patients in this age group developed severe malaria, compared to 18% of the subjects who were >40 years old (odds ratio 4.29). Moreover, all deaths occurred in the latter group. Male subjects, who are overrepresented among malaria cases, did not differ

**Table 21.5** Age-related mortality and severe disease in travelers with *P. falciparum* malaria. (Adapted from [20], [21].)

| Country | Total number of malaria cases | Mortality | Age <40 | Age >40 | OR | 95% CI |
|---|---|---|---|---|---|---|
| USA | 1760 | 3.8% | 1.7% | 7% | 4.28 | 7.44–2.46 |
| Italy | 194 | 1.5% | 0.8% | 2.6% | 3.15 | 35.37–0.28 |
| Italy | 298 | 2.3% | 1.2% | 3.6% | 2.96 | 7.57–1.16 |
| Indonesia | 1059 | 0.7% | 0.6% | 2.5% | 4.16 | 20.95–0.83 |
| Israel | 135 | 2.2% | 0% | 5.8% | — | 2.47–∞ |
| Overall: | 4146 | 2.5% | 1.1% | 5.3% | 3.97 | 6.02–2.62 |
| TropNet[a] | 1270 | 1.4% | 1.1% | 5.1% | 3.29 | 1.78–18.47 |
| Age-related severe falciparum malaria in travelers | | | | | | |
| | Total number of cases | Severe malaria | | | | |
| Israel | 165 | 9.6% | 4.7% | 17.7% | **4.29** | 1.25–14.75 |
| Italy | 194 | 8.7% | 4.4% | 19.0% | **5.13** | 1.72–15.33 |
| TropNet[b] | 1270 | 9.6% | 9.2% | 14% | 3.29 | 1.20–9.01 |

[a] The cutoff for analysis in this study was age 60.
[b] The OR results applied to cerbral complications. Cutoff age 60 as above.

from female subjects with regard to severity of the disease [20].

This high rate of severe malaria and mortality among those >40 years old is reported from other countries as well (Table 21.5) [20, 21].

The vulnerable population from endemic areas, children and pregnant women, is less represented in the travel population; thus, information is scarce. In the GeoSentinel study on malaria in travelers, 13 were known to be pregnant and none had severe or complicated malaria [6].

Severe malaria usually develops 3–7 days after the onset of symptoms. The presenting signs and symptoms are diverse and may involve a single organ or, more often, organs in combination. The WHO criteria of severe malaria are listed in Figure 21.3 [22]. In travelers, common presentations are cerebral malaria, ARDS, and acute renal failure. The number of vital organs involved and extent of vital organ impairment determine the prognosis. In a large study of severe malaria cases (although only about 60% were nonimmune travelers) done in intensive care units in France, the features that were significantly associated with death among patients admitted with severe malaria included at least three of the WHO major criteria, or even one of the following criteria: unrousable coma, pulmonary edema, metabolic acidosis, and shock [23].

### Cerebral malaria

The definition of cerebral malaria is unrousable coma, which may be of sudden onset or with short prodromal symptoms including headache, agitation, drowsiness, and seizures, followed by unconsciousness. In a returned traveler with coma associated with febrile disease and proof of malaria parasites in peripheral blood, the diagnosis of cerebral malaria is obvious. In endemic areas, parasitemia is not sufficient to exclude other pathogens (such as bacterial meningitis), which could be responsible for the clinical condition, and therefore lumbar puncture is required. Cerebral malaria by itself does not cause signs of meningeal irritation; thus, if this is present, a lumbar puncture is indicated, even in a traveler.

Cerebral malaria may cause permanent neurological deficit in children in endemic areas, but this is much less common in adults. In travelers, data are less available, but it appears that those who survive cerebral malaria do not suffer from sequelae [23].

### Respiratory distress syndrome

Respiratory distress often is insidious and may present not on admission but rather after admission and initiation of treatment (which is one of the reasons that falciparum cases should be treated in a hospital). Initial symptoms might be a dry cough, more often while recumbent, followed by shortness of breath and finally full-blown pulmonary edema. Monitoring the oxygen saturation of the patient daily is important, as it might be the first warning sign for the development of ARDS. Chest X-ray findings can range from basilar infiltrates and fluid overload to full-blown pulmonary edema and ARDS. These patients may require mechanical ventilation with advanced supportive care.

### Acute renal failure

In some case series, acute renal failure is the most common complication among travelers. The definition corresponds to laboratory findings of serum creatinine levels >30 mg/L (>265 micromol/L). In most cases, the renal failure is nonoliguric, without uremic complications. Those who have uremic complications or become oliguric need hemodialysis. Several pathogenic mechanisms interact to create the clinical manifestations. The predominant lesions are acute tubular necrosis and mild proliferative glomerulonephropathy. Although this complication is not common in populations of endemic areas, it is associated with a very high mortality rate of 45% [24]. In contrast, among travelers, renal failure is a common presentation but not associated with higher mortality [22]. In addition, these patients, even those who need dialysis, do not progress to chronic renal disease.

A unique historical feature of acute renal failure with high mortality was its association with massive intravascular hemolysis and hemoglobinuria, which colored the urine black, so that it was termed "blackwater fever". It was more commonly associated with quinine use, and in fact disappeared during the second half of the twentieth century, when chloroquine replaced quinine. It was recently described again in a report from France, where 21 cases were observed with these phenomena, although without fatalities. Only about one-third of these cases were treated with quinine; the rest were treated with mefloquine or halofantrine [25].

Other WHO criteria are less commonly met in travelers. *Shock* usually occurs if bacterial sepsis accompanies the malaria, and therefore in malaria cases presenting with shock, an investigation looking for co-infection is important.

*Anemia*, as mentioned above, is not common in travelers, unless they carry the infection for long periods or have very high parasitemia. In any case, blood transfusions are easily available in industrialized countries, which is not the case in many endemic countries.

*Hypoglycemia* is another feature that is uncommon in travelers. However, in patients who become drowsy, glucose levels should be checked before the diagnosis of cerebral malaria is made. Quinine treatment may potentiate hypoglycemia, especially in pregnant women.

*Hyperparasitemia.* There is not always a correlation between the degree of parasitemia and the severity of malaria. Many nonimmune travelers present with severe malaria and low (<1%) parasitemia. It is important to note that in falciparum infection, due to their tendency to be sequestered in the small capillaries, a large number of parasites may exist, but the percentage of infected peripheral erythrocytes may still be low. However, patients with high parasitemia (in the nonimmune >5%) are more likely to present with severe malaria. The follow-up of the patient should include daily monitoring of the level of parasitemia to assure adequate response to treatment. The role of blood exchange is discussed below.

### Severe vivax malaria

Severe and complicated vivax malaria, without co-infection with *P. falciparum,* has been documented. Its presentation may be remarkably similar to that of severe and complicated falciparum malaria and can include hyperparasitemia (density of infection can reach 10–20%), severe anemia, thrombocytopenia, cerebral malaria, ARDS, and renal failure [26]. Vivax malaria is more likely to cause splenic rupture, hematoma, and torsion than falciparum malaria is. However, in studies evaluating severe and complicated vivax malaria, the "falciparum-like" complications still occur more commonly than splenic complications [10]. The risk of death with complicated vivax malaria was 18% in one study of 11 patients in India proven to have *P. vivax* as a single infection [10]. In another study in Indonesia, risk of death with severe malaria was similar (25% vs 24%) among 36 severely ill patients with vivax malaria and 277 patients with falciparum malaria [26]. Another study performed in Papua New Guinea showed that the risk of severe malaria in children was similar: 11.7% for *P. falciparum*, 8.8% for *P. vivax* (a nonsignificant difference) [27]. The pathogenesis of severe vivax malaria is presumably due to a host inflammatory response (which is stronger in vivax infection), and not related to cytoadherence with sequestration, which has not been described in *P. vivax.*

### Mortality from malaria

In Western countries, the mortality rate among all patients with imported falciparum malaria is in the range 1.4–3.8% (Table 21.5), which is probably much higher than seen among populations in endemic countries. In many Western case series, it is not clear how many patients are actually immigrants as opposed to nonimmune travelers. In an Israeli case series of nonimmune travelers, the mortality rate among falciparum cases was 2.2% [20].

In a large US study, the estimated case-fatality rate for US travelers with imported malaria (all species) was 0.9% (range 0–4.4% by year). The case-fatality rate according to species was 1.3% for *P. falciparum*, 0.06% for *P. vivax*, 0.3% for *P. malariae*, and 0.3% for *P. ovale* [28]. These figures demonstrate that even benign forms of malaria contribute to malaria deaths. A caveat to this, however, is that in these cases there may have been co-infection with *P. falciparum*, which was missed by the microscopic diagnosis (PCR is the ultimate method of accurate species diagnosis).

Another important point suggested in this study was that most deaths (85%) were preventable [28].

The reason for this high mortality was in part poor adherence to chemoprophylaxis by travelers. However, for 66% of the persons who died, medical errors may have contributed to the fatal outcome; these errors included failure to prescribe the correct chemoprophylaxis regimen, failure to diagnose malaria on initial presentation, failure to initiate treatment promptly at diagnosis, or treatment with an antimalarial drug that was inappropriate for the infecting species or region of acquisition [28]. Similar findings were also found in a study from Canada [29].

## Treatment

### Treatment of uncomplicated *P. falciparum* malaria

*P. falciparum* infection should be considered an emergency where the patient's condition could worsen within hours. Therefore, treatment should be initiated without delay and with good medical follow-up because the situation of the patient may deteriorate after treatment initiation. There is often controversy concerning which patients should be hospitalized. These dilemmas are often related to the health policies within the country. Our policy is to hospitalize every patient with *P. falciparum* infection.

Chemotherapy of *P. falciparum* infection should be based on drugs acting on the infected erythrocytes, with rapid cidal activity. The principal drugs used are listed in Table 21.6 and include:
- Atovaquone–proguanil (Malarone)
- Artemether–Lumfantrine (Coartem or Riamet)
- Quinine + Doxycycline or + Clindamycin
- Mefloquine (Lariam or Mephaquine)
- Chloroquine.

A few guidelines may help in deciding which drug is appropriate.

### Geographical area

Because of drug resistance patterns in certain regions of the world, not every drug is appropriate.

*Chloroquine*, which was the "miracle" drug for several decades due to its high efficacy, low toxicity, and short schedule, should not be used now because of widespread *P. falciparum* resistance. It can be used in infections acquired in Central America, the Caribbean, and some Middle Eastern countries where the risk of malaria is very low. Chloroquine continues to play a major role in treating vivax malaria (next section) and other nonfalciparum infections (*P. ovale* and *P. malariae*).

*Mefloquine* should not be used in infections acquired in the Thai–Myanmar and Thai–Cambodian border regions because of significant resistance. There are reports of 50% failure with this drug.

### Breakthrough malaria

Travelers who contract malaria despite taking chemoprophylaxis might indicate a drug-resistant strain (although a subtherapeutic blood level cannot be ruled out). Therefore, it is preferable that the drug used for treatment be different from the drug used for prophylaxis.

### Contraindications

Mefloquine, because of its neuropsychiatric effects, should not be used in patients with neuropsychiatric disorders.

Atovaquone–proguanil and artemether–lumfantrine should not be used in pregnancy because data about their safety are lacking.

### Duration of treatment and tolerability

The desired drug is one with a short duration of treatment combined with a low profile of adverse events. Based on this, the old and efficacious drug quinine is unattractive. It requires the longest duration of treatment (Table 21.6) with a high occurrence of adverse events. The common adverse event is called *cinchonism*, expressed as headache, dizziness, tinnitus, impaired hearing, and nausea. Although these symptoms are transient and disappear without residua, for some patients they are intolerable.

Mefloquine, on the other hand, has the advantage of a short duration of treatment (it can be completed in less than 24 hours), but may have a high rate of adverse events, mainly neuropsychiatric effects (see Chapter 23).

### Availability

Availability of antimalarial drugs in industrialized countries can be a problem. Although all the drugs mentioned

**Table 21.6** Oral drugs used for *P. falciparum* treatment.

| Drug | Adult dose | Duration of treatment | Remarks |
|---|---|---|---|
| Atovaquone–proguanil (Malarone) | 4 tab once every 24 hours [or 2 tab × 2/day] | 3 days | Gastrointestinal adverse effects, should be taken with meal |
| Artemether–lumfantrine (Riamet) 20/120 mg combination | 4 tabs/dose (0, 8, 24, 36, 48 and 60 hours) | 3 days | Still not available in many industrialized countries |
| Quinine sulfate + doxycycline | 650 mg × 3/day 100 mg × 2/day | 5–7 days 7 days | High level of adverse events Contraindicated in pregnancy and children; |
| or clindamycin | 7 mg/kg × 3/day | 7 days | Indicated for pregnancy and children |
| Mefloquine | 750 mg + 500 mg (12 hours later) | 1 day | Not for use in infections acquired in Southeast Asia (mainly Thai–Myanmar and Cambodia borders); Contraindicated in patients with neuropsychiatric illnesses |
| Chloroquine[a] | 600 mg base (1 gr), followed by 300 mg base (0.5 gr) at 6, 24, 48 hours [Total of 1.5 gr base or 2.5 gr. salt]. | 2 days | Use only in infections of *P. falciparum* acquired in central America and Caribbean. |

[a]This schedule is also the treatment for *P. vivax, P. ovale,* and *P. malariae.*

have been used by millions of people, not all are registered in every industrialized country. In some countries, registered antimalarial drugs might be stored in a central national pharmacy, thus making them less available. This factor clearly becomes an important factor in choosing the drug.

The two most attractive options therefore seem to be atovaquone–proguanil and artemether–lumfantrine, which have short duration of treatment, low risk of adverse events, and only occasional resistance. The parasite clearance time and the fever clearance time (defervescence), which reflect the cidal activity of the drugs, are slightly different. Artemether–lumfantrine seems to act faster, with median time to parasite clearance and fever clearance in travelers of 41.5 and 36.8 hours, respectively [30]. Atovaquone–proguanil seems to be slower, with median parasite clearance time of 63 hours [31]. In another study in travelers, in the atovaquone–proguanil group, defervescence occurred after 3.7 days and parasite clearance time was 3.3 days, which was about 24 hours slower than with mefloquine treatment [32].

## Treatment of severe malaria

Severe malaria is a medical emergency and should preferably be treated in an intensive care unit. Initial management is based on treatment for any acutely and severely ill patient. The initial rapid clinical assessment should focus on airway and circulation and include assessments of the level of consciousness, respiratory status, and state of hydration. In patients with a decreased level of consciousness, hypoglycemia should be ruled out (although it is not common in travelers). Convulsions should be treated promptly with anticonvulsants, but this is not recommended as prophylaxis for all cases of cerebral malaria. Intravenous rehydration should be commenced if indicated, but fluid overload should be prevented, because it may increase the risk of pulmonary edema (ARDS). Hemodialysis might be indicated in oliguric renal failure.

### Drug therapy

Drug therapy in severe malaria (and in patients who cannot take oral treatment) should be parenteral, and should

- *Artesunate* 2.4 mg/kg given intravenously at 0, 12, and 24 hours, and then daily
- *Artemether* 3.2 mg/kg given intramuscularly as loading dose, then 1.6 mg/kg given intramuscularly daily (to total of 640 mg)
- *Quinine dihydrochloride* 20 mg salt/kg in 5% dextrose given over 4 hours intravenously on admission, then 10 mg/kg every 8 hours given over 2-4 hours.
  — Infusion rate should not exceed 5 mg salt/kg per hour
  — Maximal daily dose should not exceed 1800 mg/day
- *Quinidine gluconate* 10 mg salt/kg given intravenously in normal saline solution over 1-2 hours (maximal dose 600 mg), followed by continuous infusion of 0.02 mg/kg/min.

  For both quinine and quinidine treatment:
  — Monitor glucose level
  — Electrocardiographic monitoring during treatment
  — After 48 hours of intravenous treatment, the dose should be reduced by 30–50%
  — Switch to oral treatment when possible

---

\* Total treatment duration should be 5–7 days.

\* All of the above parenteral drugs should be accompanied by doxycycline treatment to overcome possible resistance.

**Figure 21.4** Parenteral treatment of severe malaria.

be started as soon as possible. Our current arsenal of parenteral drugs is very limited and includes the cinchona alkaloid quinine or quinidine and the relatively new artemisinin derivates; see Figure 21.4.

The cinchona alkaloid quinine has been the drug of choice for severe malaria since its discovery about 300 years ago. In the 1950s, it was supplanted by the synthetic 4-aminoquinoline antimalarial chloroquine, but with the worldwide rise of chloroquine resistance, quinine returned to widespread use in the last decades of the twentieth century. Due to its short supply in several Western countries, another cinchona alkaloid isomer, quinidine, was in use with similar results [33].

The situation is now rapidly changing once more with the discovery and development by Chinese scientists of the artemisinin derivatives, the most rapidly acting of all antimalarial drugs.

Compared with quinine, the artemisinins reduce parasite counts faster, and there is now evidence from a study in Asia that, compared to quinine, they reduce mortality in adults with severe malaria [34]. The artemisinin derivatives are rapidly parasiticidal, and unlike quinine, they kill young circulating parasites before they sequester in the deep microvasculature, a fact that may explain their advantage over quinine [35]. However, quinine and quinidine remain very effective drugs to treat severe malaria, and preferences for a particular drug should never delay treatment with one of them.

Quinidine, which was formerly used extensively in cardiac intensive care units as an anti-arrhythmic agent, was lifesaving for patients with severe malaria. However, since quinidine was replaced by new anti-arrhythmic drugs, the treatment for malaria patients has become more difficult. Even though these are lifesaving drugs, in many Western countries, they may be available only in specialist centers or stored in government-regulated pharmaceutical centers, to be purchased as needed, which obviously may delay treatment.

Intravenous artesunate has not been approved yet by the FDA, and despite its superior value for severe malaria treatment, it is not available in most Western countries. A new GMP formulation of artesunate is being developed by the U.S. Army and it is hoped that it will obtain FDA approval in the near future.

Thus, although artemisinin derivatives have become the drug of choice according to WHO policy [22], they are not available in most Western countries, and quinine or quinidine is the first line treatment. In the USA, intravenous quinine is not available; only intravenous quinidine is available through the CDC Malaria Hotline. In Europe, quinine is available and is usually the drug of choice.

Treatment with quinine or quinidine is associated with more adverse events. Quinine is more likely to cause cinchonism (discussed earlier), and quinidine cardiac toxicity with arrhythmic events. Therefore, ECG monitoring is important, with attention to the Q–T interval.

These drugs may cause hyperinsulinemia and consequently hypoglycemia, especially in children and pregnant women.

Treatment with quinine may be associated with significant hemoglobinuria (blackwater fever).

Quinine and quinidine can be used in pregnant women. Parenteral artesunate is now recommended by WHO as the drug of choice for the treatment of severe malaria in the second and third trimesters of pregnancy [22].

### Exchange transfusion

Exchange transfusion for patients with high parasitemia remains controversial. The idea behind this procedure is rapid clearance of the parasite burden. However, evidence from trials is contradictory, and a well-randomized study is unlikely, especially among travelers. Exchange transfusion is not advisable for parasitemia <10%, and at higher parasite counts the evidence is mixed. Many centers with expertise in malaria consider exchange transfusion if parasite counts are >20%, but some centers never use it [36].

### Adjunctive treatments

Even in the industrialized countries with the best medical care, the mortality of patients with severe malaria is high, reaching about 20%. In many cases, the deterioration occurs after conventional antimalaria treatment

is initiated. It should be remembered that several aspects of the disease, as well as outcomes, are caused by host immunological responses. In view of the double effects of immune responses in malaria patients (protective and immunopathological), an adjuvant therapy, immune modulator therapy, which will tip the balance toward recovery, is needed (in many ways, this is similar to bacterial sepsis with multiorgan failure). So far, all trials with such treatments have failed, including corticosteroids and mannitol for cerebral edema and heparin in cases of DIC. In addition, anti-tumor necrosis factor (TNF), iron chelators, and dichloroacetate have not been shown to be beneficial and in some instances were harmful.

### Treatment failure (recrudescence)

Drug resistance continues to pose problems, particularly with *P. falciparum* infection. It may occur in travelers taking chemoprophylaxis and in patients treated for acute malaria. Failure of complete eradication of the parasites from the blood will cause *recrudescence* of the disease, usually within one month after termination of treatment. Thus, patients should be advised upon discharge from the hospital that if fever recurs, they should be rechecked for malaria.

According to the WHO grading [22], *sensitive* strains are asexual parasites that have cleared by day 7 of treatment and have no subsequent recrudescence within the 28 days that follow. It is important to note that the presence of gametocytes alone does not cause clinical symptoms and is not considered treatment failure.

The resistance pattern is divided into three grades:

**R1** Asexual parasites seem to be cleared from the blood, but recrudescence appears within 28 days (in mefloquine treatment, the follow-up should be longer, 6 weeks).

**R2** Marked reduction in parasitemia (>75%) occurs within 48 hours, but complete clearance does not occur within 7 days.

**R3** No marked reduction occurs within 48 hours of the beginning of treatment.

Because of the possibility of falciparum resistance, even with newer drugs such as atovaquone–proguanil and artemether–lumfantrine, it is important to monitor the parasite density in daily blood smears.

Our experience with atovaquone–proguanil treatment demonstrates a slower cidal effect and a longer period of time to defervescence than with quinine. Thus, patients at the end of the 3-day treatment with atovaquone–proguanil may still be febrile but usually are without parasitemia, and this is not considered drug failure at this stage.

## Treatment of *P. vivax* infection

### Treatment of acute attack

Chloroquine has been a first-line therapy for acute attacks of vivax malaria since 1946. Early clinical investigators developed the recommended adult dose of 1.5 g base delivered over 48 hours as an effective cure for falciparum and vivax malaria. Chloroquine-resistant *P. falciparum* emerged in the late 1950s and spread worldwide, whereas chloroquine-resistant *P. vivax* emerged only in the late 1980s [37] and is a significant problem mainly in eastern Indonesia, where more than half of infections with *P. vivax* appear resistant. However, resistance has been reported from elsewhere in Southeast Asia, South Asia, and South America, although on a much smaller scale and of less clinical importance. The late appearance of chloroquine-resistant vivax infection was probably because of the dose of 1.5 g used for *P. falciparum* infection, which was five times that needed to cure *P. vivax* infections [37].

For chloroquine-sensitive *P. vivax*, standard chloroquine therapy clears the blood of asexual parasites within 72 hours (Table 21.6). Other drugs used to treat falciparum malaria, such as mefloquine and the artemisinin derivatives (ACT) or atovaquone–proguanil, have been shown to have almost 100% efficacy in areas of chloroquine-resistant vivax malaria [38].

*Recrudescence* in vivax infection is unusual but may happen in those who are treated with chloroquine for infection acquired in the Pacific islands.

*Relapse* is common in vivax and ovale infection, and is completely different from recrudescence. In relapse, a new infection emerges from hypnozoites in the liver. The liver hypnozoites are not susceptible to acute treatment with blood schizinocidal drugs, and primaquine treatment is required, as discussed below.

### Anti-relapse therapy (radical cure)

Primaquine is needed to prevent late relapses, which is, therefore, termed "radical-cure" or anti-relapse therapy.

Primaquine is an 8-aminoquinoline. It was first synthesized during World War II and was widely used during the Korean War. Unfortunately, even after more than 50 years, primaquine remains the only available drug for the prevention of relapse in vivax malaria. Its mode of action remains unknown, especially for its action against hypnozoites.

### Dosing

The standard recommended dose of primaquine for prevention of *P. vivax* relapse has traditionally been 15 mg (base) daily for 14 days since the 1950s. This schedule was extensively studied in American soldiers during the Korean War and found to be efficacious for the Korean vivax strain and safe even without checking G6PD levels [39]. Therefore, this schedule was adopted and is still quoted in textbooks. However, shortly after, in the early 1950s, it became obvious that this dose was not sufficient for the Chesson strain (the vivax strain of New Guinea), and failure rates of up to 80% were noted. Exclusively for this strain, the recommended dose in the literature is 6 mg/kg as a total dose. With rising failure rates among travelers who were treated with the standard dose, the need for re-evaluation of this recommendation became obvious.

The necessary dose depends on the geographical location, as the sensitivity of vivax to primaquine differs from one region to the other. For example, in the Pacific (Chesson strain), 6 mg/kg is needed, whereas in Ethiopia, only 4 mg/kg is needed [40].

Another key consideration in primaquine dosing is the weight of the patient. Studies have shown weight >80 kg to be a significant risk factor for relapse after primaquine therapy with 15 mg/day [40].

Thus, the best approach to treating relapse should be giving a total dose of primaquine based on the weight of the patient combined with the dose needed in the area where the infection was acquired. However, in most endemic areas this sensitivity information does not exist.

The new recommendation from some authorities of giving 30 mg daily for 14 days for vivax malaria acquired anywhere (CDC recommendation) seems to be sufficient in most cases. It means a total of 420 mg of primaquine, which translates in 80-kg patients to >5 mg/kg. For patients >80 kg acquiring the disease in the Pacific area, we recommend administering 30 mg daily to achieve a total dose of 6 mg/kg over as many days as is required (Figure 21.5).

### Schedule

The efficacy of treatment is dependent on the total dose of primaquine given and not on the number of treatment days. Good efficacy is achieved whether treatment is delivered daily over 7, 14, or 21 days or once a week for 8 weeks. Because up to 30 mg/day is well tolerated, we recommend giving this dose once daily with a meal, for as

---

## The Art of PART

•Anti-relapse therapy is needed after infection with P. vivax (radical cure), and is to be considered after leaving endemic area for malaria (terminal prophylaxis).

•Primaquine is the only drug that currently exists for this purpose.

•The most important point is the **total dose** given; 6 mg/kg seems to be adequate worldwide.

•The duration of treatment is not important, rather giving the total dose needed.

•A tolerable daily dose of primaquine is 30 mg (base).

•Thus, divide the total dose into 30 to get the number of days needed for treatment.

••An example: A patient who weighs 85 kg will need 510 mg of primaquine, which will be administered in 17 days, whereas a patient weighing 55 kg will need 330 mg, administered in 11 days.

•DO NOT FORGET TO CHECK G6PD  BEFORE TREATMENT

**Figure 21.5**  The art of PART (Presumptive Anti-Relapse Therapy).

many days as needed. For those who suffer from GI upset with this dose, it can either be divided to two doses a day (15 mg × 2) or reduced to 15 mg/day for a longer period.

### G6PD-deficient patients

Primaquine use that caused hemolysis during the 1950s led to the discovery of the inborn deficiency of glucose-6-phosphate dehydrogenase (G6PD). In studies on G6PD-deficient African-Americans, primaquine-induced hemolysis was determined to be mild and self-limited, even with continued dosing. Primaquine destroyed only senescent red blood cells in the African A-variant of G6PD (typically having >15% residual activity). These investigators found that 45 mg of primaquine given once a week for 8 weeks was better tolerated among G6PD-deficient subjects and had good efficacy [41]. Primaquine is contraindicated in individuals with variants (e.g., Mediterranean and Asian) of G6PD deficiency associated with less than 5% residual G6PD activity because of the danger of life-threatening hemolysis. Thus, in these cases, the radical cure is not recommended, but rather continued follow-up and retreatment upon relapse. The same holds true if the G6PD status cannot be determined.

### Schedule of chloroquine plus primaquine

The common schedule for treating patients with vivax malaria is giving chloroquine followed by primaquine. Primaquine theoretically can be given at any point be-

fore relapse occurs. However, some studies indicate the advantage of giving these drugs concomitantly.

When primaquine is combined with chloroquine against chloroquine-resistant P. vivax, efficacy against blood stages is dramatically improved [42]. Thus, combining these drugs is an option for treating chloroquine-resistant vivax malaria [26].

In addition, in a series of experimental challenges during the 1950s, Alving et al. demonstrated that the potent activity of primaquine against hypnozoites is apparently enhanced when it is given with either chloroquine or quinine [43].

The practical lesson from these studies is that concurrent administration of both drugs primaquine and chloroquine may enhance the activity of chloroquine against the blood stage parasites and enhance the primaquine effect against the liver stage of the parasite. Thus, starting primaquine early during the treatment course of vivax malaria (immediately after obtaining G6PD results) might be beneficial for both clearing the parasitemia and killing the hypnozoites.

### Approach to patients with suspected malaria

On one hand, malaria can be life-threatening, especially in the case of P. falciparum infection, but on the other hand, it is treatable. Delay in diagnosis and treatment is an important contribution to severe and fatal outcomes. Therefore, some guidelines will be discussed in this section to help with the diagnosis and management of patients with suspected malaria.

• Malaria is a febrile illness in nonimmune travelers (it might be a *nonfebrile* illness in immigrant populations); however, periodicity of fever is usually absent. A number of travelers have lost their lives because physicians ruled out malaria in cases where the fever was not periodic.

• Initial negative malaria smear does not rule out malaria. Detection of malaria parasites requires a minimum level of parasitemia, and therefore the test should repeated twice at 12-hour intervals. Details of diagnostic methods are thoroughly discussed in Chapter 22.

• Travel history is important. Febrile illness in a traveler returning from Sub-Saharan Africa is highly suggestive of malaria (usually *P. falciparum*).

• Basic laboratory tests may help in estimating the likelihood of malaria. Leukocytosis is hardly seen in malaria; on the other hand, normal or low leukocyte counts increase suspicion, especially when accompanied by low platelet counts. Anemia is usually not seen in malaria among travelers.

The travel period and the incubation time of malaria species may help in determining the diagnosis. All malaria species have an incubation time for the first attack of about 2 weeks from the mosquito bite until clinical symptoms appear. Malaria cannot be seen less than 7 days after exposure. Therefore:

• Febrile illnesses that begin less than 7 days after exposure are very unlikely to be malaria.

• Febrile illnesses that begin within 1 month after return could be caused by any of the malaria species, including *P. falciparum*. Therefore, if the malaria species cannot be determined by the laboratory, it should be treated as falciparum malaria (which usually covers the other species as well).

• Severe malaria that has a non-falciparum malaria diagnosis should be rechecked for verification.

• Late onset malaria (more than 2 months after return, or more than 3 months in someone who took prophylaxis) is most likely non-falciparum malaria. If the laboratory diagnosis is falciparum malaria, it should be verified. This is important to know because non-falciparum cases will need a radical cure with primaquine.

• Immigrants may present with late-onset falciparum malaria.

The best method for species diagnosis is PCR, which should be performed on whole blood taken before treatment, sent in an anticoagulant tube.

## References

1 Cox-Singh J, Davis TM, Lee KS, et al. Plasmodium knowlesi malaria in humans is widely distributed and potentially life threatening. *Clin Infect Dis* 2008 15;46:165–71.

2 Austin SC, Stolley PD, Lasky T. The history of malariotherapy for neurosyphilis. Modern parallels. *JAMA* 1992;268:516–9.

3 Schwartz E. New insights and updates on vivax malaria. Presented at the 56th Annual Meeting, American Society of Tropical Medicine and Hygiene. Philadelphia (PA); Nov 4–8, 2007.

4 Bray RS, Garnham PC. The life-cycle of primate malaria parasites. *Br Med Bull* 1982;38(2):117–22.

5 Hay SI, Guerra CA, Tatem AJ, Noor AM, Snow RW. The global distribution and population at risk of malaria: past, present, and future. *Lancet Infect Dis* 2004;4:327–36.

6 Leder K, Black J, O'Brien D, et al. Malaria in travelers: a review of the GeoSentinel surveillance network. *Clin Infect Dis* 2004;39:1104–12.

7 Wilson ME, Weld LH, Boggild A, et al. GeoSentinel Surveillance Network. Fever in returned travelers: results from the GeoSentinel Surveillance Network. *Clin Infect Dis* 2007;44:1560–68.

8 Jelinek T, Schulte C, Behrens R, Grobusch MP, Coulaud JP, Bisoffi Z, et al. Imported falciparum malaria in Europe: sentinel surveillance data from the European network on surveillance of imported infectious diseases. *Clin Infect Dis* 2002;34(5):572–6.

9 Thwing J, Skarbinski J, Newman RD, et al. Centers for Disease Control and Prevention. Malaria surveillance—United States, 2005. *MMWR Surveill Summ* 2007;56:23–40.

10 Kochar DK, Saxena V, Singh N, Kochar SK, Kumar SV, Das A. *Plasmodium vivax* malaria. *Emerg Infect Dis* 2005;11(1): 132–4.

11 Elliott JH, O'Brien D, Leder K, et al.; GeoSentinel Surveillance Network. Imported *Plasmodium vivax* malaria: demographic and clinical features in nonimmune travelers. *J Travel Med* 2004;11(4):213–17.

12 Mendis K, Sina BJ, Marchesini P, Carter R. The neglected burden of *Plasmodium vivax* malaria. *Am J Trop Med Hyg* 2001;64(1–2 Suppl):97–106.

13 Muhlberger N, Jelinek T, Gascon J, et al. Epidemiology and clinical features of vivax malaria imported to Europe: sentinel surveillance data from TropNetEurop. *Malar J* 2004;3:5.

14 Collins WE, Jeffery GM. *Plasmodium malariae*: parasite and disease. *Clin Microbiol Rev* 2007;20:579–92.

15 Hemmer CJ, Holst FG, Kern P, et al. Stronger host response per parasitized erythrocyte in *Plasmodium vivax* or *ovale* than in *Plasmodium falciparum* malaria. *Trop Med Int Health* 2006;11:817–23.

16 Genton B, D'Acremont V. Clinical features of malaria in travellers and migrants.. In: Schlagenhauf P, editor. *Travelers' Malaria*, 2nd ed. Hamilton (Ont): BC Decker; 2008. p. 134–47

17 Badiaga S, Barrau K, Parola P, Brouqui P, Delmont J. Contribution of nonspecific laboratory test to the diagnosis of malaria in febrile travelers returning from endemic areas: value of hypocholesterolemia. *J Travel Med* 2002;9:117–21.

18 Beeson JG, Brown GV. Pathogenesis of *Plasmodium falciparum* malaria: the roles of parasite adhesion and antigenic variation. *Cell Mol Life Sci* 2002;59:258–71.

19 Diagne N, Rogier C, Sokhna CS, et al. Increased susceptibility to malaria during the early postpartum period. *N Engl J Med* 2000;343:598–603.

20 Schwartz E, Sadetzki S, Murad H, Raveh D. Age as a risk factor for severe *Plasmodium falciparum* malaria in nonimmune patients. *Clin Infect Dis* 2001;33:1774–7.

21 Mühlberger N, Jelinek T, Behrens RH, et al.; TropNet-Europ; Surveillance importierter Infektionen in Deutschland Surveillance Networks. Age as a risk factor for severe manifestations and fatal outcome of falciparum malaria in European patients: observations from TropNetEurop and SIMPID Surveillance Data. *Clin Infect Dis* 2003;36: 990–95.

22 WHO. *WHO Guidelines for the Treatment of Malaria.* Geneva: WHO; 2006.

23 Bruneel F, Hocqueloux L, Alberti C, et al. The clinical spectrum of severe imported falciparum malaria in the intensive care unit: report of 188 cases in adults. *Am J Respir Crit Care Med* 2003;167:684–9.

24 Mishra SK, Das BS. Malaria and acute kidney injury. *Semin Nephrol* 2008;28:395–408.

25 Bruneel F, Gachot B, Wolff M, Régnier B, Danis M, Vachon F; Corresponding Group. Resurgence of blackwater fever in long-term European expatriates in Africa: report of 21 cases and review. *Clin Infect Dis* 2001;32:1133–40.

26 Baird JK, Schwartz E, Hoffman SL. Prevention and treatment of vivax malaria. *Curr Infect Dis Rep* 2007;9:39–46.

27 Genton B, D'Acremont V, Rare L, et al. *Plasmodium vivax* and mixed infections are associated with severe malaria in children: a prospective cohort study from Papua New Guinea. *PLoS Med* 2008;5:e127.

28 Newman RD, Parise ME, Barber AM, Steketee RW. Malaria-related deaths among U.S. travelers, 1963–2001. *Ann Intern Med* 2004;141:547–55.

29 Kain KC, Harrington MA, Tennyson S, Keystone JS. Imported malaria: prospective analysis of problems in diagnosis and management. *Clin Infect Dis* 1998;27:142–9.

30 Hatz C, Soto J, Nothdurft HD, et al. Treatment of acute uncomplicated falciparum malaria with artemetherlumefantrine in nonimmune populations: a safety, efficacy, and pharmacokinetic study. *Am J Trop Med Hyg* 2008;78: 241–7.

31 Bouchaud O, Monlun E, Muanza K, et al. Atovaquone plus proguanil versus halofantrine for the treatment of imported acute uncomplicated *Plasmodium falciparum* malaria in nonimmune adults: a randomized comparative trial. *Am J Trop Med Hyg* 2000;63:274–9.

32 Hitani A, Nakamura T, Ohtomo H, Nawa Y, Kimura M. Efficacy and safety of atovaquone-proguanil compared with mefloquine in the treatment of nonimmune patients with uncomplicated *P. falciparum* malaria in Japan. *J Infect Chemother* 2006;12:277–82.

33 Phillips RE, Warrell DA, White NJ, Looareesuwan S, Karbwang J. Intravenous quinidine for the treatment of severe falciparum malaria. Clinical and pharmacokinetic studies. *N Engl J Med* 1985;312:1273–8.

34 Dondorp A, Nosten F, Stepniewska K, Day N, White N; South East Asian Quinine Artesunate Malaria Trial (SEAQUAMAT) Group. Artesunate versus quinine for treatment of severe falciparum malaria: a randomised trial. *Lancet* 2005;366: 717–25.

35 Day N, Dondorp AM. The management of patients with severe malaria. *Am J Trop Med Hyg* 2007;77(6 Suppl):29–35.

36 Whitty CJ, Lalloo D, Ustianowski A. Malaria: an update on treatment of adults in non-endemic countries. *BMJ* 2006;333:241–5.

37 Baird JK. Chloroquine resistance in *Plasmodium vivax. Antimicrob. Agents Chemother* 2004;48: 4075–83.

38 Lacy MD, Maguire JD, Barcus MJ, et al. Atovaquone/proguanil therapy for *Plasmodium falciparum* and *Plasmodium vivax* malaria in Indonesians who lack clinical immunity. *Clin Infect Dis* 2002,35:92–5.

39 Garrison PL, Hankey DD, Coker WG, et al. Cure of Korean vivax malaria with pamaquine and primaquine. *J Am Med Assoc* 1952;149:1562–3.

40 Schwartz E, Regev-Yochay G, Kurnik D. Short report: a consideration of primaquine dose adjustment for radical cure of *Plasmodium vivax* malaria. *Am J Trop Med Hyg* 2000;62(3):393–5.

41 Alving AS, Johnson CF, Tarlov AR, et al. Mitigation of the hemolytic effect of primaquine and enhancement of its action against exoerythrocytic forms of the Chesson strain of *Plasmodium vivax* by intermittent regimens of drug administration. *Bull WHO* 1960,22:621–31.

42 Baird JK, Basri H, Subianto B, et al. Treatment of chloroquine-resistant *Plasmodium vivax* with chloroquine and primaquine or halofantrine. *J Infect Dis* 1995;171(6):1678–82.

43 Alving AS, Arnold J, Hockwald RS, et al. Potentiation of the curative action of primaquine in vivax malaria by quinine and chloroquine. *J Lab Clin Med* 1955;46:301–6.

44 Schwartz E. P. vivax malaria: prevention and treatment. In: Schlagenhauf P, editor. *Travelers' Malaria*, 2nd ed. Hamilton (Ont): BC Decker; 2008. p. 134–47.

# 22 Malaria Diagnosis in Travelers

## R. Scott Miller

Walter Reed Army Institute of Research, Silver Spring, MD, USA

## Challenges of malaria diagnosis in travelers

In a review of returned traveler visits to the GeoSentinel Surveillance Network from 1997 to 2006, malaria was the most common etiology of fever in all returned travelers, accounting for 21% of the fever etiologies (14% *P. falciparum* and 6% *P. vivax*) and 33% of the deaths [1]. Although 80–90% of travelers suffering from malaria will present for evaluation with fever [2, 3], other symptoms may develop and bring a traveler in for medical evaluation before the onset of the classic fever, chills, and rigor syndrome. Those symptoms include headache, back pain, chills, increased sweating, myalgia, nausea, vomiting, diarrhea, and cough and may lead clinicians to pursue other diagnoses. Healthy volunteers who are given an experimental infection as part of vaccine development efforts offer glimpses of early symptoms of malaria in a carefully monitored setting. Symptoms preceded a diagnostic malaria smear in over 60% of volunteers, typically consisting of headache, myalgias, and fatigue lasting 1–3 days before detection of malaria in the bloodstream [4]. Hence, it is paramount for clinicians to consider and evaluate for malaria in the differential diagnosis of febrile travelers to areas endemic for the parasite.

As evidenced by the variation in onset and in the nature of symptoms, prompt and accurate diagnosis of malaria in the traveler presents some unique challenges. The major concern is that most travelers have no or little immunity to the disease, so that the infection can multiply rapidly and progress to cause organ dysfunction after only a few life cycles of symptomatic illness. In nonimmunes, falciparum malaria should still be treated as an infectious disease emergency, because ill subjects can progress from appearing well to coma, renal failure, pulmonary edema,

and death in a few hours. Even expatriates of malarial regions now living in nonendemic areas quickly lose their immunity and compose the largest group of travelers who develop malaria. This group, commonly referred to as VFRs (visiting friends and relatives), make up >50% of malaria cases in the USA annually [5] and the largest group in Europe as well [2]. Travelers are more likely than VFRs to get severe malaria or die (RR 2.69; 95% CI 1.2–7.3), however, likely due to their complete lack of immunity or to the protective effect of hemoglobinopathies in populations from endemic regions [6].

Compounding the risk of rapid progression of illness is that many travelers are also delayed in presenting to health care. A likely cause is that they do not want to interrupt their plans and often do not know how to access reliable health services while traveling. Upon their return, if fevers do not start with the first few weeks, the relationship to travel is often obscured. Another important reason for the delay in diagnosis is the failure of clinicians, who see febrile returning travelers, to consider malaria.

The typical time to fever onset for *P. falciparum* is 11 days, whereas relapsing malaria, *P. vivax*, occurs much later, at a median of 44 days [2]. Additionally, many travelers assume that they are protected from malaria when they use bite-reduction strategies or chemoprophylaxis for malaria. Chemoprophylaxis or insect repellants can be highly effective when used properly, but even in clinical trials where adherence to drugs can be monitored, none are completely effective.

## Parasitology of malaria in travelers

The species of parasites responsible for illness in travelers reflect local malaria transmission patterns in the countries visited. In aggregate analysis of data from the USA and Europe, *P. falciparum* predominates, with the majority of cases acquired in Sub-Saharan Africa. Among Australian travelers, *P. vivax* predominates, reflecting more traveler

*Tropical Diseases in Travelers*, 1st edition. Edited by E. Schwartz.
© 2009 by Blackwell Publishing, ISBN: 978-1-4051-8441-0.

**Table 22.1** Imported malaria cases: frequency by *Plasmodium* species in returning travelers and visitors to the USA, 2002–2006.

| Plasmodium species | 2002 | 2003 | 2004 | 2005 | 2006 | Mean |
|---|---|---|---|---|---|---|
| *P. falciparum* | 52.3% | 53.4% | 49.5% | 48.6% | 39.2% | 48.6% |
| *P. vivax* | 25.4% | 22.9% | 23.8% | 22.1% | 17.6% | 22.4% |
| *P. malariae* | 2.8% | 3.6% | 3.5% | 3.5% | 2.9% | 3.4% |
| *P. ovale* | 2.8% | 2.6% | 2.0% | 2.5% | 3.0% | 2.6% |
| Mixed | 0.8% | 0.9% | 1.3% | 0.8% | 0.6% | 0.9% |
| Species undetermined | 15.9% | 16.6% | 19.8% | 22.6% | 36.6% | 22.3% |
| Total cases | 1337 | 1278 | 1324 | 1528 | 1564 | 7031 |

*Source:* Adapted from data in [5, 7].

visits to Oceania and Southeast Asia. The species of parasites detected in imported malaria cases (~75% of whom are travelers) over the past 5 years in the USA are shown in Table 22.1. Diagnostic testing capable of determining malaria species is clearly needed.

Unlike local endemic populations, it is rare for travelers to be infected by more than one type of *Plasmodium*. In the USA from 2001 to 2006, the percentage of returning travelers with mixed infections ranged from 0.6% to 1.3%. This low rate of mixed infection can reduce confounders in treatment that must be considered when treating local populations. Mixed infections remain a likely scenario for foreign nationals from endemic countries who become ill while traveling abroad.

## Tests for the diagnosis of malaria in travelers

Because of the need to tailor therapy to the species of malaria infection and to drug resistance among parasites where it was likely acquired, empirical antimalarial therapy without diagnostic tests should be avoided if at all possible. Traditionally, in the USA, treatment has been withheld until a parasitological diagnosis is confirmed. Disease progression while waiting for test results is well described, especially for *P. falciparum* infections. Availability of rapid malaria antigen testing with results in 10–15 minutes is a major breakthrough in the diagnosis of falciparum malaria [8]. If a rapid malaria test is not available, empirical treatment with newer and less toxic antimalarials, such as atovaquone–proguanil, is a sound decision while the results of the diagnostic tests are pending.

In some clinical settings, diagnostic malaria testing may not be available or reliable. Malaria smears are frequently misinterpreted in sites without strong quality control programs [9]. Even in Thailand, which can boast one of the best malaria control programs in the world, with regular quality control re-evaluation of malaria slides, the diagnostic accuracy of the clinical malaria smear in clinic settings may be as low as 80% [10]. Rapid malaria tests purchased in endemic countries may also have quality control problems, potentially yielding inaccurate results. Clinicians should recommend to the traveler that, if he or she becomes ill while still in the malaria-endemic country or at a locale where malaria diagnosis is difficult, a malaria smear should be made before treatment is started and given to the patient to take home. This can be interpreted at a later date to assess if additional therapy (e.g., anti-relapse therapy with primaquine) is needed.

The goals of malaria diagnosis are to confirm the presence or absence of parasites in the blood, and, when they are present, to determine the species and estimate the density and stage of parasitemia. Since the development of stains containing methylene blue by Ehrlich in 1899, the microscopic analysis of a malaria smear has been the standard diagnostic test for malaria diagnosis, and in the hands of a skilled microscopist readily provides the requisite information. New diagnostic malaria tests, namely immunochromatographic antigen detection tests and various nucleic amplification techniques, can also yield similar information. These will each be discussed in subsequent sections.

In travelers, malaria is occasionally surreptitiously diagnosed by analysis of blood films as part of a complete blood count. Although these are not routinely performed any more in many laboratories, detection of hemazoin (malaria pigment) may still yield presumptive diagnosis of malaria among travelers via routine hematology testing. Hemazoin, a crystalline heme byproduct of the intra-erythrocytic parasite, is produced after digestion of hemoglobin. It is often taken into phagocytes removing cellular debris after schizont rupture. Hemazoin can be measured in various automated hematology analyzers by the depolarization of the laser light passing through the flow cytometer channel. Automated hematology analyzers, such as the Cell-Dyn (CD) 3500 (Abbott-Diagnostics, Maidenhead, UK), detect malaria pigment in monocytes and neutrophils (they may also detect pigment in schizonts and gametocytes) during routine automated blood counts. In Portugal, 174 samples from 148 patients who presented to the emergency department were analyzed. Compared with microscopy, the sensitivity was 95% and the specificity was 88% [11]. Several studies have revealed sensitivities from 49% to 98% and specificity of 82–97% [12]. Not surprisingly, sensitivity is higher in patients from endemic countries, where asymptomatic malaria and delayed clinical presentation due to immunity result in more parasite turnover and increased pigment formation. Clinicians can check with their clinical laboratories to assess whether they can detect unsuspected malaria as part of routine automated hematology screening. Instruments may need to be programmed to flag suspicious samples for clinical correlation and definitive malaria evaluation.

## Microscopic examination of Giemsa-stained thick and thin blood smears

As mentioned, the microscopic detection of parasites on Giemsa-stained blood smears remains the reference standard for malaria diagnosis. A Giemsa-stained thick blood film is usually used to screen for the presence of parasites, whereas a thin blood film helps to determine the species and assists with quantitation. Thick blood films allow rapid examination of a relatively large volume of blood, enabling the detection of even scanty parasitemias of all blood parasites. With an expert microscopist, the detection limit for Giemsa-stain microscopy is 5–20 parasites/$\mu$l for thick blood films, but limits of detection rise to nearly 500 parasites/$\mu$l in less experienced hands. This limit of detection for a thick smear is only 10 times better than that for a thin blood film even though the thick blood film requires a 50 times greater volume. The reason for this is that some parasites are not seen in the thick film due to the need to focus through multiple planes.

Conventional microscopy allows the identification of all four human *Plasmodium* species through different mor-

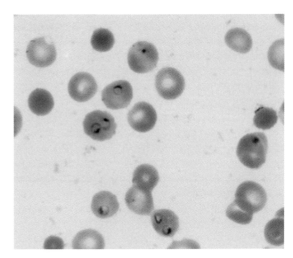

**Figure 22.1** Ring forms of *Plasmodium falciparum* in a Giemsa-stained thin smear. (Courtesy of Dr. Peter Weina.)

phologies in the parasite stages, quantification of parasites, and determination of other prognostic factors, such as the stage of the parasites in the life cycle [13]. All stages of the parasite may be seen in the peripheral blood in cases of *P. vivax*, *P. ovale*, and *P. malariae*, but generally only the small ring parasites and (in established infections) the banana-shaped gametocytes are found in *P. falciparum*. If ring forms alone are present in the smear, the determination of species or of a mixed infection is very difficult (Figures 22.1 and 22.2). The recently described fifth human parasite from Southeast Asia, *P. knowlesi*, is microscopically difficult to distinguish from *P. malariae* [14].

### Sample collection for blood films

Ideally, blood should be collected during or shortly after fever, as an indicator of schizont rupture and new RBC invasion, and before initiation of antimalarial treatment. For malaria diagnosis, blood should ideally be taken direct from the patient's finger or ear and the smears prepared at the bedside or in the clinic. Films prepared in this way adhere better to the microscope slide, leave a clearer background on thick films after lysis, and undergo minimal parasite and red cell morphological changes. Alternatively, blood may be collected from an EDTA-containing blood tube, but collection should be done quickly because EDTA will distort parasite morphology after a few hours. These smears must also be dried longer (at least 3 hours, preferably overnight) to ensure adherence to the slide.

If clinicians plan to prepare smears for routine diagnosis of malaria at the bedside, at least two thin and two thick

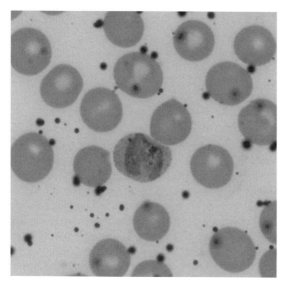

**Figure 22.2** Trophozoite of *Plasmodium vivax* in a Giemsa-stained thin smear. (Courtesy of Dr. Peter Weina.)

blood films should be made. One each of the thick and thin films, stained with Giemsa, should be adequate for detection of parasitemia and for determination of species. A second slide should always be held in reserve. If problems with diagnosis arise during staining or examination of the first film, the other slide is available for further study. In attempts to reduce time and labor with microscopy, rapid alternate techniques such as Field's stain may be employed in the laboratory at the cost of some loss of sensitivity [15]. If a rapid Field's stain will also be used in your laboratory for urgent diagnosis, a third slide will be required for that purpose.

The principle for preparation of a thick smear is to prepare an unfixed dried film, about five to six red blood cells thick, from which the hemoglobin is lysed out, either before or during the staining process. Parasites are then stained and stand out out against the relatively acellular background. Steps for preparing the thick film include the following:

• A drop of blood (3–5 mm in diameter) or 6 $\mu$l from a micropipette is placed near one end of the slide.

• It is slowly spread, with the corner of another slide or a swab stick, to cover an oval area approximately 10–15 mm diameter. The final density of the smear should allow newsprint to be just visible through it. If bubbles develop, gently stir again until no bubbles remain.

• Thoroughly dry the smear, horizontally, in an incubator at 37°C for 1 hour or longer. Smears made from

anticoagulated blood should ideally be allowed to dry overnight.

• Remember not to fix the dry film with methanol, so that the erythrocytes may be lysed in the staining process.

The principle of the thin smear is the same as for routine hematology review of cellular elements in the blood: preparation of a single layer of cells to maximize evaluation of the morphology of the cellular elements. Steps for preparing the thin film include the following:

• Collection of one drop of blood or 4 $\mu$l from a micropipette.

• Prepare thin blood film as for routine hematology using a second spreader slide to spread the blood across the slide. After the blood has spread over two-thirds of the width of the slide, it is pushed down the microscope slide in a smooth continuous motion. Ensure that the film has a good tail (known as a feathered edge) for best parasite speciation and does not reach the edges of the slide laterally.

• Allow the film to dry in air and fix with methanol for 30 to 60 seconds before staining.

For further details of specimen preparation and various staining methods, readers are referred elsewhere [13, 16].

## Examining blood films

At least 100 high-power fields (hpf, ~0.28 $\mu$l blood) should be examined on a thick smear before a slide is considered negative for malaria. For suspected low parasitemias, examination of up to 500 hpf will improve diagnostic yield by sampling a large volume of blood [13]. For thin films, examination should start with the tail, where cells are a single layer thick and not clumped. Particularly for *P. vivax* and *P. ovale*, it is important to look along the edges of the film. Generally, to avoid eye fatigue and loss of concentration, a single microscopist should read no more than 35–40 smears daily.

A parasite count or density is a useful predictor of disease severity, although in *P. falciparum* it is critical to remember that circulating parasites are an underestimate of total body burden due to parasite sequestration in the postcapillary venules. Parasites in thick film fields are counted until 200 leucocytes have been seen; counting may continue to 500 white blood cells (WBCs) for low-density parasitemias (typically, <10 parasites seen at 200 WBCs counted). A recognized rapid estimate of the parasite count per $\mu$l on thick films is to use a standard value (8000 cells/$\mu$l) for the white cell count—the parasite count is thus multiplied by 40 to give parasites per $\mu$l of blood. This does not take into account the known loss of parasites in the thick film, which suggests that it is an underestimate, but the standard white blood cell value is probably too high, which helps to cancel out this error. A more accurate count uses the most recently obtained WBC count from an automated hematology analyzer using the following formula:

$$\frac{\text{# of asexual parasites counted}}{\text{# of WBCs counted}} \times \text{WBC count (cells/}\mu l)$$
$$= \text{asexual parasites/}\mu l.$$

For higher-density parasitemias, the percentage of parasitized erythrocytes can be directly enumerated from Giemsa-stained thin films. Typically, 5000 RBCs are reviewed and the percentage of parasitized erythrocytes can be then multiplied by the measured RBC mass (cells/$\mu l$) to calculate parasite density.

## Limitations of conventional microscopy

As a diagnostic modality, conventional microscopy is time-consuming, requires technician expertise, electricity, and fragile equipment, and is limited in the diagnosis of very low parasitemias and the detection of mixed *Plasmodium* infections [8]. Tradition, the low cost of reagents, and the vast experience of experts trained during the malaria eradication campaigns in endemic countries maintain its popularity.

Accurate microscopic diagnosis is a skill still learned with training and experience, and in nonendemic countries only with imported malaria, and can be a difficult skill to master and not necessarily the "gold standard" [8]. Routine clinical microscopy cannot reliably detect very low parasitemias (<5–10 parasites/$\mu l$) or sequestered parasites, and hence a serial testing paradigm is used with repeated testing every 12 hours at least three times before malaria can be excluded as a cause of symptoms. At very low parasite densities, as typically seen in travelers at the onset of symptoms, errors increase in both detection of parasites and species diagnosis [10]. Even at higher parasitemias, mixed infections can be missed, especially with *P. malariae* and *P. ovale* [17]. Finally, even when the test is ordered, clinicians may choose not to wait for the test results or may lack confidence in the test and treat the patient despite negative microscopy [9]. These problems are magnified in nonendemic regions, where malaria microscopy is infrequently performed. Kain et al. in Toronto report that microscopy may miss 59% of cases and incorrectly identify species 64% of the time, resulting in therapeutic delays of 5.1–7.6 days [18]. As previously discussed, therapeutic delays of 3–4 days can prove fatal.

## Rapid immunochromatographic tests for malaria

Antigen detection in whole blood offers an alternate to microscopy for detecting infection, with the theoretical advantage for *P. falciparum* that antigen still circulates while many parasites are sequestered [19]. Current malaria rapid diagnostic tests (MRDTs) utilize a lateral-flow immunochromatographic technology, similar to that of many home pregnancy tests (Figure 22.3). Malaria RDTs utilize polyclonal or monoclonal antibodies directed against select target parasite antigens to fix mobile antigens when they are present in the blood, and a separate antibody conjugated to an indicator, typically colloidal gold, to produce a visible line. Although most are marketed for whole blood, antigen is readily detectable in sera as well, but performance parameters are less well defined (Miller, unpublished data). An in-depth review of malaria rapid diagnostic tests was recently published [8].

## Antigen targets

The characteristics of the malaria antigen target and the detection antibodies are paramount in understanding a given assay's diagnostic capacity. The malaria antigens currently used as diagnostic targets are either specific to a *Plasmodium* species or conserved across the human malarias (panmalarial antigens). Targets conserved across all human malarias (pan-*Plasmodium* antigens) that have been identified and successfully used include lactate dehydrogenase (pLDH) and aldolase enzymes [20, 21]. Falciparum-specific monoclonals have been successfully

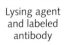

**Figure 22.3** Schematic of a malaria rapid diagnostic test. (With permission from Murray [8].)

Lysing agent and labeled antibody    Bound antibody #1    Bound antibody #2    Control    Nitrocellulose strip

deployed for histidine-rich protein-2 (HRP-2) and *P. falciparum* lactate dehydrogenase (pfLDH), whereas monoclonals specific to other malarias have undergone limited evaluation [22].

The first antigen used in a commercial assay and the target of most RDTs in the marketplace today is histidine-rich protein II (HRP-2), a water-soluble protein unique to *Plasmodium falciparum,* localized in the parasite cytoplasm and on the erythrocyte membrane. It is found in abundance in all knob-positive *P. falciparum* parasites, with increasing concentrations from ring stage to trophozoite, and it readily diffuses into the plasma [23]. It is abundantly produced in the asexual stages but is also found in young *P. falciparum* gametocytes. Hence, it can be detected at lower parasitemias than the panmalarial antigens such as aldolase [8, 24]. Many different monoclonal antibodies of both IgG and IgM have been raised and may be employed on different RDTs. Mutants with altered binding sites that escape monoclonal recognition have now been identified and may be responsible for occasional false negative HRP-2 tests [25].

Select *Plasmodium* enzymes are the other primary antigen diagnostic target. *Plasmodium* lactose dehydrogenase (pLDH), the terminal enzyme in the malaria parasite's glycolytic pathway, is an antigen target in sexual and asexual stage malaria parasites. Monoclonal antibodies have now been developed that can target a conserved element of pLDH on all human malaria species (panmalarial) or specific regions unique to each malaria species [20]. Specific monoclonals of *P. falciparum* or *P. vivax* LDH have been used in commercial products, but no evaluations of *P. ovale-* or *P. malariae*-specific antigens have been published. Aldolase, a key enzyme in the glycosis pathway in all malaria parasites, is also well conserved across all human species of *Plasmodium* and is often used as a panmalarial antigen target [21]. Other antigens have been recognized as possible components of future diagnostic tests, but none are currently available in the marketplace [26].

## Target profile for a malaria RDT in travelers

The WHO has set a target sensitivity for *P. falciparum* of 95% for malaria RDTs at 100 parasites/$\mu$l, with a focus on tests developed for use in endemic countries [22]. Ideal requirements for malaria RDTs in the traveler population who seek diagnosis in a nonendemic region require a target profile different from that of populations in endemic regions, however. Likewise, a product that may be useful by travelers for self- or buddy diagnosis will also require differing characteristics (Table 22.2).

**Table 22.2** Target characteristics for malaria RDTs in travelers.

| | Diagnosis in nonendemic countries | Self-diagnosis |
|---|---|---|
| | Assay specifications | |
| ICH GMP | Yes | Yes |
| Stable to 40°C | No (room temperature) | Yes |
| Point-of-care test (CLIA waived) | Yes | Yes |
| Individual test packaging | No | Yes |
| Packaged with gloves/lancet | No | Yes |
| Simple to perform/interpret | Ideal | Yes |
| Cost per test | $20 | $20 |
| | Assay performance characteristic | |
| Detects all human malarias | Yes | Yes |
| Separately detects Pf | Yes | Yes |
| *Plasmodium* species-specific | Ideal | Ideal |
| Lower limit detection <100 parasites/$\mu$l | Yes | Yes |
| High specificity (>98%) | Yes | Yes |

*Source:* Adapted from Murray CK, Gasser RA Jr., Magill AJ, Miller RS. Update on rapid diagnostic testing for malaria. *Clin Microbiol Rev* 2008;21:97–110.

## Performance of malaria RDTs in the marketplace in traveler populations

Rapid antigen detection tests for malaria (RDTs) have expanded dramatically in the commercial marketplace over the past decade. An estimated 12 million RDTs were produced in 2005, with nearly 100 products available (available from URL: www.wpro.who.int/sites/rdt/home).

More than 100 publications have evaluated field and lab-based performance malaria RDTs in various populations [8, 27]. Marx et al. [27] completed a meta-analysis of the accuracy of malaria RDTs in returning travelers. This summary was limited by inadequate cases of non-falciparum malaria and lack of three-band assays (dual antigen-capture assays performed on the same test), which are now commonplace. In febrile travelers returning from Sub-Saharan Africa, it obtained a typical probability of *P. falciparum* malaria of 1.1% (95% CI, 0.6–1.9%) after a negative three-band HRP-2 test result and 97% (CI, 92–99%) after a positive test result. It concluded that microscopy was still required for species identification and test confirmation. Relatively few dual-antigen products now in the marketplace have been evaluated in travelers ([pLDH/PfLDH (OptiMal, DiaMed) [28, 29]; HRP-2/Aldolase [29–32]). Overall, performance in traveler populations reveals levels of sensitivity (≥95% for Pf) similar to those for endemic populations, and improved specificity (Table 22.3). HRP-2-based antigen tests for *P. falciparum* are more sensitive than Pf LDH tests for the same species. Current panmalarial antigens (PLDH and aldolase) perform similarly for the diagnosis of *P. vivax*. As mentioned previously, the lower specificity in endemic populations is not surprising, in that residual malaria antigen (especially HRP-2) may persist for weeks after a treated infection, and such volunteers are rarely excluded from these field trials.

## Caveats to using malaria RDTs in travelers

As summarized in Table 22.3, a single malaria antigen test, similarly to thick/thin Giemsa-stained microscopy, is not adequate to exclude the diagnosis of malaria in a symptomatic traveler. All assays currently available are less sensitive for *P. vivax* (~80–85%) than for *P. falciparum*, and even less sensitive for *P. malariae* or *P. ovale* [33, 34]. None of the assays can accurately diagnose mixed infec-

tions. Even for *P. falciparum*, rare false negative HRP-2 tests have been described due to HRP-2 mutants that do not bind to the capture or signal antibodies [25], or rarely due to the prozone effect, where overwhelming antigenemia causes lack of complexing with signal antibodies [35]. Use of a three-line or dual antigen capture test may theoretically still detect panmalarial antigen in these cases, but would yield an inaccurate diagnosis of non-falciparum malaria. Although malaria rapid tests may speed diagnosis, a blood smear confirmation for detection of parasites and species identification is strongly recommended.

Although it has not been formally tested, it is certainly expected biologically that parasitemia density, and hence antigenemia, will rise in untreated infections in nonimmune or traveler populations. Hence, daily serial antigen testing may detect a malaria infection that was below the lower limits of detection of the assay on initial evaluation. In a hospital setting, serial Giemsa-stained blood smears are the preferred method for diagnostic reevaluation of febrile travelers. However, in settings where diagnostic microscopy is not available or not accurate, serial antigen testing is a rational approach.

The most common cause of false positive tests in travelers who have not premedicated is likely a true positive that is below the detection threshold of microscopy. PCR, which is a more sensitive assay, may help in the scenario. Actual false positives do occur, however, occasionally due to rheumatoid factors [37]. These occur less often with the newer generation assays that use IgM, rather than IgG, as the signal or capture antibody [22], but still occurred in 8% of rheumatoid factor positive persons tested with the second-generation BinaxNOW assay (BinaxNOW Malaria package insert, Binax Inc., 2006).

Last, it is important to remember that serial malaria antigen testing as a measurement of response to therapy is not an accurate reflection of parasite killing and should not be performed. The structural protein HRP-2, used as a target in most Pf assays, is detectable in the bloodstream for 3–4 weeks after successful treatment of infection [38]. The enzyme antigens, LDH and aldolase, revert to negative upon successful treatment, but all target antigens are also produced by gametocytes. Hence, the test may remain or revert to positive if Pf gametocytes circulate in the convalescent phase of infection, as commonly occurs despite effective treatment of the asexual stages of infection. Malaria smears should be used to monitor success of malaria treatment.

**Table 22.3** Key studies of the performance of currently available *P. falciparum* (Pf) and pan-malaria rapid diagnostic tests in travelers.

| Product | Antigens | Sensitivity Pf | Sensitivity Pv | Specificity | Reference standard | Population | Reference |
|---------|----------|----------------|----------------|-------------|--------------------|-----------|-----------|
| NOW Malaria (Binax Inc.) | Pf: HRP-2 | 96.0% | 86.7% | 98.7% | Hospital-based blinded single microscopy | Symptomatic travelers Toronto | [30] |
| | Panmalarial: aldolase | 94.3% | 86.7% | 98.7% | Blinded PCR | 106 Pf 103 non-Pf 47 negative | |
| NOW Malaria (Binax Inc.) | Pf: HRP-2 Panmalarial: aldolase | 97.5% | 100% | 98.9% | Hospital-based blinded dual microscopy | Symptomatic travelers France 80 Pf 13 Pv 457 negative | [29] |
| NOW Malaria (Binax Inc.) | Pf: HRP-2 Panmalarial: aldolase | 96.7% | n/a | 95.6% | Hospital-based expert microscopy | Italy travelers and migrants 118 Pf 11 Pv 159 negative | [32] |
| OptiMAL strip (DiaMed AG) | Pf: pfLDH Panmalarial: pLDH | 96.8% | 100% | 99.4% | Hospital-based blinded single microscopy | US travelers 32 Pf 11 non-Pf 173 negative | [28] |
| OptiMAL-IT (DiaMed AG) | Pf: pfLDH Panmalarial: pLDH | 84.3% | 84.6% | 98.4% | Hospital-based blinded dual microscopy | Symptomatic travelers France 80 Pf 13 Pv 457 negative | [29] |

*Source*: Adapted from [8] with permission.

## Special situations for travelers

There is a benefit to using RDT in verifying a diagnosis of malaria in a traveler who has begun treatment and who had the diagnosis made in the endemic country. The smear could be negative, but the RDT would still be positive, confirming the initial diagnosis of malaria (a diagnosis that is often unreliable in many endemic countries). Therefore, although the RDT period of positiveness after treatment can be a disadvantage, in this particular case the use of RDT can help.

## Use of the malaria RDT for self-diagnosis

For travelers without access to health care diagnostic services, only the malaria RDT offers hope over empiric symptom-based initiation of therapy. A febrile traveler

who carried a RDT could potentially perform and interpret the test to aid in deciding whether to start malaria therapy (standby emergency self-treatment) (Figure 22.4). The technology has yet to fulfill this promise.

Several studies have evaluated the self-diagnosis strategy using various Pf-only (two-band) RDT products. One hundred sixty healthy Swiss travelers were asked to perform ParaSight-F tests during pretravel counseling. After oral instruction, 75% performed the test correctly, which rose to 90% after written training. Interpretation of the results, however, remained disappointing at 70%, with 14% false negative results [39]. Studies in self-diagnosis of returning febrile travelers have shown variable accuracy with test performance, with worsening results based on the severity of the febrile illness [40, 41]. Although improved test design and easy-to-use instructions may overcome some of these difficulties, the more complex

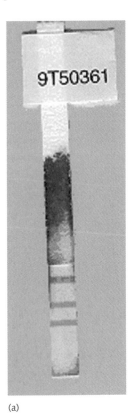

(a)

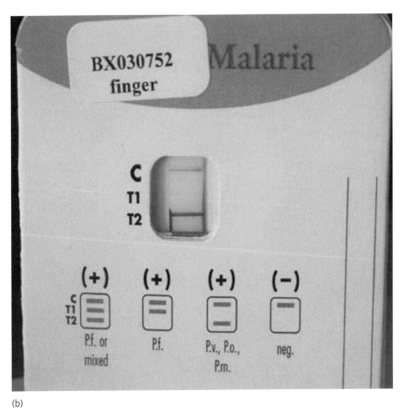

(b)

**Figure 22.4** Examples of three-band (*P. falciparum* or any malaria) tests. (a) Shows the nitrocellulose strip separated from the packaging. The three lines convey detection of the antigen to HRP-2 and the panmalarial antigen, consistent with *P. falciparum* infection. (b) Shows the BinaxNOW test, which detects the panmalarial antigen (T2) without HRP-2 (T1), indicative of a non-falciparum malaria; in this case, due to *P. vivax*. (From Clinton K. Murray, Robert A. Gasser, Jr., Alan J. Magill, R. Scott Miller. Update on Rapid Diagnostic Testing for Malaria. Copyright © American Society of Microbiology. *Clin Microb Rev* 2008: p. 97–110, with permission from American Society for Microbiology.)

three-band test design (for separate Pf and Pv diagnosis) may confuse most travelers [42]. More data on use of these tests by travelers or their companions after pretravel training with good visual aids is clearly needed.

Last, concern has been raised about heat (above 35°C) and humidity degradation of some tests currently in the marketplace, leading to inconsistent test performance [43]. For unclear reasons, pLDH tests have been more susceptible to heat degradation than HRP-2 tests. Individual packaging may reduce the problem, but until further testing, consistent performance of malaria RDTs in the rural tropics, such as experienced by some backpackers, must be questioned. In summary, use of malaria RDTs by inexperienced travelers for self-diagnosis should be very restricted with the products currently available.

## The polymerase chain reaction

In the past decade, the PCR has become a major research technique in malaria, and several validated assay methods are available to assist in the diagnosis of febrile travelers [12]. Most PCR assays were developed to detect *P. falciparum*, although many assays detect several or all four species, or even target selected drug-resistance biomarkers. None are commercially available at this time, however, as the only commercial real-time PCR assay [44] for the diagnosis of malaria (Artus RealArt Malaria PCR Kit CE, Qiagen, Germany) was removed from the market in December 2007.

Generally, PCR assays can detect fewer parasites in the blood than well-performed thick blood films, with a limit of detection 1–2 logs below that for microscopy (lower limits of reliable detection 1–5 parasites/$\mu$l). This was convincingly demonstrated by several authors who reanalyzed PCR-positive/thick-film-negative samples ("false positives") by either extensive microscopy or different nucleic acid amplification assays. This frequently confirmed that "false" positives with PCR were in fact true positives [45]. Another advantage of PCR is its significantly improved species identification in mixed infections when compared with microscopy. Although PCR can detect cases with lower parasitemias, PCR assays may miss some cases, even with high parasite numbers. Problems involve amplification inhibitors, including heme, DNA degradation, and genotypic variants [46].

The time needed to perform most traditional PCR assays prohibits their commercial use in routine diagnostic situations, although they are often used to resolve ambiguous diagnosis from conventional microscopy or rapid antigen testing. However, real-time PCR is a rapid (1 hour), efficient method for the specific diagnosis of malaria and does not require multiple complex procedures or skilled technologists [47]. These methods may have wider commercial application in the sensitive and specific diagnosis of malaria [48].

## Summary

For travelers suspected of malaria infection, microscopy of Giemsa-stained thick and thin smears remains the reference diagnostic test. This assay can confirm the presence or absence of malaria, determine the species of infection, and quantify the parasitemia. New malaria rapid diagnostic tests can markedly improve the time to test results and are very specific and quite accurate for *P. falciparum*. Performance to detection of non-falciparum malaria is not as good, and when it is used, a malaria smear should also be performed to confirm the diagnosis. PCR-based assays are increasingly replacing microscopy in research and epidemiology settings, but are not commercially available at this time. They can be very useful in resolving ambiguous test results from the other assays described.

### Disclaimer
The opinions or assertions contained herein are the private views of the author and are not to be construed as official or as reflecting the views of the US Department of the Army, the US Department of Defense, or the US government.

## References

1 Wilson ME, Weld LH, Boggild A, et al. Fever in returned travelers: results from the GeoSentinel surveillance network. *Clin Infect Dis* 2007;44:1560–68.

2 Leder K, Black J, O'Brien D, et al. Malaria in travelers: a review of the GeoSentinel surveillance network. *Clin Infect Dis* 2004;39:1104–12.

3 Jelinek T, Schulte C, Behrens R, et al. Imported falciparum malaria in Europe: sentinel surveillance data from the European network on surveillance of imported infectious diseases. *Clin Infect Dis* 2002;34:572–6.

4 Epstein JE, Rao S, Williams F, et al. Safety and clinical outcome of experimental challenge of human volunteers with *Plasmodium falciparum*-infected mosquitoes: an update. *J Infect Dis* 2007;196:145–54.

5 Mali S, Steele S, Slutsker L, et al. Malaria surveillance—United States, 2006. In: Surveillance Summaries, June 20, 2008. *MMWR Morb Mortal Wkly Rep* 2008;57(SS-5):24–39.

6 Legros F, Bouchaud O, Ancell T, et al. Risk factors for imported fatal *Plasmodium falciparum* malaria, France, 1996–2003. *Emerg Infect Dis* 2007;13:883–8.

7 Thwing J, Skarbinski J, Newman RD, et al. Malaria surveillance—United States, 2005. In: Surveillance Summaries, June 8, 2007. *MMWR Morb Mortal Wkly Rep* 2007;56(SS-6):23–38.

8 Murray CK, Gasser RA Jr., Magill AJ, Miller RS. Update on rapid diagnostic testing for malaria. *Clin Microbiol Rev* 2008;21:97–110.

9 Reyburn H, Mbatia R, Drakely C, et al. Overdiagnosis of malaria in patients with severe febrile illness in Tanzania: a prospective study. *BMJ* 2004;329(7476):1212–16.

10 McKenzie FE, Sirichaisinthop J, Miller RS, et al. Dependence of malaria detection and species diagnosis by microscopy on parasite density. *Am J Trop Med Hyg* 2003;69:372–6.

11 Hanschied T, Melo-Cristino J, Pinto BG. Automated detection of malaria pigment in white blood cells for the diagnosis of malaria in Portugal. *Am J Trop Med Hyg* 2001;64:290–92.

12 Hawkes M, Kain KC. Advances in malaria diagnosis. *Expert Rev Anti Infect Ther* 2007;5:485–95.

13 Warhurst DC, Williams JE. ACP Broadsheet no 148. July 1996. Laboratory diagnosis of malaria. *J Clin Pathol* 1996;49:533–8.

14 Cox-Singh J, Davis TM, Lee KS, et al. *Plasmodium knowlesi* malaria in humans is widely distributed and potentially life threatening. *Clin Infect Dis* 2008;46:165–71.

15 Mendiratta DK, Bhutada K, Narang R, et al. Evaluation of different methods for diagnosis of *P. falciparum* malaria. *Indian J Med Microbiol* 2006;24:49–51.

16 World Health Organization. *Basic Malaria Microscopy. Part I: Learner's Guide*. Geneva: World Health Organization; 1991.

17 Kilian AH, Metzger WG, Mutschelknauss EJ, et al. Reliability of malaria microscopy in epidemiological studies: results of quality control. *Trop Med Int Health* 2000;5:3–8.

18 Kain KC, Harrington MA, Tennyson S, Keystone JS. Imported malaria: prospective analysis of problems in diagnosis and management. *Clin Infect Dis* 1998;27:142–9.

19 Dondorp AM, Desakorn V, Pongtavornpinyo W, et al. Estimation of the total parasite biomass in acute falciparum malaria from plasma PfHRP2. *PLoS Med* 2005;2, e204. Erratum in: *PLoS Med* 2005;2,390.

20 Makler MT, Piper RC, Mihous WK. Lactate dehydrogenase and the diagnosis of malaria. *Parasitol Today* 1998;14:376–7.

21 Lee N, Baker J, Bell D, et al. Assessing the genetic diversity of the aldolase genes of *Plasmodium falciparum* and *Plasmodium vivax* and its potential effect on performance of aldolase-detecting rapid diagnostic tests. *J Clin Microbiol* 2006;44:4547–9.

22 Bell D, Peeling RW, WHO—Regional Office for the Western Pacific/TDR. 2006. Evaluation of rapid diagnostic tests: malaria. *Nat Rev Microbiol* 2006;4(9 Suppl):S34–S38.

23 Howard RJ, Uni S, Aikawa M, et al. Secretion of a malaria histidine-rich protein (Pf HRP II) from *Plasmodium falciparum*-infected erythrocytes. *J Cell Biol* 1986;103:1269–77.

24 Richter J, Goebels K, Muller-Stoever I, et al. Co-reactivity of plasmodial histidine-rich protein 2 and aldolase on a combined immuno-chromographic-malaria dipstick (ICT) as a potential semi-quantitative marker of high *Plasmodium falciparum* parasitaemia. *Parasitol Res* 2004;94:384–5.

25 Lee N, Baker J, Andrews KT, et al. Effect of sequence variation in *Plasmodium falciparum* histidine-rich protein 2 on binding of specific monoclonal antibodies: implications for rapid diagnostic tests for malaria. *J Clin Microbiol* 2006;44:2773–8.

26 Forney JR, Wongsrichanalai C, Magill AJ, et al. Devices for rapid diagnosis of malaria: evaluation of prototype assays that detect *Plasmodium falciparum* histidine-rich protein 2 and a *Plasmodium vivax*-specific antigen. *J Clin Microbiol* 2003;41:2358–66.

27 Marx A, Pewsner D, Egger M, et al. Meta-analysis: accuracy of rapid tests for malaria in travelers returning from endemic areas. *Ann Intern Med* 2005;142:836–46.

28 Palmer CJ, Bonilla JA, Bruckner DA, et al. Multicenter study to evaluate the OptiMAL test for rapid diagnosis of malaria in U.S. hospitals. *J Clin Microbiol* 2003;41:5178–82.

29 De Mondbrison F, Gerome P, Chaulet JF, et al. Comparative diagnostic performance of two commercial rapid tests for malaria in a non-endemic area. *Eur J Clin Microbiol Infect Dis* 2004;23:784–6.

30 Farcas GA, Zhong KJ, Lovegrove FE, et al. Evaluation of the Binax NOW ICT test versus polymerase chain reaction and microscopy for the detection of malaria in returned travelers. *Am J Trop Med Hyg* 2003;69:589–92.

31 Cuadros J, Martin-Rabadan P, Merino FJ, et al. Malaria diagnosis by NOW ICT and expert microscopy in comparison with multiplex polymerase chain reaction in febrile returned travellers. *Eur J Clin Microbiol Infect Dis* 2007;26:671–3.

32 Gatti S, Gramegna M, Bisoffi Z, et al. A comparison of three diagnostic techniques for malaria: a rapid diagnostic test (NOW Malaria), PCR and microscopy. *Ann Trop Med Parasitol* 2007;101:195–204.

33 Dyer ME, Tjitra E, Currie BJ, Anstey NM. Failure of the 'pan-malarial' antibody of the ICT Malaria P.f/P.v immunochromatographic test to detect symptomatic *Plasmodium malariae* infection. *Trans R Soc Trop Med Hyg* 2000;94:518.

34 Mason DP, Wongsrichanalai C, Lin K, et al. The panmalarial antigen detected by the ICT Malaria P.f/P.v immunochromatographic test is expressed by *Plasmodium malariae*. *J Clin Microbiol* 2001;39:2035.

35 Risch L, Bader M, Huber AR. Self-use of rapid tests for malaria diagnosis. *Lancet* 2000;355(9199):237.

36 Lee N, Baker J, Andrew KT, et al. Effect of sequence variation in *Plasmodium falciparum* histidine-rich protein 2 on binding of specific monoclonal antibodies: Implications for rapid diagnostic tests for malaria. *J Clin Microbiol* 2006;44:2773–8.

37 Iqbal J, Sher A, Rab A. *Plasmodium falciparum* histidine-rich protein 2-based immunocapture diagnostic assay for malaria: cross-reactivity with rheumatoid factors. *J Clin Microbiol* 2000;38:1184–6.

38 Igbal J, Siddique A, Jameel M, Hira PR. Persistent histidine-rich protein 2, parasite lactate dehydrogenase, and panmalarial antigen reactivity after clearance of *Plasmodium falciparum* monoinfection. *J Clin Microbiol* 2004;42:4237–41.

39 Trachsler M, Schlagenhauf P, Steffen R. Feasibility of a rapid dipstick antigen-capture assay for self-testing of travellers' malaria. *Trop Med Int Health* 1999;4:442–7.

40 Whitty CJM, ArmstrongM, Behrens RH. Self-testing for falciparum malaria with antigen-capture cards by travelers with symptoms of malaria. *Am J Trop Med Hyg* 2000;63:295–7.

41 Jelinek T, Amsler L, Grobusch MP, Nothdurft HD. Self-use of rapid tests for malaria diagnosis by tourists. *Lancet* 1999;354(9190):1609.

42 Grobusch MP, Ha:nscheid T, Gobels K, et al. Sensitivity of *P. vivax* rapid antigen detection tests and possible implications for self-diagnostic use. *Travel Med Infect Dis* 2003;1:119–22.

43 Chiodini PL, Bowers K, Jorgensen P, et al. The heat stability of *Plasmodium* lactate dehydrogenase-based and histidine-rich protein 2-based malaria rapid diagnostic tests. *Trans R Soc Trop Med Hyg* 2007;101:331–7.

44 Farcas GA, Zhong KJ, Mazzulli T, Kain KC. Evaluation of the RealArt Malaria LC Real-Time PCR Assay for malaria diagnosis. *Am J Trop Med Hyg* 2004;42:636–8.

45 Seeso N, Nopparat P, Hedrum A, et al. An integrated system using immunomagnetic separation, polymerase-chain reaction and colorimetric detection for diagnosis of *Plasmodium falciparum*. *Am J Trop Med Hyg* 1997;56:322–8.

46 Oliveira DA, Shi YP, Oloo AJ, et al. Field evaluation of a polymerase-chain-reaction based nonisotopic liquid hybridization assay for malaria diagnosis. *J Infect Dis* 1996;173:1284–7.

47 Rougemont M, van Saanen M, Sahli R, et al. Detection of four *Plasmodium* species in blood from humans by 18S rRNA gene subunit-based and species specific real-time PCR assays. *J Clin Microbiol* 2004;42:5636–43.

48 Vo TK, Bigot P, Gazin P, et al. Evaluation of a real-time PCR assay for malaria diagnosis in patients from Vietnam and in returned travellers. *Trans R Soc Trop Med Hyg* 2007;101:428.

# 23 Malaria—Prevention

Eli Schwartz

Chaim Sheba Medical Center, Tel Hashomer, Israel and Sackler School of Medicine, Tel Aviv University, Tel Aviv, Israel

## Introduction

Malaria prevention in travelers to endemic areas is one of the most complicated and challenging aspects of travel medicine. This stems from the fact that not only are there vast areas of the world that remain endemic (see Figure 21.2), but also the epidemiology of malaria continues to change. Moreover, data among local populations do not necessarily reflect the epidemiology of malaria in travelers, and accurate data in travelers are scarce.

Theoretically, malaria prevention could be based on a *vaccine*, on *personal protection*, or on *chemoprophylaxis*. Because a malaria vaccine is not on our near horizon, and personal protection, although an important tool, is often not sufficient, chemoprophylaxis remains the principal means of preventing malaria.

Preventive medicine is clearly a fundamental part of travel medicine, and malaria chemoprophylaxis poses several significant problems.

**A** Risk–benefit: The risk of malaria infection and the severe consequences of the disease should be weighed against the risk of the drug itself to the traveler. Several drugs have had fatal outcomes for consumers; others have caused significant adverse events and an interruption of travel due to these events. This side of the equation is not always weighed aptly by those who prescribe these drugs.

**B** Cost–benefit: With the development of malaria-resistant species, new drugs have been made available, usually at a higher cost. Thus for budget travelers, especially on long-term trips, use of these drugs becomes a burden. When the malaria risk is minimal, the benefit of such an expense is often felt not to be justified.

**C** Inadequacy of the current chemoprophylaxis: Although we use the term "malaria prophylaxis," in reality we have falciparum prophylaxis and not panmalaria pro-

phylaxis. Travelers who take the recommended prophylactic drugs may still present with late-onset vivax infection [1]. Although vivax malaria in most cases does not have a severe outcome, it remains a significant disease, and one that the traveler would like to prevent. Additionally, if a traveler contracts malaria in spite of prophylaxis, he or she may deem it useless and skip taking it for subsequent trips.

Adverse events, cost–benefit calculations, and the inadequacy of preventing late-onset vivax malaria are all probable reasons for low adherence to prophylaxis, well known to those practicing travel medicine. A survey done in our institute of travelers presenting post-travel, seeking medical advice for any reason ($n = 605$), demonstrated a significant contrast between a history of following recommendations for vaccination and adherence to malaria prophylaxis. Whereas 84% had received recommended vaccinations, only 35% adhered to malaria prophylaxis (either complete or partial) [unpublished data].

These results highlight the discrepancy between medical recommendations for malaria prophylaxis and travelers' perceptions.

## Personal protection

Personal protection refers to all measures that can be taken to reduce the risk of anopheline bites. Because the *Anopheles* mosquito is a night feeder, protection is relatively easy compared, for example, to protection from dengue mosquitoes, which are day feeders. Protective strategies include wearing clothing after sunset that covers as much bare skin as possible and using mosquito repellents on exposed skin containing about 35% *N, N*-diethyl-3-methylbenzamide (DEET) formulations. The use of insecticide-impregnated clothing can also be helpful [2]. Indoors, staying and sleeping in air-conditioned rooms and sleeping under mosquito nets provide good protection. For expatriates who live in endemic areas,

*Tropical Diseases in Travelers*, 1st edition. Edited by E. Schwartz.
© 2009 by Blackwell Publishing, ISBN: 978-1-4051-8441-0.

eradicating mosquito breeding sites around the house is important. Strict adherence to these measures reduces the chance of acquiring malaria, but they cannot be relied upon to prevent malaria in environments where anopheline mosquitoes and infected humans are present in abundance.

Malaria in many areas of the world is seasonal and usually reaches its peak at the end of the rainy season. Thus, avoiding travel during peak malaria seasons may reduce the risk.

## Principles of chemoprophylaxis: blood stage vs liver stage prophylaxis

The parasite's life cycle in humans occurs in two stages (Figure 23.1). In the initial liver stage, or exo-erythrocytic stage, parasites multiply in the hepatocytes and eventually cause them to rupture. Two species, *P. vivax* and *P. ovale*, have persistent liver stages resulting in relapse months to years later.

The second, or blood (erythrocytic) stage, occurs when the parasites are released into the bloodstream, invade erythrocytes, and cause clinical illness. This stage occurs

usually after $12 \pm 3$ days in *P. falciparum* infection and after $14 \pm 3$ days in *P. vivax* infection.

The following points should be noted.
- The malaria parasite is different in its sensitivity to drugs in each stage of its cycle. Thus, a drug that acts on the parasite during the erythrocytic stage will not necessarily act against it in its liver stage and vice versa.
- Chemoprophylaxis does not prevent the infection (as in the case of vaccine-preventable diseases), but rather has a cidal effect against the parasite, either within the erythrocytes or within the hepatocytes, thus preventing the clinical disease.

Based on the parasite's life cycle, there are two types of malaria chemoprophylaxis, depending on the site of action.

*Blood stage* prophylaxis refers to drugs that act only on parasites within the red blood cells (RBCs). These are the commonly known antimalarial drugs that have been used over the past 60 years or so. Among their disadvantages is that they must be continued for 4 weeks after travel to eliminate the parasites within the RBCs that may emerge from the liver as late as 2–4 weeks after exposure. Another major disadvantage is that because these drugs have no activity against the liver stage and development

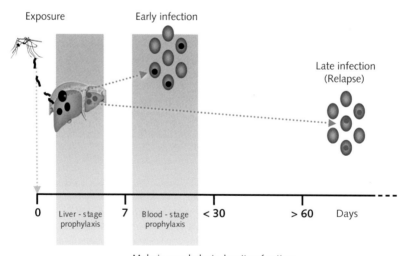

Malaria prophylaxis, by site of action

**Figure 23.1** Malaria life cycle (partial illustration).
- Blood stage prophylaxis: Drugs that act on the malaria parasites only within the erythrocytes (e.g., mefloquine, chloroquine, and amodiaquine). They have to be continued for 1 month after leaving the endemic area. As seen in the figure, late infections will not be prevented.

- Liver stage prophylaxis: Drugs that act on the malaria parasites within the hepatocytes (e.g., primaquine and Malarone). It is sufficient to continue the drug for a few days after leaving the endemic area. These may prevent all types of malaria and late infection.

of hypnozoites, they actually prevent only primary vivax (and ovale) infection, and do not have the ability to prevent relapse. They, therefore, achieve complete prevention only in the case of *P. falciparum* infection.

*Liver stage* prophylaxis refers to drugs that act on the parasite while it is invading the hepatocytes. Because these drugs kill the parasite early during the infectious process, there is no need to continue taking the drug after leaving the endemic areas. For falciparum infection, liver stage prophylaxis has the advantage of shortening the duration of prophylaxis usage. Instead of continuing medication for 1 month post-travel, there is only a need to continue for several days, which may increase compliance with the full prophylaxis schedule. In the case of vivax (and ovale) infection, liver stage prophylaxis is imperative. Only drugs that act early on the liver stage and prevent hypnozoite formation offer complete prevention of this infection. There are currently only two drugs that act on the liver stage, atovaquone–proguanil and primaquine, and only primaquine has cidal activity against hypnozoites (as will be discussed further in the vivax prophylaxis section).

## Falciparum prophylaxis

The introduction of chloroquine in the 1950s brought great hope that falciparum prevention could be easily achieved with a long-acting drug that was well tolerated and taken on a weekly basis. However, within a relatively short period of time (about one decade), drug resistance appeared, first in Southeast Asia and within a few years throughout the endemic areas. Currently, the resistance of *P. falciparum* to chloroquine is almost universal. It remains effective only in Central America, the Caribbean, and some of the Middle Eastern countries where the prevalence of *P. falciparum* is in any case very low [3].

The history of the development of chemoprophylaxis since then involves trying to find new drugs that are both efficacious and well tolerated. It should be remembered that a drug with even an infrequent severe adverse event, if used as prophylaxis for a very large volume of travelers, might quickly be seen as a harmful drug. Two drugs that were introduced after chloroquine, namely amodiaquine and sulfadoxin-pyrimethamine (Fansidar), were excluded from prophylactic use because of severe adverse events, including fatal cases. With amodiaquine, fatalities were due to agranulocytosis, and with Fansidar, they were due to fatal toxic epidermal necrolysis. Risk–benefit calculations at that time showed that in some geographical areas, the risk of fatal outcomes from these drugs was higher than that from the disease [4].

The principal drugs currently in use are mefloquine, doxycycline, and atovaquone–proguanil. In some European countries the combination of chloroquine and proguanil is still recommended [5] (Table 23.1).

### Mefloquine

Mefloquine (Lariam, Mephaquin) was developed from a quinolone–methanol compound at the Walter Reed Institute. It was found to have potent antimalaria activity, including activity against chloroquine-resistant *P. falciparum* strains. Because of its long half-life, it can

**Table 23.1** Use of antimalarial drugs for *P. falciparum* prophylaxis.

| Drug | Dose (adult) | Dose regimen | Beginning of prophylaxis (before exposure) | End of prophylaxis (after exposure) |
|---|---|---|---|---|
| Atovaquone–proguanil | 250 mg/100 mg | Daily | 1 day | 7 days |
| Mefloquine | 250 mg | Once a week | 1–3 weeks | 4 weeks |
| Doxycycline | 100 mg | Daily | 1–2 days | 4 weeks |
| Primaquine[a] | 30 mg (base) [usually = 2 tabs] | Daily | 1 day | 3–7 days |
| Chloroquine | 300 mg (base) = 500 mg salt | Once a week | 1 week | 4 weeks |
| Proguanil[b] | 200 mg [= 2 tabs] | Daily | 1 day | 4 weeks |

[a] G6PD testing is mandatory before its use.
[b] Use only in combination with chloroquine.

be taken on a weekly basis. These characteristics of the drug created optimism in the mid-1980s, when it was first introduced in Europe (and in the USA in 1990), that an ideal replacement for chloroquine had been found. In addition, long-term prophylactic usage among Peace Corps volunteers in Sub-Saharan Africa demonstrated its safety and good tolerability [6].

However, during the subsequent decades of its use, several concerns arose.

## Mefloquine resistance

Resistance was occasionally reported first from the Thai–Cambodian border, followed by reports from other parts of Asia and to a lesser extent from Africa and the Amazon region. The level of mefloquine resistance in the area of the Thai–Cambodian and Thai–Burmese borders has reached 50%, thus precluding its prophylactic use in this specific region [7]. In other regions, the resistance level currently is more anecdotal and the drug can be used.

However, the main concerns for travelers regarding the use of mefloquine are its safety and tolerability.

## Mefloquine safety and tolerability

Mefloquine's adverse side effects may include neuropsychiatric, gastrointestinal, and less commonly dermatological events.

The neuropsychiatric adverse events (AE) associated with mefloquine are the most worrisome complaints and have received a vast amount of public attention (probably more than for any other malaria prophylactic drug). The neurological disorders include headache, dizziness, confusion, vertigo, and seizures. Peripheral neuropathies such as paresthesia, tremors, and ataxia have also been reported. The psychiatric disorders may include insomnia, strange dreams, restlessness, anxiety, depression, and psychosis.

The incidence of any AE due to the drug is hard to assess because results vary and range from about 10% to 90% depending on the study design and whether a comparator was used [8]. The rate of drug withdrawal also varies, from 0.9% to 5% [9, 10].

The issue of greatest concern with chemoprophylaxis is the rate of serious AEs, resulting in possible life-threatening conditions or causing severe disability or prolonged hospitalization. Well-designed prospective studies of mefloquine's adverse events may not identify a significantly greater number of events in comparison to other antimalaria drugs, because of the small number of participants, and it is also easy to miss the relatively rare severe adverse events [9–11]. Only postmarketing surveillance

studies (with their limitations) have sample sizes large enough to capture the rare serious adverse events, making it possible to draw significant conclusions.

Results of a study done by questionnaire among mefloquine users in British soldiers showed a rate of severe AEs as 1:6000 [12], whereas a questionnaire among European travelers showed a rate of 1:10,000 [13]. Spontaneous reporting among Canadian travelers demonstrated a rate reaching 1:20,000 [8].

Mefloquine AEs are more common in women, as reported in all studies. In most cases, susceptible individuals have problems after the first 1–3 doses [14]. The recommendation therefore is to start mefloquine about two weeks before departure in order to assess any adverse effects that may necessitate the use of an alternative prophylaxis.

In a case control study among travelers with serious AEs due to mefloquine prophylaxis, no difference in the level of mefloquine in the blood was found between the patients and the control groups. Also, no significant difference was found between mefloquine levels in the blood of men and women. These results suggest that blood levels of mefloquine do not correlate with its severe adverse events [14].

### Pregnancy

One of the advantages of mefloquine is that it is the only drug that can be taken during pregnancy when traveling to chloroquine-resistant areas. It is officially recommended for the second and third trimesters of pregnancy. Limited data also suggest that its use during the first trimester is safe. Therefore, mefloquine should be recommended to a pregnant woman who cannot avoid traveling to endemic areas during her first trimester [7].

### Contraindications

Due to the possible drug-associated neuropsychiatric effects, mefloquine is contraindicated in travelers who have seizure disorders. In addition, it should not be given to travelers with active psychiatric disorders, such as depression, anxiety, psychosis, or any other major psychiatric disorders. It is advisable not to prescribe this drug to patients with a history of such psychiatric disorders, even if they are currently stable [15].

### Hypersensitivity

Because the drug is related to quinine, it should not be given to persons with known hypersensitivity to mefloquine or to quinine compounds. It is also not recommended for travelers with cardiac conduction abnormalities.

## Doxycycline

The tetracyclines are broad-spectrum antibiotics, which have antimalarial activity and hence potential for use in prevention and treatment of falciparum malaria. Doxycycline, which is the long-acting compound among them, is the most suitable for malaria prophylaxis.

In studies conducted looking at malaria prophylaxis in nonimmune populations, the dosage used was 100 mg daily, resulting in greater than 95% efficacy against *P. falciparum*, indicating that it is as efficacious as the other drugs currently available, such as mefloquine and atovaquone–proguanil [16]. Although it has some liver-stage activity, its main action is on the erythrocytic stage. Thus, 4 weeks of continuation of the drug is required after leaving an endemic area.

Malaria resistance to doxycycline has not been reported yet in any of the malaria-endemic areas.

### Tolerability

The most common adverse events associated with doxycycline are gastrointestinal complaints such as abdominal pain, nausea, vomiting, and diarrhea. A severe complication is esophageal ulceration, and therefore the recommendation is to take it in an upright position, with food or a full glass of water, and not before bedtime.

Dermatological complications include photosensitivity, which is a concern for travelers exposed to the sun in tropical countries. The dermatological complications may affect 21% of users [17], although in a four-arm multicenter randomized controlled trial comparing doxycycline, mefloquine, atovaquone–proguanil, and chloroquine–proguanil in travelers to Africa, skin reactions with doxycycline were less common than with chloroquine–proguanil [11].

An important adverse effect of the drug among female travelers is the risk of vaginal candidiasis, which is estimated to occur in 2.8% of users [18].

The requirement to take doxycycline daily and the fact that it must be continued for 1 month after leaving a malaria endemic area are also drawbacks of its use.

Extra benefits of using doxycycline for malaria prophylaxis are its preventive effect against leptospirosis, which is a common hazard in the tropics, and its potential protection against rickettsial diseases and travelers' diarrhea.

*Contraindications* are for pregnant women, breastfeeding mothers, children under 8, and those with a history of allergy to any of the tetracycline classes.

**Blood Stage Prophylaxis:**

1. Acts on infected erythrocytes.
2. Should be continued 4 weeks after leaving endemic area.
3. Prevents primary infection.
4. Complete prevention of P. *falciparum* only.

**Liver Stage Prophylaxis:** [Primaquine, Atovaquone-proguanil*]

1. Acts on hepatocytes.
2. Discontinue after leaving the area.
3. May prevent primary and late infection.
4. Potentially, complete prevention of all malaria types.*

\* Data show that A-P does not give complete prevention of vivax malaria.

**Figure 23.2** Types of malaria chemoprophylaxis.

## Atovaquone–proguanil

The spread of drug-resistant falciparum malaria and the widespread reluctance to use the known antimalaria drugs due to their side effects led to the pursuit of new antimalaria drugs. Atovaquone–proguanil (Malarone) is the latest antimalarial drug to be developed.

This drug is well tolerated and has good efficacy against resistant falciparum strains.

An added advantage of atovaquone–proguanil is that it acts on the *liver stage* of the malaria parasite, thus shortening considerably the amount of time it needs to be continued post-travel (Figure 23.2). It is therefore the first liver-stage drug since the introduction of malaria chemoprophylaxis (with the exception of primaquine, which will be discussed below).

The drug is a fixed combination of atovaquone 250 mg and proguanil 100 mg. Pediatric tablets contain the same combination with a quarter of the dose of each component (62.5/25 mg).

Atovaquone alone is a well-established drug against *Pneumocystitis carinii*. Its mode of action against the *Plasmodium* species is inhibition of the mitochondrial electron transport system, at the level of the cytochrome b complex.

Proguanil is an old antimalaria drug, which acts by inhibiting the parasite's dehydrofolate reductase.

Each of these drugs has weak antimalarial activity, but in combination there is a synergistic effect, with an efficacy of 95–100% [19]. Each of these drugs' components was tested separately in human volunteers and found to be active at the liver stage [20, 21]. The fixed combination (Malarone) was also tested in human volunteer challenge trials, where nonimmune subjects were given one tablet of Malarone daily for 8 days, starting 1 day before the mosquito challenge and continuing for 7 days after. None of the subjects ($n = 12$) who took Malarone developed malaria, whereas all ($n = 4$) who took a placebo developed falciparum malaria [22]. This clearly demonstrated that the combination of the drugs has good activity against the liver stage of *P. falciparum*. This study was the basis for recommending continuation of the drug Malarone for 7 days after leaving the endemic areas.

## Tolerability

Several studies of Atovaquone-proguanil have been conducted among travelers to evaluate its safety and tolerability in comparison to other antimalarial drugs. In a four-armed multicenter randomized controlled trial comparing the four drugs commonly used in travelers, namely mefloquine, doxycycline, chloroquine–proguanil, and atovaquone–proguanil, the last had the lowest withdrawal rate due to adverse events (2%) [11]. In other studies where only one drug was used as a comparator, either mefloquine or chloroquine–proguanil, atovaquone–proguanil had a better safety profile [10, 23].

The drug has been in use for about a decade and seems to have a very good safety and tolerability record. Its main drawback is its higher cost in comparison to the other antimalarial drugs, which obviously increases with increased length of travel.

The most common adverse events are related to gastrointestinal complaints, such as abdominal pain, nausea, or vomiting, and, therefore, it is recommended that it be taken with a meal. Dermatological complaints such as rashes and pruritus may occur, probably due to the proguanil component.

## Indications

Atovaquone–proguanil is indicated for P. *falciparum* prophylaxis. It should be taken daily, beginning 1 day before entering the endemic area, throughout the stay there, and for 7 days after leaving the area. (Its role in the treatment of falciparum malaria is discussed in Chapter 21.)

In the USA, it is indicated without a time limitation, meaning that long–term travelers, expatriates, and military personnel on long-term missions can use it. In several European countries, its use is limited to short-term travelers (30–90 days) because data on its safety with prolonged use are lacking.

It is indicated for children above 5 kg, but dose should be modified according to weight (see Appendix A).

## Contraindications

Atovaquone–proguanil is contraindicated in patients with severe renal failure (creatinine clearance <30 mL/min) and in those with known allergies to one of the drug components. The drug is contraindicated in pregnancy, because there is not sufficient information about its safety in pregnancy.

## Primaquine

Primaquine, as viewed by many clinicians, is suited only for treatment of *P. vivax* infection. However, since its introduction in the early 1950s, primaquine has been found to be active against the early liver stages of both falciparum and vivax malaria.

Primaquine is an 8-aminoquinoline and was developed in the 1940s. In a study conducted in 1954, in healthy volunteers who were inoculated with *P. falciparum* but were given primaquine, at a daily dose of 30 mg, before the sporozoite inoculation, the infection was prevented [24].

Despite the fact that primaquine was highly effective against the early liver stages of the parasites (*P. falciparum* and *P. vivax*), it never gained widespread use as chemoprophylaxis. This was most likely for two principal reasons. The first was reports of severe adverse effects, including methemoglobinemia and hemolytic anemia occurring in glucose-6-phosphate dehydrogenase (G6PD)-deficient patients [25, 26]. The second was the introduction of a new drug, chloroquine, that was relatively safe and highly potent.

In recent years, however, primaquine has made its comeback as prophylaxis (Table 23.2) and not just for the radical cure of vivax malaria (for its use as a radical cure, see Chapter 21).

The first study of primaquine use as prophylaxis was conducted in Kenya among a local population in a hyperendemic area, known to have a 90% incidence of new cases of falciparum malaria and with an estimate of nearly one infective mosquito bite per person per night. The efficacy at the end of a 3-week follow-up period was 85% for primaquine, 84% for doxycycline, 77% for mefloquine, and 54% for chloroquine/proguanil [27].

Another study was conducted in Irian Jaya (northeast Indonesia), an area endemic for both falciparum and vivax malaria, with a population of transmigrants who were most likely nonimmune. After 52 weeks, efficacy against *Plasmodium falciparum* relative to placebo was 94.5% for primaquine and 33.0% for chloroquine, and efficacy against *Plasmodium vivax* was 90.4% for primaquine and 16.5% for chloroquine [28].

**Table 23.2** Summary of studies of primaquine for malaria prophylaxis.

| Site (Ref.) | Population | Number of subjects taking primaquine | Efficacy (%) | | Withdrawals from study |
|---|---|---|---|---|---|
| | | | *P. vivax* | *P. falciparum* | |
| Kenya [27] | Children | 32 | NA | 85 | 0 |
| Indonesia [28] | Transmigrants | 43 | 90 | 95 | 0 |
| Colombia [29] | Soldiers | 122 | 85 | 94 | 3 |
| Indonesia [30] | Transmigrants | 97 | 94 | 88 | 0 |
| Israel [31] | Travelers to Ethiopia | 106 | NA | NA | 1 |
| Israel [32] | Travelers to Ethiopia | 110 | NA | NA | 0 |

NA = not assessed.

A similar study was conducted in 1997 with Colombian soldiers [29]. In the primaquine group, the protective efficacy was 94% against *P. falciparum* and 85% against *P. vivax*. Another study, again with transmigrants to Irian Jaya, showed similar results. Participants received 20 weeks of primaquine or placebo. Primaquine showed an overall protective efficacy of 93%, with > 92% protective efficacy against *P. vivax* and 88% against *P. falciparum* [30].

## Tolerability

The most common adverse effects of primaquine are gastrointestinal effects that are dose-dependent. In studies done during the early 1950s, it was found that doses of up to 30 mg/day were associated with minimal gastrointestinal upset and only doses of 45 mg/day or higher were associated with a significant rate of adverse effects [1, 4].

Recent studies have also shown minimal adverse effects. In a Colombian study [24], two subjects (2%) who were taking the drug withdrew from the study because of gastrointestinal complaints. In an Indonesian study [26], primaquine was taken daily for about 1 year, with no withdrawals from significant adverse events. Complaints were similar in the placebo and drug groups.

In the author's study among travelers [31, 32], primaquine was well tolerated. There was only one withdrawal, which was due to nausea and vomiting (a rate of 1 in approximately 200 cases) (Table 23.2).

Primaquine has gained more recognition in recent years and was listed in Canada and the USA as an option for malaria prophylaxis [7, 33]. Its role was reemphasized in a report from a CDC expert meeting on malaria chemoprophylaxis [34].

## Toxicity

Primaquine can produce marked hemolysis when the drug is administered daily to individuals with G6PD deficiency; therefore, testing for G6PD before treatment is necessary. Methemoglobinemia occurs in normal individuals, but is without clinical significance.

## Dosage and recommendation

Because primaquine is a drug that acts on the liver stage of the malaria parasite, there is no need to continue taking it for 1 month after departure from the malarious area (in contrast to most of the other antimalarial drugs mentioned above, which act on the erythrocyte stage of the malaria parasite). Therefore, the traveler should start taking it 1 day before entering the area and continue taking it daily for 3–7 days after departure. The recommended dose is 30 mg (two tablets) per day for adults. Due to the short half-life of primaquine, it must be taken daily, preferably with food to avoid gastrointestinal upset. The CDC recommends taking it for 7 days after departure [34]. Other authorities recommend it for only 3 days after cessation of exposure [35].

The pediatric dose is 0.5 mg/kg/day.

Pregnant women should not take it, mainly because of the risk of G6PD deficiency in the fetus. Lactating women can use it if the infant has been tested for G6PD.

## Special populations

Special populations that may need particular attention are pregnant women and children, for whom not all drugs mentioned above can be recommended (Table 23.3). For pediatric dose see Appendix A. Breastfeeding mothers should know that the amount of antimalaria drugs excreted in the milk is not sufficient to offer protection to the child; on the other hand, it will not likely be

**Table 23.3** Features of the main drugs used for *P. falciparum* prophylaxis.

| Drug's name | Site of action | *P. falciparum* efficacy | Adverse event profile | Use in pregnancy | Pediatric use | Reported long-term use |
|---|---|---|---|---|---|---|
| Chloroquine | Blood stage | Usually not (only Central America) | Low | Yes | Yes, all ages | 30 months |
| Mefloquine | Blood stage | + (resistance in Southeast Asia) | High mainly neuro-psychiatric | Yes, from second trimester. Limited data on first trimester | Yes, above 5 kg | 30 months |
| Doxycycline | Blood stage | + | Low GI, vaginal discharge | No, teratogenic | Yes, only >8 years old | 12 months |
| Atovaquone–proguanil (Malarone) | Liver stage | + | Low GI | No, not enough data | Yes, above 5 kg | 8 months |
| Primaquine | Liver stage | + | Low G6PD needed | No, G6PD status of fetus is unknown | Yes, all ages | 12 months |

harmful, even with drugs that are not approved for small children [7].

Another special population is long-term travelers or expatriates who remain for several years in endemic areas. Two questions arise: which drug is safe for long-term use, and what is the best approach, taking chemoprophylaxis continuously, or using only personal protection measures and seeking medical care in the case of a febrile illness [36].

Mefloquine and chloroquine (which is of no value in most areas of the world) are the only drugs that have a good long-term follow-up record [6] (Table 23.3). Atovaquone–proguanil, although recommended by the CDC for long-term use, has never been assessed for large numbers of patients, and the longest period of observation was 34 weeks [37].

The safety of doxycycline has been demonstrated in patients taking it for long periods for acne; in addition, there are reports of soldiers taking it for up to 1 year for malaria prophylaxis [38].

The safety of long-term primaquine use has been tested in Indonesia, where it was given for 52 weeks [28].

It is evident that expatriates who live for long periods of time even in Sub-Saharan Africa typically do not take malaria chemoprophylaxis continuously, but rather rely on identifying symptoms and seeking medical care (usually available and known to them) when needed.

Long-term travelers in endemic areas should be encouraged to take chemoprophylaxis continuously throughout their trips, especially in Sub-Saharan Africa.

## Vivax prophylaxis

*P. vivax* (and *P. ovale* as well) has a more complicated life cycle than *P. falciparum* due to the formation of liver hypnozoites, which can result in a clinical relapse several months after the primary infection. Therefore, complete prevention of this infection is much more challenging and can be achieved only if both primary and late infections are prevented.

The life cycle of *P. vivax* has a bimodal incubation time:
**A** The primary attack, which follows exposure to infectious sporozoites, occurs about $14 \pm 3$ days after the mosquito bite (for *P. falciparum* this incubation time is of $12 \pm 3$ days).
**B** The late infection is a relapse following activation and maturation of the dormant liver stage hypnozoite (Figure 23.1).

The chance of and incubation time for relapse largely depend upon the geographic origin of the infection. The tropical *P. vivax* strains tend to have a higher probability of relapse (>30%), a shorter period between primary attack and relapse (17–45 days), and a higher incidence

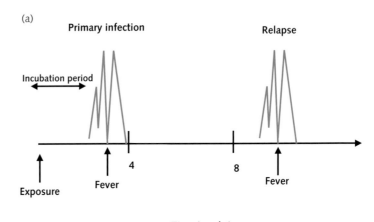

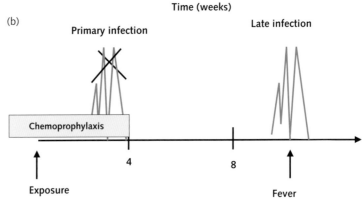

**Figure 23.3** Vivax infection— natural history. (a) In a person who did not take any prophylaxis. The primary attack will occur less than 1 month (usually ~2 weeks) after exposure, and a relapse may follow several months later. (b) In a person who took chemoprophylaxis. The primary attack is suppressed by the prophylaxis and the first clinical attack (actually a relapse) will occur several months after exposure.

of multiple relapses (> 2), whereas the temperate strains (e.g., the Korean strain) tend to have fewer relapses and a longer period before relapse, about 9 months [39]. Thus, clinicians should be alert to the possibility of vivax malaria attacks several months or even a year or more after travel to an endemic area [1].

Blood stage prophylaxis is the most common type of prophylaxis in use. Chloroquine was the first drug in this group to be extensively used. It was introduced in the early 1950s for the prevention of both falciparum and vivax malaria. Chloroquine-resistant *P. falciparum* appeared quite quickly, in the late 1950s; chloroquine-resistant *P. vivax* presented only in the late 1980s. It is a significant problem in eastern Indonesia, where more than half of infections with *P. vivax* appear to be resistant. Resistance has occasionally been reported from other areas in Southeast Asia, South Asia, and South America [40].

Mefloquine and doxycycline are also common blood stage drugs for prophylaxis and are found to be effective

against *P. falciparum* and against *P. vivax* as well. During the 1990s, well-controlled trials of all of these drugs were conducted in northeastern Indonesian New Guinea, where vivax malaria is heavily endemic and notoriously resistant to chloroquine. They demonstrated 100% protective efficacy [41]. Because these drugs have no activity against liver stages and development of hypnozoites, they actually prevent only *primary infection* and not *late relapses*. In fact, in recent years, with the increase of travel to the tropics, it has become more evident that using recommended prophylaxis, which is almost exclusively blood stage prophylaxis, only postpones the first clinical attack of malaria to several months after return (Figure 23.3). This was clearly demonstrated in a study among US and Israeli travelers, of which the majority of all imported vivax cases [60–80%] were late infections (more than 2 months after return) in travelers who took recommended prophylaxis. This clearly illustrates the deficiency of the currently recommended prophylaxis in fully preventing vivax infection [1].

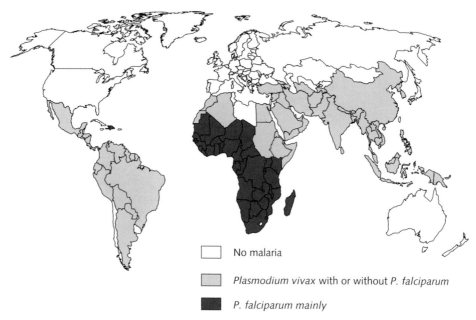

☐ No malaria

☐ *Plasmodium vivax* with or without *P. falciparum*

■ *P. falciparum* mainly

**Figure 23.4** Global distribution of *P. falciparum* and *P. vivax*.

The common recommendation of chloroquine use for vivax prevention is based on the sensitivity of vivax to chloroquine, but it ignores the fact that chloroquine cannot prevent hypnozoite formation and therefore cannot prevent late infection.

Thus, the usefulness of chloroquine or other blood stage prophylaxis in complete prevention of vivax is very limited (it might have some value only in areas where the relapse rate is very low), and it should not be regarded as a vivax prophylaxis.

To overcome this problem, there are two options (Figure 23.4). One is adding terminal prophylaxis, meaning presumptive standard treatment with primaquine upon leaving an endemic area. The term "presumptive antirelapse therapy" (PART) has been proposed to better describe this treatment strategy [34]. It is intended to kill latent liver stages of *P. vivax* and thus prevent relapse. The dose of primaquine for this purpose is under reevaluation. The common practice of dosing with 15 mg daily for 14 days is probably insufficient, especially for the large body weights of typical travelers from industrialized countries. The current preferred recommendation is a single 30-mg dose of primaquine (base) taken daily for 14 days after leaving the endemic area.

There remains with this approach a gray area regarding which travelers would benefit. Should everyone who was in a malaria endemic area where there is *P. vivax* take it,

or should it be reserved for high-risk populations, such as long-term travelers or those who have been to highly endemic vivax area (e.g., the Omo region in Ethiopia)?

The second and more convenient approach is using liver stage prophylaxis. This prophylaxis can prevent both primary attacks and relapses of *P. vivax* and can be effective for *P. falciparum* prevention as well. Primaquine is the only drug known to have this prophylactic activity against vivax malaria. Atovaquone–proguanil, despite being a known liver stage prophylaxis against falciparum malaria (as mentioned above), does not prevent late vivax infection. Studies that looked at the efficacy of the drug for vivax malaria found it to be 82% efficacious in Indonesia and 100% in Colombia [42, 43]. However, both studies evaluated its efficacy only for primary infection (a follow-up 1 month after exposure). Recent evidence from Israeli travelers to Ethiopia (Omo region) has shown the inefficacy of this drug for preventing late infection. Although during the first month post-travel the efficacy of atovaquone–proguanil was 100%, the relapse rate among users was 56% during 1 year of follow-up, similar to that for blood stage drugs [Schwartz, submitted for publication].

On the other hand, primaquine studies of the last 10 years show effective protection against primary attacks in transmigrants in Indonesia and in travelers [44]. In travelers, long-term follow-up also demonstrated its efficacy in preventing relapse [31]. Our

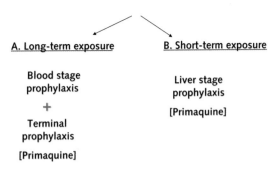

A. Long-term exposure    B. Short-term exposure

Blood stage
prophylaxis              Liver stage
+                        prophylaxis

Terminal                 [Primaquine]
prophylaxis

[Primaquine]

**Figure 23.5** Vivax prophylaxis strategy.

previously mentioned study showed that in the highly endemic area of Ethiopia, although the malaria attack rate among non-primaquine users (mefloquine, doxycycline, and atovaquone–proguanil) was about 50%, in primaquine users it was 1.4% [Schwartz, submitted for publication].

Because the early clinical trials of primaquine demonstrated its activity against falciparum malaria as well [24], it can be used as a single agent for all malaria species.

The dose and contraindications are mentioned above (Table 23.1).

In conclusion, for short-term travelers to vivax-predominant areas (Figure 23.5), a daily dose of primaquine (only if G6PD is normal) seems to be the most convenient option.

For long-term travelers, a weekly dose of chloroquine (depending on the area) or of mefloquine (if there are no contraindications), followed by terminal prophylaxis with primaquine, would be most convenient and efficacious (Figure 23.4).

## The threshold for malaria chemoprophylaxis use

The optimal drug for malaria chemoprophylaxis is not always clear, and just as important is the question of using chemoprophylaxis at all.

Clearly, malaria chemoprophylaxis should not be used in areas where there is no malaria. Therefore, the practitioner who sees travelers before departure should be familiar with the nonendemic areas. It should be remembered that even within endemic countries, there are often areas free of malaria. For example, travelers who trek in Nepal are not at risk because of the high altitude. The same holds true for travelers to high-altitude areas even within Sub-Saharan Africa, such as Addis Ababa (Ethiopia), Asmara ( Eritrea), Nairobi (Kenya), and Harare (Zimbabwe).

In the endemic areas, the risk for travelers varies significantly. The highest risk for falciparum malaria is in West Africa, estimated to be 2.4% per month of stay, whereas in East Africa it is 1.5% per month of stay. Risk is also high in travelers to the Pacific islands (Solomons and Papua New Guinea), but is 10–20 times less in travelers to Asia, and 30–40 times less in travelers to Latin America [45].

Thus, the more complicated issue is the decision about malaria chemoprophylaxis in those who travel to low-risk areas, and what should be the threshold (if any) for using chemoprophylaxis. There is no consensus yet about this issue. According to the policy of the US CDC, the world is "all or none" in regard to chemoprophylaxis; one should either take it or not [7]. The WHO introduced another category for certain areas of the world where the recommended policy is personal protection only (named type 1 prophylaxis) [15]. The problem with the WHO recommendation is that in areas with type 1 recommendations there is almost zero risk. In fact, these are areas where even the CDC does not recommend any chemoprophylaxis (e.g., Morocco and Algeria).

The real challenge in travel medicine is making recommendations for low-risk malaria areas such as Central and South America and parts of East Asia. In these regions, the risk of malaria definitely exists and there are cases of imported malaria from those areas. However, the overall risk for travelers is low. Part of the calculation should be based on an equation, where one side reflects the level of severe and fatal outcomes from the prophylactic agents and the other side represents the risk of severe and fatal outcomes from falciparum malaria in a particular area. The problem is that good and accurate data for both sides of the equation are lacking. A recent study from Europe suggests that the risk of adverse events from chemoprophylaxis is likely to be significantly higher than the risk of acquiring malaria in the most popular tourist destinations in Central and South America. In these areas, the malaria attack rate is low and mostly due to *P. vivax* rather than *P. falciparum* infection [3]. The benefit of chemoprophylaxis in preventing *P. vivax* is very limited, as discussed above.

Two of the highest-risk countries, as reported by the Pan American Health Organization (PAHO), French Guiana and Surinam, are places where visitors are also at high risk of malaria, and chemoprophylaxis would be appropriate for travel to the risk areas within these countries, but not to other Latin America countries [3].

A similar conclusion came from an analysis of malaria imported into eight European countries from the Indian subcontinent (ISC) (India, Pakistan, Bangladesh, and

Sri Lanka) [46]. The proportion of cases from the ISC ranged from 1.4% to 4.6% of total imported cases, and again *P. falciparum* cases accounted for only 13% of all cases from the region. Thus, the calculated risk of malaria in UK residents visiting the region was < 1 case per 1000 years of exposure [46].

An Israeli study that looked at the importation of malaria cases from East Asia (including India) during a 6-year period (2000–2005) found an overall estimated malaria attack rate of 4.7 per 100,000 travelers, whereas the attack rate caused by *P. falciparum* was 1.59 cases per 100,000 travelers. The breakdown of the two most popular destinations showed the attack rate for *P. falciparum* to be 3.4/100,000 travelers to India and 0.39/100,000 in Thailand. In Thailand, the calculated attack rate was 1 per 9000 years of travel within the country. A parallel survey among Israeli travelers to East Asia found that only about 15% of travelers took malaria prophylaxis. Thus, our data show that ~60,000 travelers have to take prophylaxis to prevent 1 case of *P. falciparum* malaria [47].

We, therefore, advocate revising the current CDC and WHO general recommendations on malaria prophylaxis for tourists to Asia, identifying the hot spots of high risk for malaria in this region, and recommending chemoprophylaxis only for these areas.

Although patterns of travel can differ according to countries of origin, the accumulated Israeli data and data from the European countries support this finding of reduced risk in many popular tourist destinations. In fact, the TropNet group recommends that the nonselective prescribing of chemoprophylaxis for visitors to the India subcontinent should be dropped [46].

An alternate strategy adopted by a number of European countries, such as Switzerland [48], is to provide travelers with emergency standby treatment if malaria symptoms occur during travel. This ensures treatment of life-threatening attacks of falciparum malaria and avoids adverse events associated with excessive chemoprophylaxis. It has the disadvantage of cost, because all travelers would have to purchase therapy.

There is no consensus about the use of standby therapy. However, the strategy of bite prevention remains important, as these measures are effective and safe and have the added benefit of reducing other vector-borne diseases. In addition, travelers have to be educated to seek medical advice in the case of a febrile illness.

Although there is not yet a consensus among world and national health authorities concerning the correct use of chemoprophylaxis, it seems that travelers have created

their own policy and have voted against indiscriminate use of chemoprophylaxis.

# References

1 Schwartz E, Parise M, Kozarsky P, Cetron M. Delayed onset of malaria–implications for chemoprophylaxis in travelers. *N Engl J Med* 2003;349(16):1510–16.

2 Soto J, Medina F, Dember N, Berman J. Efficacy of permethrin-impregnated uniforms in the prevention of malaria and leishmaniasis in Colombian soldiers. *Clin Infect Dis* 1995;21(3):599–602.

3 Behrens RH, Carroll B, Beran J, et al.; TropNetEurop. The low and declining risk of malaria in travellers to Latin America: is there still an indication for chemoprophylaxis? *Malar J* 2007;6:114.

4 Peto TE, Gilks CF. Strategies for the prevention of malaria in travellers: comparison of drug regimens by means of risk–benefit analysis. *Lancet* 1986;1:1256–61.

5 Chen LH, Wilson ME, Schlagenhauf P. Controversies and misconceptions in malaria chemoprophylaxis for travelers. *JAMA* 23;297(20):2251–63.

6 Lobel HO, Miani M, Eng T, Bernard KW, Hightower AW, Campbell CC. Long-term malaria prophylaxis with weekly mefloquine. *Lancet* 1993;341:848–51.

7 CDC. *CDC Health Information for International Travel, 2008.* Atlanta: CDC; 2007.

8 Schlagenhauf P. Mefloquine. In: Schlagenhauf P, editor. *Travelers' Malaria.* 2nd ed. Hamilton (Ont): BC Decker; 2008. p. 134–47.

9 Peragallo MS, Sabatinelli G, Sarnicola G. Compliance and tolerability of mefloquine and chloroquine plus proguanil for long-term malaria chemoprophylaxis in groups at particular risk (the military). *Trans R Soc Trop Med Hyg* 1999;93(1): 73–7.

10 Overbosch D, Schilthuis H, Bienzle U, et al. Atovaquone–proguanil versus mefloquine for malaria prophylaxis in nonimmune travelers: results from a randomized, double-blind study. *Clin Infect Dis* 2001;33:1015–21.

11 Schlagenhauf P, Tschopp A, Johnson R, et al. Tolerability of malaria chemoprophylaxis in non-immune travellers to Sub-Saharan Africa: multicentre, randomised, double blind, four arm study. *BMJ* 2003;327:1078–81.

12 Croft AM, World MJ. Neuropsychiatric reactions with mefloquine chemoprophylaxis. *Lancet* 1996 Feb 3;347(8997):326.

13 Steffen R, Fuchs E, Schildknecht J, et al. Mefloquine compared with other malaria chemoprophylactic regimens in tourists visiting East Africa. *Lancet* 1993;341:1299–1303.

14 Schwartz E, Potasman I, Rotenberg M, Almog S, Sadetzki S. Serious adverse events of mefloquine in relation to blood level and gender. *Am J Trop Med Hyg* 2001;65:189–92.

15 World Health Organization. *International Travel and Health: 2007.* Geneva: World Health Organization; 2007.

16 Ohrt C, Richie TL, Widjaja H, et al. Mefloquine compared with doxycycline for the prophylaxis of malaria in Indonesian soldiers: a randomized, double-blind, placebo-controlled trial. *Ann Intern Med* 1997;126:963–72.

17 Sánchez JL, DeFraites RF, Sharp TW, Hanson RK. Mefloquine or doxycycline prophylaxis in US troops in Somalia. *Lancet* 1993;341:1021–2.

18 Smith K, Leyden JJ. Safety of doxycycline and minocycline: a systematic review. *Clin Ther* 2005;27(9):1329–42.

19 Ling J, Baird JK, Fryauff DJ, et al. Randomized, placebo-controlled trial of atovaquone/proguanil for the prevention of *Plasmodium falciparum* or *Plasmodium vivax* malaria among migrants to Papua, Indonesia. *Clin Infect Dis* 2002;35:825–33.

20 Shapiro TA, Ranasinha CD, Kumar N, Barditch-Crovo P. Prophylactic activity of atovaquone against *Plasmodium falciparum* in humans. *Am J Trop Med Hyg* 1999;60:831–6.

21 Editorial. More about Paludrine. *Br Med J* 1946;1: 919–20.

22 Berman JD, Nielsen R, Chulay JD, et al. Causal prophylactic efficacy of atovaquone–proguanil (Malarone) in a human challenge model. *Trans R Soc Trop Med Hyg* 2001;95:429–32.

23 Høgh B, Clarke PD, Camus D, et al.; Malarone International Study Team. Atovaquone–proguanil versus chloroquine-proguanil for malaria prophylaxis in non-immune travellers: a randomised, double-blind study. Malarone International Study Team. *Lancet* 2000;356:1888–94.

24 Arnold J, Alving AS, Hockwald RS, et al. The antimalarial action of primaquine against the blood and tissue stages of falciparum malaria. *J Lab Clin Med* 1955;46:391–7.

25 Cohen RJ, Sachs JR, Wicker DJ, Conrad ME. Methemoglobinemia provoked by malarial chemoprophylaxis in Vietnam. *N Engl J Med* 1968;279:1127–31.

26 Georg JN, Sears DA, McCurdy PR, et al. Primaquine sensitivity in caucasians: hemolytic reactions induced by primaquine in G-6-PD deficient subjects. *J Lab Clin Med* 1967;70:80–93.

27 Weiss WR, Oloo AJ, Johnson A, et al. Daily primaquine is effective for prophylaxis against falciparum malaria in Kenya: comparison with mefloquine, doxycycline, and chloroquine plus proguanil. *J Infect Dis* 1995;171:1569–75.

28 Fryauff DJ, Baird JK, Basri H, et al. Randomised placebo-controlled trial of primaquine for prophylaxis of falciparum and vivax malaria. *Lancet* 1995;346:1190–93.

29 Soto J, Toledo J, Rodriguez M, et al. Primaquine prophylaxis against malaria in nonimmune Colombian soldiers: efficacy and toxicity. *Ann Intern Med* 1998;129:241–4.

30 Baird JK, Lacy MD, Basri H, et al. Randomized, parallel placebo-controlled trial of primaquine for malaria prophylaxis in Papua, Indonesia. *Clin Infect Dis* 2001;33:1990–97.

31 Schwartz E, Regev-Yochay G. Primaquine as prophylaxis for malaria for nonimmune travelers: A comparison with mefloquine and doxycycline. *Clin Infect Dis* 1999;29(6): 1502–6.

32 Schwartz E. New approach to malaria prophylaxis. Presented at the 48th Annual Meeting of the American Society of Tropical Medicine and Hygiene. Washington DC; Nov 1999.

33 Committee to Advise on Tropical Medicine and Travel (CATMAT). 2004 Canadian recommendations for the prevention and treatment of malaria among international travellers. *Can Commun Dis Rep* 2004;30(Suppl 1):1–62.

34 Hill DR, Baird JK, Parise ME, Lewis LS, Ryan ET, Magill AJ. Primaquine: report from CDC expert meeting on malaria chemoprophylaxis. *Am J Trop Med Hyg* 2006;75:402–15.

35 Baird JK, Fryauff DJ, Hoffman SL. Primaquine for prevention of malaria in travelers. *Clin Infect Dis* 2003;37:1659–67.

36 Chen LH, Wilson ME, Schlagenhauf P. Prevention of malaria in long-term travelers. *JAMA* 2006;296:2234–44.

37 Overbosch D. Post-marketing surveillance: adverse events during long-term use of atovaquone/proguanil for travelers to malaria-endemic countries. *J Travel Med* 2003;10 Suppl 1:S16–20; discussion S21–3.

38 Shanks GD, Roessler P, Edstein MD, Rieckmann KH. Doxycycline for malaria prophylaxis in Australian soldiers deployed to United Nations missions in Somalia and Cambodia. *Mil Med* 1995;160:443–5.

39 Bray RS, Garnham PC. The life-cycle of primate malaria parasites. *Br Med Bull* 1982;38(2):117–22.

40 Baird JK. Chloroquine resistance in *Plasmodium vivax. Antimicrob Agents Chemother* 2004;48:4075–83.

41 Baird JK, Schwartz E, Hoffman SL. Prevention and treatment of vivax malaria. *Curr Infect Dis Rep* 2007;9:39–46.

42 Ling J, Baird JK, Fryauff DJ, et al. Randomized, placebo-controlled trial of atovaquone/proguanil for the prevention of *Plasmodium falciparum* or *Plasmodium vivax* malaria among migrants to Papua, Indonesia. *Clin Infect Dis* 2002;35:825–33.

43 Soto J, Toledo J, Luzz M, Gutierrez P, Berman J, Duparc S. Randomized, double-blind, placebo-controlled study of malarone for malaria prophylaxis in non-immune colombian soldiers. *Am J Trop Med Hyg* 2006;75:430–33.

44 Baird JK, Hoffman SL. Primaquine therapy for malaria. *Clin Infect Dis* 2004;39(9):1336–45.

45 Steffen R. Strategies of malaria prevention in nonimmune visitors to endemic countries. In: Schlagenhauf P, editor. *Travelers' Malaria.* 2nd ed. Hamilton (Ont.): BC Decker; 2008. p. 107–14.

46 Behrens RH, Bisoffi Z, Bjorkman A, et al. Malaria prophylaxis policy for travellers from Europe to the Indian sub continent. *Malar J* 2006;5:1–7.

47 Stienlauf S, Goldman D, Meltzer E, Anis E, Schwartz E. Malaria incidence in Israeli travelers to Asia: an implication for malaria chemoprophylaxis ? Presented at the Joint International Tropical Medicine Meeting and the 6th Asia–Pacific Travel Health Conference. Bangkok, Thailand; Nov 2006.

48 Hatz CF, Beck B, Blum J,et al. Supplementum 1: Malariaschutz fur Kurzzeitaufenthalter. Available from URL: http://www.bag.admin.ch/themen/medizin/00682/00684/02535/index.html?lang=de.

# 24 Schistosomiasis

## Eli Schwartz

Chaim Sheba Medical Center, Tel Hashomer, Israel and Sackler School of Medicine, Tel Aviv University, Tel Aviv, Israel

## Introduction

Schistosomiasis, also named bilharziasis (after the German physician Theodore Bilharz who worked in Egypt during the nineteenth century and was the first to discover the life cycle of the parasite), is one of the most prevalent infectious diseases in the world. It is endemic in more than 76 countries, mainly in the less developed countries, and is estimated to place about 20% of the endemic population at risk. Thus, the number of people affected is estimated to be ∼200 million [1].

The schistosomes are a group of trematodes (flukes), some of which are pathogenic to humans. The principal parasites that affect humans are *Schistosoma haematobium, S. mansoni*, and *S. japonicum;* less prevalent are *S. intercalatum* in Africa and *S. mekongi* in the Far East. Figure 24.1 presents the global distribution of schistosome species. Schistosomiasis is most prevalent in Africa, where *S. haematobium* and *S. mansoni* dominate.

In the recent decades, schistosomiasis has been gaining attention in developed countries because increasing numbers of returning travelers have been presenting at medical facilities with a variety of symptoms due to schistosomiasis. In most cases, the disease was acquired in Sub-Saharan Africa. Back in the developed world, it becomes a medical challenge to Western doctors less familiar with the disease.

Schistosomiasis is an excellent example of the differences between morbidity in local populations and morbidity in travelers. The differences exist in clinical manifestations, in diagnosis, and in treatment (Table 24.1), increasing the challenge of diagnosis and management of returning travelers.

*Tropical Diseases in Travelers*, 1st edition. Edited by E. Schwartz.
© 2009 by Blackwell Publishing, ISBN: 978-1-4051-8441-0.

## Epidemiology

Schistosomiasis ranks second only to malaria among the parasitic diseases in the number of people infected and of those at risk. According to the World Heath Organization (WHO), approximately 200 million people are infected with *Schistosoma* species and another 790 million people are at risk for infection. This estimate reflects an increase of about 10% over the last comprehensive estimates made a decade before [1]. Schistosomiasis is endemic in at least 76 countries in Africa, the Middle East, Asia, South America, and the Caribbean.

Approximately 85% of those infected are believed to live in Sub-Saharan Africa, with the highest prevalence and infection intensity usually found in school-age children, adolescents, and young adults [1].

## Epidemiology in travelers

Three large case series published recently have shown that among travelers, schistosomiasis is acquired almost exclusively in Africa. These are the data of the GeoSentinel group, the TropNetEurope surveillance network, and an Israeli nationwide study. In all of these studies, Africa was the source for the infection in about 90% of all cases [2–4]. The absence of cases from other regions of high endemicity may be due to the fact that schistosomiasis is often a focal disease; perhaps the specific locations frequented by travelers in South America and the Far East are often not infected. Laos, which opened up for international travelers during the 1990s, has become popular among travelers, and an important part of tourist activity in the country is water recreational activities on the Mekong River and its tributes. We have recently seen an increasing number of travelers with *S. mekongi* infection [unpublished data].

The incidence of schistosomiasis among travelers can only be guessed at from circumstantial evidence. The

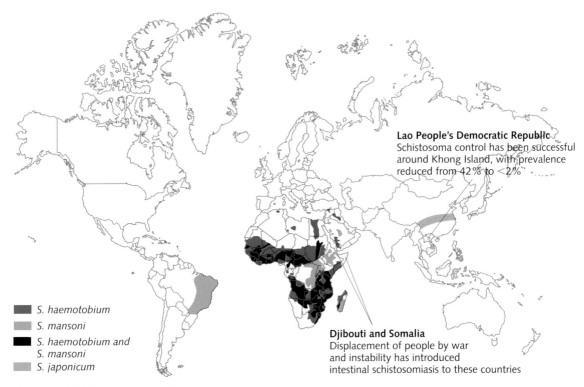

**Lao People's Democratic Republic**
Schistosoma control has been successful around Khong Island, with prevalence reduced from 42% to <2%

**Djibouti and Somalia**
Displacement of people by war and instability has introduced intestinal schistosomiasis to these countries

- ■ *S. haemotobium*
- ■ *S. mansoni*
- ■ *S. haemotobium and S. mansoni*
- ■ *S. japonicum*

**Figure 24.1** Global distribution of schistosomiasis.

**Table 24.1** Comparison of schistosomiasis in travelers and endemic populations.

|  | Travelers | Populations of endemic areas |
|---|---|---|
| Main clinical presentation | Acute schistosomiasis | Chronic schistosomiasis |
| Time of onset of symptoms (after exposure) | Weeks (4–8) | Years |
| Pathogenesis | Immune-complex disease | Granuloma formation |
| Principal clinical manifestations | Cough, fever, rash eosinophilia | Genitourinary and or hepatic–intestinal manifestations |
| Species specific cause | All species | *S. haematobium*—genitourinary All other species—hepatic–intestinal |
| Diagnosis | Mainly through serology Ova occasionally found in stool/urine | Presence of ova in stool/urine or in affected tissue Serology is not helpful |
| Treatment: Steroid | Effective | Not effective |
| Praziquantel | Effective | Effective |
| Artemether | May play a role | Probably not effective |
| Outcome | Reversible | May cause irreversible fibrotic changes, secondary malignancy |

GeoSentinel database shows that schistosomiasis is one of the leading causes of morbidity among travelers, accounting for 4% of cases for Sub-Saharan Africa [5]. Other data point to schistosomiasis as a significant cause of morbidity among travelers to Africa who had contact with fresh water bodies. A study at Lake Malawi, one of the major infected fresh water lakes, showed that there was a correlation between the rate of infection and the number of days of exposure, with an estimate of up to 90% infection of travelers who stayed longer than 10 days [6].

Infection with *Schistosoma* spp. is often focal and or seasonal, and therefore an exposure in the same place will not necessarily result in infection. However, when exposure occurs in infected water, the result may be a very high infection rate.

For example, it is reported that several rafting tours in African rivers resulted in 55%–100% of travelers becoming infected [7].

A recent report of safari travelers who were exposed in a natural pond at a frequently visited luxury hotel in Tanzania showed an 80% infection rate [8]. This report highlights two aspects of *Schistosoma* infection. First, all fresh water in endemic areas (especially in Africa) is a potential source for infection, even if it used to be considered safe. Second, there was a high attack rate among people who were exposed to the same body of water. This attack rate, which may approach 100%, is rarely seen in other infectious diseases.

## *Schistosoma* life cycle

The life cycle of *Schistosoma* involves two hosts: humans and snails (Figure 24.2). An infected human sheds the schistosome eggs into fresh water via urine or feces. Snails,

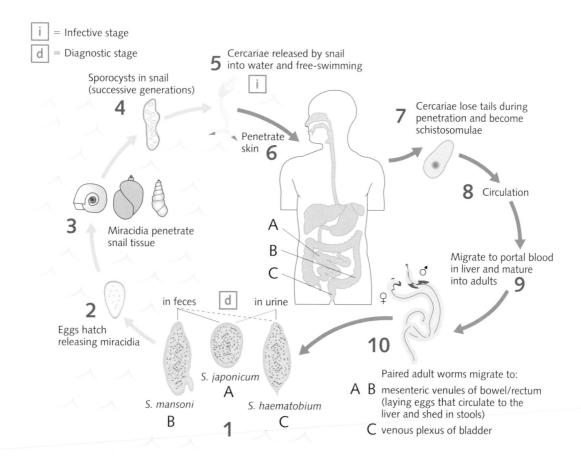

**Figure 24.2** *Schistosoma* life cycle.

the intermediate hosts, ingest the eggs that subsequently hatch and go through a number of cycles of multiplication. They are then excreted into the water as cercariae, the infective form. Cercariae have the ability to penetrate human skin or, if ingested, to penetrate the gut. Travelers mostly are infected while swimming in contaminated water.

In the process of invading human skin, the cercariae lose their tails and change into the juvenile form, called schistosomules. The schistosomules migrate first to the lungs and, within 1 week, reach the liver. After about 6 weeks, they mature into adult flukes that mate and descend via the venules to their final habitat: the vesicle beds in *S. haematobium* infection and the mesenteric beds in *S. mansoni* and *S. japonicum* infection.

The life span of the adult fluke is a matter of controversy, but it is known to be several years, even up to 30 years.

Most of the eggs that an adult fluke lays are excreted by the host either via urine in *S. haematobium* or via feces in the other species. From the public health point of view, these eggs are important because they are the cause of the spread of the disease. A minority of the eggs will remain stuck in the host tissue, causing granuloma formation.

These granulomas are what cause the clinical symptoms of schistosomiasis.

## Clinical manifestations

The clinical manifestations can be divided into three major stages, which correspond to the three important phases in the human host (Figure 24.3).

The first phase, *swimmer's itch* or *cercarial dermatitis*, which occurs within 24 hours after skin penetration by the cercariae, is manifested as a transient (hours) itchy eruption, appearing soon after exposure.

The second phase, *acute schistosomiasis* (AcS) or *Katayama syndrome*, occurs during schistosomule tissue migration and maturation, within 2–8 weeks after exposure. This phase is associated with transient (days or weeks) hypersensitivity manifestations.

The last phase, *chronic schistosomiasis*, appears months to years after infection and is associated with target organ damage (genitourinary, gastrointestinal, or ectopic migration to other organs) that results from granuloma formation around schistosome eggs retained in the tissues.

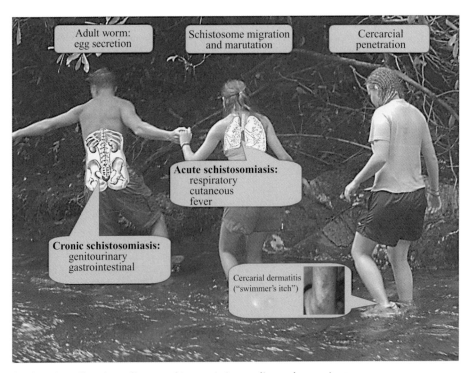

**Figure 24.3** The clinical manifestations of human schistosomiasis according to the parasite stage.

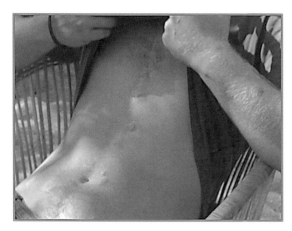

**Figure 24.4** Swimmer's itch. [Courtesy of Dr. G. Artom.]

## Swimmer's itch (cercarial dermatitis)

Invasion of the skin by the cercariae gives rise to a pruritic papular rash that appears a few hours after exposure and usually lasts less than 48 hours (Figure 24.4). This symptom can also occur after infestation with a nonhuman schistosome (e.g., avian schistosomes, which are seen around freshwater lakes in the northern United States), and in these cases because the cercaria is trapped in the skin and does not have the ability to penetrate into the body, the skin symptoms appear more frequently and are more intense.

In fact, in travelers infected with schistosomiasis, only a minority can recall a history suggestive of swimmer's itch. The occurrence of cercarial dermatitis ranges between 7% and 36% [4, 9]. However, in many cases, data were collected a long time after the exposure, and travelers may have forgotten such transient phenomena. The absence of a history of swimmer's itch can by no means be used to exclude a diagnosis of schistosomiasis.

## Acute schistosomiasis (Katayama syndrome)

Acute schistosomiasis is the phase most commonly seen in travelers, and the one that underscores the major difference from local populations. In a large Israeli cohort, it was noted in 66% of infected travelers. In outbreak investigations where there is more precise investigation and follow-up, the rate of symptomatic infection may reach more than 80% [8].

AcS is considered a severe immunological reaction to the parasite. One theory postulates that as the flukes begin to lay eggs, soluble antigens leak out from the eggs into the bloodstream. At this stage antibody production lags behind antigen release, and excess antigen prevails. This imbalance causes the immune complex disease, and because the antigen is soluble, the effect is systemic. Recovery takes place after antigen–antibody balance is achieved [10]. However, data in travelers show clearly that this syndrome may occur well before oviposition takes place [11, 12]. Thus, the symptoms are probably the result of an immunological reaction to a variety of circulating antigens at different stages in the life cycle of the parasite. The clinical symptoms are a form of serum sickness or antigen–antibody complex disease [13].

Local populations that are constantly exposed to the pathogen do not have this clinical presentation (although they might have had it during their childhood). Travelers are markedly different from local people and immigrants in this respect.

It is still occasionally suggested in textbooks that AcS is a syndrome typically encountered in heavy infestations with *S. japonicum* or *mansoni*, but rarely if ever caused by *S. haematobium* [14]. Findings among travelers suggest that this is not the case, and rather that this syndrome appears with all species. It is an immune phenomenon, and not species-specific, and can develop after infection with each of the schistosomes that infect humans. The reason that some species have rarely been reported in the literature as causing AcS (e.g., *S. mekongi* and *S. intercalatum*) may merely reflect the lack of traveler exposure.

In addition, this phenomenon seems to be idiosyncratic and not related to the dose of inoculum of the parasites. Therefore, the length of exposure in water is not a factor determining the clinical presentation of AcS [8].

### Clinical symptoms

The acute symptom complex usually appears 2–8 weeks after exposure. The common symptoms are fever, cough, malaise, and headache, accompanied by hepatosplenomegaly and marked eosinophilia. Figures 24.5 and 24.6 show the frequency of symptoms, the mean time of appearance after exposure, and the mean duration based on a prospective evaluation of group of travelers [8]. Historically this complex was first described in 1847 in the Katayama district near Hiroshima, Japan by Fujii [15], and is often referred to as Katayama fever. Data in travelers show that fever occurs in about 70% of AcS cases [4, 8], and, therefore, the term "acute schistosomiasis" or "Katayama syndrome" is more accurate than "Katayama fever".

*Fever* in AcS is usually high, with alternating spikes of fever and chills, and can mimic malaria. Fever might be the first symptom of the disease and can be accompanied

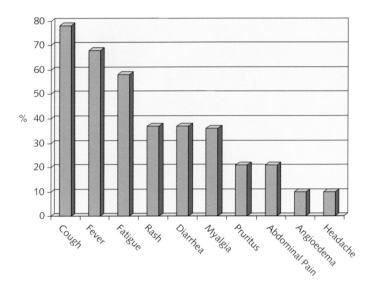

**Figure 24.5** Symptom distribution among patients.

by urticarial rash and angioedema, which may offer a clue that it is not malaria.

The median time for the febrile episode is about 11 days [8], although it may relapse after several days. In most cases, eosinophilia will accompany the fever, which strongly suggests a diagnosis of schistosomiasis (with the correct epidemiological background). Eosinophilia can help in ruling out malaria, a disease in which eosinophils almost completely disappear from the peripheral blood.

*Pulmonary symptoms* during acute schistosomiasis were neglected phenomena in previous descriptions of the disease, but seem to be one of the prominent features. These symptoms are frequently reported among ill travelers. For example, in a detailed follow-up of patients with AcS, 78% suffered from respiratory symptoms [8]. They have also been found to be one of the prolonged symptoms of the disease, with a median of 22 days, and in some patients may last for several months [4, 8]. Patients with pulmonary schistosomiasis report shortness of breath, wheezing, and dry cough, mainly while recumbent. Reports show that in some cases, the pulmonary symptoms coincide with febrile illness [16]. However, most patients presented with these symptoms several weeks after the fever had subsided. Many patients can recall having had a febrile disease before the onset of pulmonary symptoms, but the pulmonary symptoms continued for weeks

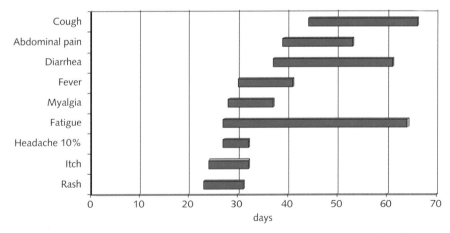

**Figure 24.6** Time line of symptoms, appearance after exposure, and mean duration of symptoms. (Adapted from Leshem E, Maor Y, Meltzer E, Assous M, Schwartz E. Acute Schistosomiasis outbreak: clinical features and economic impact. *Clin Inf Dis* 2008;1499–1506, with permission from the University of Chicago Press.)

after the fever subsided [11, 17]. The physical examination is usually unremarkable, although in some patients prolonged expiration may be noted. The fact that respiratory symptoms tend to follow a protracted course may lead to a misdiagnosis of allergy and/or asthma, unless a thorough history is taken that reveals recent exposure to fresh water in endemic areas.

Pulmonary involvement can be divided into three forms [18]:

1 Symptomatic cases with radiological findings (either chest X ray or CT scan). The radiological findings may be evident at presentation, or, not uncommonly, may appear after antischistosomal treatment. In either case, cough may persist for several weeks, despite treatment.

2 Symptomatic cases without radiological findings. In some patients, the clinical course is similar to the one state above, but radiological findings (either chest X ray or CT scan) are absent. This may be due either to the small dimensions of the findings, making them invisible by conventional methods, or to their transient nature.

3 Asymptomatic cases with radiological findings. Cases in which there are pulmonary findings without a current history of pulmonary symptoms are rare. The incidence of these cases is unknown, since radiology is usually not performed for asymptomatic patients. However, we were able to identify such cases, since we performed chest X rays as part of the evaluation of patients who were diagnosed with a suspicion of early schistosomiasis.

Pulmonary involvement begins about one month after exposure. The pulmonary infiltrates therefore cannot be attributed to schistosomule migration through the lungs, which occurs typically 5–7 days after penetration, nor can they be attributed to granuloma formation around schistosomal eggs, because this process starts before oviposition is expected to take place. It is most likely that the pulmonary pathology is immunologically mediated and similar to that seen in other forms of eosinophilic pneumonias, where the inciting agent exists elsewhere in the body (e.g., the intestines), but the eosinophils are sequestered in the pulmonary capillaries. Indeed, in cases in which transbronchial biopsy was done, eosinophilic infiltration was found without evidence for larva or eggs [10, 11]. Additional support for the immunological theory is the observation that some patients developed radiological findings only after antischistosomal treatment was initiated. Treatment is a known factor in antigenic stimulation [19] and may be accompanied by transient clinical deterioration [20].

The most common *dermatological finding* at this stage of the disease is urticarial rash (Figure 24.7), which some-

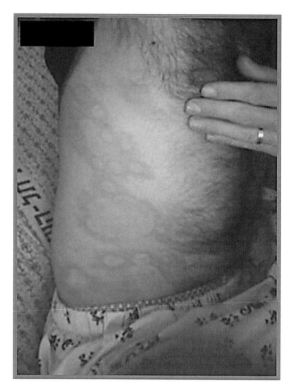

**Figure 24.7** Urticarial rash in a patient with acute schistosomiasis.

times is associated with angioedema. This is usually the first symptom and sign that appears in AcS (Figure 24.6). The urticarial rash appears in about 30–50% of patients [8, 21] and may last for about eight days. It is a diffuse migratory rash, which often prompts patients to seek immediate medical care, at which time the patient may be diagnosed as having "allergic reactions" and treated with antihistamines or glucocorticoids, without further evaluation.

Significant fatigue, which is the longest-lasting symptom (an average of 6 weeks) [8], may accompany the syndrome of AcS, and may lead to a significant loss of work, school, and leisure time [8].

Other symptoms may include headaches, athralgias, and often severe neck pain.

Gastrointestinal complaints, such as abdominal pain and diarrhea, may occur in about one-third of the cases.

### Physical findings

The physical examination, with the exception of dermatological findings, is usually unremarkable. Occasionally mild hepatosplenomegaly occurs.

## Laboratory findings

Laboratory findings in AcS are significant for eosinophilia in most patients (∼70%). The eosinophil count in the majority of cases is very high, with an average of 3000/mm³. The eosinophil counts gradually normalize following praziquantel treatment; however, some patients may have a very slow response, showing persistently high eosinophil counts despite antischistosoma treatment and with no evidence for other helminthic infections.

Other abnormalities may include mildly abnormal liver function tests (transaminase up to twice normal range) and in about 10% of cases, thrombocytopenia [8].

## Imaging

Abnormal imaging during the acute stage of the disease may be found in the chest. The most common radiographic chest abnormalities observed are small, nodular lesions with ill-defined borders (Figure 24.8a). Less common are reticulonodular patterns (Fig. 24.8b). Chest CT reveals more nodular lesions than are apparent on chest X rays, with ill-defined nodules (Figure 24.9). In rare cases, a bilateral, diffuse ground glass pattern has been demonstrated. Neither pleural effusion nor lymphadenopathy is evident. In about 25% of our cases, the radiographic abnormalities appeared only after praziquantel therapy [17, 18].

## Diagnosis

In general, the diagnosis of early schistosomiasis in travelers still poses a challenge, and has to be based initially on clinical judgment. The traditional test, examining stool and urine for parasite eggs, has low sensitivity in travelers. Further, it must be emphasized that nonimmune patients may be acutely ill with manifestations of acute schistosomiasis well before oviposition by the adult flukes has begun, and stool or urine exams performed at this time will be unrevealing.

Thus, serologic tests are the methods of choice. However, they are not routinely used, and in some places are performed only in research laboratories. In addition, the sensitivity and specificity of the tests vary with the antigen used. The laboratory at the Centers for Disease Control and Prevention (CDC, Atlanta, USA) uses FAST-ELISA as the initial step in diagnosis. Confirmation and speciation of positive ELISA results is performed with an enzyme-linked immunoelectrotransfer blot (EITB) that provides almost 100% specificity in confirming the presence of *Schistosoma* species [6]. This method has proved to be highly sensitive and specific, and usually becomes positive relatively early, 4–6 weeks after exposure. Other

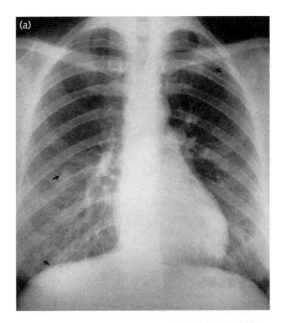

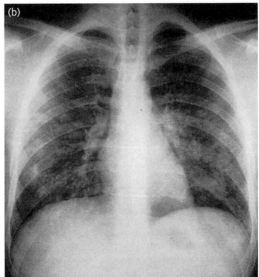

**Figure 24.8** Chest X ray of acute schistosomiasis. (a) A chest radiograph that reveals several small round lesions in both lungs (arrows). (b) A chest X ray that reveals diffused, increased lung markings, and prominent hilum with ill-defined nodules.

methods may be less sensitive and specific and may become positive at a later time. In any case, a negative initial serology result, when it is obtained within 3 months after exposure, should be repeated after this 3 month period.

There are two major limitations of the serology test. One is that it stays positive for many years after infection

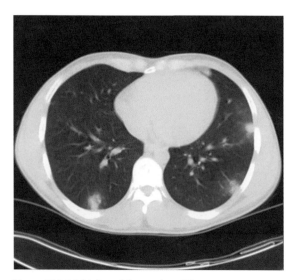

**Figure 24.9** Multiple nodules on chest CT.

(even if efficacious treatment was given); thus, it is of no value for determining re-exposure, or for evaluating the success or failure of treatment. Therefore, a serology test is not the tool for diagnosis of current schistosome infection among local populations or among immigrants (but rather detection of ova in stool or urine). The other is that symptoms of AcS may appear before serology becomes positive. Therefore, for the clinician, the most important factor is obtaining a good travel history of the patient, especially regarding exposure to fresh water in endemic areas. The high eosinophilic counts that occur during the acute stage of the disease may be a very useful indication for diagnosis.

Methods of antigen detection in blood are strongly needed for diagnosis and evaluation of the disease in travelers. These should be based on circulating cercarial antigen (and not on adult worm antigen). An animal model validating this approach was reported nearly 20 years ago, but was not developed further [22].

## Treatment

Acute schistosomiasis is immunological by nature, and thus corticosteroids may be an effective therapy. Patients with severe manifestations either at presentation or following praziquantel treatment should get short courses of steroids. The dose and the length of steroid treatment have never been assessed systematically. We have found that 0.5 mg/kg of prednisone is usually sufficient. It is given for 1 week and then tailored to the patient's condi-

tion. In many cases, one course will be enough. Some will relapse upon cessation of the drug and will need a longer course.

The role of praziquantel treatment during the acute stage is uncertain. Although this is the drug of choice for treating all schistosome species (see *Treatment*, below), it is known to be effective only against the adult fluke [23]. Thus, its role in acute schistosomiasis has not been proven because at that stage of the disease, the fluke may not have fully matured. In some cases, praziquantel treatment may even aggravate the symptoms of AcS (urticarial rash, increased cough, etc.). If praziquantel is given during the acute stage, it should be repeated several weeks later (at least 3 months from the exposure), when the fluke has matured enough to be killed by the drug. Without repeated treatment in these cases, patients may present later on with chronic schistosomiasis [4, 21].

Based on the pathophysiology of the disease at this stage, the treatment of early, acute schistosomiasis at presentation can be with corticosteroids alone, followed by praziquantel later on, 3 months from last exposure, to ensure eradication of the adult flukes. Controlled studies comparing these two options are very difficult to perform because of the small numbers of patients seen at each clinic, and because we do not have a good tool to assess eradication of the flukes.

The new promising antischistosomal drugs are the artemisinin derivates. Artemether, a Chinese drug that originally was developed as an antimalarial agent, has been shown to have antischistosomal activity on the juvenile forms of the schistosome [24], in contrast to praziquantel, which acts on the mature form. Thus, theoretically, artemether may play a role in treating the acute stage of *Schistosoma* infection. However, these studies have not yet been done.

In summary, the most common form of the disease in travelers is acute schistosomiasis. Management of this population has never been assessed systematically.

## Chronic schistosomiasis

The late stage, or chronic schistosomiasis (ChS), appears months to years after infection and results from granuloma formation around the schistosome eggs retained in the tissues. *S. haematobium* infection affects the urinary system and may cause painless hematuria (usually terminal hematuria), dysuria, and, later, obstructive uropathy. It may even cause squamous cell carcinoma of the bladder in untreated long-term infection.

*S. mansoni* and *S. japonicum* affect the gastrointestinal system; infection may cause chronic diarrhea, abdominal discomfort, and colonic polyposis. Severe and longstanding infection may cause hepatic fibrosis (Symmer's pipestem fibrosis) with portal hypertension and splenomegaly.

As mentioned, the chronic phase of the disease is the common presentation among local populations. It is estimated that the disease causes an annual loss of between 1.7 and 4.5 million disability adjusted life years (DALYs) [1]. Immigrants to developed countries will seek medical care for chronic complications, sometimes many years after their migration.

Among travelers, only a minority will present with ChS, as was observed in a large Israeli cohort of *Schistosoma* patients where only 20% presented with ChS [4]. Among them, genitourinary problems are much more common, and may include hematuria, unresolved dysuria, or hematospermia. Failure to obtain a proper travel history may lead to unnecessary invasive procedures. The typical scenario is of a patient who is evaluated for urological complaints. Ultrasound may reveal a tumor–like lesion in the bladder. This "tumor" is subsequently removed with cystoscopy. The pathological result will show *Schistosoma* eggs within the tissue, and at this point the travel history is ascertained.

Obstructive uropathy is not expected to be seen in travelers, as it is a sequela of heavy and repeated infection. The same holds true for the late gastrointestinal sequelae such as cirrhosis and portal and pulmonary hypertension, which are all the aftermath of heavy/repeated infection typical of local populations, and not of travelers. This is in contrary to AcS symptoms, which are not dose-related.

### Ectopic migration of schistosomal eggs

The schistosomes are blood flukes residing in the vesicle beds or in the mesenteric beds (depending on the species). Thus, during oviposition, ectopic migration of the eggs can occur through the veins to tissues out of their usual habitats, such as the brain, spinal cord, or skin.

### Central nervous system involvement

Neuroschistosomiasis, which is due to ectopic eggs migrating into the CNS, is the most worrisome complication of late schistosome infection. It is likely to occur with all schistosome species. This may involve the brain or the spinal cord. In brain involvement, S. *japonicum* is the main culprit and, in spinal involvement, S. *mansoni* [25]. Both spinal and brain involvement due to schistosomiasis have been reported in travelers [26, 27].

With spinal cord involvement, myelopathy may present clinically as acute transverse myelitis or as subacute myelo-radiculopathy. Acute transverse myelitis is the most common neurological complication of *Schistosoma* infection. In transverse myelitis, patients typically present with rapidly evolving weakness and sensory disturbance of both lower limbs, typically associated with sphincter dysfunction. The conus medullaris and cauda equina are the most common sites of involvement [25].

CNS schistosomiasis is most common with S. *japonicum* infection, occurring in as many as 2–5% of infections and accounting for high rates of epilepsy in endemic areas. Symptoms are focal or generalized seizures, focal neurological deficits, signs of increased intracranial pressure due to the mass effect, and diffuse encephalitis.

Early recognition of neuroschistosomiasis is important so that early medical intervention can be initiated in an attempt to avoid severe disability. Diagnosis is achieved by detecting blood eosinophilia or CSF pleocytosis (with or without eosinophilia) and by MRI of the spine showing cord swelling [25].

For treatment of these cases, a longer course of praziquantel (usually of 5 days) with steroids should be considered. The minimally symptomatic or asymptomatic individual may be treated with praziquantel alone. However, adjunctive therapy with corticosteroids should be considered for patients with prominent neurological symptoms or CNS mass lesions with evidence of surrounding edema [25].

### Hematospermia

Infection of the genital organs is not infrequent in endemic areas. Most reports deal with female genital involvement. Evidence from field studies indicates that the incidence of male genital involvement in schistosomal infection is higher than previously appreciated [28]. The presentation of hematospermia seems to be rare among travelers, with only three previous reports [29–31], which probably does not reflect the real magnitude of the problem.

Patients may seek medical attention after they notice bloody sperm (hematospermia), or patients may complain of lower abdominal pain, perineal dull tension, testicular hyperesthesia, and coital discomfort. In some cases, a history of frank hematuria before hematospermia had begun may be recalled.

### Physical examination and laboratory findings

Physical examination is usually unremarkable, without prostate enlargement or tenderness (only the minority have mild pain on prostate palpation). This nonfinding may differentiate this form of prostatic infection from other etiologies of prostatitis.

Because this infection does not occur in the early stages of the schistosomal infection, the blood count is usually within normal limits, without significant eosinophilia. Mild eosinophilia (absolute count 500–1000/mm$^3$) may exist, and in these cases it can be another hint of schistosomal infection. Other laboratory tests are normal, and the prostate-specific antigen (PSA) that has been tested in a limited number of patients is also normal.

Urinalysis may be normal, or with microscopic hematuria.

Transrectal ultrasonography has been reported normal in some cases [31]. In other cases, series hyperechoic zones or calcification were found [30].

### Diagnosis

Schistosome eggs may be found in semen specimens, or sometime in prostate biopsies (Figure 24.10). Despite the absence of hematuria, urine collection may show eggs of *S. haematobium*.

It is important to note that *S. mansoni*, which usually resides in mesenteric vessels, has also been reported to be a cause of hematospermia [30].

Infection of the female genital organs is more frequent in endemic areas than infection of male genital organs (and the consequences of genital involvement in terms of morbidity and fertility are unclear).However, in travelers, female genital infection is very rare [32].

### Appendicitis

Appendicitis is considered an unusual complication of schistosomiasis, although in highly endemic areas, schistosomiasis is reported to account for approximately 5% of appendicitis cases. Interestingly, the association has been noted most often with *S. haematobium*. Two patterns have been proposed for acute appendicitis associated with schistosomiasis [33]: *Obstructive acute appendicitis* is described as severe fibrosis accompanied by many calcified eggs, and is a complicated chronic infection. *Granulomatous acute appendicitis* is characterized by eosinophilic infiltration and tissue necrosis due to a newly acquired infection causing acute appendicitis. This form is more likely to occur in travelers [34].

### Asymptomatic infection

Travelers seem to know that there is a risk of schistosomiasis from exposure to fresh water in endemic countries. Although more often than not, this knowledge will not keep them from enjoying recreational activities in the water, it may lead them subsequently to seek medical advice concerning screening. Another common scenario might be that an individual's diagnosis with schistosomiasis leads other travelers from the group with similar exposure to inquire about the need to be screened. In fact, in the GeoSentinal study, about 35% of *Schistosoma* sufferers sought medical advice for asymptomatic screening [3].

Screening is recommended because late complications may occur in initially asymptomatic patients. As shown in the Israeli study, 26% of initially asymptomatic cases went on to develop ChS. These data suggest that a quarter

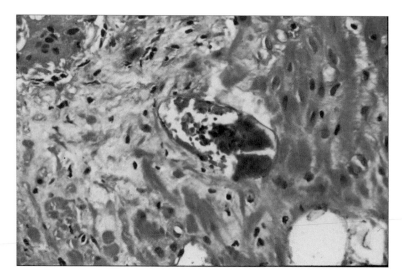

**Figure 24.10** *S. haematobium* egg in prostate biopsy. (Magnification ×400.)

of asymptomatic travelers may later develop ChS, which provides strong support for the recommendation to screen and treat [4].

## Diagnosis

Laboratory findings in the chronic schistosomiasis stage might show only minor changes. Blood count may reveal mild eosinophilia, usually less than the total eosinophil count 1000/mm$^3$.

Unexplained liver function test abnormalities in a traveler who returned from an endemic area may be due to occult *Schistosoma* infection.

In cases of *S. haematobium* infection, abnormal urine sediment findings are hematuria (usually microhematuria) and leukocyturia, with negative urine culture.

A definitive diagnosis is made by recovering the schistosome eggs in the urine or stool, or in the affected ectopic organ. However, the sensitivity of stool or urine examinations, even when performed on three separate occasions, is limited by the sporadic passage of eggs by the adult flukes and the low fluke burden usually found in travelers. Rectal biopsy may increase the sensitivity of the test to some extent.

Thus, serological testing is potentially much more sensitive and valuable even in ChS.

As mentioned earlier, for AcS, some serology tests can give species-specific results, whereas most commercial tests will give only genus-specific results (indicating if any *Schistosoma* species is present or not).

A major limitation of serology tests is that they stay positive for many years despite efficacious treatment, thus preventing their use in confirming recent exposure or in evaluating the success or failure of treatment. Therefore, serology testing is unsuited to assessing local populations or immigrants from endemic areas.

## Treatment

The drug of choice for all schistosome species infections is praziquantel. The recommended schedule is 2 doses of 20–30 mg/kg over 12 hours (the higher dose is recommended for *S. japonicum* and *S. mekongi*).

The drug should be taken with liquids during a meal. Adverse events are rare and usually include gastrointestinal complaints such as vomiting, nausea, and abdominal discomfort.

Praziquantel resistance, although reported in local populations, is rarely seen in travelers, although cases of treatment failure have been reported in travelers [35, 36]. Our experience with patients with hematospermia who received the conventional treatment was that they had a relapse after several months [31]. This treatment failure might be peculiar to hematospermia, taking into consideration that pharmacologically, the prostate is known to be hostile to many antimicrobials, and the levels of praziquantel attained in the prostate may not be adequate for parasite eradication. For this complication, higher doses at the outset or a longer course of treatment are desirable [31].

In dealing with chronic infection with fibrotic sequelae in immigrant populations, one may assume that the changes are irreversible. Interestingly, several prospective studies have shown that praziquantel treatment reverses mild to moderate changes in the liver and urinary system [37, 38]. The author recommends that chronic patients be given drug therapy, regardless of the severity of their symptoms, because the spectrum of side effects of the drug is mild and because the treatment is targeted at killing the adult flukes, thus stopping egg shedding and halting the progression of the disease.

## Prevention

Control and prevention of the disease in endemic countries is beyond the scope of this chapter. Among travelers to endemic areas, mainly Africa, prevention of the disease is primarily achieved by avoiding contact with fresh water lakes and rivers. (There is no risk of contracting schistosomiasis in salt water.) Our experience with travelers shows that this advice is often not followed, as water entertainment (e.g., diving in Lake Malawi or rafting on rivers in Africa) is too enticing.

Using a repellent before swimming, such as DEET (*N,N*-diethyl-toluamide), the active ingredient for mosquito repelling, may give some protection [39]. Another approach is vigorous towel drying immediately after exposure [40]. The assumption is that these procedures will kill the cercariae that are still entrapped in the skin. These methods have never been studied systematically but are anecdotal reports [41].

Recent research has found artemether, the Chinese antimalarial drug, to be active against the juvenile forms of schistosome. Thus, it may play a role in treating people soon after exposure and blunting future clinical symptoms [42].

A controlled study was done in China during a flood and showed that people exposed to schistosomes who were treated with arthemether had significantly fewer episodes of acute schistosomiasis [43]. Further studies in nonimmune populations are needed before a conclusion about the role of this drug can be reached.

## Conclusions

*Schistosoma* infection is one of the most common infectious diseases, limited in the past to endemic countries. With the enormous increase in migration and travel, we encounter more and more cases in developed, nonendemic countries. Although the disease has been known for many years from studies in endemic countries, the new patient population of nonimmune travelers present with a different clinical pattern that needs further investigation. One of the features of the disease in the nonendemic population is acute schistosomiasis, which appears to be much more common than had previously been suspected.

Clinicians in the Western countries have a higher chance of encountering the early (acute) form of the disease, although some travelers, and especially immigrants from endemic countries, may present with late (chronic) schistosomiasis. Thus, physicians should be acquainted with both forms of the disease.

## References

1 Steinmann P, Keiser J, Bos R, Tanner M, Utzinger J. Schistosomiasis and water resources development: systematic review, meta-analysis, and estimates of people at risk. *Lancet Infect Dis* 2006;6:411–25.

2 Grobusch MP, Muhlberger N, Jelinek T, et al. Imported schistosomiasis in Europe: sentinel surveillance data from TropNetEurope. *J Travel Med* 2003;10:164–7.

3 Nicolls DJ, Weld L, Schwartz E, Reed C, Sonnenburg F, Kozarsky P, for the GeoSentinel Surveillance Network. Schistosomiasis in travelers: a review of patients reported to the GeoSentinel Surveillance Network. *Am J Trop Med Hyg*, in press.

4 Meltzer E. Meltzer E, Artom G, et al. Schistosomiasis among travelers: new aspects of an old disease. *Emerg Infect Dis* 2006;12(11):1696–1700.

5 Freedman DO, Weld LH, Kozarsky PE, Fisk T, Robins R, von Sonnenburg F, et al. Spectrum of disease and relation to place of exposure among ill returned travelers. *N Engl J Med* 2006;354(2):119–30.

6 Cetron MS, Chitsulo L, Sullivan JJ, et al. Schistosomiasis in Lake Malawi. *Lancet* 1996;348:1274–8.

7 Schwartz E, Kozarsky P, Wilson M, Cetron M. Schistosome infection among river rafters on Omo River, Ethiopia. *J Travel Med* 2005;12(1):3–8.

8 Leshem E, Maor Y, Meltzer E, Assous M, Schwartz E. Acute schistosomiasis outbreak: morbidity and economic impact. *Clin Infect Dis* 2008;47(12)1499–506.

9 Visser LG, Polderman AM, Stuiver PC. Outbreak of schistosomiasis among travelers returning from Mali, West Africa. *Clin Infect Dis* 1995;20:280–85.

10 Davidson BL, el-Kassimi F, Uz-Zaman A, et al. The "lung shift" in treated schistosomiasis. Bronchoalveolar lavage evidence of eosinophilic pneumonia. *Chest* 1986;89:455–7.

11 Schwartz E, Rozenman J, Perelman N. Pulmonary manifestations of early *Schistosoma* infection among nonimmune travelers. *Am J Med* 2000;109:718–22.

12 Walt F. The Katayama syndrome. *S Afr Med J* 1954;28:89–93.

13 Hiatt RA, Ottesen EA, Sotomayor ZR, et al. Serial observations of circulating immune complexes in patients with acute schistosomiasis. *J Infect Dis* 1980;142:665–70.

14 Maguire JH. Trematodes (schistosomes and other flukes). In: Mandell GL, Bennett JE, Dolin R, editors. *Principles and Practice of Infectious Diseases*, 6th ed. Philadelphia (PA): Churchill Livingstone; 2005. p. 3276–85.

15 Ishii A, Tsuji M, Tada I. History of Katayama disease: schistosomiasis japonica in Katayama district, Hiroshima, Japan. *Parasitol Int* 2003;52:313–19.

16 Doherty JF, Moody AH, Wright SG. Katayama fever: an acute manifestation of schistosomiasis. *BMJ* 1996;313:1071–2.

17 Cooke GS, Lavlani A, Gleeson FV, Conlon CP. Acute pulmonary schistosomiasis in travelers returning from lake Malawi, sub-Saharan Africa. *Clin Infect Dis* 1999;29:836–9.

18 Schwartz E. Pulmonary schistosomiasis. *Clin Chest Med* 2002;23(2):433–43.

19 Harnett W, Kusel JR. Increased exposure of parasite antigens at the surface of adult *Schistosoma mansoni* exposed to praziquantel *in vitro*. *Parasitology* 1986;93: 401–5.

20 Harris AD, Cook GC. Acute schistosomiasis (Katayama fever): clinical deterioration after chemotherapy. *J Infect* 1987;14:159–61.

21 Grandiere-Perez L, Ansart S, Paris L, et al. Efficacy of praziquantel during the incubation and invasive phase of *Schistosoma haematobium* schistosomiasis in 18 travelers. *Am J Trop Med Hyg* 2006;74(5):814–18.

22 Hayunga EG, Mollegard I, Duncan JF, Sumner MP, Stek M Jr, Hunter KW Jr. Development of circulating antigen assay for rapid detection of acute schistosomiasis. *Lancet* 1986;2: 716–18.

23 Xiao S, Catto BA, Webster LT. Effects of praziquantel on different developmental stages of *Schistosoma mansoni in vitro* and *in vivo*. *J Infect Dis* 1985;151:1130–37.

24 Shuhua X, Binggui S, Chollet J, et al. Tegumental alterations in juvenile *S. hematobium* harboured in hamsters following artemether treatment. *Parasitol Int* 2001;50:175–83.

25 Carod-Artal FJ. Neurological complications of Schistosoma infection. *Trans R Soc Trop Med Hyg* 2008;102:107–16.

26 Centers for Disease Control. Acute schistosomiasis with transverse myelitis in American students returning from Kenya. *MMWR Morb Mortal Wkly Rep* 1984;33(31):445–7.

27 Houston S, Kowalewska-Grochowska K, Naik S, McKean J, Johnson ES, Warren K. First report of *Schistosoma mekongi* infection with brain involvement. *Clin Infect Dis* 2004;38(1): e1–6.

28 Leutscher P, Ramarokoto C-E, Reimert C, et al. Community-based study of genital schistosomiasis in men from Madagascar. *Lancet* 2000;355:117–18.

29 Torresi J, Sheori H, Ryan N, Yung A. Usefulness of semen microscopy in the diagnosis of a difficult case of *Schistosoma haematobium* infection in a returned traveler. *J Travel Med* 1997;4:46–7.

30 Corachan M, Valls ME, Gascon J, et al. Hematospermia: a new etiology of clinical interest. *Am J Trop Med Hyg* 1994;5:580–84.

31 Schwartz E, Pick N, Shazberg G, Potasman I. Hematospermia due to schistosome infection in travelers: diagnostic and treatment challenge. *Clin Infect Dis* 2002;35;1420–24.

32 Landry P, Favrat B, Raeber PA.Genital schistosomiasis after a missed diagnosis of Katayama syndrome. *J Travel Med* 1996;3(4):237–8.

33 Satti MB, Tamimi DM, Al Sohaibani MO, Al Quorain A. Appendicular schistosomiasis: a cause of clinical acute appendicitis? *J Clin Pathol* 1987;40:424–8.

34 Weber G, Borer A, Zirkin HJ, Riesenberg K, Alkan M. Schistosomiasis presenting as acute appendicitis in a traveler. *J Travel Med* 1998;5:147–8.

35 Alonso D, Munoz J, Gascon J, Valls ME, Corachan M. Failure of standard treatment with praziquantel in two returned travelers with *Schistosoma haematobium* infection. *Am J Trop Med Hyg* 2006;74(2): 342–4.

36 Herwaldt BL, Tao LF, van Pelt W, Tsang VC, Bruce JI. Persistence of *Schistosoma haematobium* infection despite multiple courses of therapy with praziquantel. *Clin Infect Dis* 1995;20(2):309–15.

37 Homeida MA, El Tom I, Nash T, et al. Association of the therapeutic activity of praziquantel with reversal of Symmers' fibrosis induced by *S. mansoni*. *Am J Trop Med Hyg* 1991;45:360–65.

38 Ohamae H, Tanaka M, Hayashi M, et al. Improvement of ultrasonographic and serologic changes in *S. japonicum* infected patients after treatment with praziquantel. *Am J Trop Med Hyg* 1992;46:99–104.

39 Jackson F, Doherty JF, Behrens RH. Schistosomiasis prophylaxis *in vivo* using *N,N*-diethyl-m-toluamide (DEET). *Trans R Soc Trop Med Hyg* 2003;97(4):449–50.

40 Centers for Disease Control and Prevention. Schistosomiasis among river rafters—Ethiopia. *MMWR Morb Mortal Wkly Rep* 1983;32(44):585–6.

41 Ramaswamy K, et al. Topical application of DEET for schistosomiasis. *Trends Parasitol* 2003;19(12):551–5.

42 Utzinger, J, et al. Oral artemether for prevention of *Schistosoma mansoni* infection: randomised controlled trial. *Lancet* 2000;355(9212):1320–25.

43 Song Y, et al. Preventive effect of artemether on schistosome infection. *Chin Med J* 1998;111(2): 123–7.

# 25 Filarial Infections

## Thomas B. Nutman

National Institutes of Health, Bethesda, MD, USA

## Introduction

Filarial worms are nematodes or roundworms that dwell in the subcutaneous tissues and the lymphatics. Although eight filarial species commonly infect humans, four are responsible for most of the pathology associated with these infections. These are (1) *Brugia malayi*, (2) *Wuchereria bancrofti*, (3) *Onchocerca volvulus*, and (4) *Loa loa*. The distribution, biological features, vectors, and primary pathology of each of the filarial parasites of humans are given in Table 25.1.

In general, each of the parasites is transmitted by biting arthropods. Each goes through a complex life cycle that includes an infective larval stage carried by the arthropods and an adult worm stage that resides in humans, either in the lymph nodes or adjacent lymphatics or in subcutaneous tissue. The offspring of the adults, the *microfilariae* (200–250 µm long and 5–7 µm wide), either circulate in the blood or migrate through the skin. The microfilariae then can be ingested by the appropriate biting arthropod and develop over 1–2 weeks into infective larvae that are capable of initiating the life cycle over again. A generalized schematic is shown in Figure 25.1. Adult worms are long-lived, whereas the life spans of microfilariae range from 3 months to 3 years, depending on the filarial species [1]. Infection is generally not established unless exposure to infective larvae is intense and prolonged. Furthermore, clinical manifestations of these diseases develop rather slowly.

There are significant differences between patients native to the endemic areas and those who are travelers or recent arrivals to filariasis-endemic regions of the world in the clinical manifestations of the various filarial infections (Figure 25.2) [2]. Characteristically, the disease in previously unexposed individuals (e.g. travelers or trans-

migrants) is more acute and intense than in natives of the endemic region. Moreover, in travelers, extended exposure (typically more than 30 days) is usually required, as most of the vectors that transmit filariae are relatively inefficient. Also, the interval between exposure and onset of symptoms may be prolonged. Finally, standard parasitological assessments may be negative, so that other (and often more indirect) tests are frequently required for diagnosis.

Among travelers, the filarial diseases most commonly acquired are onchocerciasis and loiasis, with lymphatic filariasis being a distant third. In the most comprehensive study of filarial infections in travelers [2], ~75% were acquired during travel to Africa, with an additional 10% acquired in South America [2].

## Lymphatic filariasis

There are three lymphatic-dwelling filarial parasites of humans: *B. malayi*, *B. timori*, and *W. bancrofti*. Adult worms usually reside in either the afferent lymphatic channels or the lymph nodes. These adult parasites may remain viable in the human host for decades.

### Epidemiology

#### *B. malayi* and *B. timori*

The distribution of brugian filariasis is limited primarily to China, India, Indonesia, Korea, Japan, Malaysia, and the Philippines. In both brugian species, two forms of the parasite can be distinguished by the periodicity of their microfilariae (Mf). Nocturnally periodic forms have Mf present in the peripheral blood primarily at night, whereas subperiodic forms have Mf present in the blood at all times, but with maximal levels in the afternoon.

The nocturnal form of brugian filariasis is more common and is transmitted in areas of coastal rice fields (by mansonian and anopheline mosquitoes), whereas the

*Tropical Diseases in Travelers*, 1st edition. Edited by E. Schwartz.
© 2009 by Blackwell Publishing, ISBN: 978-1-4051-8441-0.

**Table 25.1** Epidemiological and biological features of the human filariases.

| Species | Endemic areas | Vector | Microfilariae | Adult worm location | Primary pathology |
|---|---|---|---|---|---|
| *Brugia malayi* | China, India, Malaysia, and some Pacific island groups | Mosquitoes, including *Anopheles*, *Aedes*, and *Mansonia* spp. | Blood-borne, sheathed, nocturnally periodic, or subperiodic | Lymphatics | Lymphedema, adenolymphangitis |
| *B. timori* | Southeastern Indonesia | *Anopheles barbirostris* | Blood-borne, sheathed, nocturnally periodic | Lymphatics | Lymphedema, adenolymphangitis |
| *Loa loa* | Western and Central Africa | *Chrysops* spp. | Blood-borne, sheathed, diurnally periodic | Subcutaneous tissues, including subconjunctiva | Allergic |
| *Mansonella ozzardi* | Central and South America, Caribbean | *Culicoides* spp. and *Simulium amazonicum* | Skin and blood-borne, unsheathed, nonperiodic | Thoracic and peritoneal cavities, lymphatics | ??? |
| *M. perstans* | Sub-Saharan Africa, northern coast of South America, Tunisia and Algeria | *Culicoides* spp. | Blood-borne, unsheathed, nonperiodic | Serous cavities, mesentery, perirenal, and retroperitoneal tissues | ??? |
| *M. streptocerca* | Western and Central Africa | *Culicoides grahamii* | Skin, unsheathed, nonperiodic | Dermis | Dermal |
| *Onchocerca volvulus* | Sub-Saharan Africa, Latin America, and the Arabian peninsula | *Simulium* spp. | Skin, unsheathed, nonperiodic | Subcutaneous nodules | Dermal, ocular |
| *Wuchereria bancrofti* | Sub-Saharan Africa, Southeast Asia, western Pacific, Caribbean, northern coast of South America | Mosquitoes, including *Anopheles*, *Aedes*, and *Culex* species | Blood-borne, sheathed, nocturnally periodic, or subperiodic | Lymphatics, lymph nodes | Lymphedema, adenolymphangitis, hydrocele |

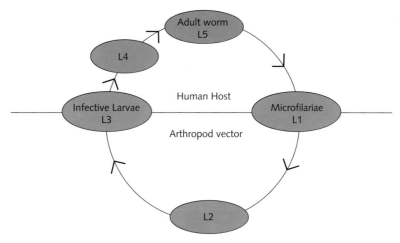

**Figure 25.1** General life cycle of the filarial parasites in humans. Microfilariae (L1) are produced by the adult worms (L5). L2 and L3 are larval development stages in the arthropod vector. L3 larval forms are infective for humans. L4 develop from the newly arrived infective larval (L3) forms.

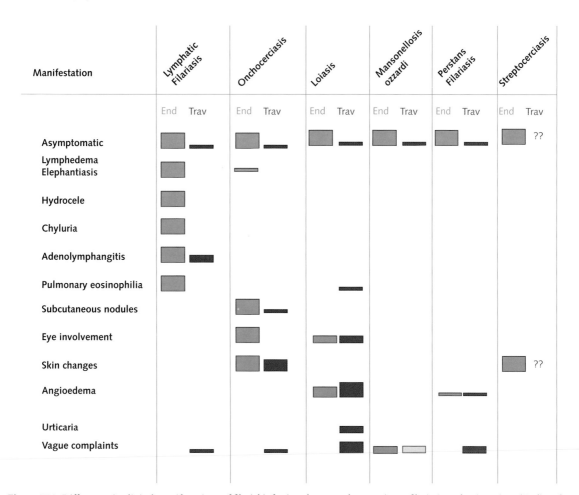

**Figure 25.2** Differences in clinical manifestations of filarial infections between those native to filariasis-endemic regions (End) and travelers to or temporary residents of filariasis-endemic regions (Trav). Height of the bar relates to frequency of the manifestation relative to the other group. Absence of a bar indicates a manifestation not described.

subperiodic form is found in the swamp forests (manso-nian vector). Although humans are the common host, *B. malayi* can be a natural infection of cats.

### *W. bancrofti*

Bancroftian filariasis is found throughout the tropics and subtropics, including Asia and the Pacific islands, Africa, areas of South America, and the Caribbean basin. Humans are the only definitive host for this parasite and are therefore the natural reservoir for infection. Like brugian filariasis, there are both a *periodic* and a *subperiodic* form of the parasite. Generally, the subperiodic form is found only in the Pacific islands (including the Cook and Ellis Islands, Fiji, New Caledonia, the Marquesas, Samoa, and the Society Islands); elsewhere, *W. bancrofti* is nocturnally periodic. The natural vectors are *Culex fatigans* mosquitoes in urban settings and usually anopheline or acdean mosquitoes in rural areas.

There is a paucity of epidemiological data on lymphatic filariasis in travelers. Very sustained exposure to infective larvae is required; most commonly the diagnosis of lymphatic filariasis is made on an incidental finding of a parasite in tissue samples.

### Clinical manifestations of those native to the endemic region

The three most common presentations of the lymphatic filariases are asymptomatic (or subclinical) microfilaremia, adenolymphangitis (ADL), and lymphatic obstruction.
**1** Patients with *asymptomatic microfilaremia* rarely come to the attention of medical personnel except through the incidental finding of Mf in the peripheral blood during surveys in endemic regions. Such asymptomatic persons are clinically unaffected by the parasites, although lymphoscintigraphic evaluation of these individuals suggests that lymphatic dysfunction (and tortuosity) is common [3], as is scrotal lymphangiectasia (detectable by ultrasound) in men with *W. bancrofti* infections [4, 5].
**2** *Acute filarial ADL* is characterized by high fever (and shaking chills), lymphatic inflammation (lymphangitis and lymphadenitis), and transient local edema. The lymphangitis is retrograde, extending peripherally from the lymph node draining the area where the adult parasites reside. Regional lymph nodes are often enlarged, and the entire lymphatic channel can become indurated and inflamed. Concomitant local thrombophlebitis can occur as well. In brugian filariasis, a single local abscess may form along the involved lymphatic tract and subsequently rupture to the surface. Lymphadenitis and lymphangitis occur in both the upper and the lower extremities with

both bancroftian and brugian filariasis, but involvement of the genital lymphatics occurs almost exclusively with *W. bancrofti* infection. Genital involvement can be manifested by funiculitis, epididymitis, scrotal pain, and tenderness.

In endemic areas, another type of acute disease, dermatolymphangioadenitis (DLA) [6], is recognized as a syndrome that is associated with high fever, chills, myalgia, and headache. Edematous inflammatory plaques clearly demarcated from normal skin are seen. Occasionally, vesicles, ulcers, and hyperpigmentation may also be noted. There is often a history of trauma, burns, radiation, insect bites, punctiform lesions, or chemical injury. Entry lesions, especially in the interdigital area, are common.
**3** Chronic manifestations of lymphatic filariasis develop in only a small proportion of the filarial-infected population. If lymphatic damage progresses, transient lymphedema can develop into *lymphatic obstruction* and the permanent changes associated with elephantiasis. Brawny edema follows the early pitting edema, and thickening of the subcutaneous tissues and hyperkeratosis occur. Fissuring of the skin develops, as do hyperplastic changes. Superinfection of these poorly vascularized tissues becomes a problem. In bancroftian filariasis, when genital involvement is evident, scrotal lymphedema or hydrocele formation occurs. Furthermore, if there is obstruction of the retroperitoneal lymphatics, renal lymphatic pressure can increase to the point at which they rupture into the renal pelvis or tubules, so that chyluria is seen. The chyluria is characteristically intermittent and is often prominent in the morning just after the patient arises.

### Clinical manifestations in travelers or in new arrivals to endemic areas

As mentioned previously, there are significant differences in the clinical manifestations of filarial infection, or at least in the time course over which they appear, between individuals who have recently entered the endemic areas (travelers or transmigrants) and those who are native to these areas.

Given sufficient exposure to the vector (typically months, not weeks), patients often present with the signs and symptoms of acute lymphatic or scrotal inflammation. Urticaria and localized angioedema are common. Lymphadenitis of the epitrochlear, axillary, femoral, or inguinal nodes is often followed by lymphangitis, which is retrograde. Occasionally, transient (and typically reversible) lymphedema occurs early in the infection [7–9].

Acute attacks are short-lived and, in contradistinction to filarial ADL seen in native patients, are generally not accompanied by fever. If allowed to continue (by chronic exposure to infected mosquitoes), these attacks become increasingly severe and quickly (compared with the indigenous population) lead to permanent lymphatic inflammation and obstruction. However, early removal of the patients from continued reexposure seems to hasten the end of the clinical syndrome [7].

## Diagnosis

Diagnosis of filarial diseases can be problematic, because these infections most often require parasitological techniques to demonstrate the offending organisms [10]. In addition, satisfactory methods for definitive diagnosis in amicrofilaremic states can be extremely difficult. The diagnostic procedures, however, should take advantage of the periodicity of each organism, as well as its characteristic morphological appearance. The following techniques may be used for examining blood or other fluids, such as chyle, urine, and hydrocele fluid.

### Direct examination

A small volume of fluid is spread on a clean slide. The slide is then air-dried, stained with Giemsa stain, and examined microscopically.

### Nuclepore filtration

A known volume of anticoagulated blood is passed through a polycarbonate (Nuclepore) filter with 3-μm pores. A large volume (~30 ml) of distilled (or filtered) water is passed through the filter device (the water will lyse or break open the red cells, leaving the worms intact and more easily visible). The filter is then air-dried, stained with Wright's or Giemsa stain, and examined by microscopy. For studies in the field, 1 ml of anticoagulated blood can be added to 9 ml of a solution of 2% formalin/10% Teepol and stored for up to 9 months before filtration [10].

### Knott's concentration technique

In Knott's concentration technique, 1 ml of anticoagulated blood is placed in 9 ml of 2% formalin. The tube is centrifuged. The sediment is spread on a slide and dried thoroughly. The slide is then stained with Wright's or Giemsa stain and examined microscopically.

### Indirect measures

### Detection of circulating parasite antigen

Assays for circulating antigens of *W. bancrofti* permit the diagnosis of microfilaremic and cryptic (amicrofi-laremic) infection. Two tests are currently commercially available, an enzyme-linked immunosorbent assay (Trop-Ag *W. bancrofti,* manufactured by JCU Tropical Biotechnology Pty. Ltd, Townsville, Queensland, Australia), and a rapid-format card test (marketed by Inverness Medical, Scarborough, ME). Both assays have reported sensitivities that range from 95–100% and specificities that approach 100%. There are currently no tests for circulating antigens in brugian filariasis.

### Serodiagnosis using parasite extract

Development of serodiagnostic assays of sufficient sensitivity and specificity for routine use has proven difficult, primarily because of poor specificity. As is the case for serodiagnosis of most infectious diseases, it is difficult to differentiate previous infection or exposure to the parasite (aborted infection) from currently active infection, as serology typically remains positive after treatment. Indeed, most residents of filariasis-endemic regions are antibody-positive and remain so over their lifetimes (even if removed from the endemic region). Nevertheless, serologic assays have a definite place in diagnosis, as a negative assay result effectively excludes past or present filarial infection.

### Molecular diagnostics

PCR-based assays for DNA of *W. bancrofti* and *B. malayi* in blood have also been developed. In a number of studies evaluating PCR-based diagnosis, the method has shown sensitivity equivalent to or greater than that of parasitological methods, detecting patent infection in almost all infected subjects.

### Imaging studies

In cases of suspected *W. bancrofti* infection, examination of the scrotum or female breast using high-frequency ultrasound in conjunction with Doppler techniques may result in the identification of motile adult worms within dilated lymphatics. Worms may be visualized in the lymphatics of the spermatic cord in up to 80% of infected men with *Wuchereria bancrofti.* Live adult worms have a distinctive pattern of movement within the lymphatic vessels (termed the *filaria dance sign*). In *B. malayi* infection, adult worm nests have been found in the breast, the thigh, and the calf and in or near inguinal and epitrochlear lymph nodes [11, 12]. This technique may be useful in monitoring the success of antifilarial chemotherapy, by watching for the disappearance of the dance sign.

Radionuclide lymphoscintigraphic imaging of the limbs reliably demonstrates widespread lymphatic abnormalities both in asymptomatic microfilaremic persons and in those with clinical manifestations of lymphatic pathology. Although of potential utility in the delineation of anatomical changes associated with infection, lymphoscintigraphy is unlikely to assume primacy in the diagnostic evaluation of individuals with suspected infection.

### Approach to diagnosis in travelers

If lymphatic filariasis is suspected, antifilarial antibody testing (available both commercially and in reference laboratories around the world) is recommended. If negative, this should exclude the diagnosis. If positive, it indicates that a search for a more specific diagnosis should be made by doing an assay for circulating filarial antigen (only for *W. bancrofti*) or by demonstrating the parasite (in peripheral blood) or the parasite DNA (by PCR).

### Treatment

With newer definitions of clinical syndromes in lymphatic filariasis and new tools for assessing clinical status (e.g., ultrasound, lymphoscintigraphy, circulating filarial antigen assays), approaches to treatment based on infection status and pathogenesis have been proposed.

#### Microfilaria-positive individuals

A growing body of evidence indicates that although they may be asymptomatic, virtually all persons with *W. bancrofti* or *B. malayi* microfilaremia have some degree of subclinical disease (hematuria, proteinuria, abnormalities on lymphoscintigraphy). Thus, early treatment of asymptomatic persons is recommended to prevent further lymphatic damage. Diethylcarbamazine (DEC), which has both macrofilaricidal and microfilaricidal properties, is the drug of choice.

#### Microfilaria-negative antigen-positive individuals

Because lymphatic disease is associated with the adult worm, treatment with DEC is recommended for microfilaria-negative adult worm carriers (persons who are microfilaria-negative but filaria antigen- or ultrasound-positive).

#### Acute manifestations of lymphatic filariasis

*Filarial adenolymphangitis (ADL)*
Supportive treatment is recommended for ADL, including rest; postural drainage, particularly if the lower limb is affected; cold compresses at the site of inflammation; and antipyretics and analgesics for symptomatic relief. During the acute episode, treatment with antifilarial drugs is not recommended, because it may provoke additional adult worm death and exacerbate the inflammatory response. After the acute attack has resolved, if the patient remains microfilaria- or antigen-positive, DEC can be given to kill the remaining adult worms.

For patients with ADL secondary to bacterial or fungal infections, cold compresses, antipyretics, and analgesics are recommended. The patient should remain at rest, with the affected limb elevated. Antibiotic therapy must be initiated while awaiting results of cultures of blood or tissue aspirates. The bacteria isolated during these attacks are sensitive to most systemic antibiotics, including penicillin.

#### Chronic manifestations of lymphatic filariasis

Chronic manifestations of lymphatic filariasis include lymphedema and urogenital disease. Although antifilarial drug therapy is rarely, if ever, the definitive treatment for these conditions, such treatment is indicated if the patient has evidence of active infection (e.g., detection of microfilaria or filarial antigen in the blood, or of the filaria dance sign on ultrasound examination). Not infrequently, the inflammatory response secondary to treatment-induced death of the adult worm exacerbates manifestations of chronic disease.

#### Lymphedema

Careful attention must be paid to the management of lymphedema once it has occurred. Elevation of the affected limb, elastic stockings, and local foot care will ameliorate some of the symptoms associated with lymphedema. Data indicate that filarial elephantiasis and lymphedema of the leg may be partially reversible with a treatment regimen that emphasizes hygiene, prevention of secondary bacterial infections, and physiotherapy. This regimen is similar to that now recommended for treatment of lymphedema from most nonfilarial causes, which is known by a variety of names, including complex decongestive physiotherapy and complex lymphedema therapy. Surgical decompression using a nodovenous shunt may provide improvement in extreme cases. Hydroceles can be drained repeatedly or managed surgically.

#### Treatment options and dosage

The recommended course of DEC treatment (12 days; total dose, 72 mg/kg) has remained the standard for many years and has both macrofilaricidal and microfilaricidal activity. Regimens that utilize combinations of single doses of albendazole (400 mg) and either DEC (6 mg/kg) or ivermectin (200 μg/kg) have each been demonstrated to have a sustained microfilaricidal effect, but their effect on adult worms has been variable. Interestingly, either 6 weeks of daily doxycycline (200 mg/day) [13]—a regimen that targets an intracellular, Rickettsia-like *Wolbachia* endosymbiont)—or a 7-day course of DEC (6 mg/kg)/albendazole (400 mg) has significant macrofilaricidal activity and sustained microfilaricidal activity [14].

Side effects of DEC treatment include fever, chills, arthralgias, headaches, nausea, and vomiting. Both the development and the severity of these reactions are directly related to the number of Mf circulating in the bloodstream and may represent an acute hypersensitivity reaction to the antigens released by dead and dying parasites. To avoid these side effects, one can either initiate treatment with a very small dose of DEC and increase the dose to the full level over a few days, or premedicate the patient with corticosteroids. Ivermectin has a side-effect profile similar to that of DEC when used in lymphatic filariasis. Albendazole (when used in single-dose regimens) has relatively few side effects associated with its use in lymphatic filariasis.

DEC is not commercially available in the United States, but is available in many countries throughout the world. Albendazole, ivermectin, and doxycycline are all available commercially.

### Prevention and control

For travelers, personal protective measures to prevent mosquito bites are useful. Impregnated bed nets have been shown to have a salutary effect. Weekly or monthly DEC can kill developing forms of filarial parasites and has been shown to be useful as a prophylactic agent in humans, although controlled trials have not been performed.

Community-based intervention is the current approach to control of lymphatic filariasis. The underlying tenet of this approach is that mass annual distribution of albendazole with either DEC (for all areas except those where onchocerciasis is coendemic) or ivermectin will profoundly suppress microfilaremia. If the suppression is sustained, then transmission can be interrupted.

### Tropical eosinophilia syndrome

Tropical eosinophilia syndrome, or tropical pulmonary eosinophilia (TPE; reviewed in [15]), was recognized as being of filarial etiology only in the late 1950s or early 1960s, when it was noted that the antifilarial drug DEC was effective in this syndrome and that patients with TPE had extraordinarily high levels of antifilarial antibodies

in their blood. Although circulating microfilariae were never found, lung and lymph node biopsies occasionally revealed trapped microfilariae.

A majority of reported cases have been from India, Pakistan, Sri Lanka, Southeast Asia, Guyana, and Brazil. Well-documented cases in travelers have not been described.

### Clinical features

The main features of this syndrome, besides a history of residence in a filariasis-endemic region, include paroxysmal cough and wheezing (usually nocturnal), occasional weight loss, low-grade fever, adenopathy, and extreme peripheral blood eosinophilia ($>3000/mm^3$). Chest radiographs may be normal but generally show increased bronchovascular markings, diffuse miliary lesions, or mottled opacities primarily involving the mid and lower lung fields. Pulmonary function testing often shows restrictive abnormalities, which may be accompanied by obstructive defects.

This syndrome is associated with marked elevations of antifilarial antibodies, as well as extremely elevated levels of total serum IgE. Furthermore, in the absence of successful treatment, permanent pulmonary damage (interstitial fibrosis) can develop.

### Treatment

DEC is the drug of choice for treatment of TPE. Treatment for tropical eosinophilia is DEC at a dose of 6 mg/kg per day for 14 days. Symptoms usually resolve between days 4 and 7 of therapy. Characteristically, respiratory symptoms resolve rapidly after treatment with DEC. Despite dramatic initial improvement after conventional treatment with DEC, symptoms recur in approximately 20% of patients 12–24 months after treatment, and a majority of patients continue to have subtle clinical, radiographic, and functional abnormalities. Repeat treatment may be necessary to prevent pulmonary fibrosis, a serious sequela of TPE if it is left untreated. Ivermectin has not been shown to be effective in TPE.

## Onchocerciasis

### Epidemiology

Onchocerciasis, or "river blindness," is caused by infection with *O. volvulus,* a subcutaneous-dwelling filarial worm. Approximately 18 million people are infected, mostly in Equatorial Africa, the Sahara, Yemen, and parts of Central and South America (Guatemala, Venezuela, Mexico, Ecuador, Colombia, and Brazil). The infection is transmitted to humans through the bites of blackflies of the genus *Simulium*, which breed along fast-flowing rivers in the previously mentioned tropical areas. Among travelers, the most common destinations associated with acquisition of onchocerciasis most recently have been Liberia, Sierra Leone, and Ethiopia.

## Clinical features

The major disease manifestations of onchocerciasis are localized to the skin, lymph nodes and lymphatics, and eyes.

### Skin

Pruritus is the most frequent manifestation of onchocercal dermatitis. This pruritus may be accompanied by the appearance of localized areas of edema and erythema that are characteristically evanescent. If the infection is prolonged, lichenification and pigment changes (either hypopigmentation or hyperpigmentation) can occur; these often lead to atrophy, "lizard skin," and mottling of the skin. These skin changes can also become superinfected, particularly in the presence of excoriation or trauma. An immunologically hyperreactive form of dermatitis (commonly termed *sowda* or localized onchodermatitis) can occur; the affected skin becomes darker as a consequence of the profound inflammation that occurs as microfilariae in the skin are being cleared.

The subcutaneous nodules contain the adult worms. In the Central American form of the disease, nodules tend to be distributed on the upper part of the body, particularly on the head, neck, and shoulders. In Africa, the onchocercomata tend to be found over bony prominences, such as the coccyx, femoral trochanter, iliac crests, lateral aspects of the knee and elbow, and head. It is thought that for every palpable nodule, there are probably at least five deeper nodules.

### Lymph nodes

Lymphadenopathy is frequently found, particularly in the inguinal and femoral areas. As the glands enlarge, they can come to lie within areas of loose skin (so-called hanging groins), which predisposes the affected patients to hernias. Scarring in lymph nodes may lead to regional lymphedema.

### Eyes

Onchocercal eye disease can take many forms, and most can lead to severe vision loss or blindness. Usually seen in persons with moderate or heavy infections, the ocular disease spares no part of the eye. Conjunctivitis, anterior uveitis, iridocyclitis leading to secondary glaucoma, scle-

rosing keratitis, optic atrophy, and chorioretinal lesions can be found.

## Clinical manifestations in travelers or in new arrivals to endemic areas

In travelers, the dermatitis is maculopapular, evanescent, and often restricted to one area of the body and rarely leads to chronic skin disease. Lymphedema is more commonly a presenting symptom in travelers with onchocerciasis. The risk of ocular disease, typically related to microfilarial burden, is exceedingly low in travelers to onchocerca-endemic regions of the world, in large part because travelers most commonly have light infections [16, 17].

## Diagnosis

Definitive diagnosis depends on finding an adult worm in an excised nodule or, more commonly, microfilariae in a skin snip.

### Skin snip

A small piece of skin is elevated by the tip of a needle or skin hook held parallel to the surface, and a razor or scalpel blade is used to shave off the skin area stretched across the top surface of the needle. Alternatively, a corneoscleral punch can be used to obtain a blood-free circular skin specimen.

Skin snips are generally obtained from an area of affected skin or from the scapular, gluteal, and calf areas (in the African form) or the scapular, deltoid, and gluteal areas (in the Central American form). Once obtained, the skin snips are incubated in a physiological solution (such as normal saline); the emergent microfilariae can be seen under a microscope after 1–4 hours. Occasionally, in light infections, overnight incubation is necessary.

### Serodiagnosis

Although a rapid format card test [18] specific for onchocerciasis has been developed, only standard antifilarial antibody testing is widely available. As for lymphatic filariasis, serology in travelers is useful only when negative because it excludes onchocerciasis as a diagnostic possibility. Because onchocerciasis is often coendemic with other filariae, positive serology would not be sufficiently specific for presumptive therapy.

### Molecular diagnosis

Highly specific and sensitive PCR-based assays have been developed for the detection of *O. volvulus* DNA in skin snips that are microscopically negative [19]. This has proven useful in the detection of very low infection levels, but requires expensive equipment and reagents, as well as rigorous training and quality control, and is not widely available.

## Treatment

The major goals of therapy are to prevent irreversible lesions and to alleviate bothersome symptoms. Surgical excision of nodules is recommended when the nodules are located on the head because of the proximity of the microfilaria-producing adult worms to the eye, but chemotherapy is the mainstay of treatment.

Ivermectin, a semisynthetic macrocyclic lactone, is considered first-line therapy for onchocerciasis. It is given orally in a single dose of 150 µg/kg [20]. It is characteristically given annually or semiannually. With treatment, most patients have a mild or no reaction. Pruritus, cutaneous edema, and/or a maculopapular rash occur in approximately 1–10% of treated individuals. Significant ocular complications are extremely rare, as is hypotension (1 in 10,000). Contraindications to treatment include pregnancy, breastfeeding, age < 5 years, and CNS disorders that might increase the penetration of ivermectin into the CNS (e.g., meningitis).

Although treatment with ivermectin results in a marked drop in microfilarial density, its effect can be short-lived (much less than 6 months in some cases). Thus, it is occasionally necessary to give ivermectin more frequently for persistent symptoms. A 6-week course of doxycycline has been demonstrated to be macrofilaristatic (rendering the female adult worms sterile for long periods), thereby providing sustained microfilarial suppression [21].

## Prevention

Vector control has been beneficial in highly endemic areas in which breeding sites are vulnerable to insecticide spraying, but most onchocerciasis-endemic areas are not suited to this type of control. Community-based administration of ivermectin every 6–12 months is now being used to interrupt transmission in endemic areas. This measure, in conjunction with vector control, has already helped to reduce the prevalence of the disease in endemic foci in Africa and Latin America [22]. No drug has proven useful for prophylaxis of O. volvulus infection in travelers, nor have truly effective personal protective measures been identified.

## Loiasis

The distribution of L. loa is limited to the rain forests of West and Central Africa. Tabanid flies (deerflies) of the genus Chrysops are the intermediate hosts. The adult parasite lives in the subcutaneous tissues in humans; then microfilariae circulate in the bloodstream with diurnal periodicity.

## Clinical manifestations

L. loa infection may be present as asymptomatic microfilaremia, with the infection being recognized only after subconjunctival migration of an adult worm (the so-called eye worm). Other patients have episodic Calabar swellings. If the associated inflammation extends to the nearby joints or peripheral nerves, corresponding symptoms (e.g., entrapment neuropathy or arthritis) can develop. Nephropathy, encephalopathy, and cardiomyopathy can occur, but rarely.

## Clinical manifestations in travelers or in new arrivals to endemic areas

There appears to be a difference between the presentation of loiasis in those native to the endemic area and visitors [23]. The latter tend to have a greater predominance of allergic symptomatology. The episodes of Calabar swellings tend to be more frequent and debilitating, and such patients rarely have microfilaremia. In addition, visitors have extreme elevation of eosinophils in the blood, as well as marked increases in antifilarial antibody titers.

Typically, acquisition of loiasis requires exposure in a loa-endemic region of Africa (limited regions of West and Central Africa) for more than a month [2].

## Diagnosis

Definitive diagnosis is made through parasitological examination, either by finding microfilariae in the peripheral blood, or by isolating the adult worm from the eye (or in subcutaneous biopsy material following treatment). Molecular diagnostics (PCR) can be used for definitive diagnosis as well. However, the diagnosis must often be made on clinical grounds, particularly in travelers (usually amicrofilaremic) to the endemic region.

## Treatment

DEC (8–10 mg/kg per day for 21 days) is effective against both the adult and the microfilarial forms of L. loa, but multiple courses are frequently necessary before the loiasis resolves completely. In heavy microfilaremia, allergic or other inflammatory reactions can take place during treatment, including CNS involvement with coma and encephalitis. Heavy infections can be treated initially with apheresis to remove the microfilariae and with glucocorticoids (40–60 mg of prednisone per day) followed by doses of DEC (0.5 mg/kg per day). If antifilarial treatment has no adverse effects, the prednisone dose can be rapidly tapered off and the dose of DEC gradually increased to 8–10 mg/kg per day. Albendazole or ivermectin (although neither is approved for this use by the Food and Drug Administration) has been shown to be effective in reducing microfilarial loads, but ivermectin has been associated with severe adverse reactions (including death) in heavily microfilaremic patients with loiasis [24].

## Prevention

DEC (300 mg weekly) has been shown to be an effective prophylactic regimen for loiasis [25]. Typically, this should be reserved for people traveling to highly endemic countries (e.g., Cameroon, Nigeria, Gabon) for stays longer than a month.

## *Mansonella ozzardi* infection

The distribution of *Mansonella ozzardi* is restricted to Central and South America and certain Caribbean islands. The parasite is transmitted to the human host by biting midges *(Culicoides furens)* and blackflies *(S. amazonicum).* Although adult worms have only twice been recovered from humans, studies on the microfilariae show that they circulate in the bloodstream with little periodicity. The pathology of *M. ozzardi* infection is poorly characterized. Many consider it to be nonpathogenic [26]. However, headache, articular pain, fever, pulmonary symptoms, adenopathy, hepatomegaly, and pruritus have been ascribed to infection with this organism [27]. Eosinophilia accompanies *M. ozzardi* infection as well. Diagnosis is made by demonstrating the characteristic microfilariae in the peripheral blood. DEC has little or no effect on this infection, but ivermectin has been shown to be effective in reducing symptoms and circulating microfilariae.

## Perstans filariasis

*M. perstans* is distributed across the center of Africa and in northeastern South America. The infection is transmitted to humans through the bites of midges *(Culicoides* spp.). The adult worms reside in the body cavities (pericardial, pleural, peritoneal), as well as in the mesentery and the perirenal and retroperitoneal tissues. The microfilariae circulate in the blood without periodicity. As with *M. ozzardi* (see preceding discussion), the pathology relating to this infection is ill defined [28].

Although most patients appear to be asymptomatic, clinical manifestations of this infection include transient angioedematous swellings of the arms, face, or other body parts (not unlike the Calabar swellings of *L. loa* infection); pruritus; fever; headache; arthralgias; neurological or psychological symptoms; and right upper quadrant pain. Occasionally, pericarditis and hepatitis occur.

The diagnosis is made through parasitological evaluation by finding the microfilariae in the blood or in other body fluids (serosal effusions). Perstans filariasis is often associated with peripheral blood eosinophilia and antifilarial antibody elevations.

Although most studies have failed to demonstrate the efficacy of standard antifilarial regimens in reducing Mp microfilarial levels, recent data suggest that combination therapy with DEC and mebendazole may be more effective. Doxycycline is also effective in the treatment of this infection in those regions where the *Mansonella perstans* contains *Wolbachia* (e.g., Mali, Cameroon).

## Streptocerciasis

*M. streptocerca (Dipetalonema streptocerca, Tetrapetalonema streptocerca)* is largely found in the tropical forest belt of Africa from Ghana to Zaire. It is transmitted to the human host by biting midges (*Culicoides* spp.).

The pathology of streptocerciasis is both dermal and lymphatic [29]. In the skin, there are hypopigmented macules (and occasionally papular rashes) that are thought to be secondary to inflammatory reactions around microfilariae. The distribution of the parasite in the skin of the human host tends to be across the shoulders and upper torso. Lymph nodes of affected individuals may show chronic lymphadenitis with scarring.

The major clinical manifestations are related to the skin pruritus, papular rashes, and pigmentation changes. Most infected individuals also show inguinal lymphadenopathy; however, many patients are completely asymptomatic.

The diagnosis is made after finding the characteristic microfilariae on skin-snip examination. DEC is particularly effective in treating infection by both the microfilarial and the adult form of the parasite. The recommended dosage is 6 mg/kg per day in divided doses for 21 days. After treatment, as in onchocerciasis, the following symptoms often present: urticaria, arthralgias, myalgias, headaches, and abdominal discomfort. Ivermectin at a dose of 150 µg/kg has a salutary microfilaricidal effect and is likely to achieve primacy in the treatment of this infection [30].

## References

1 Nutman TB. Experimental infection of humans with filariae. *Rev Infect Dis* 1991;13(5):1018–22.

2 Lipner EM, Law MA, Barnett E, et al. Filariasis in travelers presenting to the GeoSentinel surveillance network. *PLoS Negl Trop Dis* 2007;1(3):e88.

3 Freedman DO, de Almeida Filho PJ, Besh S, Maia e Silva MC, Braga C, Maciel A. Lymphoscintigraphic analysis of lymphatic abnormalities in symptomatic and asymptomatic human filariasis. *J Infect Dis* 1994;170:927–33.

4 Amaral F, Dreyer G, Figueredo-Silva J, et al. Live adult worms detected by ultrasonography in human Bancroftian filariasis. *Am J Trop Med Hyg* 1994;50:753–7.

5 Dreyer G, Noroes J, Rocha A, Addiss D. Detection of living adult *Wuchereria bancrofti* in a patient with tropical pulmonary eosinophilia. *Braz J Med Biol Res* 1996;29:1005–8.

6 Dreyer G, Medeiros Z, Netto MJ, Leal NC, de Castro LG, Piessens WF. Acute attacks in the extremities of persons living in an area endemic for bancroftian filariasis: differentiation of two syndromes. *Trans R Soc Trop Med Hyg* 1999;93(4):413–17.

7 Wartman WB. Filariasis in American armed forces in World War II. *Medicine* 1947;26:332–92.

8 Moore TA, Reynolds JC, Kenney RT, Johnston W, Nutman TB. Diethylcarbamazine-induced reversal of early lymphatic dysfunction in a patient with bancroftian filariasis: assessment with use of lymphoscintigraphy. *Clin Infect Dis* 1996;23:1007–11.

9 Dondero TJ Jr, Mullin SW, Balasingam S. Early clinical manifestations in filariasis due to *Brugia malayi*: observations in man. *Southeast Asian J Trop Med Publ Health* 1972;3:569–75.

10 Eberhard ML, Lammie PJ. Laboratory diagnosis of filariasis. *Clin Lab Med* 1991;11:977–1010.

11 Shenoy RK, Suma TK, Kumaraswami V, et al. Doppler ultrasonography reveals adult-worm nests in the lymph vessels of children with brugian filariasis. *Ann Trop Med Parasitol* 2007 Mar;101(2):173–80.

12 Mand S, Supali T, Djuardi J, Kar S, Ravindran B, Hoerauf A. Detection of adult *Brugia malayi* filariae by ultrasonography in humans in India and Indonesia. *Trop Med Int Health* 2006 Sep;11(9):1375–81.

13 Taylor MJ, Makunde WH, McGarry HF, Turner JD, Mand S, Hoerauf A. Macrofilaricidal activity after doxycycline treatment of *Wuchereria bancrofti*: a double-blind, randomised placebo-controlled trial. *Lancet* 2005;365(9477):2116–21.

14 El Setouhy M, Ramzy RM, Ahmed ES, et al. A randomized clinical trial comparing single- and multi-dose combination therapy with diethylcarbamazine and albendazole

for treatment of bancroftian filariasis. *Am J Trop Med Hyg* 2004;70(2):191–6.

15 Ottesen EA, Nutman TB. Tropical pulmonary eosinophilia. *Annu Rev Med* 1992;43:417–24.

16 McCarthy JS, Ottesen EA, Nutman TB. Onchocerciasis in endemic and nonendemic populations: differences in clinical presentation and immunologic findings. *J Infect Dis* 1994;170:736–41.

17 Pryce D, Behrens R, Davidson R, Chiodini P, Bryceson A, McLeod J. Onchocerciasis in members of an expedition to Cameroon: role of advice before travel and long term follow up. *BMJ* 1992;304:1285–6.

18 Weil GJ, Steel C, Liftis F, et al. A rapid-format antibody card test for diagnosis of onchocerciasis. *J Infect Dis* 2000;182:1796–9.

19 Zimmerman PA, Guderian RH, Aruajo E, et al. Polymerase chain reaction-based diagnosis of onchocerca volvulus infection: improved detection of patients with onchocerciasis. *J Infect Dis* 1994;169:686–9.

20 Greene BM, Taylor HR, Cupp EW, et al. Comparison of ivermectin and diethylcarbamazine in the treatment of onchocerciasis. *N Engl J Med* 1985;313:133–8.

21 Hoerauf A, Volkmann L, Hamelmann C, et al. Endosymbiotic bacteria in worms as targets for a novel chemotherapy in filariasis. *Lancet* 2000;355(9211):1242–3.

22 Thylefors B, Alleman M. Towards the elimination of onchocerciasis. *Ann Trop Med Parasitol* 2006;100(8):733–46.

23 Klion AD, Massougbodji M, Sadeler B-C, Ottesen EA, Nutman TB. Loiasis in endemic and non-endemic populations: immunologically mediated differences in clinical presentation. *J Infect Dis* 1991;163:1318–25.

24 Chippaux JP, Boussinesq M, Gardon J, Gardon-Wendel N, Ernould J-C. Severe adverse reaction risks during mass treatment with ivermectin in loiasis-endemic areas. *Parasitol Today* 1996;12:448–50.

25 Nutman TB, Miller KD, Mulligan M, et al. Diethylcarbamazine prophylaxis for human loiasis. Results of a double-blind study. *N Engl J Med* 1988;319:752–6.

26 McNeeley DF, Raccurt CP, Boncy J, Lowrie RC Jr. Clinical evaluation of *Mansonella ozzardi* in Haiti. *Trop Med Parasitol* 1989;40:107–10.

27 Marinkelle CJ, German E. Mansonelliasis in the Comisaria del Vaupes of Colombia. *Trop Geogr Med* 1970;22:101–11.

28 Stott G. Pathogenicity of *Acanthocheilonema perstans*. *J Trop Med Hyg* 1962;65:230–32.

29 Meyers WM, Connor DH, Harman LE, Fleshman K, Moris R, Neafie RC. Human streptocerciasis. A clinico-pathologic study of 40 Africans (Zairians) including identification of the adult filaria. *Am J Trop Med Hyg* 1972;21:528–45.

30 Fischer P, Bamuhiiga J, Buttner DS. Treatment of human *Mansonella streptocerca* infection with ivermectin. *Trop Med Int Health* 1997;2:191–9.

# Human Trypanosomiasis: African and American Trypanosomiasis (Chagas Disease)

Johannes A. Blum

Swiss Tropical Institute, Basel, Switzerland

## Human African trypanosomiasis or sleeping sickness

Human African trypanosomiasis (HAT), or sleeping sickness, is caused by the protozoan parasites *Trypanosoma brucei gambiense* (*T. b. gambiense*, the West African form) and *Trypanosoma brucei rhodesiense* (*T. b. rhodesiense*, the East African form), both transmitted by the bite of the tsetse fly, *Glossina* sp.

The disease appears in two stages, the early or hemolymphatic and the late or meningoencephalitic. The latter is characterized by invasion of the CNS by trypanosomes.

*T. b. gambiense* HAT is characterized by a chronic progressive course, lasting months to years, leading to death if left untreated. *T. b. rhodesiense* HAT, however, is usually acute and death occurs within weeks or months.

HAT seems to be a re-emerging infection in Sub-Saharan Africa, and in the last decade, increasing reports in travelers have been documented.

## Epidemiology

### Epidemiology in endemic countries

In Africa, an estimated 50,000–70,000 individuals are infected with HAT and 17,000–37,000 new cases are diagnosed per year. Sixty million people are at risk of contracting the disease in over 36 countries. The distribu-

tion of the disease is in tropical Africa between 15°N and 20°S latitude. Areas most affected are parts of the Democratic Republic of Congo (DRC), Angola, and South Sudan (Figure 26.1). In endemic countries, *T. b. gambiense* infections are currently responsible for over 96% of all reported HAT cases. HAT is commonly transmitted in rural regions. Nevertheless, a recent description of HAT among urban residents of Kinshasa (DRC) and Daloa (Ivory Coast) demonstrates that residents of periurban belts can also be affected.

### Epidemiology of HAT in travelers

HAT due to *T. b. gambiense* is very rare among short-term tourists, but has been reported in immigrants, refugees, and long-term expatriate residents living in rural settings. Because of its long incubation time and chronicity, HAT has to be considered even if the last visit to an endemic region occurred many years before.

In contrast, *T. b. rhodesiense* HAT may be seen in short-term tourists traveling to East African game reserves, mainly in Tanzania [1, 2], but also in Botswana, Rwanda, Kenya, Zambia, and Malawi. A cluster of nine tourists traveling to Serengeti and Tarangire National Parks in Tanzania acquired *T. b. rhodesiense* HAT in 2001 [1].

## Clinical presentation

The clinical presentation of HAT (see Table 26.1) is different in local populations and immigrants when compared to travelers or expatriates returning from Africa. Therefore, the two groups are described separately here.

*Tropical Diseases in Travelers*, 1st edition. Edited by E. Schwartz.
© 2009 by Blackwell Publishing, ISBN: 978-1-4051-8441-0.

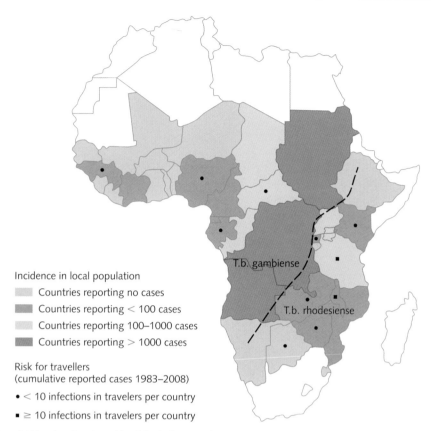

**Figure 26.1** Map of Africa showing the epidemiological status of countries considered endemic for human African trypanosomiasis. (Courtesy of Pere P. Simarro, WHO, PloS Medicine.)

### *T. b. gambiense* HAT in local populations

The incubation period of *T. b. gambiense* HAT is not well defined, but can be months or years. The disease may progress for months or years before the correct diagnosis is established. A trypanosomal chancre (local reaction at the location of the tsetse fly bite) is rarely seen. Chronic and intermittent fever, headache, pruritus, lymphadenopathy, and, to a lesser extent, hepatosplenomegaly are the leading signs and symptoms of the first stage. After several months, with the invasion of the CNS by the trypanosomes, sleep disturbances and neuropsychiatric disorders dominate the clinical presentation and fever is rarely seen. The most important symptoms and signs are as follow:

- Pruritus and sensory disorders such as hyperesthesia or paresthesia are often severe, long-lasting, and accompanied by scratch marks on the skin.
- Lymphadenopathy is characterized by enlarged lymph nodes, which are commonly small (1–2 cm), painless,

mobile, numerous, and typically localized in the neck region.
- Sleep disorder is the leading symptom after which sleeping sickness is named, already observed in the nineteenth century. Patients with sleeping sickness have frequent short episodes of sleep during the day and night. The total time of sleep is equal to that of healthy people. Lhermitte described this sleep as follows:

> Sleep overcomes the patient in a rapid and brutal way: sleep occurs during a conversation without finishing the sentence or during meals with a full mouth; the head sinks to the breast and the sleep is complete. During the first crisis it is possible to awake the patient, but in repeated crisis attempts to awake the patient are fruitless.

Somnographic studies have since confirmed these historic findings and demonstrated that the disease causes

**Table 26.1** Signs and symptoms according to stage and population affected.

| | | HAT (*T. b. gamb.*) Early stage | HAT (*T. b. gamb.*) Late stage | HAT (*T. b. rhod.*) Early stage | HAT (*T. b. rhod.*) Late stage |
|---|---|---|---|---|---|
| Chancre at inoculation site | Locals | <5% | | 5–20% | |
| | Travelers | 21–50% | | 51–80% | |
| Trypanosomal rash | Locals | 0 | | 0 | |
| | Travelers | Unknown | | 21–50% | |
| Fever | Locals | 21–50% | 5–20% | 51–80% | 51–80% |
| | Travelers | > 80% | > 80%[a] | > 80% | > 80% |
| Lymphadenopathy | Locals | 51–80% | 51–80% | | 51–80% |
| | Travelers | > 80%, satellite to inoculation site | | > 80% (satellite to inoculation site) | 51–80%[a] |
| Sleeping disorder | Locals | 20–80%[a] | 20–80% | < 5% | 51–80% |
| | Travelers | Unknown[a] | Unknown[a] | | |
| Laboratory findings | Locals | Usually normal | Usually normal | Unknown[a] | Unknown[a] |
| | Travelers | Leukopenia, thrombopenia, anemia, elevated CRP, abnormal liver and renal function[a] | Unknown | Leukopenia thrombopenia, anemia, elevated CRP, abnormal liver and renal function | Leukopenia thrombopenia, anemia, elevated CRP, abnormal liver and renal function[a] |
| Pruritus | Locals | 51–80 % | 21–50% | <5% | 21–50% |
| | Travelers | Unknown | | <5% | <5%[a] |
| Headache | Locals | 51–80% | 51–80% | 51–80% | 51–80%[a] |
| | Travelers | > 80%[a] | Unknown[a] | > 80% | > 80% |
| Hepatomegaly, splenomegaly | | 51–80% | 21–50% | 5–50% | 5–50% |
| Neurological signs | Locals | <20% | 20–80% | <5% | 21–50% |
| | Travelers | Unknown[a] | 50–80%[a] | <5% | Unknown[a] |

[a] Only a limited number of patients.

dysregulation of the circadian rhythm of the sleep/wake cycle and a fragmentation of the sleeping pattern, characterized by the occurrence of sleep-onset rapid-eye-movement (SOREM), rather than the frequently reported "inversion of sleep" [3].
- The neurological symptoms include tremor, general motor weakness, paralysis of an extremity, hemiparesis, akinesia, and abnormal movements, such as dyskinesia, chorea–athetosis, Parkinson-like movements due to muscular hypertension, unspecific movement disorders, and speech disorders. These disorders are rarely seen during the first stage and increase with the duration of the disease, reflecting the severity of the affliction. Abnormal archaic reflexes can also be observed.
- Psychiatric symptoms such as psychotic reactions, aggressive behavior, or inactivity with apathy may

dominate the clinical picture. In Europe, immigrants have been wrongly hospitalized in psychiatric clinics.
- Cardiac involvement documented by ECG alterations is frequently seen, but rarely of clinical relevance. The most frequent ECG changes are depolarization changes and low voltage, but not—in contrast to Chagas heart disease—conduction problems and blocks [4].
- Endocrine disorders, comprising hypo- and hyperfunction of the thyroid and adrenal cortex, rarely demand specific treatment [5]. The circadian rhythm of secretion of prolactin, renin, growth hormone, and cortisol levels disappears in severe cases [3].

### T. b. rhodesiense HAT

*T. b. rhodesiense* is a more acute disease. Patients progress within a few weeks to the second stage, and death occurs within 6 months. The clinical presentation is similar, but trypanosomal chancres are more often seen, the localization of enlarged lymph nodes is submandibular, axillary, and inguinal rather than nuchal, and edemas are more frequently observed. Enlargement of lymph nodes can be in the draining area of the trypanosomal chancre or can be generalized. Compared to *T. b. gambiense* HAT, thyroid dysfunction, adrenal insufficiency, and hypogonadism are more frequently found, and myocarditis is more severe and may even be fatal [6].

### Clinical presentation in travelers (T. b. gambiense and T. b. rhodesiense HAT)

The symptomatology of travelers is markedly different from the usual textbook descriptions of African HAT patients, and is similar for *T. b. gambiense* and *T. b. rhodesiense* HAT [7, 8]. The onset of the disease is almost invariably acute and of the febrile type, with temperatures of up to 40–41°C [9, 10], regardless of where the infection was acquired. A chancre at the inoculation side is frequent and a trypanosomal rash may be observed on the white skin. Headache is a common sign of *T. b. rhodesiense*. Routine laboratory tests are more seriously disturbed.

*T.b. rhodesiense* HAT has a short incubation period of a few days in tourists (<3 weeks) and is acute, life-threatening with high fever, headache, and a trypanosomal chancre as the leading signs and symptoms [1,2,8].

The most important symptoms and signs include the following:
- According to most case reports, acute high *fever* is the leading symptom and a diagnosis is often made at this stage. If left untreated, the pyrexial episodes become irregular (*T.b. gambiense* and *T.b. rhodesiense*). Each at-

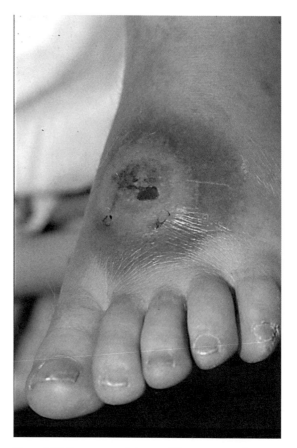

**Figure 26.2** Trypanosomal chancre. (Photo courtesy of A. Moore, E. Ryan.)

tack may last from a day to a week and attacks may be separated by from a few days to month-long intervals [7]. Hyperpyrexia is a common, but not constant feature and is more likely to appear in the early phase of the illness.
- A trypanosomal chancre (Figure 26.2) consists of a tender, purplish area of induration, which develops at the infecting tsetse bite. The lesion develops within 5–15 days, may ulcerate, and is often accompanied by a satellite lymphadenopathy. Within a few weeks, the chancre disappears without leaving a trace. It is seen in about two-thirds of *T. b. rhodesiense* HAT patients and a quarter of *T. b. gambiense* HAT patients.
- Trypanosomal rash (Figure 26.3), which may appear at any time after the first febrile episode, consists of blotchy irregular erythematous macules with a diameter of up to 10 cm. A large proportion of the macules develop a central area of normal-colored skin, giving the rash a circinate or

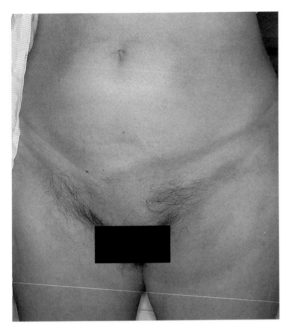

**Figure 26.3** Trypanosomal rash. (Photo courtesy of Ezzedine K. From Ezzedine K, Darie H, Le Bras M, Malvy D. Skin features accompanying imported human African trypanosomiasis: hemolymphatic *Trypanosoma gambiense* infection among two French expatriates with dermatologic manifestations. *J Travel Med* 2007 May–Jun;14(3):192–6.

serpiginous outline. The trunk is chiefly affected and the erythema is seldom marked. The rash is evanescent, fading in one place and reappearing in another over a period of several weeks. It is not tender and does not itch [7, 9].
• Severe headache may be associated with the febrile attacks.
• Enlargement of lymph nodes can occur in the draining area of the trypanosomal chancre or can be generalized.
• Psychiatric alterations include behavior abnormalities even in the first stage and severe sleeping disturbances or psychotic reactions in the second stage.
• Nonspecific gastrointestinal symptoms such as nausea, vomiting, or diarrhea may accompany HAT [1].
• Cardiac signs include ECG alterations due to myopericarditis (ST-T wave changes) and conduction problems such as transient AV block III, supraventricular tachycardia and ventricular premature captures (class Lown IV b) and transient second-degree heart block.

## Laboratory findings
One can observe slight anemia and impaired renal function among *T. b. gambiense* HAT patients [4, 5]. However,

liver enzymes, lactate dehydrogenase, creatinine kinase, and blood sugar are mostly normal [11]. In tourists with *T. b. rhodesiense* HAT, the routine chemistry is more seriously disturbed: severe hematological disorders such as thrombopenia, leukopenia, and anemia, severely impaired renal function, electrolyte disturbances, and highly elevated levels of C reactive protein, liver enzymes, bilirubin, and lactate dehydrogenase have been described [2, 8].

## Radiological findings
Because CT scan may be normal, magnetic resonance imaging (MRI) is usually preferred. The understanding of MRI alterations in HAT patients is based on a few case reports. The alterations are multifarious and include symmetrical, focal lesions, diffuse hyperintensity, brain edema with demyelination and brain atrophy, and multiple abnormal signals. The alterations were localized in the brainstem, basal ganglia, white matter, and central gray matter. The lesions shown on MRI disappear after treatment.

## Diagnosis
The diagnosis is based on visualization of the parasite in lymph node aspirate, peripheral blood, or CSF, PCR technology, and serological tests.

Often, because of the high and constant parasitemia in tourists affected by *T. b. rhodesiense*, the visualization of the parasite in the blood smear poses no problem. In contrast, the number of parasites in the peripheral blood in *T. b. gambiense* HAT can be very low, less than 100 trypanosomes/ml, which is below the detection limit of the most sensitive methods in use today. Failure to demonstrate parasites, therefore, does not necessarily exclude infection. Microscopic examination of wet blood films, Giemsa stained thin blood films, or thick blood films has a detection limit as high as 5000–10,000 trypanosomes/ml. The sensitivity can be improved by using more sophisticated concentration methods such as microhematocrit centrifugation techniques or quantitative buffy coat (detection limit: 450–500 trypanosomes/ml). The mini-anion-exchange centrifugation technique enables the detection of less than 100 trypanosomes/ml, but is not available in most laboratories. The sensitivity of parasitological examination of the lymph node aspirate varies between 40% and 80% [12].

A delay between sampling and examination can lead to a false negative result since trypanosomes do not survive a long time after sampling. Additionally, the sample should be sent to the laboratory at a temperature of 2–8°C (not frozen), be protected from sunlight, and be tested within 12 hours. Recognition of the parasite, mainly in thick blood smears and lymph node aspirates, requires experienced laboratory technicians. Detection by PCR is sensitive, but has not yet been fully validated and is not yet routinely available.

The Card Agglutination Test for Trypanosomiasis (CATT/*T. b. gambiense*) is a cost-efficient screening method for mass screening for West African HAT. In most endemic regions, its sensitivity varies from 87% to 98%. However, the CATT test is not sensitive for *T. b. rhodesiense*. For *T. b. rhodesiense* HAT, a serological test (IFAT) is performed at the Institut voor Tropische Geneeskunde (Klinik Leopold II, Antwerp). However, not all serological tests for HAT are validated in travelers, their sensitivity varies from region to region, and their specificity can be as low as 61%.

The invasion of the CNS by the parasite brings about the second stage of the disease and is defined by changes in the CSF determined mainly by an elevated white blood cell count (WBC; $> 5/mm^3$) or the presence of trypanosomes. Unfortunately, the limited sensitivities of these analyses may lead to incorrect identification of the stage of HAT. The presence of intrathecal immunoglobulin M (IgM) or interleukin 10 reflects the stage significantly better than the WBC count in the CSF [13], but is not yet completely validated and commercially available.

## Treatment

The choice of drug is directed by the species and the stage of the disease. During the second stage, only drugs with the capacity to pass the blood–brain barrier should be applied. Treatment recommendations are summarized in Table 26.2. However, often the limited availability of drugs outside of endemic regions, as well as time constraints, determines the choice of drug. Thus, in patients with first stage *T. b. rhodesiense* HAT, pentamidine was used until suramin became available.

**Table 26.2** Treatment of HAT according to stage.

|  | *T. b. gambiense* | *T. b. rhodesiense* |
| --- | --- | --- |
| First or early stage | Pentamidine | Suramin |
| Second or late stage | Eflornithine, Melarsoprol | Melarsoprol |

In endemic regions, a pretreatment of highly endemic concomitant diseases is traditionally recommended that includes treatment against malaria and worms. HAT patients co-infected with malaria have a prolongation of the QTc time (Bazett formula: $QTe = QT/SQR (RR)$) with a theoretical risk of arrhythmia [4]. In travelers, the exclusion of malaria and treatment of proven coexisting infection is ideal before treatment of HAT. However, in the case of *T. b. rhodesiense* HAT, the advantage of such treatment has to be balanced against the risk of progression to the second stage because of the risks associated with the delay of HAT treatment.

Because of the paucity of HAT outside Africa, treatment recommendations are based on studies conducted in endemic regions. National guidelines for dosages and schedules vary and have never been compared with each other. Only melarsoprol and eflornithine treatment schedules are based on international trials [14].

Recent data suggest that the combination of nifurtimox for 10 days with eflornithine for 7 days is better tolerated than eflornithine alone in *T.b. gambiense* HAT patients. However, the limited availability of nifurtimox hampers its use, and the treatment is not yet fully validated or formally recommended. A short-course melarsoprol treatment (daily injections of 2.2 mg/kg for 10 days) is established for *T. b. gambiense* HAT. For *T. b. rhodesiense* HAT, it is under evaluation, and preliminary results show no inferiority to the classical schedule.

In second-stage *T. b. rhodesiense* HAT, a pretreatment with suramin is proposed in some national guidelines to reduce parasitemia before the initiation of melarsoprol.

Treatment schedules, adverse effects, and their management are summarized in Table 26.3. The most feared complications of sleeping sickness treatment with melarsoprol are encephalopathic syndromes comprising convulsions, progressive coma, and psychotic reactions. They occur more frequently in *T. b. rhodesiense* HAT (10%) than in *T. b. gambiense* HAT (5%) and have a fatality rate of about 50%. It is impossible to predict the risk of developing an encephalopathic syndrome based on the signs and symptoms before treatment initiation. The prophylactic use of prednisone reduces both the incidence and the mortality of the syndrome. In the absence of controlled trials, there are currently no guidelines for treatment of encephalopathic syndromes. However, dexamethasone 0.5–0.6 mg/kg/day divided into 4–6 doses against cerebral edema, anticonvulsive treatment in the presence of convulsions, correction of electrolyte dysbalance, and vasoactive substances to control arterial hypotension are recommended.

**Table 26.3** Treatment schedules, adverse effects, and their management.

| Drug | Adverse effect | Management/follow up |
|---|---|---|
| Pentamidine<br>4 mg/kg at 24-hourly intervals<br>for 7 days i.m. (or as i.v. short infusion) | Aseptic abscess (accidental contact of pentamidine with the subcutaneous tissue) | Pentamidine has to be injected slowly and strictly intramuscularly with a long needle (50 mm). |
| | Diabetes, hypoglycemia, proteinuria | Fasting glycemia and urine for proteinuria and glycosuria have to be checked before every injection and 3 weeks and 2 months after the last injection |
| | Rhabdomyolysis | Creatinine kinase in case of clinical signs of rhabdomyolysis such as myalgia or kidney failure |
| | Hypotension | Blood pressure and heart rate have to be measured before and after the injection (every 15 minutes for 1 hour) |
| | Subjective complaints, myalgia, nausea and gustative abnormalities, headache, pain on the injection side, abdominal pain | |
| Suramin<br>Test dose of 200 mg i.v.<br>20 mg/kg days 1, 3, 7, 14, and 21 | Immediate reactions:<br>Gastrointestinal: nausea, vomiting, colic pain<br>Allergic reactions: anaphylactic shock (less than 1/2000), urticaria | Slow i.v. injection<br>Facilities for treatment of anaphylactic shock should be available |
| | Late reactions (3–48 hours):<br>Febrile reaction, mainly after the first injection (due to lysis of the trypanosomes), photophobia, lacrimation, hyperesthesia | |
| | Delayed reactions:<br>Common: kidney damage, proteinuria (usually mild)<br>Rare: allergic dermatitis, polyneuropathia agranulocytosis, hemolytic anemia | Urine and kidney function before each administration<br>Red and white blood cell count before each administration<br>Neurological examination |
| Melarsoprol<br>*T. b. gambiense*:<br>2.2 mg/kg i.v. 10 daily doses<br>*T. b. rhodesiense* (Tanzania):<br>(Pretreatment with suramin:<br>day 1: 0.5 g, day 2 and 3: 1 g)<br>3 series of 3 days with 1-week interval:<br>  day 1: 2.16 mg/kg<br>  day 2: 2.52 mg/kg<br>  day 3: 2.88 mg/kg; interval of 7 days<br>  day 4: 2.88 mg/kg<br>  day 5: 3.24 mg/kg<br>  day 6: 3.6 mg /; interval of 7 days<br>  days 7–9: 3.6 mg/kg | Encephalopathic reaction: convulsions, progressive coma | Prevention: concomitant administration of prednisone (1 mg/kg) [19]<br><br>Treatment: dexamethasone 0.5–0.6 mg/kg/day divided in 4–6 doses, anticonvulsive and vasoactive medication if needed<br><br>Treatment may be restarted after disappearance of symptoms [20]. |

**Table 26.3**  (*Continued*)

| Drug | Adverse effect | Management/follow up |
|---|---|---|
| | Skin reactions: Maculopapular or bullous eruptions, exfoliative dermatitis | Stop treatment, corticosteroids Treatment may be restarted after disappearance of rash |
| | Polyneuropathy (motor and sensitivity) | |
| | Diarrhea, hypotension | Daily control of blood pressure and pulse rate |
| | Cardiac involvement: arrhythmia, ECG alterations [4], cardiac failure | Daily control of blood pressure and pulse rate ECG days 0, 3, 7 Arrhythmia: corticosteroids |
| | Phlebitis at injection site | Local antiphlogistic treatment |
| Eflornithine [21]: 100 mg/kg short infusions at intervals of 6 h for 14 days | Convulsions 2–7% | Anticonvulsive medication; treatment may be continued |
| | Bone marrow toxicity, anemia, leucopenia, thrombopenia, risk of secondary bacterial infections [21] | Hemoglobin, WBC, and platelets twice weekly Rapid treatment of bacterial infections |
| | Gastrointestinal: diarrhea, nausea, vomiting, abdominal pain | Symptomatic treatment |

## Prognosis in travelers

The prognosis depends on the disease stage. Whereas most patients diagnosed during the early stage have a favorable outcome, in tourists with late-stage HAT severe disease with renal failure demanding hemodioalysis [8], multiorgan failure, disseminated intravascular coagulation, and coma [1] is commonly reported and 10–20% die [1]. Therefore, rapid diagnosis and treatment are crucial.

## Prevention

No vaccine is available, and chemoprophylaxis is not recommended, because of the toxicity of the available drugs and the low risk of infection. The only preventive measure is the reduction of tsetse fly bites. The flies are attracted to bright or contrasting colors, particularly blue, as well as to the dust and motion of vehicles. They can bite through thin clothes, and insect repellents provide only partial protection. As routine preventive measures, travelers should avoid known areas of tsetse fly infestation, travel in cars with screened or closed windows in endemic foci, use insect repellent, and wear wrist- and ankle-length clothes.

After a tsetse fly bite, the patient has to be observed. The risk of infection is low. In the case of a chancre, fever, or other symptoms, trypanosomes have to be looked for in an aspirate of the chancre, in the blood, and, eventually, in a lymph node aspirate.

## American trypanosomiasis (Chagas disease)

Chagas disease is caused by the protozoan parasite *T. cruzi*. It is transmitted by deposits of infected feces of reduviid bugs on the skin, which are rubbed into skin lesions or into the conjunctiva, and by the oral ingestion of uncooked food that has been contaminated with infected reduviid feces. Congenital and nosocomial transmission is also observed. Chagas disease develops in phases. The acute phase presents with fever, myalgia, headache, and the Romaña sign (unilateral painless periorbital edema at the site of parasite entry). The acute phase is followed by an asymptomatic, indeterminate phase. Only 10–30% of patients develop chronic Chagas disease with cardiomyopathy or chronic gastrointestinal disease.

## Epidemiology

### Endemic countries

Chagas disease occurs mainly in Latin America, where over 20 million people were thought to be infected during the 1980s. Since then, Latin American countries have made an enormous effort to control the infection, and current estimates suggest that fewer than 8 million people remain infected.

### Chagas in the Western world

The risk of Chagas disease is minimal in returning travelers, and no cases have yet been reported in travelers. However, because of the length of the indeterminate phase, Chagas has to be considered in Latin American immigrants even if they left the endemic country decades before.

According to estimates, the prevalence of *T. cruzi* in Latin American immigrants is 16 per 1000, 9 per 1000, 25 per 1000, and 8–50 per 1000 in Australia, Canada, Spain, and the USA, respectively [15]. The transmission of Chagas disease is no longer confined to the Americas because it is transmitted through blood transfusions and organ transplants. Since 2007, the screening of blood for Chagas disease has been proposed in the USA and is under discussion in Europe.

### Chagas heart disease

Only 10–30% of patients develop chronic Chagas cardiopathy, characterized by chronic inflammation with mononuclear cell infiltration, loss of myocardial cells, and diffuse fibrosis affecting the cardiac muscle and the conduction system. Right bundle branch block or left anterior hemiblock precedes other manifestations of chronic heart disease in the majority of cases. Progression of the disease leads to cardiac dilatation and biventricular failure. Prominent features of advanced Chagas heart disease include left ventricular apical aneurism and combinations of complex ventricular arrhythmias, sinus bradyarrhythmias, and intraventricular or atrioventricular conduction blocks. The most common causes of death are sudden death due to arrythmia, progressive heart failure, and, to a lesser extent, embolism of mural thrombi to the brain or other organs [16]. Thromboembolic stroke may be the first manifestation of Chagas heart disease.

### Extracardiac Chagas disease

Neurological findings are rare in Chagas disease. Meningoencephalitis occurs mainly in acute Chagas disease in children under the age of 2, including congenital cases, and in immunosuppressed patients. HIV-infected patients with chronic Chagas disease may present with acute and severe illness, in particular meningoencephalitis and myocarditis. The intestinal form of Chagas disease usually manifests as megaesophagus and megacolon and may or may not be associated with the cardiac form. Its frequency varies between 10% and 20% [17].

### Diagnosis

Serological testing is the standard diagnostic tool. PCR is indicated in acute Chagas disease, in Chagas patients with immunosuppression, and in neonates from mothers with positive Chagas serology. The indication for diagnostic testing is summarized in Table 26.4.

### Treatment

Treatment of congestive heart failure is the principal treatment in Chagas disease. The effect of antiparasitic treatment is still debated and depends on the age of the patient.

**Table 26.4** Chagas disease: indications for serologic testing.

- Latin American immigrant or person who received blood or an organ by a Latin American immigrant
- *and* one of the following clinical criteria
  - Cardiac failure, cardiac arrhythmia
  - ECG: right bundle branch block or left anterior hemiblock
  - Stroke without cardiovascular risk factor
  - Immunosuppression
  - Pregnancy (risk of congenital transmission 1–10%)
  - Blood donation or organ transplantation

According to recent recommendations, antitrypanosomal treatment is suggested for all cases of acute and congenital Chagas disease and for children 18 years or younger. For adults aged 19–50 years without advanced Chagas disease cardiomyopathy, drug treatment should generally be offered. It is optional for those more than 50 years of age because of the higher risk of adverse advents than for younger adults [18]. The management of chagasic congestive heart failure is in general the same as with other heart diseases. A recent review article on the management of Chagas disease written by Bern et al. can be recommended to clinicians with special interest [18].

## Prevention

The use of bed nets in houses possibly infected with reduviids (poorly constructed houses), the avoidance of uncooked food and drinks, and the screening of blood for Chagas disease are proposed as preventive measures.

## Acknowledgments

I thank Christian Burri, Gabriele Pohlig, and Christoph Hatz for their valuable comments.

## References

1 Jelinek T, Bisoffi Z, Bonazzi L, van Thiel P, Bronner U, de Frey A, et al. Cluster of African trypanosomiasis in travelers to Tanzanian national parks. *Emerg Infect Dis* 2002;8(6):634–5.

2 Moore AC, Ryan ET, Waldron MA. Case records of the Massachusetts General Hospital. Weekly clinicopathological exercises. Case 20-2002. A 37-year-old man with fever, hepatosplenomegaly, and a cutaneous foot lesion after a trip to Africa. *N Engl J Med* 2002;346(26):2069–76.

3 Buguet A, Bourdon L, Bisser S, Chapotot F, Radomski MW, Dumas M. [Sleeping sickness: major disorders of circadian rhythm]. *Med Trop (Mars )* 2001;61(4–5):328–39.

4 Blum JA, Burri C, Hatz C, Kazumba L, Mangoni P, Zellweger MJ. Sleeping hearts: the role of the heart in sleeping sickness (human African trypanosomiasis). *Trop Med Int Health* 2007;12(12):1422–32.

5 Blum JA, Schmid C, Hatz C, Kazumba L, Mangoni P, Rutishauser J, et al. Sleeping glands?—The role of endocrine disorders in sleeping sickness (*T. b. gambiense* human African trypanosomiasis). *Acta Trop* 2007;104(1):16–24.

6 Reincke M, Arlt W, Heppner C, Petzke F, Chrousos GP, Allolio B. Neuroendocrine dysfunction in African trypanosomiasis. The role of cytokines. *Ann N Y Acad Sci* 1998;840:809–21.

7 Duggan AJ, Hutchinson MP. Sleeping sickness in Europeans: a review of 109 cases. *J Trop Med Hyg* 1966;69(6):124–31.

8 Oscherwitz SL. East African trypanosomiasis. *J Travel Med* 2003;10(2):141–3.

9 Ezzedine K, Darie H, Le Bras M, Malvy D. Skin features accompanying imported human African trypanosomiasis: hemolymphatic *Trypanosoma gambiense* infection among two French expatriates with dermatologic manifestations. *J Travel Med* 2007;14(3):192–6.

10 Iborra C, Danis M, Bricaire F, Caumes E. A traveler returning from Central Africa with fever and a skin lesion. *Clin Infect Dis* 1999;28(3):679–80.

11 Bisser S, Bouteille B, Sarda J, Stanghellini A, Ricard D, Jauberteau MO, et al. [Contribution of biochemical tests in the diagnosis of the nervous phase of human African trypanosomiasis]. *Bull Soc Pathol Exot* 1997;90(5):321–6.

12 Chappuis F, Loutan L, Simarro P, Lejon V, Buscher P. Options for field diagnosis of human African trypanosomiasis. *Clin Microbiol Rev* 2005;18(1):133–46.

13 Lejon V, Buscher P. Review article: cerebrospinal fluid in human African trypanosomiasis: a key to diagnosis, therapeutic decision and post-treatment follow-up. *Trop Med Int Health* 2005;10(5):395–403.

14 Schmid C, Richer M, Bilenge CM, Josenando T, Chappuis F, Manthelot CR, et al. Effectiveness of a 10-day melarsoprol schedule for the treatment of late-stage human African trypanosomiasis: confirmation from a multinational study (Impamel II). *J Infect Dis* 2005;191(11):1922–31.

15 Schmunis GA. Epidemiology of Chagas disease in nonendemic countries: the role of international migration. *Mem Inst Oswaldo Cruz* 2007;102(Suppl 1): 75–85.

16 Maguire JH. Chagas' disease—can we stop the deaths? *N Engl J Med* 2006;355(8):760–61.

17 Barrett MP, Burchmore RJ, Stich A, Lazzari JO, Frasch AC, Cazzulo JJ, et al. The trypanosomiases. *Lancet* 2003;362(9394):1469–80.

18 Bern C, Montgomery SP, Herwaldt BL, Rassi A Jr, Marin-Neto JA, Dantas RO, et al. Evaluation and treatment of Chagas disease in the United States: a systematic review. *JAMA* 2007;298(18):2171–81.

19 Pepin J, Tetreault L, Gervais C. [The use of oral corticosteroids in the treatment of human African trypanosomiasis: a retrospective survey in Nioki, Zaire]. *Ann Soc Belg Med Trop* 1985;65(1):17–29.

20 Blum J, Nkunku S, Burri C. Clinical description of encephalopathic syndromes and risk factors for their occurrence and outcome during melarsoprol treatment of human African trypanosomiasis. *Trop Med Int Health* 2001;6(5):390–400.

21 Chappuis F, Udayraj N, Stietenroth K, Meussen A, Bovier PA. Eflornithine is safer than melarsoprol for the treatment of second-stage *Trypanosoma brucei gambiense* human African trypanosomiasis. *Clin Infect Dis* 2005;41(5):748–51.

# 27 Cystic Echinococcosis

Enrico Brunetti

University of Pavia and IRCCS S. Matteo Hospital Foundation, Pavia, Italy

## Introduction

Cystic echinococcosis (CE), also known as hydatidosis, is an infection caused by the larval stage (metacestode) of *Echinococcus granulosus*. In humans, it may result in a wide spectrum of clinical manifestations, ranging from asymptomatic infection to severe, even fatal disease. *E. granulosus* has a worldwide distribution; areas of highest prevalence are those where sheep are grazed using dogs.

In recent times, CE is increasingly seen in immigrants from endemic areas to Western countries where either the disease is virtually unknown or its prevalence is low. It is rarely reported as a travel-related disease, that is, in short-term travelers to endemic areas, partly because the hydatid cyst typically grows slowly and may long remain clinically silent.

Of three forms of echinococcosis occurring in humans, cystic echinococcosis (CE) and alveolar echinococcosis, the latter caused by *E. multilocularis*, are of special importance because of their wide geographic distribution and their medical and economic impact. Alveolar echinococcosis will not be discussed in this chapter, given its limited relevance in travel medicine. Polycystic echinococcosis (caused by *E. vogeli* and *E. oligarthrus*) is less frequent and is restricted to Central and South America.

## General epidemiology

*E. granulosus* has a broad geographic range, in all continents and in circumpolar, temperate, subtropical, and tropical zones. The highest prevalence of the parasite is found in parts of Eurasia, Africa, Australia, and South America (Figure 27.1). Within the endemic zones, the prevalence of the parasites varies from sporadic to high, but only a few countries can be regarded as being free of *E. granulosus*.

The true incidence is difficult to determine because of the slow growth and variable clinical presentation. In addition, most epidemiological reports are based on hospital- and surgery-based surveys that greatly underestimate the actual rates of infection, especially in low socioeconomic groups with limited access to diagnosis and treatment. Thus, the public health importance of this zoonosis remains underappreciated [1].

Since the mid-1980s, however, mass community-based surveys using portable ultrasound scanners have been conducted in many remote, rural areas of the world, including Tunisia, Libya, Tanzania, Kenya, Sudan, Ethiopia, Argentina, Uruguay, and China. The sensitivity and specificity of ultrasound have also been shown to be superior to those of serology in prevalence surveys [2]. These studies showed the real burden of the disease, uncovering infection rates of up to 6.6% [3].

Numerous studies have provided evidence that *E granulosus* exists as a complex of different strains, which differ in a wide variety of aspects that have an impact on the epidemiology, pathology, and control of CE. To date, 10 distinct genotypes (G1–G10) have been identified. The great majority of *E. granulosus* isolates from human patients thus far characterized by genotype have been of the sheep genotype (G1).

Comparative maturation and growth rates of most of the genotypic variants are currently not available: further studies in this area might provide information about possible differences in the clinical presentation of CE acquired in different parts of the world. What we know applies primarily to genotype G1 in sheep and canid hosts.

The adult intestinal form of *E. granulosus* is a small tapeworm 3–6 mm long, attached to the small intestines of the definitive canid hosts (dogs, coyotes, wolves). Cysts occur in herbivore intermediate hosts (sheep, cattle, goats).

*Tropical Diseases in Travelers*, 1st edition. Edited by E. Schwartz.
© 2009 by Blackwell Publishing, ISBN: 978-1-4051-8441-0.

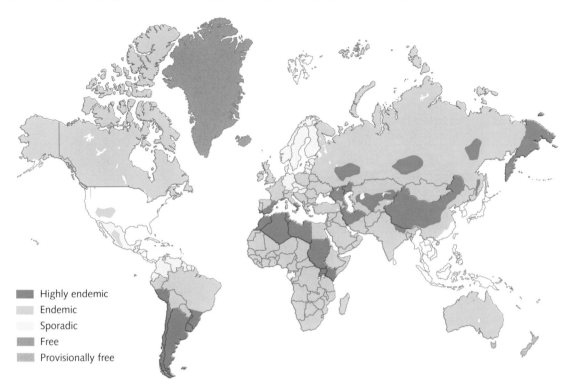

**Figure 27.1** Geographic distribution of *E. granulosus*. (From Eckert J, Gemmell MA, Meslin F-X, and Pawlowski ZS, editors, *WHO/OIE Manual on Echinococcosis in Humans and Animals: a Public Health Problem of Global Concern*. Paris (France): World Health Organization; 2001.)

In the typical dog–sheep cycle, *Echinococcus* eggs are passed in the feces of an infected dog and may be ingested by grazing sheep. They hatch into embryos in the intestine, penetrate the intestinal mucosa, and are carried by the blood to the major filtering organs, the liver and lungs. After the developing embryos localize in a specific organ or site, they transform into cysts. The cysts contain small tapeworm heads, or protoscoleces.

Protoscoleces are infective to dogs that may ingest viscera containing echinococcal cysts because of the habit in endemic countries of feeding dogs viscera of home-slaughtered sheep or other livestock. Protoscoleces attach to the dog's intestinal mucosa, where they develop into mature adult tapeworms, capable of starting the life cycle over.

Humans may become infected by ingesting tapeworm eggs passed from an infected carnivore (Figure 27.2). This occurs most frequently when individuals handle or contact infected dogs or other infected carnivores or inadvertently ingest food or drink contaminated with fecal material containing tapeworm eggs.

## Epidemiology in travelers

Most cases of CE in nonendemic countries—and increasingly in Western European countries that are endemic in certain areas—are seen in immigrants from endemic countries [4, 5]. Reports of travelers from nonendemic areas who travel frequently to highly endemic areas and have become infected during these trips are exceptional [6].

In a world where the frequency of international travel is reaching levels previously unknown, control programs and prevention are crucial not only for the resident populations but also for international travelers to these areas, and hence to health systems geographically remote from endemic areas. Infectious diseases and travel medicine consultants should add CE to the list of very rare diseases that can be acquired during international travels.

There appear to be no differences between CE in local residents and travelers. However, as very little is known about the influence of genotypic strains (see above) and

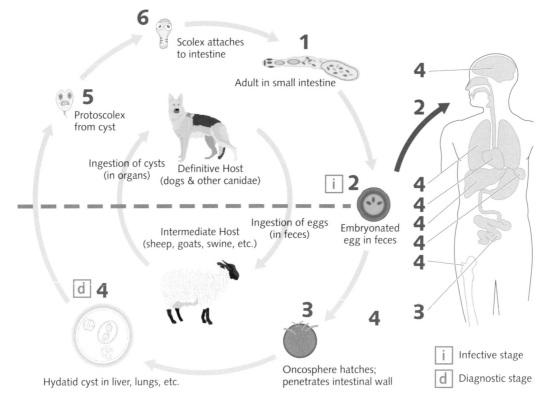

**6** Scolex attaches to intestine

**1** Adult in small intestine

**5** Protoscolex from cyst

Ingestion of cysts (in organs)

Definitive Host (dogs & other canidae)

**4**

**2**

|i| **2** Embryonated egg in feces

Ingestion of eggs (in feces)

Intermediate Host (sheep, goats, swine, etc.)

**4**
**4**
**4**
**4**
**4**

|d| **4**

**3** Oncosphere hatches; penetrates intestinal wall

**4**

**3**

Hydatid cyst in liver, lungs, etc.

|i| Infective stage

|d| Diagnostic stage

**Figure 27.2** Life cycle of *E. granulosus*. (From CDC Web site. Available from URL: http//www.dpd.cdc.gov/dpdx/html/echinococcosis.htm.)

host factors [7] on the development of the cysts, future studies might advance our knowledge on the subject.

## Clinical aspects

The liver is the organ most frequently involved in CE (approximately two-third of patients); the second most often involved organ is the lung.

In each anatomic site, cysts are surrounded by the peri-parasitic host tissue (pericyst), which encompasses the endocyst of larval origin. The endocyst has an outer, acellular laminated layer and an inner, or germinative, layer that gives rise to brood capsules and protoscoleces (Figures 27.3 and 27.4). The cyst is filled with clear fluid, numerous brood capsules and protoscoleces. Some cysts may also harbor daughter cysts of variable size. The growth rate of the cysts is variable. The average increase of cyst diameter is thought to be of order 1 cm/year, but data on natural history are scarce.

The presentation of human CE is protean. Patients come to the clinician's attention for different reasons, such as when a large cyst has some mechanical effect on organ function or rupture of a cyst causes acute hypersensitivity reactions. Often, the cyst is diagnosed accidentally during radiographic examination, body scanning, or surgery or for other clinical reasons.

Common symptoms are upper abdominal discomfort and pain, poor appetite, and a mass in the abdomen. Physical findings are hepatomegaly, a palpable mass if on the surface of the liver or other organs, and abdominal distention. If cysts in the lung rupture into the bronchi, an intense cough may develop, followed by vomiting of hydatid material and cystic membranes.

Cysts in the liver should be included in the differential diagnosis of several conditions, such as jaundice, colic-like pains, liver abscess, portal hypertension, ascites, compression of the inferior vena cava, and Budd–Chiari syndrome. Cysts in the lung should be included in the differential diagnosis of tumor of the chest, chest pain, chronic cough,

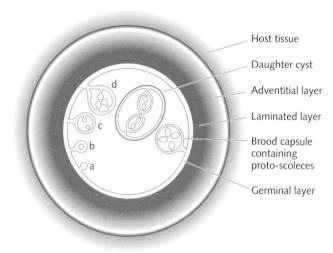

Host tissue

Daughter cyst

Adventitial layer

Laminated layer

Brood capsule
containing
proto-scoleces

Germinal layer

**Figure 27.3** Diagrammatic representation of the metacestode of *E. granulosus*. (From Eckert J, Gemmell MA, Meslin F-X, and Pawlowski ZS, editors, *WHO/OIE Manual on Echinococcosis in Humans and Animals: a Public Health Problem of Global Concern.* Paris (France): World Health Organization; 2001.)

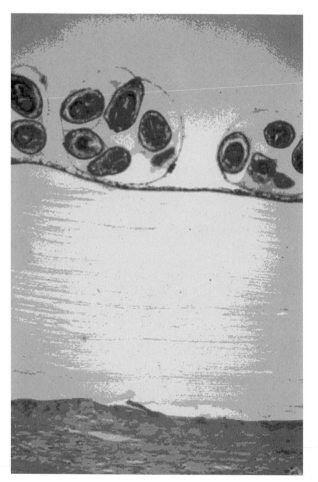

**Figure 27.4** Cross-section of echinococcal cyst showing (bottom up) pericyst, laminated layer, and germinal layer with brood capsules, each containing protoscoleces. (From Busilacchi P, Rapaccini L, editors, *Ecografia Clinica*, Naples (Italy): Idelson-Gnocchi; 2006; Courtesy Professor HM Seitz, Dept. of Parasitology, University of Bonn, Bonn, Germany.)

pneumothorax, eosinophilic pneumonitis, pleural effusion, parasitic lung embolism, hemoptysis, and biliptysis.
Cysts in the heart can cause a cardiac mass, pericardial
effusion, and embolism. Cysts in the breast need to be
differentiated from neoplasms. Cysts located in the spine
and in the brain can cause serious neurological symptoms,
including paralysis and seizures.

Acute infection in humans has never been documented
[8], so all we know about it comes from experimental
studies in animal intermediate hosts. Cavity formation
and development of both germinal and laminated layers of
the cyst wall occur 10–14 days post-infection. Formation
of brood capsules and protoscoleces requires a longer time
period (10 months to 4 years in sheep).

## Diagnosis

The diagnosis of CE is based mainly on imaging methods
and on serology, with the latter having a minor, confirmatory role. *E. granulosus* eggs are shed with the feces by
the definitive hosts (canids) but not by intermediate hosts
(Figure 27.2). Therefore, direct diagnosis in human intermediate hosts is only possible through demonstration of
viable protoscoleces in the cyst, which can be obtained at
surgery or by percutaneous aspiration. The latter cannot
be performed routinely for technical and safety reasons
(see section on percutaneous treatments below).

Routine laboratory tests do not show specific results.
In patients with rupture of the cyst in the biliary tree,
marked and transient elevation of cholestatic enzyme levels occurs, often in association with hyperamylasemia and
eosinophilia (up to 60%). In most cases, eosinophilia is
limited (<15%) or absent.

## Imaging
The introduction of modern imaging tools (ultrasound
and CT and, to a lesser extent, MRI) has revolutionized
the diagnosis and clinical management of CE.

Ultrasound is the procedure of choice for diagnosing asymptomatic cystic echinococcosis because it is safe,
noninvasive, and relatively inexpensive. Cysts in every part
of the abdomen and in muscles can be imaged with ultrasonography.

Ultrasound is useful in longitudinal studies, such as
monitoring the response of cysts to treatment and recording cyst growth rate.

Various classifications exist of ultrasonographic pictures in cystic echinococcosis, the most widely used being the one proposed by Gharbi et al. in the early 1980s
[9]. In 2003, the World Health Organization Informal
Working Group on Echinococcosis (WHO-IWGE) proposed a standardized ultrasound classification based on
the active–transitional–inactive status of the cyst, as suggested by its sonographic appearance [10] (Figure 27.5).
The standardized classification scheme is intended to promote uniform standards of diagnosis and treatment and
may be applied to the clinical treatment of patients as well
as to field diagnostic surveys.

In this classification, six cyst stages have been defined
and assigned to three clinical groups. The active group includes developing cysts, which may be unilocular (CE1) or
multivesicular with daughter cysts (class CE2) and which
are usually found to be viable. The transitional group
(class CE3) contains cysts that are usually starting to de-
generate (internal membrane detachment and predominantly solid cysts with daughter cysts), which may be
either viable or nonviable by light microscopy. The inactive group (classes CE4 and CE5) exhibit involution and
signs of solidification of cyst content with increasing degrees of calcification and are nearly always found to be
nonviable.

The WHO classification provides a rational basis
for choosing an appropriate CE treatment scheme and
follow-up: surgery, percutaneous treatment, such as PAIR
(puncture– aspiration–injection–reaspiration), benzimidazole chemotherapy, or simply "watch and wait." The
WHO classification recognizes two basic types of morphology for CE3: the *water-lily sign* for floating membranes, which is now known as subclass CE3a, and predominantly solid cysts with daughter cysts, or subclass
CE3b. This subdivision has been proposed based on their
different responses to PAIR and albendazole, which is generally good for CE3a and poor for CE3b. A recent study
has used nuclear magnetic resonance spectroscopy to shed
some light on the metabolic reasons for this different behavior [11].

Radiographic examination is useful for cysts in the
lungs, bone, and muscle and for detecting calcified cysts.

Echocardiography may be used to detect cardiac
lesions.

CT scanning has the advantage of inspecting any organ (lung cysts can be explored with ultrasonography
only if they are superficially located), detecting smaller
cysts located outside the liver, locating cysts precisely,
and sometimes differentiating parasitic from nonparasitic

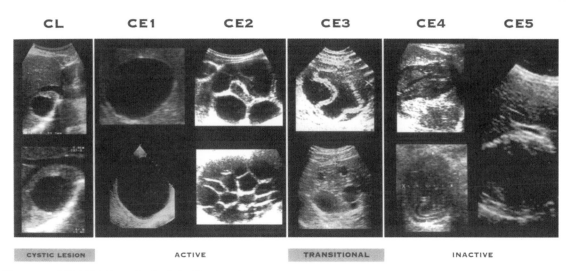

**Figure 27.5** WHO/IWGE standardized classification of echinococcal cysts. (From WHO-IWGE, http://whqlibdoc.who.int/hq/2001/WHO_CDS_CSR_APH_2001.6.pdf.)

cysts. However, the cost of CT scanning is not affordable in several endemic countries.

MRI may have some advantages over CT scanning in the evaluation of postsurgical residual lesions, recurrences, and selected extrahepatic infections, such as cardiac infections [12].

Cystic echinococcosis is one of the few parasitic infections in which the basis for *laboratory* diagnosis is primarily serology and not direct search for the parasite in stool or organs.

## Serology

Serological tests are useful for confirming presumptive imaging diagnoses; however, the limitations of serodiagnosis in CE must be borne in mind to interpret the findings correctly. False positive reactions, which occur relatively frequently in persons with other helminthic infections, cancer, and chronic immune disorders, may be misleading. False negative test results may occur in 50% of patients with solitary lung cysts.

Detectable immune responses have been associated with the location, integrity, and vitality of the larval cyst. Hepatic cysts are more likely to elicit an immune response than pulmonary cysts. Regardless of localization, antibody detection tests are least sensitive in patients with intact endocysts (CE1).

Serological tests are usually positive when the endocyst is detached (CE3a) and in the active (CE2) or transitional (CE3b) stage. With few exceptions, serological tests are negative in patients with inactive cysts (CE 4 and CE 5). Although no longitudinal, prospective studies exist on this subject, serological titers slowly decrease when a cyst becomes inactive (CE4, CE5) and after radical surgery. Titers may long remain positive after conservative surgery, in which the antigen source (the germinal layer) is not completely removed.

Serotiters usually increase immediately after medical or percutaneous treatments because of the mobilization of the antigen following disruption of cyst integrity, and slowly decrease several months after treatment, provided it has been successful (permanent solidification of the cyst has been obtained).

Cysts in the lungs, brain, and spleen are associated with lower serodiagnostic reactivity, whereas those in bone appear to stimulate detectable antibody more regularly. Cysts of the brain or eye and calcified cysts often induce no or low antibody titers. Children aged 3–15 years may produce minimal serological reactions. In other words, it appears that the sensitivity of serological tests is inversely related to the degree of sequestration of the hydatid antigens inside cysts, regardless of the location.

Given the complexity of clinical pictures, especially when cysts at different stages are simultaneously present in the same liver, it is very difficult to use serology to assess response to treatment. This difficulty is compounded by false positive tests in patients who have undergone radical surgery (with complete removal of the antigen source) and whose serological tests nonetheless remain constantly positive [13]). Research is needed to clarify these issues and avoid overtreatment.

The indirect hemagglutination (IHA) test and enzyme-linked immunosorbent assay (ELISA) are the most widely used methods for detection of anti-*Echinococcus* antibodies (immunoglobulin G, IgG).

Specific confirmation of reactivity can be obtained by demonstrating echinococcal antigens by immunoblot assays (8-, 16-, and 21-kD bands). These are the most *E. granulosus*–specific tests described, but they may be detected in serum of patients with other forms of echinococcosis (e.g., alveolar echinococcosis, caused by *E. multilocularis*, whose prognosis and treatment are different from those of *E. granulosus*) and 5% to 10% of patients with *Taenia solium* cysticercosis [14].

### Other diagnostic procedures

Fine-needle aspiration biopsy of a cyst performed under ultrasonographic guidance, with a transhepatic approach, under anthelmintic coverage, is generally safe and useful for differentiation of cystic echinococcosis, malignancy, abscesses, and nonparasitic cysts. The procedure must be carried out in the presence of an anesthesiologist ready to manage the rare, but possible, anaphylactic reaction.

Fine-needle aspiration biopsy may be particularly helpful in cases with no detectable anti-*Echinococcus* serum antibodies and inconclusive imaging appearance. The hooks are usually numerous and can be found even in bacteriologically infected and/or degenerating cysts.

### Treatment

Until recently, surgery was the only option for treatment of echinococcal cysts. However, in the past 20 years, chemotherapy with benzimidazole compounds and, more recently, cyst puncture and percutaneous treatments have been introduced and, increasingly, are supplementing or even replacing surgery as the preferred treatment. Experienced clinicians also increasingly choose expectant management, or "watch and wait," for uncomplicated inactive (CE4 and CE5) liver cysts.

### Surgery

Surgical procedures can be conservative or radical. Conservative surgery aims at the sterilization and evacuation of cyst content and partial removal of the cyst. This is carried out by puncture of the cyst, partial aspiration of the content to permit introduction of the scolecidal agent,

and total aspiration thereafter. The risks are anaphylactic shock; chemical cholangitis or alveolar/bronchial damage, if the cyst communicates with the biliary or bronchial tree, and spillage of cyst content and secondary echinococcosis. Relapse rates of up to 20% are reported after surgery of liver cysts [15] and up to 11% for lung cysts [16].

Radical surgery aims at complete removal of the cyst with or without hepatic or lung resection. Peripherally located lung cysts of any size and small to medium-sized centrally located cysts can be excised without sacrificing lung parenchyma. Standard radical procedures are wedge resection of lung parenchyma of less than one segment, and for liver and lung cysts, segmentectomy and lobectomy. Total cystectomy is the ideal procedure [15] to reduce complication and relapse rates.

Radical procedures bear greater intraoperative risks, with fewer postoperative complications and relapses [15, 17].

Conservative procedures are preferred for lung cysts, with radical procedures such as segmentectomy and lobectomy required for extended parenchymal involvement, severe pulmonary suppuration, and complications such as pulmonary fibrosis, bronchiectasis, or severe hemorrhage [16].

In patients with complicated cysts (rupture, cystobiliary and most cases of cystobronchial fistula, compression of vital organs and vessels, hemorrhage, secondary bacterial infection), surgery maintains its place as the treatment of choice [18].

### Medical therapy

Benzimidazole carbamates (mebendazole and albendazole) are anthelmintic drugs that have proved effective against the larval stages of *E. granulosus*. Since the early 1980s, chemotherapy has been used for treatment of human echinococcosis. Mebendazole was introduced first, but albendazole became the drug of choice because of its better absorption and better clinical results. Drugs were given in 3-month cycles interrupted for 2 weeks after 28 days, but this scheme appeared to be parasitostatic rather than parasitocidal. Therefore, continuous daily treatment for a 3-month period was introduced.

In a study with the largest series published to date, patients with one single cyst were treated with mebendazole or albendazole for a period of 3–6 months. At 22 (12–170) months follow-up, success rate (i.e., cyst "solidification" rate; Figure 27.6) was 74% in all patients.

The efficacy of albendazole (82%) was superior to that of mebendazole (56%). Relapse rate was 25% in both treatment groups. Most relapses (78%) occurred within

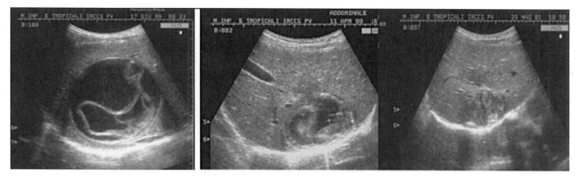

**Figure 27.6** Progressive decrease in size and solidification of a CE3a cyst after treatment with albendazole over 2 years. The cyst goes from CE3a to CE4 stage. (From Busilacchi P, Rapaccini L, editors, *Ecografia Clinica*, Naples (Italy): Idelson-Gnocchi; 2006.)

2 years after the end of treatment. More than 90% of these cysts responded well to additional courses of benzimidazoles.

Extended post-treatment monitoring is crucial to assess the success rate: 22% of relapses occurred between 2 to 8 years following treatment.

Multivesicular cysts, hepatic cysts, and cysts in older patients responded less well to treatment than univesicular cysts, pulmonary cysts, and cysts in younger patients (< 30 years of age), respectively [19].

The natural course of pulmonary hydatid cysts was prospectively studied by comparing albendazole treatment with a placebo. The efficacy of albendazole was superior to that of the placebo (71% of the cysts improved in the treatment group compared to 15.4 % in the placebo group) [20].

Benzimidazoles are also important for perioperative administration. This is done with the intent of softening the cyst before the intervention, thus reducing the risk of spillage and secondary echinococcosis following seeding of the peritoneal cavity [21]. Although the efficacy of perioperative prophylaxis has never been properly studied, it is generally adopted as a cautionary measure.

Contraindications to chemotherapy include chronic hepatic disease and bone marrow depression. Because benzimidazole drugs are teratogenic, they should never be administered to pregnant women.

Albendazole is generally safe and well tolerated, but it is important to monitor patients on a monthly basis during treatment. Rises in hepatic enzymes may be observed, but they are thought to be the result of immunological responses (damage and immune uncloaking of the parasite by the drug), leading to local inflammation, rather than the expression of drug toxicity. These effects are tempo-

rary and, if rise of transaminases is higher than seven- to eightfold, treatment can be stopped for a month, allowing enzymes to go back to normal. On resumption of treatment, this effect is generally either absent or less marked.

Some clinical evidence [22] suggests that the addition of praziquantel to albendazole may be helpful. One potential advantage is that praziquantel and albendazole interact, producing increased plasma concentrations of both drugs [23].

## Percutaneous treatment

Percutaneous treatment for abdominal CE was introduced in the mid-1980s following the diffusion of minimally invasive procedures made possible by the widespread use of new imaging tools, particularly CT and ultrasound. Initially received with skepticism by some, it developed into an attractive alternative to surgery and benzimidazole derivatives for certain cyst stages.

These treatment modalities aim to destroy the germinal layer with scolecidal agents or to evacuate the entire endocyst.

The most popular method in the first group is PAIR (short for Puncture, Aspiration, Injection of a scolecidal agent, and Reaspiration), whereas several modified catheterization techniques belong to the second, and are generally reserved for cysts that are difficult to drain, or tend to relapse after PAIR (multivesicular cysts or cysts with predominantly solid content and daughter cysts). They are based on the aspiration of the solid contents of the cyst, the germinal and the laminated layer, through a large-bore catheter or device. Two types of approaches are currently in use, the catheterization technique and the modified catheterization techniques, in particular PEVAC

(Percutaneous EVACuation), MoCaT (Modified Catheterization Technique), and DMFT (Dilatable Multi Function Trocar).

The puncture of echinococcal cysts has long been discouraged because of risks of anaphylactic shock and spillage of the fluid; however, as experience with ultrasonography-guided intervention has increased since the early 1980s, a growing number of articles have reported its effectiveness and safety in treating abdominal, especially liver, echinococcal cysts. At least 4209 cysts have been punctured, either for diagnostic or for therapeutic purposes, and 16 cases of anaphylactic shock (2 of them lethal, = 0.047%) have been reported. Peritoneal seeding has never been reported [24].

Under albendazole coverage, cysts are punctured under ultrasonographic or CT guidance either with a needle or with a catheter, according to their size. Albendazole is given to prevent secondary echinococcosis in case of intraperitoneal spillage, but has no role in avoiding anaphylactic shock. The presence of an anesthesiologist who can intervene in case of allergic manifestations or anaphylactic shock is mandatory. Usually, a small quantity of fluid is first aspirated and examined by light microscopy to observe for the presence of viable protoscoleces (Figure 27.7). If they are present, the cyst is aspirated completely.

At this point, contrast medium is injected into the cavity to exclude connections of the cyst with the biliary tree and the cyst is viewed by fluoroscopy. If no connections are evident, a scolecidal agent, usually hypertonic sodium chloride solution or ethanol, is injected, left for a variable period (usually 5–30 min), and then reaspirated. The destruction of protoscoleces can be observed in fluid samples aspirated after the injection of a scolecidal agent.

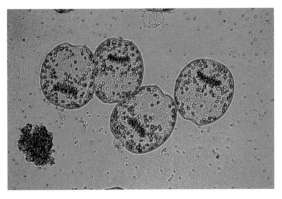

**Figure 27.7** Viable protoscoleces seen under light microscopy examination after aspiration from a CE1 cyst.

As happens with drug therapy, positive responses include both a decrease in cyst size and a progressive change in echo pattern (generally solidification) (Figure 27.6).

PAIR is a valuable alternative to surgery in terms of cost containment and hospitalization time. In CE1 and CE3a echinococcal cysts, PAIR is an effective therapeutic tool. The use of PAIR should be reserved to referral or specialized centers where teams are well prepared to deal with possible complications.

## Clinical decision-making

The treatment of CE is difficult for a number of reasons. Locations as different as liver, brain, muscle, and bone present different sets of problems with respect to surgical or percutaneous access. CE is a dynamic condition, with cyst stages changing over time from active to transitional or to inactive, either spontaneously or following treatment other than radical surgery. Biologically active stages may be clinically silent, whereas inactive cysts can produce serious complications.

There are currently three treatment options that have evolved over decades without adequate evaluation of efficacy, effectiveness, rate of adverse reactions, relapse rate, and cost.

Evidence for clinical decisions is generally at the level of expert opinion. Growing experience with classifying and following up echinococcal cysts with ultrasound is enabling clinicians to assign treatment options to cyst stages, especially for cysts located in the liver.

Although reliable data and confidence intervals for effectiveness, relapse rates, adverse events, and cost effectiveness are still lacking, clinical experience from referral centers supports the following conclusions. Active CE1 or transitional CE3a cysts < 5 cm tend to respond well to ABZ; cysts from 5 to 10 cm and > 10 cm respond to PAIR plus albendazole. Catheterization techniques are more effective in giant cysts. CE2 and CE3b should be treated with catheterization techniques because they respond poorly to both PAIR and ABZ. Uncomplicated CE4 and CE5 located in the liver can be followed up at regular intervals without any treatment ("watch and wait") (Table 27.1).

## Prevention

Current control programs are predominantly based on control of dog populations, regular dosing of dogs with praziquantel or arecoline hydrobromide to eliminate *E. granulosus*, improved control of animal slaughter, and

**Table 27.1** Suggested treatment for uncomplicated echinococcal cysts of the liver.

|      | S   | M                     | L             |
| ---- | --- | --------------------- | ------------- |
| CE1  | ABZ | PAIR + ABZ fine needle | PAIR catheter |
| CE2  |     | Large-bore catheter   |               |
| CE3a | ABZ | PAIR + ABZ fine needle | PAIR catheter |
| CE3b |     | Large-bore catheter   |               |
| CE 4 |     | Watch and wait        |               |
| CE 5 |     | Watch and wait        |               |

S < 5cm
M 5–10 cm
L > 10 cm

improved sanitation and health education (avoidance of contact with dog feces, hand washing, etc.). Control programs are costly and may require more than 30 years for substantial control to be achieved, depending on the control strategy employed in a given area.

Despite ongoing control efforts, few countries have been able to substantially reduce or eradicate CE [25].

Interruption or disruption of control programs can have disastrous consequences for the health of citizens of the country in which this occurs [26] and in the long term for travelers to the area [6].

Recent evidence points to a reemergence of CE as a public health problem of increasing concern in a number of countries where control programs have been reduced because of economic problems and lack of resources, or have yet to be fully instigated.

It is likely that, unless government health authorities prioritize the disease and instigate appropriate control methods, *E. granulosus* will persist or reemerge in many endemic areas worldwide, causing severe disease and considerable economic loss.

# References

1 Budke CM. Global socioeconomic impact of cystic echinococcosis. *Emerg Infect Dis* 2006;12(2):296–303.

2 MacPherson CN, Romig T, Zeyhle E, Rees PH, Were JB. Portable ultrasound scanner versus serology in screening for hydatid cysts in a nomadic population. *Lancet* 1987;2(8553): 259–61.

3 Schantz PM, Wang H, Qiu J, Liu FJ, Saito E, Emshoff A, et al. Echinococcosis on the Tibetan Plateau: prevalence and risk factors for cystic and alveolar echinococcosis in Tibetan populations in Qinghai Province, China. *Parasitology* 2003;127 Suppl:S109–20.

4 Yuan WH, Lee RC, Chou YH, Chiang JH, Chen YK, Hsu HC. Hydatid cyst of the liver: a case report and literature review. *Kaohsiung J Med Sci* 2005;21(9):418–23.

5 Chrieki M. Echinococcosis—an emerging parasite in the immigrant population. *Am Fam Physician* 2002;66(5):817–20.

6 Brunetti E, Gulizia R, Garlaschelli AL, Filice C. Cystic echinococcosis of the liver associated with repeated international travels to endemic areas. *J Travel Med.* 2005;12(4):225–8.

7 Azab ME, Bishara SA, Ramzy RM, Oteifa NM, El-Hoseiny LM, Ahmed MA. The evaluation of HLA-DRB1 antigens as susceptibility markers for unilocular cystic echinococcosis in Egyptian patients. *Parasitol Res* 2004;92(6):473–7.

8 Brunetti E, Garlaschelli AL, Filice C, Schantz P. Comment on "Acute echinococcosis: a case report." *J Clin Microbiol* 2003;41(1):523.

9 Gharbi HA, Hassine W, Brauner MW, Dupuch K. Ultrasound examination of the hydatic liver. *Radiology* 1981;139(2):459–63.

10 International classification of ultrasound images in cystic echinococcosis for application in clinical and field epidemiological settings. *Acta Trop* 2003;85(2):253–61.

11 Hosch W, Junghanss T, Stojkovic M, Brunetti E, Heye T, Kauffman GW, et al. Metabolic viability assessment of cystic echinococcosis using high-field 1H magnetic resonance spectroscopy of cyst contents. *NMR Biomed* 2008;21(7): 734–54.

12 Heye T, Lichtenberg A, Junghanss T, Hosch W. Cardiac manifestation of cystic echinococcosis: comparison of dual-source cardio computed tomography and cardiac magnetic resonance imaging and their impact on disease management. *Am J Trop Med Hyg* 2007;77(5):875–7.

13 Galitza Z, Bazarsky E, Sneier R, Peiser J, El-On J. Repeated treatment of cystic echinococcosis in patients with a long-term immunological response after successful surgical cyst removal. *Trans R Soc Trop Med Hyg* 2006;100(2): 126–33.

14 Eckert J, Deplazes P. Biological, epidemiological, and clinical aspects of echinococcosis, a zoonosis of increasing concern. *Clin Microbiol Rev* 2004;17(1):107–35.

15 Atmatzidis KS, Pavlidis TE, Papaziogas BT, Mirelis C, Papaziogas TB. Recurrence and long-term outcome after open cystectomy with omentoplasty for hepatic hydatid disease in an endemic area. *Acta Chir Belg* 2005;105(2):198–202.

16 Ramos G, Orduna A, Garcia-Yuste M. Hydatid cyst of the lung: diagnosis and treatment. *World J Surg* 2001;25(1):46–57.

17 Daradkeh S, El-Muhtaseb H, Farah G, Sroujieh AS, Abu-Khalaf M. Predictors of morbidity and mortality in the surgical management of hydatid cyst of the liver. *Langenbecks Arch Surg* 2007;392(1):35–9.

18 Menezes da Silva A. Hydatid cyst of the liver-criteria for the selection of appropriate treatment. *Acta Trop* 2003;85(2):237–42.

19 Franchi C, Di Vico B, Teggi A. Long-term evaluation of patients with hydatidosis treated with benzimidazole carbamates. *Clin Infect Dis* 1999;29(2):304–9.

20 Keshmiri M, Baharvahdat H, Fattahi SH, Davachi B, Dabiri RH, Baradaran H, et al. A placebo controlled study of albendazole in the treatment of pulmonary echinococcosis. *Eur Respir J* 1999;14(3):503–7.

21 Cobo F, Yarnoz C, Sesma B, Fraile P, Aizcorbe M, Trujillo R, et al. Albendazole plus praziquantel versus albendazole alone as a pre-operative treatment in intra-abdominal hydatisosis caused by *Echinococcus granulosus*. *Trop Med Int Health* 1998;3(6):462–6.

22 Mohamed AE, Yasawy MI, Al Karawi MA. Combined albendazole and praziquantel versus albendazole alone in the treatment of hydatid disease. *Hepatogastroenterology* 1998;45(23):1690–94.

23 Homeida M, Leahy W, Copeland S, Ali MM, Harron DW. Pharmacokinetic interaction between praziquantel and albendazole in Sudanese men. *Ann Trop Med Parasitol* 1994;88(5):551–9.

24 Brunetti E, Troia G, Garlaschelli AL, Gulizia R, Filice C. Twenty years of percutaneous treatments for cystic echinococcosis: a preliminary assessment of their use and safety. *Parassitologia* 2004;46(4):367–70.

25 McManus DP, Zhang W, Li J, Bartley PB. Echinococcosis. *Lancet* 2003;362(9392):1295–1304.

26 Torgerson PR, Shaikenov BS, Baitursinov KK, Abdybekova AM. The emerging epidemic of echinococcosis in Kazakhstan. *Trans R Soc Trop Med Hyg* 2002;96(2):124–8.

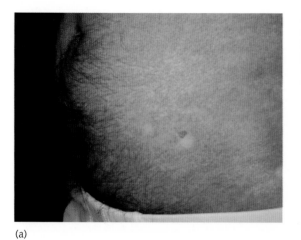
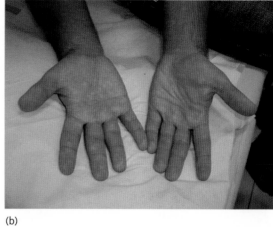

(a)                                                        (b)

**Plate 7.3**  Dengue rash (a) with island sparing and (b) involving the palms.

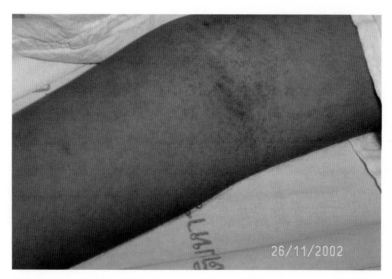

**Plate 7.5**  Tourniquet test. The test is performed by inflating a blood pressure cuff on the upper arm to a point midway between systolic and diastolic blood pressures for 5 minutes. A test is considered positive when 20 or more petechiae per square inch are observed. (Courtesy of Dr. Ann McCarthy, Tropical Medicine and International Health Clinic, Ottawa Hospital, Canada.)

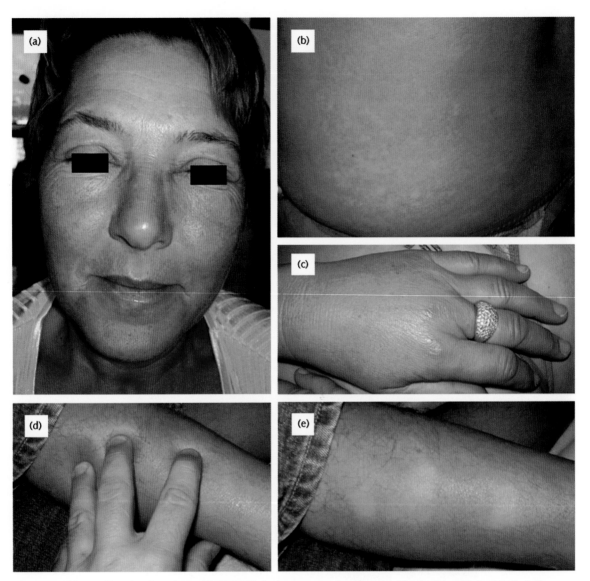

**Plate 11.2** Skin manifestations in patients with CHIKV infection returning from Reunion Island to Marseille in 2006, including a 45-year-old woman with a rash of the face (a) and abdomen (b) and edema of the face (a) and hand (c), and a 36-year-old man with a rash on the right arm that blanches with pressure (d, e). (From [14] with permission.)

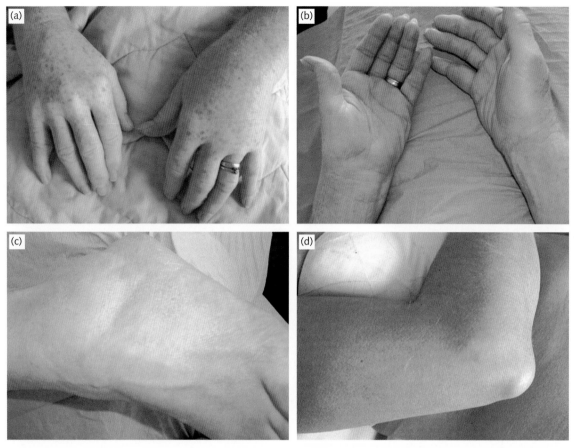

**Plate 11.3** Joint manifestations in patients with CHIKV infection returning from Reunion Island to Marseille in 2006, including bilateral tenosynovitis of extensors of wrists and fingers (a) and of wrist flexors (b), tenosynovitis of peroneus longus and brevis muscles (c), and elbow hygroma (d).

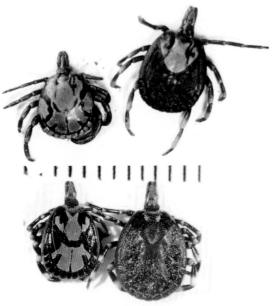

**Plate 18.1** Principal tick vectors of *R. africae*: *A. hebraeum*, male and female (upper panel), and *A. variegatum*, male and female (lower panel). Scale is millimetric.

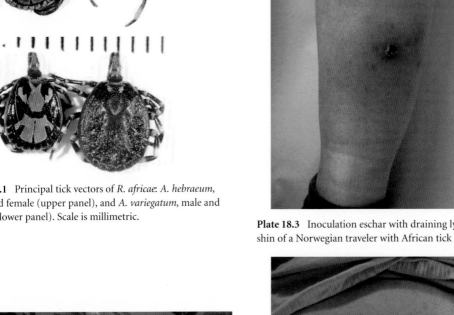

**Plate 18.3** Inoculation eschar with draining lymphangitis on shin of a Norwegian traveler with African tick bite fever.

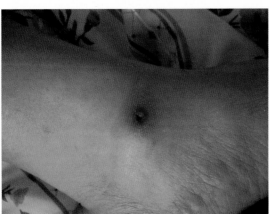

**Plate 18.2** Inoculation eschar on medial aspect of the left ankle in a Norwegian traveler with African tick bite fever.

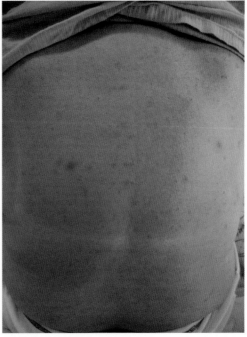

**Plate 18.4** Vesicular rash on the back of a Norwegian traveler with African tick bite fever.

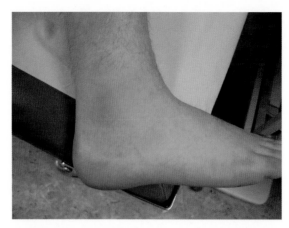

**Plate 18.5** Reactive arthritis of right ankle in a Norwegian traveler with African tick bite fever.

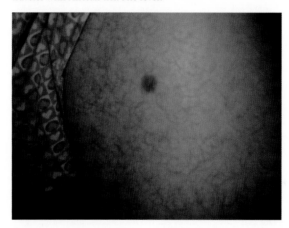

**Plate 19.1** Typical tick bite of *Ornithodoros*.

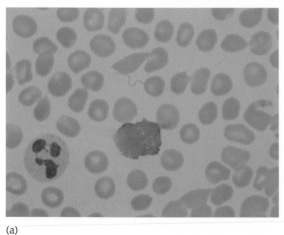

(a)

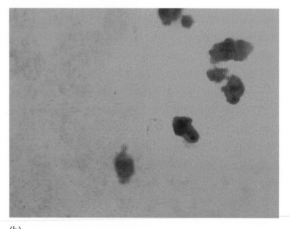

(b)

**Plate 19.3** Spirochetes on a Wright–Giemsa-stained smear of peripheral blood showing the spiral shape of the borrelia. (a) In a thin blood smear (see arrow). (b) In a thick blood smear (see arrow). (Courtesy of Dr. G. Smollen, Department of Clinical Microbiology. Chaim Sheba Medical Center, Israel.)

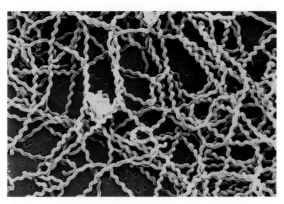

**Plate 20.1** *Leptospira*. (From Centers for Disease Control and Prevention. Content provider: CDC/NCID/Rob Weyant. Photo credit: Janice Haney Carr.)

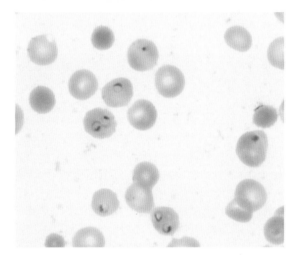

**Plate 22.1** Ring forms of *Plasmodium falciparum* in a Giemsa-stained thin smear. (Courtesy of Dr. Peter Weina.)

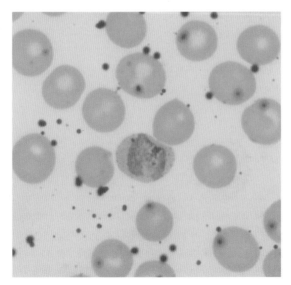

**Plate 22.2** Trophozoite of *Plasmodium vivax* in a Giemsa-stained thin smear. (Courtesy of Dr. Peter Weina.)

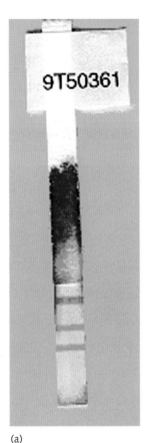

(a)

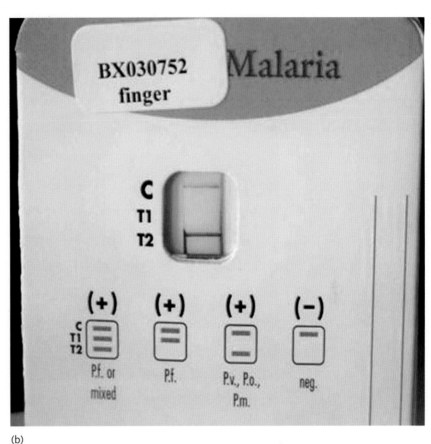

(b)

**Plate 22.4** Examples of three-band (*P. falciparum* or any malaria) tests. (a) shows the nitrocellulose strip separated from the packaging. The three lines convey detection of the antigen to HRP-2 and the panmalarial antigen, consistent with *P. falciparum* infection. (b) Shows the BinaxNOW test, which detects the panmalarial antigen (T2) without HRP-2 (T1), indicative of a non-falciparum malaria, in this case case due to *P. vivax*. (From Clinton K. Murray, Robert A. Gasser, Jr., Alan J. Magill, R. Scott Miller. Update on Rapid Diagnostic Testing for Malaria. Copyright © American Society of Microbiology. *Clin Microb Rev* Jan. 2008, p. 97–110, with permission from American Society for Microbiology.)

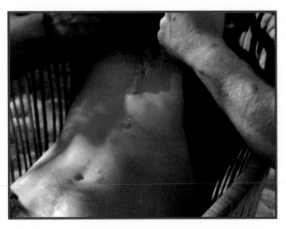

**Plate 24.4** Swimmer's itch. (Courtesy of Dr. G. Artom.)

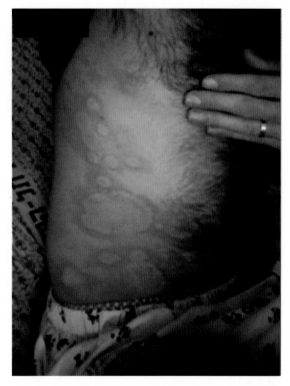

**Plate 24.7** Urticarial rash in patient with acute schistosomiasis.

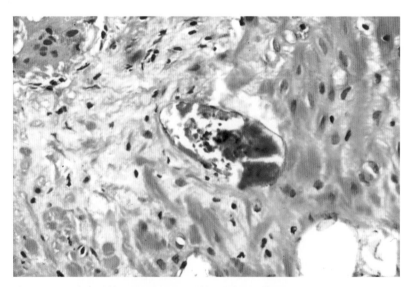

**Plate 24.10** *S. haematobium* egg in prostate biopsy. (Magnification ×400.)

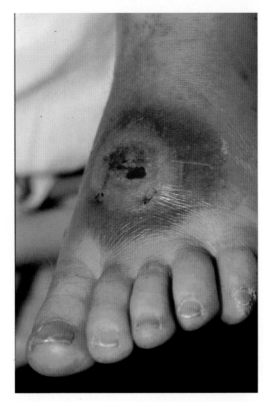

**Plate 26.2** Trypanosomal chancre. (Photo Courtesy of A. Moore, E. Ryan.)

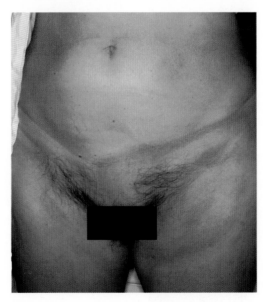

**Plate 26.3** Trypanosomal rash. (Photo courtesy of Ezzedine K. From Ezzedine K, Darie H, Le Bras M, Malvy D. Skin features accompanying imported human African trypanosomiasis: hemolymphatic *Trypanosoma gambiense* infection among two French expariates with dermatologic manifestations. *J Travel Med* 2007 May–Jun;14(3):192–6.

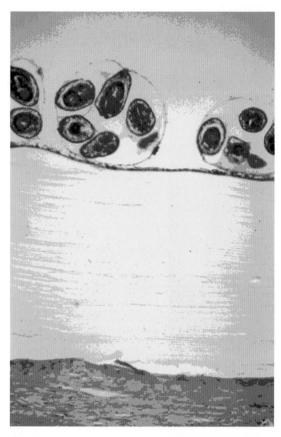

**Plate 27.4** Cross-section of echinococcal cyst showing (bottom up) pericyst, laminated layer, and germinal layer with brood capsules, each containing protoscoleces. [From Busilacchi P, Rapaccini L, editors, *Ecografia Clinica*, Naples (Italy): Idelson-Gnocchi, 2006; Courtesy Professor HM Seitz, Dept. of Parasitology, University of Bonn, Bonn, Germany.]

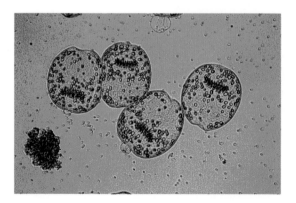

**Plate 27.7** Viable protoscoleces seen under light microscopy examination after aspiration from a CE1 cyst.

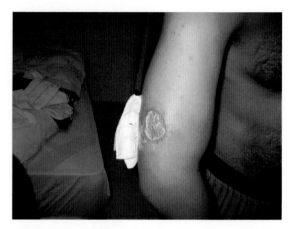

**Plate 32.5** CL due to *L. (V.) braziliensis* acquired in Bolivia; note the swollen arm (axillary lymphadenopathy was palpable).

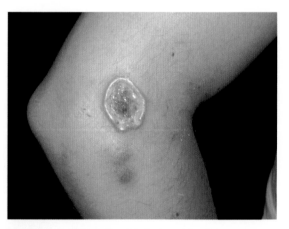

**Plate 32.6** *L. (V.) braziliensis* infection with subcutaneous nodules, sporotrichosis distribution below the lesion, and red lymphangitis spread above it.

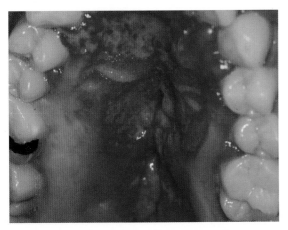

**Plate 32.7** Mucosal lesion due to *L. (V.) braziliensis* infection; note the deep ulcer in the upper palate.

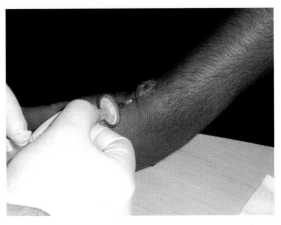

**Plate 32.10** Intralesional injection of pentostam in *L. major* lesion.

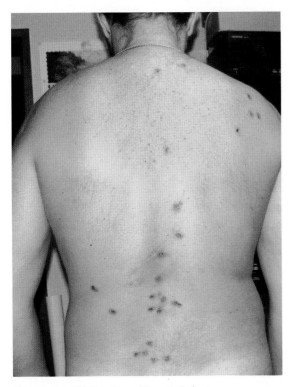

**Plate 32.9** Multiple lesions of *L. major* infection.

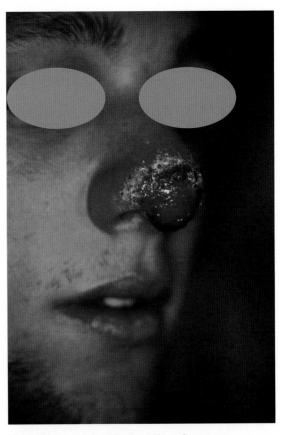

**Plate 32.11** *L. tropica* infection with erythematous–squamous type lesion.

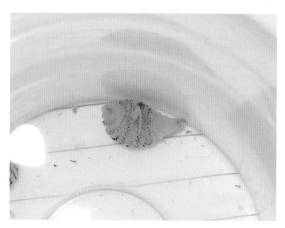

**Plate 33.1** Cutaneous lesion typical of furuncular myiasis.

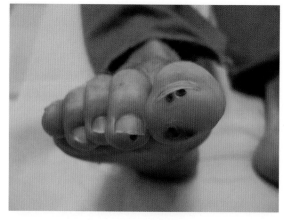

**Plate 33.4** Tunga lesion on the tip of a toe.

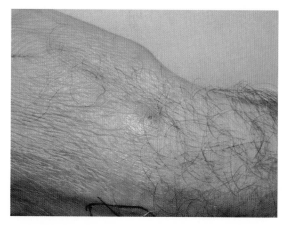

**Plate 33.2** *D. hominis* larvae.

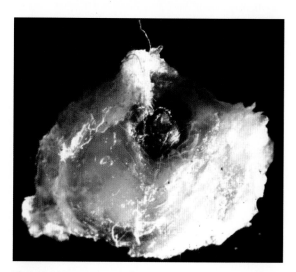

**Plate 33.5** Focus on tunga lesion.

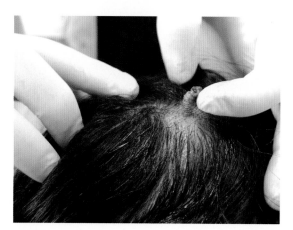

**Plate 33.3** Extraction of *D. hominis* from the scalp.

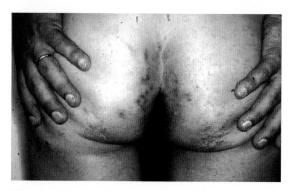

**Plate 33.6** Cutaneous lesions of the buttocks secondary to itching in a patient with scabies.

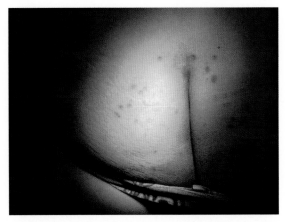

**Plate 34.1** Ground itch. (Courtesy of Eli Schwartz.)

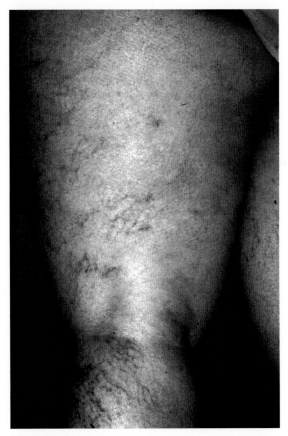

**Plate 34.2** Larva currens associated with *S. stercoralis* infection in a woman from the French West Indies.

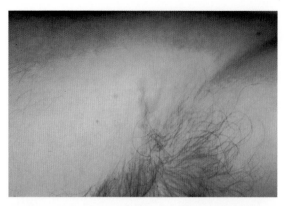

**Plate 34.3** Creeping dermatitis in the axillary area revealing loiasis in a French expatriate working in the forest industry in Gabon.

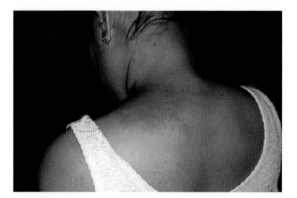

**Plate 34.4** Eosinophilic panniculitis revealing cutaneous gnathostomiasis in a woman from Southeast Asia.

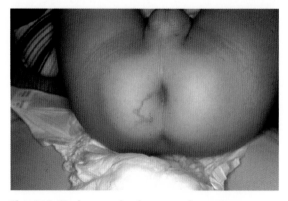

**Plate 34.5** Hookworm-related cutaneous larva migrans revealed by creeping dermatitis in a child coming back from the Caribbean.

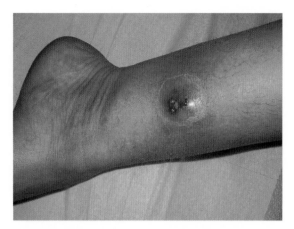

**Plate 38.1** Abscess due to Panton–Valentine positive methicillin-resistant *S. aureus* in a traveler returning from Senegal.

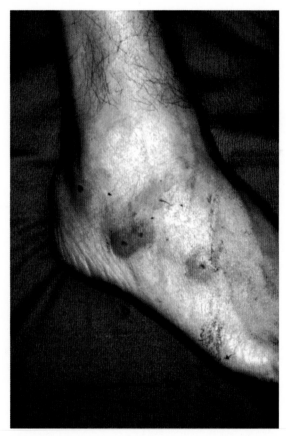

**Plate 38.2** Acute prurigo after walking accidentally into an anthill in Niger.

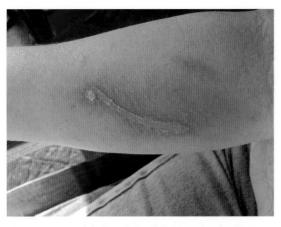

**Plate 38.3** Vesiculobullous lesion following a bite by the Nairobi fly, a poisonous beetle of the species *Paederus crebinpunctatis.* or *Paederus sabaeus* in an Israeli traveler. (Courtesy of Eli Schwartz.)

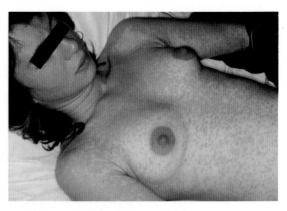

**Plate 38.5** Exanthema associated with measles in a patient returning from Southeast Asia.

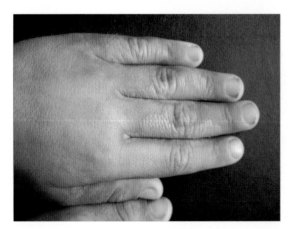

**Plate 38.4** Phytophotodermatitis associating postbullous lesions and hyperpigmented well-delimited hyperpigmented plaques in a child returning from the French West Indies (Guadeloupe).

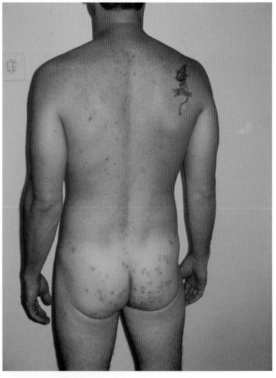

**Plate 39.3** Acute hookworm infection. A fixed papullar pruritic rash, after exposure to a sandy beach in Thailand—typical of acute hookworm dermatitis.

# 28 Neurocysticercosis

Eli Schwartz

Chaim Sheba Medical Center, Tel Hashomer, Israel and Sackler School of Medicine, Tel Aviv University, Tel Aviv, Israel

## Introduction

Cysticercosis is a human infestation, which is considered the most common parasitic disease of the human nervous system and is endemic in the less developed countries[1]. It is caused by *Taenia solium*, the pork tapeworm, although humans are the definitive host. The infection includes the course of two life cycles: one cycle in which pigs are involved, and one cycle in which transmission occurs between humans. Thus, *T. solium* can cause two different types of disease: one is a gastrointestinal infection, which is usually mild, and the other is a disease mainly of the CNS, neurocysticercosis (NCC), with severe neurological manifestations that can be fatal. Both the mode of transmission and the approach to prevention of these two diseases are different.

Humans are carriers of the adult worms, which reside in their gastrointestinal (jejunal) tracts. The adult worm consists of a head (also known as a scolex), a neck, and a segmented body (also known as a proglottid), which typically measures at least 5 m long. The proglottids contain a large number of eggs. In taeniasis, the distal segments can bud off from the rest of the body and these, or the eggs they contain, can be passed rectally. When fecally contaminated food or water is ingested by an intermediate host (pigs, in the case of *T. solium*), the eggs rupture in the intestine and release embryos that pass through the intestinal wall, travel to striated muscle (or other organs), and develop into cysticerci within the pig.

Ingestion of contaminated pork results in human taeniasis, in which larvae develop out of the cysticerci to mature worms in the small intestine (Figure 28.1A). The worm attaches to the small intestinal mucosa, causing mild inflammation with symptoms such as abdominal discomfort, nausea, and diarrhea (see chapter 31). About

*Tropical Diseases in Travelers*, 1st edition. Edited by E. Schwartz.
© 2009 by Blackwell Publishing, ISBN: 978-1-4051-8441-0.

2 months after infection, gravid proglottids begin to be excreted in the feces. The host is usually unaware of the infection or the presence of proglottids in the stools. Excretion of the eggs continues the cycle and poses a public health problem, especially in countries where hygienic infrastructure is lacking.

Humans who are carriers of adult worms excrete the eggs into the environment. Ingestion of *T. solium* eggs by the fecal–oral route can occur via contaminated food or water, or directly via hands contaminated with fecal material. Following the ingestion of eggs, the worm embryos are released in the bowel, and then by crossing the bowel wall, they are carried in the blood stream to the host tissues. (Figure 28.1B). When the embryos reach the target tissue, they form cysts. Many organs may be infected, including the CNS, the eyes, the skeletal muscles, and the spine [2]. However, the most common site of infection is the CNS, resulting in NCC. The clinical manifestations of NCC depend on the location of the cysts, their size, and their number. The most common symptom is epileptic seizures, but motor deficits and psychiatric symptoms have also been reported.

## Epidemiology

*T. solium* is a common parasite in Central and South America, Africa, parts of Asia, and Eastern Europe. It is estimated that more than 20 million people are suffering from this disease worldwide [3].

Although the disease is ancient, known from the prehistoric period, as discovered in Egyptian mummies [4], only since the second half of the twentieth century has it gained significant medical attention when NCC was diagnosed in British troops returning from India and its etiology was discovered. It is now clear that it is a major health problem in many developing countries. WHO estimates that over 50,000 deaths are due to NCC annually [5], and there is

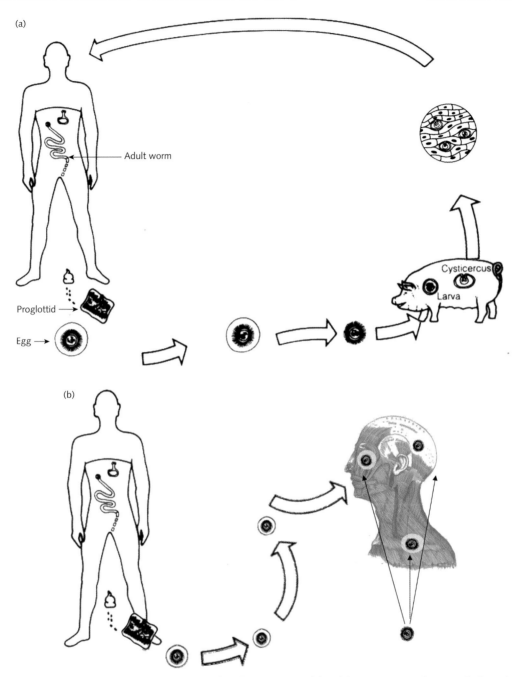

**Figure 28.1** (a) Taeniasis: a human-to-pig-to-human cycle. A human carrier of the adult worm excretes the eggs, which are then ingested by the pig and which consequently develop into cysticerci. Eating raw pork can result in taeniasis in humans.
(b) Cysticercosis: a human-to-human transmission. A human carrier of adult worms excretes the eggs into the environment. After human ingestion (fecal–oral transmission route) of *T. solium* eggs, worm embryos are released in the bowel; these cross the bowel wall and are carried by the blood stream to the host tissues, resulting in cysticercosis. The most common organs that are infected are the central nervous system, eyes, and skeletal muscles.

**Table 28.1** NCC in travelers – review of the literature.

| Country | Number of patients | Gender | Presentation | Acquired in |
|---------|-------------------|--------|--------------|-------------|
| Italy | 1 | Male | Hemianopsia, headache | Central America |
| Australia | 5 | Males | N/A | Southern Asia |
| Australia | 1 | Male | seizures | Bali |
| Denmark | 1 | Female | N/A | Far East |
| Australia | 2 | Males | Dysphasia, focal seizures | Southern Asia |
| Israel | 8 | Males-7 | 7- seizures 1-visual disturbances | 5-S.E Asia, 2-India, 1-S. America, |
| **Total** | 18 | Males =16/18 | Seizures-9/12 | Asia-16/18, Americas-2/18 |

*Source*: (From [8]).

an even higher rate of active cases of epilepsy, which has tremendous social and economic implications. In some endemic areas in South America, community-based sero-prevalence studies have shown rates as high as 24% and adult seizure disorder rates of 9.1% among seropositive persons [6].

The estimate is that in Latin America alone there are approximately 75 million people who live in areas where cysticercosis is endemic, and approximately 400,000 have symptomatic disease. Overall, NCC is the most common cause of symptomatic epilepsy worldwide [7].

## Epidemiology in travelers and in developed countries

NCC has become an emerging infectious disease in developed countries due to massive immigration from endemic countries, and to a much lesser extent, to importation by international travelers. It is estimated that the number of imported cases in the USA is the highest among all developed countries [7]. In fact, a multicenter survey in the USA revealed that 2% of people presenting at emergency rooms with convulsive disorders have radiological evidence of NCC [3].

In a large case series published in the USA, 1496 cases were identified during the period from 1980 to 2004 [7]. This is in comparison to a period of about 100 years (1857–1954), in which only 54 cases were detected. Among the 1496 patients, the vast majority were Hispanic immigrants. However, 76 cases of NCC were likely acquired within the USA during this period. A higher risk for acquiring NCC has been documented in patients who are of Hispanic ethnicity and have contact with *T. solium* tapeworm carriers. Interesting to note is that five cases occurred among ultra-orthodox Jewish members of a Jewish

community in New York, who were probably infected via housekeepers from Latin America.

The other interesting observation is that in this case series, only three US-born patients had traveled to endemic regions that might have been the source of the infection.

A search of the literature on travel-associated NCC during the last 25 years revealed that NCC is not commonly encountered among travelers [8]. Most reported cases were Australian (eight cases) and only two were European (Table 28.1).

A nationwide Israeli study in which all cases of NCC were investigated found that during the years 1994–2007, 13 cases were diagnosed in different Israeli hospitals. Eight of the cases were in Israelis who had traveled to endemic areas, whereas the other cases were in immigrants. The destinations of the travelers were India (2 patients), Southeast Asia (5 patients), and South America (1 patient). Based on these data and the estimated number of Israeli travelers to endemic countries, our estimation of attack rate was 1:275,000 clinical diseases per journey [8]. This is a very low rate, taking into account that NCC is a fecal–oral disease, which is the most common mode of disease transmission in travelers.

Underdiagnosis of symptomatic NCC patients is unlikely because it is a severe disease and brain imaging is done routinely with these symptoms. It is more likely that clinical disease occurs less frequently in travelers, either because of a lower burden of infective eggs, or because of different immunological responses.

Thus, it can be assumed that the number of seropositive individuals in travelers is much greater than the number of clinically diagnosed cases. One report in the literature on a serosurvey of 73 Peace Corps volunteers in Madagascar found a positivity rate of 8.2% without clinical disease [9].

It is interesting to note that in the early twentieth century, among British troops who were sent for duty in

India, approximately 450 had seizures upon return, and evidence of NCC was found in 75% of them [5]. Although the attack rate is not known, it seems to be much higher than we see in travelers. The reason might be a different lifestyle, longer periods of exposure, or perhaps lower living standards among the soldiers at that time.

## Gender

In the Israeli series of eight cases, seven were males. The low female representation is surprising because women make up nearly half of the total number of travelers in Israel.

Among the 10 other cases reported in the literature, 9 were males. In a summary reviewing the largest case series reported in the USA, in 9 out of 10 studies males were predominant [7]. It is possible that male travelers take risks more often than female travelers (e.g., neglecting food precautions) because several reports from endemic countries do not show male predominance in NCC in investigated communities [6].

## Clinical presentation

As mentioned above, following the ingestion of eggs, the worm embryos are released in the bowel, and then cross the bowel wall and are carried in the bloodstream to the host tissues. The target tissues are the CNS, including the spine; the eyes; the skeletal muscles; and subcutaneous tissues. Clinical disease will be related to the tissue in which cyst formation (cysticercosis) occurs.

The CNS is the most common tissue to be infected. Although NCC can cause almost any neurological symptom, the most common presentations are convulsions and intracranial hypertensive symptoms, and less often psychiatric disorders.

The symptoms of NCC result from a combination of factors including the number, stage, and localization of the parasites within the nervous system, as well as the robustness of the host's immune response against the parasites. Seizures occur in about 70% of patients and may be focal or generalized, sporadic or causing status epilepticus. Cysticercosis has become the leading cause of epilepsy in endemic countries. The convulsive disorders are usually due to cortical invasion by the parasites. Location of a cyst in the ventricular or subarachnoid space in the skull base produces severe symptomatology, due to an increase in intracranial pressure, which may lead to severe headaches, vomiting, and visual disturbances. Mental dis-

orders can develop either together with the convulsion or independently, leading to mental confusion, apathy, and dementia.

Ocular cysticercosis is the most common form after cerebral involvement. The common cyst localizations are in the vitreous, subretinal tissue and rarely may involve the anterior chamber of the eye.

Spinal cord cysticercosis is another form of NCC, caused usually by intramedullary invasion rather than subarachnoidal localization, resulting in motor or sensory manifestations.

Invasion of subcutaneous tissue gives rise to palpable, asymptomatic nodules.

Similarly, invasion of the muscles is also usually asymptomatic, causing calcifications in the muscles, which may be helpful in establishing the diagnosis of cysticercosis. In a study of patients having calcified brain cysts who underwent CT scan of their thighs, one or more muscle calcifications were seen in 52% of them [10]. Thus, some clinicians opt for X rays of the thigh as another clue to a NCC diagnosis.

Myocardial involvement in massive infection has been described, too, but is without clinical significance.

## In travelers

The natural history of NCC cannot be evaluated in the setting of endemic areas, where exposure may be continuous. However, travelers who have been to endemic areas and returned to nonendemic areas can demonstrate the natural history of the disease. Among British troops who served in India, the neurological symptoms began 2–5 years after their return, which clearly shows that the disease has a long incubation period [5].

Whereas in populations in endemic areas, a skull X ray or CT scan may show numerous calcified cysticerci, travelers both in our experience and in the reported literature usually have a single lesion. That probably reflects a much smaller infection burden in travelers.

The presentation in travelers is of cerebral disease in almost all cases, with focal or generalized seizures as the presenting symptom. Symptoms of intracranial hypertension are usually not seen. Interestingly, similar differences were found in endemic areas (in Mexico), where a comparison was made between the clinical presentation of pediatric populations and of adults. The pediatric populations were similar to the traveler population, in whom a single lesion in the brain was the most common finding, and seizures were the leading symptom in more than 80%, with only a small minority presenting with intracranial hypertension [11].

Ocular involvement is also documented in travelers. However, neither muscle calcification nor subcutaneous nodules have been seen in travelers.

## Diagnosis

New proposals for diagnostic criteria were established and published in 2001 [12]. According to these criteria, a definitive diagnosis is made when there is histological proof or direct visualization of the parasite. The major criteria are highly suggestive cysticercosis by radiology (CT or MRI), positive serology, or resolution of the lesion(s) over time, with or without antiparasitic treatment.

In endemic countries, the diagnosis is typically made on the basis of neuroimaging studies and confirmatory serology. High sensitivity and specificity (almost approaching 100%) of enzyme-linked immunoelectrotransfer blot (EITB) assay and of ELISA have been reported. However, these results apply to patients with multiple lesions. In the case of travelers, who usually have a single lesion, the sensitivity is far less. One study found that only 28% of patients with a single lesion had positive enzyme-linked immunoelectrotransfer blot assay results [13].

Thus, in travelers, a history of being in endemic countries (in all of our cases it was for a long period of several months, backpacking), with a new onset of convulsive disorders, should raise the possibility of NCC. With typical radiological findings (Figure 28.2), a clinical diagnosis can be made. MRI in travelers usually shows one or two intracortical cysts and varying degrees of wall enhancement and surrounding edema. Usually, there is no need for a brain biopsy; however, with lack of awareness and lack of experience of the treating physicians, and the availability of experienced neurosurgeons in most Western countries, patients may undergo this invasive procedure. Indeed, our first two cases had brain biopsies to rule out a suspected tumor, and the biopsy showed the parasite.

### Laboratory tests
Peripheral eosinophilia is absent in most patients (85%) with NCC, and when it exists, it is usually mild. High-grade eosinophilia in a patient with cysticercosis should encourage the physician to search for another etiology of the eosinophilia. CSF eosinophilia was reported to be high in more than 50% of cases. Serological tests can also be performed on the CSF.

### Treatment

Despite the fact that there are good and effective drugs against *T. solium* and against cysticercosis, namely albendazole and praziquantel, there is a long historical debate as to whether NCC should be treated with antiparasitic drugs [3]. The controversy arose from the concern that the inflammation that follows the cidal effect of the drug against the worm will trigger seizures and other neurological manifestations. Furthermore, the outcomes of patients with no treatment show the resolution of cortical lesions. On the other hand, there is an argument for rapid degeneration of the cysts to cut down on the duration of seizures and avoid new seizures.

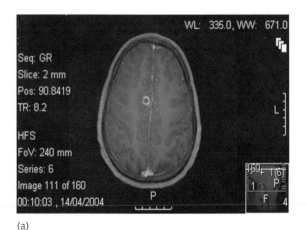

(a)

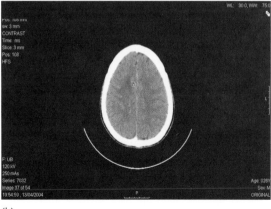

(b)

**Figure 28.2** (a) MRI showing enhancing brain lesion in a 26-year-old man with focal seizures after returning from S. America. (b) CT Scan showing a calcified brain lesion in the same patient.

Various studies have examined two aspects of outcomes. One aspect was the clearance of radiological findings with or without treatment. Results showed that in cases with only a few cysts, treatment enhances radiological clearance. With a heavy burden of infection, the effect of the drug is less pronounced [14]. Because, in travelers, the burden of cysts is usually a single one, it appears that treatment is beneficial for travelers, based on this finding.

Seizure outcome, a more meaningful clinical measure, has been assessed in only three randomized, placebo-controlled trials of anticysticercal treatment. One study did not find any difference in seizure-free individuals over 2 years [15]. However, a study of patients with a solitary cysticercus granuloma (which is more similar to a traveler's situation) found a trend toward favorable seizure outcomes with albendazole treatment [16].

Recently, Garcia and colleagues reported the outcome of a randomized, double-blind, placebo-controlled trial of albendazole plus dexamethasone treatment for 10 days in patients with active parenchymal cysticercosis. They reported a significant reduction in the number of generalized seizures in the treated group compared with controls over a 30-month follow-up period [17]. These studies also support the benefit of treating travelers with antiparasitic drugs.

Praziquantel is another effective drug against cysticercosis (a common regimen is 50 mg/kg/day for 15 days). A critical review of the available data from comparative trials suggests that albendazole is more effective than praziquantel in clinically important outcomes in patients with NCC [18]. However, the small number of comparative studies prevents a firm conclusion about the best regimen; thus these two drugs are still both options (depending also on availability and cost).

Our recommended policy is as follows:
**1** Anticonvulsive treatment until patient is stabilized.
**2** Albendazole treatment in a dose of 400 mg b.i.d. for 7–14 days.
**3** Dexamethazone in a dosage of 6 mg/day corresponding to the period of albendazole treatment.

We prefer to have the patients hospitalized during the first few days of antiparasitic treatment, although so far we have not encountered any complications during treatment.

## Outcomes

Infected travelers, who are back in their nonendemic home countries, may reveal by long-term follow up the natural history of the disease (usually of a nonheavy infection). In our experience, after antiparasitic treatment within 1–2 years, lesions disappear and cessation of the antiepileptic drugs is harmless.

Two of our patients who refused antiparasitic treatment also cleared their lesions. However, it is too early to draw conclusions as to whether treatment hastens the process of radiological disappearance of the lesions.

## Prevention

Prevention of NCC in endemic areas is beyond the scope of this chapter.

For travelers, it should be kept in mind that the severe disease of NCC is a fecal–oral transmissible disease and not related to eating raw pork. Therefore, routine precautions to prevent travelers' diarrhea also apply.

In developed countries, there are several reports of transmission of the disease from a housekeeper or cook who emigrated from an endemic area, via contaminated hands. Therefore, personal hygiene rules for housekeepers should be observed. This was clearly demonstrated in an orthodox Jewish community in New York who do not consume pork at all and probably were infected by their housekeeper [18].

## References

1 Carpio A. Neurocysticercosis: an update. *Lancet Infect Dis* 2002;2:751–62.
2 Rahalkar MD, Shetty DD, Kelkar AB, Kelkar AA, Kinare AS, Ambardekar ST. The many faces of cysticercosis. *Clin Radiol* 2000;55:668–74.
3 Singh G, Sander JW. Anticysticercal treatment and seizures in neurocysticercosis. *Lancet Neurol* 2004;3:207–8.
4 Bruschi F, Masetti M, Locci MT, Ciranni R, Fornaciari G. Cysticercosis in an Egyptian mummy of the late Ptolemaic period. *Am J Trop Med Hyg* 2006;74:598–9.
5 Garcia HH, Del Brutto OH; Cysticercosis Working Group in Peru. Neurocysticercosis: updated concepts about an old disease. *Lancet Neurol* 2005;4:653–61.
6 Fleury A, Morales J, Bobes RJ, et al. An epidemiological study of familial neurocysticercosis in an endemic Mexican community. *Trans R Soc Trop Med Hyg* 2006;100:551–8.
7 Wallin MT, Kurtzke JF. Neurocysticercosis in the United States: review of an important emerging infection. *Neurology* 2004;63:1559–64.
8 Kliers I, Karplus R, Gomori M, Nir S, Schwartz E. Neurocysticercosis in Israeli travelers. Submitted for publication.
9 Leutscher P., Andriantsimahavandy A. Cysticercosis in Peace Corps volunteers in Madagascar. *N Engl J Med* 2004;350:311–12.

10 Bustos JA, Garcia HH, Dorregaray R, et al. Detection of muscle calcifications by thigh CT scan in neurocysticercosis patients. *Trans R Soc Trop Med Hyg* 2005;99:775–9.

11 Saenz B, Ruiz-Garcia M, Jimenez E, et al. Neurocysticercosis: clinical, radiologic, and inflammatory differences between children and adults. *Pediatr Infect Dis J* 2006;25: 801–3.

12 Del Brutto OH, Rajshekhar V, White AC Jr, et al. Proposed diagnostic criteria for neurocysticercosis. *Neurology* 2001;57:177–83.

13 Wilson M, Bryan RT, Fried JA, et al. Clinical evaluation of the cysticercosis enzyme-linked immunoelectrotransfer blot in patients with neurocysticercosis. *J Infect Dis* 1991;164(5):1007–9.

14 Matthaiou DK, Panos G, Adamidi ES, Falagas ME. Albendazole versus praziquantel in the treatment of neurocysticerco-sis: a meta-analysis of comparative trials. *PLoS Negl Trop Dis* 2008;2:e194.

15 Carpio A, Santillan F, Leon P, et al. Is the course of neurocysticercosis modified by treatment with anthelminthic agents? *Arch Intern Med* 1995;155:1982–8.

16 Baranwal AK, Singhi PD, Khandelwal N, et al. Albendazole therapy in children with focal seizures and single small enhancing computerized tomographic lesions: a randomized, placebo-controlled, double-blind trial. *Pediatr Infect Dis J* 1998;17:696–700.

17 Garcia HH, Pretell EJ, Gilman RH, et al. A trial of antiparasitic treatment to reduce the rate of seizures due to cerebral cysticercosis. *N Engl J Med* 2004;350:249–58.

18 Schantz PM, Moore AC, Munoz JL, et al. Neurocysticercosis in an Orthodox Jewish community in New York City. *N Engl J Med* 1992;327(10):692–5.

# 29 Histoplasmosis and Other Endemic Fungal Infections

## Michael J. Segel[1] and Eli Schwartz[1,2]

[1] Chaim Sheba Medical Center, Tel Hashomer, Israel

[2] Sackler School of Medicine, Tel Aviv University, Tel Aviv, Israel

## Introduction

Endemic mycoses are invasive fungal infections endemic to certain geographical areas. Although more severe in immunocompromised hosts, the endemic mycoses commonly affect immunocompetent hosts as well. The more common endemic mycoses are histoplasmosis, blastomycosis, coccidiodomycosis, and paracoccidiodomycosis. Rarer diseases are penicilliosis and lobomycosis.

Among returning travelers, histoplasmosis has been reported most commonly, followed by coccidiodomycosis. The other endemic mycoses are reported rarely in travelers. With the exception of lobomycosis, all the endemic mycoses share certain common features (Table 29.1).

## Histoplasmosis

### General epidemiology

Human histoplasmosis is caused by *Histoplasma capsulatum*, a dimorphic fungus existing in soil as a mold, and in the yeast form in infected human or animal hosts. *H. capsulatum var. capsulatum* is the etiological agent of classical or American-type histoplasmosis; *H. capsulatum var. duboisii* causes African-type histoplasmosis.

Bird and bat droppings seem to encourage the growth of *Histoplasma* in the environment. Although birds may carry *H. capsulatum* spores on the feet and wings, they are not infected by the fungus. In contrast, bats as well as numerous other mammalian species have been shown to be infected with histoplasmosis. The difference between the classes is probably that the normal body temperature of birds is too high to support the growth of *H. capsulatum* [1]. Migration of birds and bats may explain the spread of *H. capsulatum* and the establishment of new environmental foci.

Classical histoplasmosis is most common in North, Central, and South America. The largest endemic areas of *H. capsulatum var. capsulatum* are the Ohio and Mississippi river valleys in the USA, virtually all of Central America, and a region including Uruguay, the southern tip of Brazil, southern Paraguay, and part of Argentina. Smaller endemic regions in South America (subject to limitations of surveillance and reporting) are the lower Amazon River valley in Brazil, the majority of Venezuela, parts of Guyana, French Guiana, and Suriname, the Bolivia–Chile border region, the Pacific coast of Colombia, and parts of the border regions of Peru with Brazil and Venezuela. Two clusters of cases have been reported in institutions (a prison and a medical campus) in nonendemic areas of the USA. Both were linked to exposure to bird droppings [2, 3]. Outside the Americas, apparently endemic cases have also been reported from Africa (West and Central Africa, Uganda, and Zimbabwe) [4], the Indian subcontinent, Southeast Asia, China, and Japan [1, 5, 6] (Table 29.2), as well as a small number of autochthonous cases from Europe, particularly Italy (Table 29.3).

Much of what is known about the epidemiology of histoplasmosis has been learned from the study of outbreaks, mostly in the endemic areas of the United States. However, outbreaks account for only a small proportion of cases of histoplasmosis [1]. Furthermore, outbreaks represent situations of heavy exposure to the fungus, and thus the distribution of clinical manifestations and immunological responses in outbreaks may differ from that in sporadic cases.

*Tropical Diseases in Travelers*, 1st edition. Edited by E. Schwartz.
© 2009 by Blackwell Publishing, ISBN: 978-1-4051-8441-0.

**Table 29.1** Common features of endemic mycoses.*

All are caused by dimorphic fungi that exist as molds in the environment, converting to the yeast form in host tissues.

Infection is generally by inhalation of spores present in the soil.

Primary infection occurs in the lungs and disseminates through the reticuloendothelial system.

Human-to-human transmission has not been documented.

Severe disease in immunocompromised hosts and, therefore, should avoid exposure to these pathogens.

*Including histoplasmosis, coccidiodomycosis, blastomycosis, paracoccidiodomycosis, and, probably, penicilliosis, but not lobomycosis.

The higher the inoculum of spores inhaled, the greater the likelihood and severity of symptomatic infection. Most outbreaks have been associated with major soil disruption such as construction or demolition in urban settings or farm work in rural outbreaks. However, many infections with *H. capsulatum* do not involve major disturbance of the soil. In most sporadic cases, sources of infection in the environment are not detected, indicating that exposure may be slight.

During outbreaks, most reported cases of histoplasmosis occur in young adults (age 15–34 years) [1]. Young adults tend to participate in activities that result in greater exposure to the fungus. In addition, older persons native to endemic areas may be relatively immune to histoplasmosis as a result of previous exposure; it has been shown that the frequency of skin test positivity increases with age, reaching a peak of 70% in those over 35 years old living in endemic disease areas [7].

*H. capsulatum var. duboisii* is apparently endemic only in Africa between the Tropics of Cancer and Capricorn (23.5° North and 23.5° South, respectively) and on the island of Madagascar [1]. Notably, both variants, *capsulatum* and *duboisii*, are endemic to Africa.

Except for very rare instances of cutaneous inoculation (e.g., in laboratory workers), natural infection by *H. capsulatum* is acquired by inhalation of spores. Transmission of disease from host to host, whether animal or human, has not been described [1].

## Epidemiology in travelers

Travel destinations of returning travelers diagnosed with histoplasmosis are listed in Table 29.2. Intriguingly, relatively few cases have been reported in travelers returning from trips in the United States. This is the case in large

national and multinational surveys [5, 6], as well as individual reports, and thus is unlikely to result from publication bias.

Surveys from Japan [5] and Europe [6] found a male predominance in cases of imported histoplasmosis. However, this may well reflect travel patterns rather than a true sex difference in susceptibility, since sex equality was reported in outbreaks [8, 9].

In travelers, the epidemiology of classical histoplasmosis (*H. capsulatum var capsulatum*) parallels that in the endemic setting: numerous sporadic cases have been reported, but also several large outbreaks. Many cases of classical histoplasmosis in travelers are associated with exploration of caves, particularly caves inhabited by bats.

Outside of Africa, African histoplasmosis (*H. capsulatum var duboisii*) has been reported largely in immigrants from Central Africa or in individuals who spent extended periods in the endemic region. A majority (14 out of 17) of cases of African-type histoplasmosis reported in a European survey occurred in hosts who did not have AIDS [10]. However, infection was disseminated in only one of the non-AIDS patients, as opposed to three of three AIDS patients. All cases were contracted in Africa.

## Clinical aspects

The clinical manifestations of classical histoplasmosis (Table 29.4) depend on three major factors: (a) the quantity of spores inhaled, (b) the general immune status of the patient, and (c) the specific immune status of the patient for *Histoplasma* [11]. Differences between travelers and natives of endemic areas, to the extent that they exist, probably reflect these factors. For example, travelers less commonly have specific immunity, which is acquired by previous exposure.

**Table 29.2** Travel destinations associated with classical histoplasmosis (*H.capsulatum var capsulatum*).

United States
Central America and Caribbean Islands
   Dominican Republic
   Honduras
   Martinique
   Guatemala
   Costa Rica
   Belize
   Cuba
   Mexico
     Yucatan
     Acapulco
   Nicaragua
   El Salvador
   Guadeloupe
   Panama
South America
   Ecuador
   Brazil
     Manaus
   Bolivia
   Argentina
   Peru
     Mato Grosso
   French Guiana
Asia
   India
   Pakistan
   Myanmar (previously Burma)
   China
   Thailand
   Indonesia
Oceania
   Australia
   New Caledonia
Africa
   Ghana
   Gambia
   Guinea-Bissau
   Ivory Coast
   Nigeria
   Congo
   Central African Republic
   Uganda
   Democratic Republic of Congo (Zaire)
   Zimbabwe

*Sources.* From [4–6, 8, 11, 16, 44–51].

**Table 29.3** European countries in which apparently autochthonous histoplasmosis has been reported.

Italy (Po River valley)
Hungary
Romania
Portugal
Great Britain
USSR (former)
Germany
Turkey

*Sources.* From [6, 11, 52].

**Table 29.4** Clinical manifestations of histoplasmosis.

**Acute pneumonitis**
Common symptoms:
   Headache, fever, cough, dyspnea
Radiological findings:
   Reticulonodular infiltrates
   Ipsilateral hilar/mediastinal lymphadenopathy
     ± calcification
Complications:
   Pericarditis
   Obstructive pneumonia
   Broncholithiasis
   Hemoptysis
   Dysphagia
   Superior vena cava syndrome
   Mediastinal fibrosis
   Pulmonary hypertension
   Rheumatological syndromes: arthralgia, erythema
     nodosum, erythema multiforme

**Chronic cavitary pulmonary histoplasmosis**
Primarily complicating pre-existing lung disease

**Disseminated histoplasmosis**
Primarily in immunocompromised hosts

- Progressive disseminated histoplasmosis
  May be acute/subacute/chronic/reactivation
  Clinical features:
  Hepatosplenomegaly
  Anemia, leukopenia, thrombocytopenia
  Septic shock
  ARDs
- CNS histoplasmosis
  Meningitis, CNS histoplasmoma
- Dissemination to other organs:
  Endocarditis, pharyngitis, laryngitis

**Table 29.5** Common symptoms of acute histoplasmosis.

| Frequency | |
| --- | --- |
| Headache | 87–95% |
| Fever | 75–79% |
| Myalgia | 71–78% |
| Cough | 71–73% |
| Chest pain | 66–71% |
| Dyspnea | 44–55% |
| Arthralgia | 52% |
| Night sweats | 44% |
| Diarrhea | 37% |
| Rash | 8% |

Low-level exposure to *H. capsulatum* in a healthy host most commonly leads to asymptomatic infection. In most such cases, chest radiology remains normal. However, in some asymptomatic (or perhaps minimally symptomatic) cases, typical radiological features of histoplasmosis may develop.

The incubation time for acute histoplasmosis is typically 1–3 weeks, but may be less in cases of reinfection [1]. It manifests as a flu-like illness: malaise, high fever, chills, headache, dry cough, and pleuritic chest pain. The systemic symptoms are almost invariably present, even more commonly than the respiratory symptoms (Table 29.5). Sometimes acute infection may be disseminated by hematogenous infection, leading to hepatosplenomegaly and bone marrow suppression. Hepatic transaminases may be elevated, and in rare cases blood cultures may be positive. With or without dissemination, the acute illness is usually self-limited, lasting up to 3 weeks, though fatigue may persist longer.

Radiological studies typically reveal bilateral diffuse reticulonodular infiltrates, sometimes with mediastinal lymphadenopathy. Splenic calcifications, not uncommon in natives of endemic regions, may reflect prior histoplasmosis with dissemination.

In some cases, low-level exposure causes a subacute pulmonary infection—cough, fever, malaise, and fatigue that may persist for weeks or even months. In these subacute cases, the chest radiograph typically shows hilar and mediastinal lymphadenopathy and patchy or sometimes focal infiltrates [11].

Chronic pulmonary histoplasmosis occurs in individuals with underlying chronic lung disease who fail to clear the infection. Chest radiography may show the findings seen in acute disease, but in addition frank consolidation, cavitation, and fluid-filled emphysematous bullae may be present. Chronic histoplasmosis will not resolve spontaneously, but rather progresses and gradually destroys the affected lungs.

Progressive disseminated histoplasmosis (PDH) is most commonly seen in immunocompromised hosts with impaired T-cell immunity, such as patients with AIDS or Hodgkin's disease or transplant recipients. The natural history of PDH in immunosuppressed hosts is a rapidly progressive disease following acute infection. PDH may present as a late reactivation of histoplasmosis in patients who acquire an immunodeficiency. A more chronic, slowly progressive course is seen in patients who have no underlying disease or mild immunodeficiency. Clinical features of PDH reflect the spread of infection through the reticuloendothelial system and may include fever, anorexia, weight loss, fatigue, respiratory symptoms, hepatosplenomegaly, and lymphadenopathy, but in many cases fever and progressive weight loss are the only findings. CNS involvement—lymphocytic meningitis sometimes accompanied by parenchymal lesions (histoplasmomas) of the brain or spinal cord—occurs in 10% of cases. Rarely, the skin, gastrointestinal system, and adrenal glands may be involved. Laboratory findings are hepatic enzyme and LDH elevation, anemia, leukopenia, and thrombocytopenia. Chest X rays are abnormal in the majority of cases, showing diffuse reticulonodular infiltrates or a miliary pattern.

Mediastinal syndromes result from mediastinal lymphadenopathy, a cardinal feature of histoplasmosis, which may be massive. Calcification of the enlarged lymph nodes is typical. Rarely, fibrosing mediastinitis develops as a consequence of histoplasmosis. The dense fibrotic tissue causes obstruction of mediastinal organs. Impingement of enlarged lymph nodes on the trachea or main bronchi or fibrotic compression may cause coughing or airway obstruction presenting as dyspnea or obstructive pneumonia. Erosion of calcified tissue into the bronchial lumen may cause broncholithiasis or hemoptysis. Esophageal compression by enlarged nodes or mediastinal fibrosis may cause dysphagia. The most dangerous features of fibrosing mediastinitis are superior vena cava syndrome and pulmonary hypertension caused by occlusion of large pulmonary arteries or veins.

Inflammatory syndromes represent an inflammatory or immune response to histoplasma rather than a direct effect of the fungus on the affected tissues. These syndromes include arthralgia, arthritis, and erythema nodosum. Pericarditis is probably a reaction to adjacent lymphadenitis.

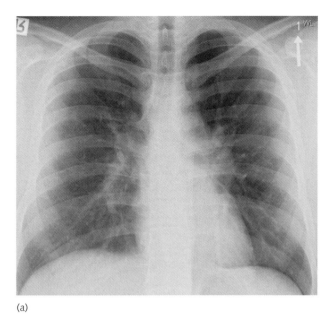
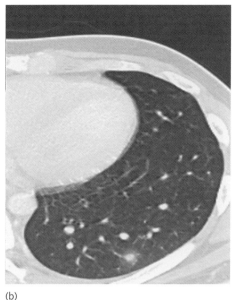

(a)                                                            (b)

**Figure 29.1** A 22-year-old male was seen after recent travel to South America. He had not visited any caves, but 10–14 days before onset of symptoms he had visited the Amazon jungles of Bolivia. He complained of 1 week of fever and severe headache, but no cough or dyspnea. A chest X ray showed a prominent left hilum and ill-defined opacities in the left lower lung field (a). Computed tomography revealed left hilar lymphadenopathy and several pulmonary nodules (b). Serological tests were positive for *H. capsulatum*.

African-type histoplasmosis typically presents as skin nodules or ulcers or osteolytic bone lesions. Biopsies show caseating granulomata. In some cases, particularly in immunocompromised hosts, the infection may disseminate to the lymph nodes, lungs, abdomen, skin, bones, and joints.

Clinical features of histoplasmosis in returning travelers generally fit one of the common forms of the disease: asymptomatic infection, incidental radiological abnormalities, acute pulmonary histoplasmosis, or PDH.

Acute pulmonary histoplasmosis usually presents within 3 weeks of exposure [8, 12], which would tend to be during travel or shortly after the traveler's return. The clinical presentation is as described above and in Table 29.5. (For illustration, see Figure 29.1.) Some returning travelers may suffer from subacute infection lasting up to a few months.

Strong evidence for the existence of asymptomatic histoplasmosis comes from rigorous epidemiological surveys triggered by outbreaks among travelers [8, 12]. In these studies, 20–30% of those who had serological evidence of infection were asymptomatic.

Incidental findings on chest radiology, presumably reflecting a past (asymptomatic or undiagnosed) infection, may be seen weeks to decades after travel. The importance

of this is that a careful travel history should be taken in individuals with multiple pulmonary nodules or mediastinal lymphadenopathy, particularly if calcified. A history of travel to an endemic region, particularly in conjunction with positive serology for histoplasma, may obviate the necessity for biopsy in an asymptomatic patient.

Rarely, PDH may be diagnosed in returning travelers even years after travel to an endemic region. Most travelers with PDH suffer from AIDS, but a few cases have been reported in apparently immunocompetent patients with a remote history of travel to Central Africa [13, 14].

A few reports have been published of returning travelers with chronic pulmonary histoplasmosis [6], erythema nodosum, rheumatological manifestations complicating acute pulmonary disease [15], and even laryngeal [16] and oral [17] histoplasmosis, which are very rare even in endemic areas.

## Diagnosis

The diagnostic strategy for suspected histoplasmosis depends greatly on the clinical context. Available diagnostic tests include fungal culture, histopathology, serological tests for antibodies, and antigen detection. Histoplasmin is no longer commercially available for skin testing. Molecular detection methods are currently under development.

The sensitivity and specificity of these tests depend on the time elapsed since infection, the immune status of the host, and the load of infectious organisms.

Fungal culture is probably the most specific tests for histoplasmosis, but it is insensitive, and growth may take as long as 4 weeks. Culture is most likely to be positive in disseminated or chronic pulmonary disease.

Histopathological examination of tissue samples enables rapid diagnosis but is positive in less than 50% of cases.

Standard serological tests for *H. capsulatum* include a complement fixation (CF) assay and an immunodiffusion (ID) assay. Antibody titers of 1:32 or more on the CF assay are considered diagnostic in the appropriate clinical context. However, lower titers should not always be disregarded, particularly in individuals who do not live in endemic regions. The ID test identifies two precipitin bands, of which the M band is more sensitive than the H band. ID is less sensitive than CF and converts more slowly in acute infections [18]. Only rarely is ID positive when CF is negative. The serological tests are 90–100% sensitive in cases of acute nondisseminated histoplasmosis and in chronic pulmonary infection. Two-thirds of patients with a mediastinal syndrome will be seropositive. A major limitation of serological testing is that antibodies develop only 2–6 weeks after exposure, thus limiting the utility of the test in severe acute infections, where timely treatment hinges on the diagnosis. Another limitation is that antibody response is impaired in immunocompromised hosts, and thus the sensitivity of serological testing (CF and ID in combination) for disseminated infection is only 67–82%. Cross-reactivity with other fungi is significant [18]—up to 40% in paracoccidioidomycosis, aspergillosis, and blastomycosis, though much less with candidiasis and coccidiodomycosis. More important is that serological tests for histoplasma may be positive in nearly 30% of patients with tuberculosis. Notably, ID is much more specific for histoplasma than CF.

In travelers with a history of travel to an endemic location and a clinical syndrome consistent with histoplasmosis, a single positive specimen is generally sufficient to establish the diagnosis. In endemic areas a positive serological test may persist from a previous infection; thus, a fourfold rise in convalescent titer is needed for conclusive diagnosis.

In returning travelers with incidentally discovered radiological abnormalities suggestive of histoplasmosis, the travel history together with positive serology may help to establish the diagnosis. However, it should be taken into account that antibody response may have waned over time.

Antigen detection is an important complement to serological tests. Antigen may be detected before seroconversion, enabling early diagnosis. Sensitivity is highest in the urine, and antigenemia is rare in the absence of antigenuria. Antigen detection is more likely when the load of the pathogen is high and in immunosuppressed hosts. Antigen can be detected in the urine in 80% of cases of disseminated histoplasmosis in immunocompetent hosts, but in as many as 95% of disseminated infections in patients with AIDS. The sensitivity is lower in acute nondisseminated infection (the common form in travelers) and very low in chronic pulmonary and mediastinal disease. There is a cross-reaction with other mycoses such as blastomycosis, paracoccidiodomycosis, and penicilliosis, but not with coccidiodomycosis.

CNS infection (meningitis, histoplasmoma) poses a particular diagnostic problem [11], particularly when the CNS is the only clinically apparent site of infection. Rapid diagnosis is of paramount importance. Stains of the CSF identify histoplasma in only 10% of cases, and cultures are positive in only about 25% of cases. When meningitis is part of a disseminated infection, urine antigen detection and culture of samples from infected sites outside the CNS have 70% and 50% sensitivity, respectively, but these tests are of little utility in isolated CNS infection. Thus, in such cases, it is prudent to stain and culture CSF (10–20 mL should be cultured). CSF (undiluted) and serum should be tested serologically for antibodies against histoplasma, and CSF should be tested for the presence of antigen. In rare cases when all of these tests are negative and the diagnosis of isolated CNS histoplasmosis is still being entertained, meningeal or brain biopsy should be considered.

## Treatment

Guidelines for the treatment of histoplasmosis have been published [19]. Most infections with histoplasma are asymptomatic or mildly symptomatic and self-limited and do not require treatment (Table 29.6). Whether therapy could hasten recovery in such cases is unknown. If a patient with acute pulmonary histoplasmosis is hypoxemic or otherwise severely ill, treatment should be initiated with amphotericin B (3–5 mg/kg/day of a liposomal formulation or 0.7–1.0 mg/kg/day of a deoxycholate formulation) for 1–2 weeks and until clinical improvement is achieved. Adding methylprednisolone (0.5–1.0 mg/kg/day) is recommended in patients with severe respiratory compromise. Thereafter, treatment can be completed with 200 mg itraconazole twice daily for a total of 12 weeks. Alternatively, in patients intolerant of oral

**Table 29.6** Indications for antifungal treatment of histoplasmosis.

**Treatment indicated**
Acute pulmonary infection, moderately severe/severe symptoms
Chronic cavitary pulmonary histoplasmosis
Progressive disseminated histoplasmosis
CNS infection

**Uncertain indications**
Acute focal pulmonary infection, infiltrates or symptoms persisting for >1 month
Mediastinal lymphadenitis or granuloma
Inflammatory syndromes treated with corticosteroids

**Treatment not indicated**
Acute focal pulmonary infection, duration <1 month, mild or moderate symptoms
Mediastinal fibrosis
Inflammatory syndromes not requiring treatment with corticosteroids
Broncholithiasis
Pulmonary nodule
Presumed ocular histoplasmosis syndrome

*Source.* From [19].

medication, treatment can be completed with amphotericin B to a total dose of no more than 35 mg/kg.

Treatment of subacute pulmonary histoplasmosis is generally not indicated unless symptoms persist for more than a month. Itraconazole (200 mg three times daily for 3 days followed by 200 mg once or twice daily for 6–12 weeks) is recommended in these cases. There is no good evidence that treatment of acute or subacute pulmonary infection prevents progression to PDH, fibrosing mediastinitis, or chronic pulmonary disease, but it is reasonable to treat those patients with underlying emphysema or immunosuppression.

Chronic pulmonary histoplasmosis will progress and lead to destruction of the lungs if untreated, and treatment is therefore recommended in all cases. Itraconazole for milder cases and amphotericin B for more severe cases are used as in acute infections, but treatment should be continued for 12–24 months [19], and preferably until radiographic abnormalities have been stable for at least 3 months [11]. Blood levels of itraconazole should be obtained after 2 weeks of therapy to ensure adequate drug exposure.

PDH can be treated according to the same principles as acute infection, though prompt initiation of therapy is obviously of greater urgency. A study in AIDS patients showed a trend favoring liposomal amphotericin B (Ambisome) over the standard formulation for induction therapy in PDH [20]. After 2 weeks of amphotericin, if clinical improvement is observed, a shift to oral itraconazole is reasonable. Here, too, blood levels of itraconazole should be obtained after 2 weeks of therapy. Treatment should continue for 6–18 months in immunocompetent hosts. In patients with ongoing immunosuppression, indefinite antifungal therapy (itraconazole 200 mg/day) may be necessary to prevent relapse. However, discontinuation of maintenance therapy is safe if antiretroviral therapy for AIDS causes the CD4 count to rise above 150 cells/μl [21]. Urine histoplasma antigen levels may be used to monitor response to therapy of disseminated histoplasmosis and for early detection of relapse.

Treatment of CNS histoplasmosis presents a particular challenge because penetration of brain tissue and CSF by some antifungal agents is poor. CNS infection has only rarely been described in returning travelers, and the reader is referred to a recent review [22] and guidelines [19] for discussion of this entity.

## Prevention
Exposure of travelers to histoplasmosis can be anticipated in endemic areas. Heavy exposure is likely in any cave located in an endemic region, particularly if it is infested by bats. Travelers with AIDS or other forms of significant immunosuppression should be warned of the hazards of *Histoplasma* infection in endemic destinations, and visiting caves likely to be contaminated should be strongly discouraged. Use of face masks should be considered in all travelers who plan to visit caves where heavy exposure to *Histoplasma* is likely. Simple paper masks are not

adequate protection [12]. Detailed information on protective equipment is available in a CDC publication available online [23].

## Coccidiodomycosis

Coccidiodomycosis, sometimes called valley fever, is caused by the tissue dimorphic fungus *Coccidiodes immitis*. Human infection occurs as a result of inhalation of spores that are found in the soil of endemic areas. *C. immitis* is endemic to an arid region of the southwestern USA, including central and southern California, Arizona, New Mexico, western Texas, and part of Utah, and a contiguous area in northern Mexico. Smaller regions of endemicity have been reported in Argentina and Paraguay and foci have been found in Central America as well.

Coccidiodomycosis has been reported in travelers returning from California, Arizona, and Mexico. Two outbreaks have been reported among travelers native to nonendemic areas of the USA returning from Mexico [24, 25]. In both cases, the groups were involved in construction work during their trips. Another outbreak occurred among participants in an international convention that took place in Flying Hills, California, a location highly endemic for *C. immitis*. In the weeks and months after the convention, cases among participants were confirmed in Britain, Finland, Australia, and New Zealand [26].

### Clinical features

Clinical features of coccidiodomycosis have many similarities to those of histoplasmosis. The majority of infections are asymptomatic, but perhaps 40% of infected individuals develop an acute flu-like illness, typically 1–3 weeks after exposure. Common symptoms are fever, malaise, headache, rash, myalgia, and dry cough. The rash is most commonly a macular erythematous eruption that appears early in the course of the illness. Erythema nodosum and erythema multiforme are less common skin manifestations associated with coccidiodomycosis.

The common radiologic appearance of acute *C. immitis* infection is patchy infiltrates. Ipsilateral lymph node enlargement may occur. Occasionally, mediastinal lymphadenopathy may appear without significant parenchymal involvement. The primary infection usually heals quite rapidly. Cavitation may occur, generally as part of the healing process.

The acute infection is generally self-limited, but progressive lung disease occasionally develops. Fever and cough persist, weight loss occurs, and radiological progression is observed.

Commonly used indicators of severity in acute infection are weight loss of >10%, intense night sweats persisting for >3 weeks, bilateral lung infiltrates or unilateral infiltrates involving more than one-half of the lung, prominent or persistent hilar adenopathy, concentrations of CF antibody to *C. immitis* of >1:16, failure to develop dermal hypersensitivity to coccidiodal antigens, inability to work, or symptoms that persist for 12 months [27].

Progressive pulmonary infection often leads to dissemination. Dissemination generally occurs within months of the primary pulmonary infection. Risk factors for progressive pulmonary disease and dissemination are similar—primarily immunosuppressed patients, especially those with AIDS, and recipients of solid organ transplants. Curiously, race plays a role in risk for dissemination—African Americans, Filipinos, and Native Americans are at higher risk than whites. Other risk factors are male sex, extremes of age, diabetes, and advanced (third trimester) pregnancy. Dissemination may involve any organ, but skin involvement and osteomyelitis are the most common. The most lethal dissemination is meningitis. Symptoms of coccidiodal meningitis may be minimal; thus, lumbar puncture is recommended in all cases of disseminated infection [28].

### Diagnosis

Pulmonary *Coccidiodes* infection can often be diagnosed by microscopic examination of respiratory tract specimens for the characteristic fungal spherules. The main distinguishing feature of *Coccidiodes* spherules is the presence of endospores. Useful special stains are PAS, KOH, Papanicolau, methenamine silver, and calcofluor white, and at least one of these should be employed if the standard smear is negative. Culture provides the most definitive diagnostic test. Culture presents a significant occupational hazard to laboratory personnel; thus, handling of mycelial cultures should be performed under rigorous biohazard precautions. The sensitivity of bronchoalveolar lavage cytology and culture is much greater than that of sputum samples (53% vs 20%) [29].

Serological tests are useful for the diagnosis of coccidiodomycosis. The two most widely used assays currently available are an immunodiffusion tube precipitin test (IDTP) and a complement fixation (CF) assay. The IDTP detects IgM and is very sensitive for the detection of recent infection—positive titer appears 1–3 weeks after the onset of acute illness, but tends to wane within a few months. The CF assay detects IgG and thus converts later in the course of disease than IDTP, but persists longer. The threshold titer for a positive result is generally 1:8. A titer higher than 1:32 or a rising titer in sequential samples may indicate worsening or disseminated disease, but dissemination should never be diagnosed by serology alone. Any positive titer in a CSF sample should be considered diagnostic of CNS coccidiodomycosis, assuming the CSF was not contaminated by peripheral blood in a traumatic tap, or by infected paraspinal tissues. The sensitivity of CSF culture for the detection of coccidiodomycosis meningitis is less than 50%, whereas that of serology (CF) is over 75% [30].

Recently, ELISA has been used to detect IgG and IgM antibodies against *C. immitis*. In one study, the sensitivity, specificity, positive predictive value, and negative predictive value were 100%, 99%, 82%, and 100%, respectively [31].

The utility of serology in monitoring the response of coccidiodomycosis to treatment is not known.

Antigen assays for coccidiodomycosis are not available. A PCR-based assay for coccidiodal DNA is currently under development [32].

## Treatment

Treatment of coccidiodomycosis should follow published guidelines [27]. Although some authorities advocate treatment of all symptomatic cases of acute coccidiodomycosis, the majority favor limiting treatment to infections in immunocompromised hosts, severe cases, and perhaps infections of those at risk for dissemination, such as women in the third trimester of pregnancy. Whether or not a decision is made to treat, the management of acute coccidiodomycosis should routinely include monitoring the patient for 1–2 years, either to document resolution or to identify, as early as possible, evidence of pulmonary or extrapulmonary complications.

Treatment with an oral azole (ketoconazole, 400 mg/d; fluconazole, 400–800 mg/d; or itraconazole, 200 mg b.i.d.) for 3–6 months is recommended for most acute infections. In a pregnant patient, amphotericin B is the drug of choice because of concerns of teratogenicity with azoles. When bilateral reticulonodular or miliary infiltrates are present, an underlying immunodeficiency state is likely. Diffuse pneumonia due to *C. immitis* is usually a manifestation of fungemia and, therefore, patients should be evaluated for dissemination. Therapy should be initiated with amphotericin B (0.5–0.7 mg/kg/day). Once clinical improvement is achieved, which may take several weeks, an oral azole can be substituted for the amphotericin B, and treatment should be continued for a total of 1 year. In patients with ongoing immunosuppression, permanent secondary prophylaxis is recommended.

In the absence of meningitis, disseminated infection can also be treated with an oral azole, but infection that is rapidly progressive or not responsive to treatment should be treated with amphotericin B for several weeks until there is clear evidence of improvement, and thereafter with an azole, to complete at least 1 year of antifungal treatment. If coccidiodal meningitis is diagnosed, oral fluconazole should be commenced at 800–100 mg/day. Itraconazole (400–600 mg/day) has also been used with comparable results. Patients who respond to azoles should be treated indefinitely, although a shift to more conventional doses (400 mg/day) is acceptable after clinical improvement has been achieved.

In the absence of immunosuppression, an asymptomatic or completely resected pulmonary nodule does not require antifungal treatment.

Surgery may be advisable for refractory lesions or those complicated by hemoptysis.

## Penicilliosis

Penicilliosis, caused by the thermally dimorphic *Penicillium marneffei*, is an emerging mycosis endemic to Southeast Asia. The vast majority of cases have been reported in AIDS patients from Thailand. Other areas known to be endemic include Vietnam, Laos, Singapore, Malaysia, Burma, Thailand, Indonesia, Hong Kong, and the Guangxi province in southern China [33]. A few cases have been reported in travelers, mostly immunosuppressed, who visited the endemic areas [34, 35]. Notably, two cases have been reported in patients native to Africa who had never traveled to Southeast Asia [36, 37]. In one of the two [36], laboratory exposure was postulated but not proved. These cases raise the possibility of endemicity of *P. marneffei* in Africa.

The only known natural hosts are bamboo rats and humans. *P. marneffei* can be isolated from the soil around the rats' burrows, but only rarely from other environmental sources. The exact route of acquisition in humans is unknown, but it is thought unlikely to be from direct contact with the rats and is presumed to be via inhalation and, rarely, inoculation [38]. There is no evidence of person-to-person spread.

Penicilliosis is an AIDS-defining illness. The infection occurs late in the course of AIDS; one series reported a CD4 cell count ranging from 1 to 110 cells/μl [34]. Penicilliosis appears to be very unusual or perhaps nonexistent in

HIV-infected individuals successfully treated with highly active antiretroviral therapy. Infections have been reported in non-AIDS immunosuppressed hosts and, rarely, in apparently immunocompetent individuals.

Common clinical features of penicilliosis include fever (present in 89–98% of cases), anemia (75–78%), weight loss (67–76%), skin lesions (53–71%), diffuse lymphadenopathy (33–58%), and hepatomegaly (36–51%) [34, 39, 40]. Skin lesions are characteristic and are therefore an important clue to the diagnosis. Papules, pustules, abscesses, nodules, or ulcers are most commonly distributed over the face, upper trunk, and extremities. In AIDS patients, the typical skin lesions are umbilicated papules very similar to molluscum contagiosum, whereas in individuals not infected with HIV, skin abscesses are more common [41].

The diagnosis of penicilliosis is confirmed by microscopic examination of skin biopsies and cultures of bone marrow, skin biopsy, and peripheral blood.

Severe cases of penicilliosis should be treated with intravenous amphotericin B (0.6 mg/kg/day) for 2 weeks, followed by 10 weeks of itraconazole (400mg/day) [42]. Voriconazole and ketoconazole are alternative azoles. Patients with ongoing immunosuppression should be maintained on 200 mg/day of itraconazole as long as immunosuppression is present, in order to prevent relapse, which will occur in a majority of patients without prophylaxis [43].

Immunosuppressed individuals, particularly those with active AIDS, should be strongly discouraged from travel to areas endemic for *P. marneffei*. If travel is undertaken nevertheless, primary prophylaxis with itraconazole should be considered.

## Endemic mycoses not reported in travelers

*Paracoccidiodomycosis*, sometimes called *South American blastomycosis*, is caused by *Paracoccidiodes brasiliensis*, a thermally dimorphic fungus endemic to the subtropical areas of Central and South America. Paracoccidiodomycosis has not been reported in tourists returning from the endemic region. All cases diagnosed outside the endemic area have occurred in individuals who lived in the endemic area for long periods, usually years. For example, in a comprehensive review of cases diagnosed in Japan [5], 16 of 17 cases affected individuals native to Brazil or descendants of Japanese emigrants to Brazil. The only Japanese citizen with paracoccidioidomycosis had lived in Brazil for five years beforedeveloping the disease. Thus, paracoccidioidomycosis seems to be limited to natives of or immigrants from the endemic region and is very unlikely to be seen in the short-term traveler.

*Blastomycosis* is endemic to an area of North America very similar to that of *Histoplasma* but extending further north, as far as the Canadian provinces of Ontario and Manitoba. Blastomycosis is much less common than histoplasmosis even within the endemic area, and has not been reported in travelers from nonendemic countries who visited the area of endemicity.

*Lobomycosis*, also known as Lobo's disease or lacaziosis, is caused by *Lacazia loboi* (previously *Loboa loboi*). The pathogen is endemic to parts of Latin America, including Bolivia, Brazil, Colombia, Costa Rica, Ecuador, French Guiana, Guyana, Mexico, Panama, Peru, Suriname, and Venezuela. The clinical features differ greatly from those of the other endemic mycoses. Lobomycosis is a localized infection of the skin characterized by keloid-like ulcerated or verrucous nodular or plaque-like lesions developing over months or even years. Systemic symptoms are absent. In many cases, infection occurs at the site of a local trauma, suggesting local invasion through the compromised skin barrier. Several hundred human cases have been described in the endemic areas. Only a handful of cases have been reported outside the endemic region. Intriguingly, in one case in Holland, infection was seen in the caregiver of a dolphin, the only other species known to be infected with *L. loboi*. The fungus has never been successfully cultured, and diagnosis is based largely on the typical morphology in tissue—spherical or lemon-shaped cells 6–12 μm in diameter, commonly arranged in chains of budding cells connected by thin, tubular bridges. Lobomycosis is poorly responsive to antifungal therapy, and the treatment of choice is surgical resection, preferably with a wide margin.

## References

1  Cano MV, Hajjeh RA. The epidemiology of histoplasmosis: a review. *Semin Respir Infect* 2001;16(2):109–18.

2  Morse DL, Gordon MA, Matte T, Eadie G. An outbreak of histoplasmosis in a prison. *Am J Epidemiol* 1985;122(2):253–61.

3  Luby JP, Southern PM Jr, Haley CE, Vahle KL, Munford RS, Haley RW. Recurrent exposure to *Histoplasma capsulatum* in modern air-conditioned buildings. *Clin Infect Dis.* 2005;41(2):170–76.

4  Antinori S, Magni C, Nebuloni M, Parravicini C, Corbellino M, Sollima S, et al. Histoplasmosis among human immunodeficiency virus-infected people in Europe: report

of 4 cases and review of the literature. *Medicine (Baltimore)* 2006;85(1):22–36.

5 Kamei K, Sano A, Kikuchi K, Makimura K, Niimi M, Suzuki K, et al. The trend of imported mycoses in Japan. *J Infect Chemother* 2003;9(1):16–20.

6 Ashbee HR, Evans EG, Viviani MA, Dupont B, Chryssanthou E, Surmont I, et al. Histoplasmosis in Europe: report on an epidemiological survey from the European Confederation of Medical Mycology Working Group. *Med Mycol* 2008;46(1):57–65.

7 Wheat LJ, Slama TG, Eitzen HE, Kohler RB, French ML, Biesecker JL. A large urban outbreak of histoplasmosis: clinical features. *Ann Intern Med* 1981;94(3):331–7.

8 Morgan J, Cano MV, Feikin DR, Phelan M, Monroy OV, Morales PK, et al. A large outbreak of histoplasmosis among American travelers associated with a hotel in Acapulco, Mexico, spring 2001. *Am J Trop Med Hyg* 2003;69(6):663–9.

9 Chamany S, Mirza SA, Fleming JW, Howell JF, Lenhart SW, Mortimer VD, et al. A large histoplasmosis outbreak among high school students in Indiana, 2001. *Pediatr Infect Dis J* 2004;23(10):909–14.

10 Manfredi R, Mazzoni A, Nanetti A, Chiodo F. Histoplasmosis capsulati and duboisii in Europe: the impact of the HIV pandemic, travel and immigration. *Eur J Epidemiol* 1994;10(6):675–81.

11 Wheat LJ. Histoplasmosis: a review for clinicians from non-endemic areas. *Mycoses* 2006;49(4):274–82.

12 Lyon GM, Bravo AV, Espino A, Lindsley MD, Gutierrez RE, Rodriguez I, et al. Histoplasmosis associated with exploring a bat-inhabited cave in Costa Rica, 1998–1999. *Am J Trop Med Hyg* 2004;70(4):438–42.

13 Desmet P, Vogelaers D, Afschrift M. Progressive disseminated histoplasmosis 10 years after return out of Africa in an immunocompetent host. *Acta Clin Belg* 2004;59(5):274–8.

14 Mahvi A, Nachega J, Piron A, Blomme C, Deneys V, Provoost N, et al. Chronic disseminated histoplasmosis in an apparently immuno-competent Belgian patient. *Acta Clin Belg* 2004;59(2):102–5.

15 Alonso D, Munoz J, Letang E, Salvado E, Cuenca-Estrella M, Buitrago MJ, et al. Imported acute histoplasmosis with rheumatologic manifestations in Spanish travelers. *J Travel Med* 2007;14(5):338–42.

16 Smeets LC, Lestrade PJ, de Visscher AV, Schneeberger PM. [Hoarseness in a recent visitor to the tropics through infection of the larynx by *Histoplasma capsulatum*]. *Ned Tijdschr Geneeskd* 2005;149(12):657–9.

17 Chauvet E, Carreiro M, Berry A, Tohfe M, Ollier S, Sailler L, et al. [Oral histoplasmosis 34 years after return of Africa]. *Rev Med Interne* 2003;24(3):195–7.

18 Wheat J, French ML, Kamel S, Tewari RP. Evaluation of cross-reactions in *Histoplasma capsulatum* serologic tests. *J Clin Microbiol* 1986;23(3):493–9.

19 Wheat LJ, Freifeld AG, Kleiman MB, Baddley JW, McKinsey DS, Loyd JE, et al. Clinical practice guidelines for the management of patients with histoplasmosis: 2007 update by the Infectious Diseases Society of America. *Clin Infect Dis* 2007;45(7):807–25.

20 Johnson PC, Wheat LJ, Cloud GA, Goldman M, Lancaster D, Bamberger DM, et al. Safety and efficacy of liposomal amphotericin B compared with conventional amphotericin B for induction therapy of histoplasmosis in patients with AIDS. *Ann Intern Med.* 2002;137(2):105–9.

21 Goldman M, Zackin R, Fichtenbaum CJ, Skiest DJ, Koletar SL, Hafner R, et al. Safety of discontinuation of maintenance therapy for disseminated histoplasmosis after immunologic response to antiretroviral therapy. *Clin Infect Dis* 2004;38(10):1485–9.

22 Wheat LJ, Musial CE, Jenny-Avital E. Diagnosis and management of central nervous system histoplasmosis. *Clin Infect Dis* 2005;40(6):844–52.

23 Lenhart SW, Schafer MP, Singal M, Hajjeh RA. Histoplasmosis—Protecting Workers at Risk. US Department of Health and Human Services, National Institute for Occupational Safety and Health Publication No. 2005-109; 2005.

24 Cairns L, Blythe D, Kao A, Pappagianis D, Kaufman L, Kobayashi J, et al. Outbreak of coccidioidomycosis in Washington state residents returning from Mexico. *Clin Infect Dis* 2000;30(1):61–4.

25 Coccidioidomycosis in travelers returning from Mexico–Pennsylvania, 2000. *MMWR Morb Mortal Wkly Rep* 2000;49(44):1004–6.

26 Coccidioidomycosis among persons attending the world championship of model airplane flying—Kern County, California, Oct 2001. *MMWR Morb Mortal Wkly Rep* 2001;50(49):1106–7.

27 Galgiani JN, Ampel NM, Catanzaro A, Johnson RH, Stevens DA, Williams PL. Practice guideline for the treatment of coccidioidomycosis. Infectious Diseases Society of America. *Clin Infect Dis* 2000;30(4):658–61.

28 Hage CE, Sarosi GA. Endemic mycosis. In: Sharma OP, editor. *Tropical Lung Disease*, 2nd ed. New York: Taylor & Francis; 2006; p. 397–429.

29 Wallace JM, Catanzaro A, Moser KM, Harrell JH, 2nd. Flexible fiberoptic bronchoscopy for diagnosing pulmonary coccidioidomycosis. *Am Rev Respir Dis* 1981 Mar;123(3): 286–90.

30 Anstead GM, Graybill JR. Coccidioidomycosis. *Infect Dis Clin North Am* 2006;20(3):621–43.

31 Crum NF, Lederman ER, Stafford CM, Parrish JS, Wallace MR. Coccidioidomycosis: a descriptive survey of a reemerging disease. Clinical characteristics and current controversies. *Medicine (Baltimore).* 2004;83(3):149–75.

32 Bialek R. Amplification of coccidioidal DNA in clinical specimens by PCR. *J Clin Microbiol* 2005;43(3):1492–3.

33 Panackal AA, Hajjeh RA, Cetron MS, Warnock DW. Fungal infections among returning travelers. *Clin Infect Dis* 2002;35(9):1088–95.

34  Antinori S, Gianelli E, Bonaccorso C, Ridolfo AL, Croce F, Sollima S, et al. Disseminated *Penicillium marneffei* infection in an HIV-positive Italian patient and a review of cases reported outside endemic regions. *J Travel Med* 2006;13(3): 181–8.

35  Carey J, Hofflich H, Amre R, Protic J, Perlman DC. *Penicillium marneffei* infection in an immunocompromised traveler: a case report and literature review. *J Travel Med* 2005;12(5):291–4.

36  Hilmarsdottir I, Coutellier A, Elbaz J, Klein JM, Datry A, Gueho E, et al. A French case of laboratory-acquired disseminated *Penicillium marneffei* infection in a patient with AIDS. *Clin Infect Dis* 1994;19(2):357–8.

37  Lo Y, Tintelnot K, Lippert U, Hoppe T. Disseminated *Penicillium marneffei* infection in an African AIDS patient. *Trans R Soc Trop Med Hyg* 2000;94(2):187.

38  Ustianowski AP, Sieu TP, Day JN. *Penicillium marneffei* infection in HIV. *Curr Opin Infect Dis* 2008;21(1):31–6.

39  Supparatpinyo K, Khamwan C, Baosoung V, Nelson KE, Sirisanthana T. Disseminated *Penicillium marneffei* infection in southeast Asia. *Lancet* 1994;344(8915):110–13.

40  Duong TA. Infection due to *Penicillium marneffei*, an emerging pathogen: review of 155 reported cases. *Clin Infect Dis* 1996;23(1):125–30.

41  Wortman PD. Infection with *Penicillium marneffei*. *Int J Dermatol* 1996;35(6):393–9.

42  Sirisanthana T, Supparatpinyo K. Epidemiology and management of penicilliosis in human immunodeficiency virus-infected patients. *Int J Infect Dis* 1998;3(1):48–53.

43  Supparatpinyo K, Perriens J, Nelson KE, Sirisanthana T. A controlled trial of itraconazole to prevent relapse of *Penicillium marneffei* infection in patients infected with the human immunodeficiency virus. *N Engl J Med* 1998;339(24):1739–43.

44  Hatakeyama S, Kashiyama T, Takechi A, Sasaki S, Akamatsu E. [Cave-associated acute pulmonary histoplasmosis in two Japanese returning from Mexico]. *Nihon Kokyuki Gakkai Zasshi* 2001;39(4):293–7.

45  Hunt PJ, Harden TJ, Hibbins M, Pritchard RC, Muir DB, Gardner FJ. *Histoplasma capsulatum*. Isolation from an Australian cave environment and from a patient. *Med J Aust* 1984;141(5):280–83.

46  Nasta P, Donisi A, Cattane A, Chiodera A, Casari S. Acute histoplasmosis in spelunkers returning from Mato Grosso, Peru. *J Travel Med* 1997;4(4):176–8.

47  Suzaki A, Kimura M, Kimura S, Shimada K, Miyaji M, Kaufman L. [An outbreak of acute pulmonary histoplasmosis among travelers to a bat-inhabited cave in Brazil]. *Kansenshogaku Zasshi* 1995;69(4):444–9.

48  Bonnet D, Balandraud P, Lonjon T, Rey P, Van de Walle JP, Cador L, et al. [Round pulmonary lesions after returning from French Guyana. Six cases of American pulmonary histoplasmosis]. *Med Trop (Mars)* 1995;55(1):55–60.

49  El Guedj M, Couppie P, Pradinaud R, Aznar C, Carme B, Clity E, et al. [Histoplasmosis due to *Histoplasma capsulatum capsulatum* and HIV infection]. *Rev Med Interne* 2000;21(5):408–15.

50  Drouhet E, Dupont B. [Histoplasmosis and other imported mycoses in 1989]. *Rev Prat* 1989;39(19):1675–82.

51  Larrabee WF, Ajello L, Kaufman L. An epidemic of histoplasmosis on the Isthmus of Panama. *Am J Trop Med Hyg* 1978;27(2 Pt 1):281–5.

52  Farina C, Gnecchi F, Michetti G, Parma A, Cavanna C, Nasta P. Imported and autochthonous histoplasmosis in Bergamo province, Northern Italy. *Scand J Infect Dis* 2000;32(3):271–4.

# 30 Intestinal Protozoa: *Giardia, Amebiasis, Cyclospora, Blastocystis hominis, Dientamoeba fragilis,* and *Cryptosporidium parvum*

## Karin Leder

Royal Melbourne Hospital, University of Melbourne and Monash University, Victoria, Australia

## Introduction

This chapter focuses on common intestinal protozoal infections that occur among travelers. Protozoa are single-celled organisms that replicate within the infected host. This is in contrast to helminths, which are multicellular organisms that often cannot complete all steps of their complex life cycles within humans (see Chapter 31). There are four distinct groups of protozoa: the amebae, the flagellates, the ciliates, and the sporozoa. These groups contain several pathogenic species, but many nonpathogenic intestinal protozoa are also reported in feces, such as *Entamoeba coli, Endolimax nana, Iodamoeba bütschlii, Trichomonas hominis,* and *Chilomastix mesnili,* which will not be discussed (Table 30.1).

Most intestinal protozoal infections are transmitted by ingestion of contaminated food or water, and travelers have an increased risk of acquiring these infections when they visit areas with poor hygienic conditions or insufficient water treatment facilities. Intestinal protozoa account for only 1–3% of acute travelers' diarrhea but for up to 30% of cases of chronic diarrhea [1]. They inhabit different parts of the gastrointestinal tract (Figure 30.1). The clinical presentations are generally relatively similar for most intestinal protozoal infections, usually involving symptoms such as diarrhea, nausea, and abdominal pain.

*Tropical Diseases in Travelers*, 1st edition. Edited by E. Schwartz.
© 2009 by Blackwell Publishing, ISBN: 978-1-4051-8441-0.

General advice given to reduce the risk of travelers' diarrhea also applies to prevention of these protozoal infections (see Chapter 17). In areas where sanitation is inadequate, all raw foods (including salads, uncooked vegetables, and rare meat, fish, and shellfish) and untreated water should be avoided, as they pose a high risk. Protozoal cysts of *Giardia lamblia* and *Entamoeba histolytica,* as well as oocysts of *Cryptosporidium,* are resistant to chlorination, but boiling water will render it safe. Previous gastric surgery and reduced gastric acidity are risk factors for acquisition of these protozoal infections.

## Giardia

*Giardia lamblia* (also known as *G. duodenalis* or *G. intestinalis*) is among the commonest parasite infection acquired by humans. It is transmitted via person-to-person spread by hand-to-mouth transmission of cysts, by the food-borne route, or via fecally contaminated water.

### Epidemiology of *Giardia* in travelers

Giardiasis is not unique to travelers, as infection can be acquired in all countries of the world. However, infection occurs with increased frequency in areas where there are poor hygienic conditions and insufficient water treatment facilities, so giardiasis is a common cause of food- and water-borne diarrhea among travelers visiting developing

**Table 30.1** Classification and primary drug treatment for the most common intestinal protozoa.

| Classification | Organism | Primary agent used for treatment |
|---|---|---|
| Amebae | *Entamoeba histolytica* | Metronidazole or tinidazole |
| | *Entamoeba coli* | Nonpathogenic |
| | *Endolimax nana* | Nonpathogenic |
| | *Iodamoeba bütschlii* | Nonpathogenic |
| Flagellates | *Giardia lamblia* | Metronidazole or tinidazole |
| | *Dientamoeba fragilis* | Metronidazole or tetracyclin |
| | *Trichomonas hominis* | Nonpathogenic |
| | *Chilomastix mesnili* | Nonpathogenic |
| Sporozoa (coccidian) | *Cyclospora cayetanensis* | Trimethoprim–sulfamethoxazole |
| | *Isospora belli* | Trimethoprim–sulfamethoxazole |
| | *Cryptosporidium parvum* | Nitazoxanide |
| Sporozoa | Microsporidiosis | Albendazole (response varies with species) |
| Ciliate | *Balantidium coli* | Tetracycline |
| Protozoan-like | *Blastocystis hominis* | Likely nonpathogenic, but often trial of metronidazole or tinidazole is given |

countries [2]. In developed countries, approximately 40% of giardiasis cases are reported among travelers. Giardiasis is the commonest identified cause of travelers' diarrhea that has persisted for 2 weeks or more and is estimated to account for approximately 5% of travelers' diarrhea overall [3]. The attack rate among travelers varies with destination and behavioral factors, but one study estimated that 7 cases occur per 1000 months abroad [4]. Another study found that the overall risk of being notified with giardiasis in returning travelers from any destination was 5.3 out of 100,000, with the highest incidences in travelers from the Indian subcontinent (628 out of 100,000), East Africa (358 out of 100,000), and West Africa (169 out of 100,000) [5].

## Clinical aspects

Ingestion of as few as 10–25 cysts can lead to giardiasis. Symptoms usually develop after an incubation period of 1–2 weeks. The spectrum of the clinical disease ranges from asymptomatic infection to self-limited acute giardiasis and to chronic infection with symptoms lasting weeks or months. Common symptoms include diarrhea, which is often watery initially but may become fatty and foul-smelling, as well as abdominal cramps/bloating, flatulence, nausea, malaise, and dyspepsia. Travelers often also complain of foul-smelling burps. Occasionally, infection is associated with a low-grade fever. Weight loss occurs in more than half of patients and can be significant (10% of body weight, averaging 4.5 kg in adults).

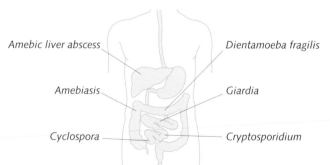

**Figure 30.1** Site of infection of the main human protozoa.

Malabsorption of fats, sugars, carbohydrates and vitamins may occur. Acquired lactose intolerance occurs in up to 20–40% of cases and can take many weeks to normalize even after clearance of the parasite [6]. Chronic giardiasis can also be associated with profound fatigue.

Why the severity of clinical disease is variable is not known, but the variation may be related to the virulence of the giardial isolate, the parasite load, and host determinants. Among children, infection with *Giardia* more often is asymptomatic, whereas in adults, it can be a debilitating disease. Chronic exposure to *Giardia* may induce partial immunity, and travelers to endemic areas seem to have higher rates of symptomatic disease than long-term residents.

## Diagnosis
Historically, diagnosis of giardiasis relied on microscopy of stool samples for ova and parasite (O&P) examination. Because *G. lamblia* is excreted intermittently, it will be detected in approximately 50–70% of cases with a single specimen and in 90% after three specimens [7]. Immunodiagnostic antigen detection assays are now available for the detection of *Giardia* and are being used with increased frequency, particularly because they are more sensitive than conventional microscopy (generally reported to have 90–100% sensitivity). However, antigen testing should not replace stool O&P examination for travelers with diarrhea, as microscopy can also reveal other pathogens. Duodenal sampling methods (e.g., string test, duodenal aspiration, or duodenal biopsy) are more invasive and are generally reserved for confusing cases in which noninvasive tests have been unrevealing. Although a range of histopathology may be found in patients with giardiasis, most commonly the duodenal mucosa appears normal.

## Treatment
Asymptomatic patients discovered to have giardia in their feces do not necessarily require treatment. However, those at risk of transmitting infections to others (e.g., children who have returned from travel and will be attending a day care center, or food handlers) should be treated. Patients with symptoms should always receive specific therapy. As *G. lamblia* is a common cause of chronic diarrhea among returned travelers, it is reasonable to give all travelers with persistent symptoms and no confirmed diagnosis a trial of empiric therapy against *Giardia*. There is no need to repeat a stool examination to check for parasite clearance in individuals who improve symptomatically.

The commonest agents used to treat giardia are metronidazole (recommended doses vary, but are usually between 250 and 400 mg t.i.d., although some authorities recommend up to 750 mg t.i.d. [usually 15–30 mg/kg/day in 3 doses in children] for between 5–7 days) or tinidazole (single 2-g dose, or 50 mg/kg for children). Isolates with decreased susceptibility to metronidazole have been described, and tinidizole is often preferred, because its efficacy is at least as good and there are fewer associated side effects [8, 9]. Albendazole (usually given at a dose of 400 mg or 22.5 mg/kg daily for 5 days), furazolidone 100 mg (1.5 mg/kg) q.i.d. for 7–10 days, and nitazoxanide 500 mg b.i.d. (100–200mg b.i.d. in children] for 3 days are alternative agents. Quinacrine 100 mg (2 mg/kg in children) t.i.d. for 5 days is another alternative. This drug has excellent activity against *Giardia* and used to be the drug of choice, but is no longer available in many countries. During pregnancy, paromomycin (25–35 mg/kg per day in 3 divided doses for 7 days) can be used.

Malabsorptive symptoms may persist following antiparasitic therapy because regeneration of functioning intestinal mucosa requires time. Recurrent diarrhea may also occur following treatment and may be due to relapsed infection or lactose intolerance. Avoidance of diary products, which often exacerbate symptoms, can be recommended. In a microbiologically proven relapse after therapy, a different treatment agent or combination regimen can be administered.

## Prevention
Food-borne spread can be prevented by adequate cooking and water-borne spread by boiling the water, as heat kills *Giardia* cysts. Iodine-based water treatment and high-quality water filtration units (pore sizes < 1 μm) can also be used.

## Amebiasis

Amebiasis is caused by the protozoan *Entamoeba histolytica*. The parasite exists in two forms, a cyst stage, which is the infective form, and a trophozoite stage, which is the form that causes invasive disease. Amebiasis is transmitted by fecal–oral spread, and infection occurs following ingestion of food or water contaminated with amebic cysts.

### Epidemiology of amebiasis in travelers
Amebiasis is a worldwide disease, but developing countries have significantly higher prevalence rates because of poorer socioeconomic conditions and sanitation levels. Areas that have high rates of amebic infection include India, Africa, Mexico, and parts of Central and South

America. In developed countries, amebiasis is mainly seen in migrants from and travelers to endemic countries. However, infection with *E. histolytica* is not a common cause of travelers' diarrhea, as the risk for an ordinary charter tourist is low and infection is uncommon in travelers who have spent less than 1 month in endemic areas [10]. Studies of German travelers to the tropics have suggested that pathogenic *E. histolytica* infection occurs in approximately 0.3% [4, 11]. It is nevertheless an important infection with the potential to cause intestinal and extraintestinal complications.

## Clinical aspects

Over the last two decades, it has been recognized that intestinal amebae with identical morphology can be one of three species, *E. histolytica*, *E. dispar*, or *E. moshkovskii*. This is important because *E. dispar* and *E. moshkovskii* are nonpathogenic. Approximately 90% of *E. histolytica* infections are asymptomatic, too, but intestinal amebiasis, amebic liver abscess, and rarely other extraintestinal manifestations can occur. The strain of *E. histolytica*, as well as host factors such as genetic susceptibility, age, and immunocompetence, ultimately determines whether infection is asymptomatic or leads to invasive disease. Both travelers and locals in endemic countries can develop clinical symptoms following infection, but there are typical presentations seen more commonly among travelers.

*E. histolytica* can cause a number of intestinal syndromes, usually after an incubation period of 7–21 days [3]. It can be associated with symptoms ranging from mild diarrhea to severe dysentery with production of bloody, mucoid stools. In travelers with intestinal amebiasis, the typical presentation is with chronic, nondysenteric diarrhea, often associated with weight loss and abdominal pain. Symptoms can last for months to years and may be clinically indistinguishable from other intestinal protozoal infection.

Other presentations can occur, although they are uncommon in travelers. Patients can present with *amebic colitis*, usual symptoms of which include diarrhea, bloody diarrhea, abdominal pain, fever, weight loss, and tenesmus. These cases may have symptoms similar to those of patients with inflammatory bowel disease. Fulminant necrotizing colitis leading to perforation and peritonitis may occur and can be associated with high (>50%) mortality. Toxic megacolon can also result. Localized colonic infection resulting in a mass of granulation tissue forming a tender palpable mass known as an "ameboma" is another possible presentation, which is important because it can mimic colon cancer, but is very rare in travelers.

## Diagnosis

The main commercially available diagnostic tools are microscopy, antigen detection assays, and serology. Stool specimens will be positive for microscopic (and often macroscopic) blood when invasive intestinal amebic disease is present. For diagnosis of intestinal amebiasis, microscopy may demonstrate cysts or trophozoites in the stool, but cannot differentiate between *E. histolytica* and the nonpathogenic amoebic strains. However, if trophozoites are found ingesting red blood cells, this is suggestive of colitis secondary to *E. histolytica* infection. Organism excretion can vary, so it is recommended that a minimum of three specimens on separate days should be sent to detect 85–95% of infections.

If colonoscopy is performed on patients with amebic colitis, typical flask-shaped abscesses may be seen. The appearance can be confused with that of inflammatory bowel disease, but it is vital to differentiate the two disorders, because outcomes can be catastrophic if patients with amebic colitis are mistakenly treated with steroids. The conditions can be differentiated histopathologically by demonstrating amebic trophozoites in the specimen.

Fecal antigen detection assays are considered superior to microscopy for diagnosis because they are sensitive, specific, rapid, and easy to perform and can distinguish between the different species. Serologic tests are also available, and antibodies will usually be detectable within 5–7 days of acute infection. Serology is less useful in endemic populations, because the test remains positive for years and thus cannot distinguish between acute infection and past exposure to the parasite in these individuals. However, it is a very useful tool among travelers for diagnosis of invasive disease (meaning that amebic colitis or an amebic liver abscess has developed).

## Treatment

The goals of antibiotic therapy for both intestinal and extraintestinal amebiasis are to eliminate invading trophozoites and to eradicate intestinal carriage of the organism and thereby prevent future invasion with any remaining cysts. Therefore, both tissue and luminal agents are used.

### Eradication of trophozoites

Metronidazole 500 to 750 mg t.i.d. for 7–10 days (35 to 50 mg/kg per day in 3 doses for children) is the usual treatment for invasive colitis. The cure rate is approximately 90%. An alternative therapy, which is much better tolerated, is tinidazole 2 g daily for 3 days (50 mg/kg in children), which has a cure rate of over 90% for amoebic colitis. Other alternative therapies (if available) are ornidazole and nitazoxanide.

## Eliminating luminal cysts

Following therapy to eradicate invasive trophozoites, treatment is required to eliminate intraluminal encysted organisms. This should also be given when treating amebic liver abscess, even if stools were negative for organisms. Intraluminal infection is most commonly managed with paromomycin (25–30 mg/kg per day orally in three divided doses for 7 days). Alternative agents (if available) include iodoquinol at a dose of 650 mg orally t.i.d. (30–40 mg/kg per day in 3 divided doses for children) for 20 days or diloxanide furoate at a dose of 500 mg t.i.d. (20 mg/kg per day in 3 divided doses for children) for 10 days. In some countries, none of these agents are readily available, so cysticidal therapy is not given.

Parasitological cure rates are approximately 85–90%. Follow-up stool examinations are required after completion of the therapy because no regimen is completely effective. Asymptomatic patients with *E. histolytica* should be treated (with an intraluminal agent alone) because of the risk of developing invasive disease and the risk of spread to family members [12].

## Extraintestinal amebiasis

Extraintestinal manifestations such as liver, pulmonary, cardiac, brain, or dermal involvement can occur, but they are rarely seen in travelers.

The most common extraintestinal manifestation of amebiasis is amebic liver abscess, which occurs when infective trophozoites migrate hematogenously mostly to the right lobe of the liver. Although amebic infections are not common in travelers, amebic liver abscesses have been reported after travel exposures as short as 4 days [13]. In one study, 35% of travelers with amebic liver abscess had spent less than 6 weeks in an endemic area [14]. For travelers returning from an endemic area, presentation is usually within 8–20 weeks (median 12 weeks) of their return and will be within 5 months in 95% of patients, although a longer lag (sometimes years) has been reported [14].

Patients with amebic liver abscess usually present acutely with a few days of fever and right upper quadrant pain. Very occasionally, patients have a more chronic presentation with months of fever, weight loss, and abdominal pain. Concurrent diarrhea is present in less than one-third of patients, and jaundice occurs in less than 10% [15]. However, it has been suggested that jaundice in amebic abscess might be due to co-infection with hepati-

tis A, because both diseases are spread by the fecal–oral route [16].

## Diagnosis

Laboratory findings in patients with amebic liver abscess often reveal neutrophilia and elevated alkaline phosphatase [17]. Imaging of the liver with ultrasound, CT, or MRI is the major method for diagnosing amebic liver abscess. A single abscess in the right lobe of the liver will be found in 70–80% of cases, although multiple lesions can be present. The imaging findings will disappear slowly (within several months), whereas clinical response is usually within days.

Needle aspiration is not usually required or recommended, but if performed will be culture-negative, thereby distinguishing amebic from bacterial infection. In amebic liver abscess, the typical aspirate findings are of acellular, proteinaceous debris and an "anchovy paste" chocolate-colored fluid consisting predominantly of necrotic hepatocytes. Trophozoites are seen on microscopy of the aspirate in fewer than 20% of cases. Indications for surgical drainage of an amebic abscess include large abscess dimensions, pain relief, impending rupture, location in the left lobe, or lack of therapeutic response to medical therapy [1].

In travelers, serology is a very useful and important tool for diagnosis of amebic liver abscess. Indirect hemagglutination is the most sensitive method. Serum antibodies will be detectable in 92–97% of patients at the time of presentation, but occasionally may be negative in the first 7 days and so may need to be repeated [18]. However, as mentioned above, serology is less useful in endemic populations, because the test remains positive for years. Thus, differentiating between a pyogenic and an amebic liver abscess in the local population is challenging, but in a returning traveler with a liver abscess and positive amebic serology, amebic liver abscess is the most likely diagnosis.

Fecal microscopy will be positive for amebae in less than 20% of hepatic abscess cases [19]. Thus, its role in diagnosis is minimal.

## Treatment

Metronidazole 500–750 mg t.i.d. (35–50 mg/kg per day in 3 doses for children) for 7–10 days is recommended. An alternate therapy, which is better tolerated, is with tinidazole 2 g (50 mg/kg in children) for 5 days, which has a cure rate of almost 100% for amebic liver abscess. Because the source of the infection is always the gastrointestinal tract, treatment for elimination of luminal cysts is needed even when stool is negative for cysts. Treatment is with paromomycin, iodoquinol, or diloxanide furoate at doses mentioned above.

## Prevention

Prevention of amebic infection in travelers involves avoiding of drinking unboiled or unbottled water in endemic areas. Uncooked food such as fruit and vegetables that may have been washed in local water should also not be consumed. Amebic cysts are resistant to chlorine at the levels used in water supplies, but disinfection with iodine may be effective. Ingestion of a single cyst is sufficient to cause disease. There is currently no vaccine available.

## Cyclospora

*Cyclospora cayetanensis* is a protozoan parasite with a wide geographic distribution. Transmission is thought to be by the fecal–oral route and by the ingestion of contaminated water. Large outbreaks of food-borne illness associated with contaminated berries and contaminated vegetables, including lettuce and snow peas, have been reported.

## Epidemiology in travelers

*Cyclospora* infections have commonly been reported from Southeast Asia, Papua New Guinea, Indonesia, India, Pakistan, Nepal, the Middle East, North Africa, the Caribbean, and Latin America (especially Peru and Guatemala). However, the true prevalence of this parasite in any population is unknown. Aside from outbreaks related to importation of contaminated foods, most reports of *Cyclospora* infection in developed countries have occurred among returned travelers who have visited endemic countries and have developed travelers' diarrhea [20, 21]. Seasonal fluctuations in infection incidence have been suggested, with the highest infection rates occurring during the summer and rainy months of the year [22].

## Clinical aspects

Following ingestion of infectious oocysts, there is an incubation period of about 7 days before symptoms develop. Although some hosts with cyclosporiasis remain asymptomatic, common symptoms include watery diarrhea, nausea, anorexia, flatulence, abdominal pain, bloating, weight loss, profound fatigue, and occasionally fever [23]. A waxing and waning course lasting for weeks or months occurs relatively commonly, and typically lasts 6–12 weeks if left untreated [3]. Therefore, *Cyclospora* can be a cause of prolonged travelers' diarrhea [20, 24–27].

## Diagnosis

The diagnosis is usually made by detecting oocysts in the stool via a modified acid-fast stain or by fluorescence microscopy.

## Treatment

The recommended therapy for cyclosporiasis is trimethoprim–sulfamethoxazole (160 mg/800 mg b.i.d. [trimethoprim 5 mg/kg/sulfamethoxazole 25 mg/kg b.i.d.]) for 7–10 days. For patients allergic to sulfa-containing drugs, ciprofloxacin or nitazoxanide (500 mg b.i.d. for 3 days) can be tried.

## Prevention

Because cyclosporiasis is a food- and water-borne infection most prominent in developing countries, the usual advice regarding safe foods and avoiding untreated tap water should be adhered to, to minimize the risks of infection.

## Blastocystis hominis

*Blastocystis hominis* is a protozoan-like organism and is one of the most common microbes detected in stool specimens. However, there is considerable controversy about whether it represents a commensal or a true pathogen, because it is frequently reported in human fecal samples from both symptomatic and asymptomatic patients. It is presumed to be spread by the fecal–oral route; contaminated water may also be a source of infection [28–30].

## Epidemiology in travelers

*B. hominis* is found worldwide but is more commonly found in the tropics and developing countries. Its prevalence in stool samples is estimated to be 10–15% among healthy asymptomatic individuals in developed countries and 30–50% in developing countries. It is commonly found in the stool of returned travelers from developing countries [28, 31, 32]. In one study among travelers and expatriates in Nepal, the prevalence from almost 2000 stool specimens was 30% [33]. In a study of 795 European patients returning from developing countries, 73 (9.1%) had *B. hominis* identified in their stool [34].

## Diagnosis

The diagnosis is made by examination of stool specimen(s) by light microscopy of stained smears or wet mounts.

## Clinical aspects and treatment

Symptoms that have been reported to be associated with *B. hominis* infection include watery diarrhea, nausea, anorexia, abdominal cramps, bloating, flatulence, and fatigue. However, there remains debate regarding whether *B. hominis* is a true pathogen. Many experts doubt there is a correlation between *B. hominis* and gastrointestinal symptoms [35–37]; it is often suggested that, rather than being a pathogen itself, *B. hominis* in a stool specimen from a symptomatic individual may reflect ingestion of contaminated food or water and should serve as a marker for another unidentified pathogen. In support of this, a report among travelers and expatriates in Nepal determined that diarrhea was no more common among individuals with a high concentration of *B. hominis* in their stools (4%) than among asymptomatic controls (5%) [33]. This suggests that *B. hominis* is not a cause of travelers' diarrhea even if it is identified in the stool of travelers. However, other studies dispute this [31]. There seems to be extensive genetic diversity among *B. hominis* isolates, and it is not clear whether virulence varies among the different strains. It is also uncertain whether the concentration of organisms in stool has any effect on symptoms. The controversy regarding the pathogenicity of *B. hominis* is further exacerbated by the fact that some laboratories do not report *B. hominis* at all, making evaluation of its potential role in asymptomatic and symptomatic individuals even more difficult. Additionally, there are no properly controlled prospective studies of the pathogenicity of *B. hominis* or the effects of specific therapy.

A common clinical approach in returned travelers with gastrointestinal symptoms for whom fecal specimens reveal only *B. hominis* is to search thoroughly to exclude other pathogens or other causes of gastrointestinal disease. If no other cause is found, it is reasonable to initiate therapy using an empirical trial of metronidazole or tinidizaole, which will be effective for other commonly acquired parasite infections such as giardiasis. If this fails, trimethoprim–sulfamethoxazole or albendazole can be tried. Asymptomatic patients found to have *B. hominis* do not require therapy.

## Dientamoeba fragilis

*Dientamoeba fragilis* is another protozoan parasite for which a role as a causative diarrheal agent is somewhat controversial. Some people believe it does not cause diarrhea, but the potential of *D. fragilis* to cause symptomatic intestinal illness is being recognized, and experts increasingly recommend specific treatment in symptomatic patients for whom no other etiology is found [38–40].

## Epidemiology and clinical aspects

*D. fragilis* has a worldwide distribution and is transmitted by the fecal–oral route, but exact means by which this parasite is acquired have not been fully defined. Asymptomatic carriers exist, but *D. fragilis* is also not uncommonly found in returned travelers with mild to moderate diarrhea, abdominal pain, flatulence, fatigue, and anorexia. In a recent review of patients with travelers' diarrhea associated with *D. fragilis*, symptoms lasted from 5 days to over 4 weeks [41].

## Diagnosis and treatment

Diagnosis relies on microscopy of appropriately fixed and stained stool samples. If found in asymptomatic individuals, no treatment is required. For those with symptoms, agents that can be tried include metronidazole 500–750 mg t.i.d. (20–40 mg/kg/day in 3 doses for children) for 10 days, tetracycline 500 mg q.i.d. (40 mg/kg/day in 4 doses for children) for 10 days, or paromomycin 25–35 mg/kg per day in 3 divided doses for 7 days.

## Cryptosporidium parvum

*Cryptosporidium parvum* is an intracellular protozoan parasite transmitted via the fecal–oral route from an infected person or animal, or from a fecally contaminated environment such as a food or water source.

## Epidemiology and clinical aspects

*C. parvum* infections occur worldwide but are more common in countries with increased crowding and poor sanitary conditions. Clinical infection occurs primarily in children in developing countries, in immunocompromised patients, in waterborne outbreaks in developed countries, and among travelers. Travelers are often infected via contaminated drinking or swimming water. In one report, cryptosporidiosis was present in 2.8% of 795 international travelers with diarrhea [34].

## Clinical manifestations and diagnosis

The incubation period for *C. parvum* is usually 1–2 weeks. In those who develop gastrointestinal symptoms, watery diarrhea with crampy abdominal pain, nausea, and anorexia are typical. The diarrhea can be severe, sometimes with an average of 12 stools per day [3]. In immunocompetent hosts, the disease is self-limiting and generally lasts 10–14 days, but it can be more protracted and severe in immunocompromised patients, including those with HIV. *Cryptosporidium* infection can be diagnosed by microscopy using an acid-fast stain, but this has low sensitivity, and it is now more common for enzyme immunoassays to be used.

## Treatment and prevention

In immunocompetent hosts, including travelers, the disease is self-limited and no therapy is required. No definitive treatment exists, but agents that have been tried in immunocompromised patients include paromomycin, azithromycin, and nitazoxanide. Prevention of cryptosporidiosis is difficult, as few oocysts (10–50) are needed to cause disease, and *C. parvum* oocysts in drinking water are refractory to chlorine disinfection. Water filters less than 1 μm may be effective, but boiling water before drinking it is most reliable. Individuals with HIV and low CD4 T-cell counts should exert particular caution when traveling abroad to prevent cryptosporidiosis and should avoid drinking water that has not been boiled.

## References

1 Okhuysen PC. Traveler's diarrhea due to intestinal protozoa. *Clin Infect Dis* 2001;33:110–4.

2 Musher DM, Musher BL. Contagious acute gastrointestinal infections. *N Engl J Med* 2004;351:2417–27.

3 Katz DE, Taylor DN. Parasitic infections of the gastrointestinal tract. *Gastroenterol Clin North Am* 2001;30:797–815.

4 Steffen R, Rickenbach M, Wilhelm U, Helminger A, Schar M. Health problems after travel to developing countries. *J Infect Dis* 1987;156:84–91.

5 Ekdahl K, Andersson Y. Imported giardiasis: impact of international travel, immigration, and adoption. *Am J Trop Med Hyg* 2005;72:825–30.

6 Farthing MJ. Giardiasis. *Gastroenterol Clin North Am* 1996; 25:493–515.

7 Hiatt RA, Markell EK, Ng E. How many stool examinations are necessary to detect pathogenic intestinal protozoa? *Am J Trop Med Hyg* 1995;53:36–9.

8 Speelman P. Single-dose tinidazole for the treatment of giardiasis. *Antimicrob Agents Chemother* 1985;27:227–9.

9 Gardner TB, Hill DR. Treatment of giardiasis. *Clin Microbiol Rev* 2001;14:114–28.

10 Pehrson PO. Amoebiasis in a non-endemic country. Epidemiology, presenting symptoms and diagnostic methods. *Scand J Infect Dis* 1983;15:207–14.

11 Weinke T, Friedrich-Janicke B, Hopp P, Janitschke K. Prevalence and clinical importance of *Entamoeba histolytica* in two high-risk groups: travelers returning from the tropics and male homosexuals. *J Infect Dis* 1990;161:1029–31.

12 Haque R, Huston CD, Hughes M, Houpt E, Petri WA Jr. Amebiasis. *N Engl J Med* 2003;348:1565–73.

13 Aucott JN, Ravdin JI. Amebiasis and "nonpathogenic" intestinal protozoa. *Infect Dis Clin North Am* 1993;7:467–85.

14 Knobloch J, Mannweiler E. Development and persistence of antibodies to *Entamoeba histolytica* in patients with amebic liver abscess. Analysis of 216 cases. *Am J Trop Med Hyg* 1983;32:727–32.

15 Stanley SL Jr. Amoebiasis. *Lancet* 2003;361:1025–34.

16 Schwartz E, Piper-Jenks N. Simultaneous amoebic liver abscess and hepatitis A infection. *J Travel Med* 1998;5:95–6.

17 Ravdin JI. Amebiasis. *Clin Infect Dis* 1995;20:1453–64; quiz 1465–6.

18 Patterson M, Healy GR, Shabot JM. Serologic testing for amoebiasis. *Gastroenterology* 1980;78:136–41.

19 Irusen EM, Jackson TF, Simjee AE. Asymptomatic intestinal colonization by pathogenic *Entamoeba histolytica* in amebic liver abscess: prevalence, response to therapy, and pathogenic potential. *Clin Infect Dis* 1992;14:889–93.

20 Kansouzidou A, Charitidou C, Varnis T, Vavatsi N, Kamaria F. Cyclospora cayetanensis in a patient with travelers' diarrhea: case report and review. *J Travel Med* 2004;11:61–3.

21 Shields JM, Olson BH. Cyclospora cayetanensis: a review of an emerging parasitic coccidian. *Int J Parasitol* 2003;33:371–91.

22 Sherchand JB, Cross JH. Emerging pathogen *Cyclospora cayetanensis* infection in Nepal. *Southeast Asian J Trop Med Public Health* 2001;32 Suppl 2:143–50.

23 Ortega YR, Sterling CR, Gilman RH, Cama VA, Diaz F. Cyclospora species—a new protozoan pathogen of humans. *N Engl J Med* 1993;328:1308–12.

24 Hoge CW, Shlim DR, Rajah R, et al. Epidemiology of diarrhoeal illness associated with coccidian-like organism among travellers and foreign residents in Nepal. *Lancet* 1993;341:1175–9.

25 Crowley B, Path C, Moloney C, Keane CT. Cyclospora species—a cause of diarrhoea among Irish travellers to Asia. *Ir Med J* 1996;89:110–12.

26 Lontie M, Degroote K, Michiels J, Bellers J, Mangelschots E, Vandepitte J. Cyclospora sp.: a coccidian that causes diarrhoea in travellers. *Acta Clin Belg* 1995;50:288–90.

27 Petry F, Hofstatter J, Schulz BK, Deitrich G, Jung M, Schirmacher P. Cyclospora cayetanensis: first imported infections in Germany. *Infection* 1997;25:167–70.

28 Kain KC, Noble MA, Freeman HJ, Barteluk RL. Epidemiology and clinical features associated with *Blastocystis hominis* infection. *Diagn Microbiol Infect Dis* 1987;8:235–44.

29 Nimri L, Batchoun R. Intestinal colonization of symptomatic and asymptomatic schoolchildren with *Blastocystis hominis*. *J Clin Microbiol* 1994;32:2865–6.

30 Leelayoova S, Rangsin R, Taamasri P, Naaglor T, Thathaisong U, Mungthin M. Evidence of waterborne transmission of *Blastocystis hominis*. *Am J Trop Med Hyg* 2004;70:658–62.

31 Jelinek T, Peyerl G, Loscher T, von Sonnenburg F, Nothdurft HD. The role of *Blastocystis hominis* as a possible intestinal pathogen in travellers. *J Infect* 1997;35:63–6.

32 Doyle PW, Helgason MM, Mathias RG, Proctor EM. Epidemiology and pathogenicity of *Blastocystis hominis*. *J Clin Microbiol* 1990;28:116–21.

33 Shlim DR, Hoge CW, Rajah R, Rabold JG, Echeverria P. Is *Blastocystis hominis* a cause of diarrhea in travelers? A prospective controlled study in Nepal. *Clin Infect Dis* 1995;21:97–101.

34 Jelinek T, Lotze M, Eichenlaub S, Loscher T, Nothdurft HD. Prevalence of infection with *Cryptosporidium parvum* and *Cyclospora cayetanensis* among international travellers. *Gut* 1997;41:801–4.

35 Senay H, MacPherson D. *Blastocystis hominis*: epidemiology and natural history. *J Infect Dis* 1990;162:987–90.

36 Markell EK, Udkow MP. *Blastocystis hominis*: pathogen or fellow traveler? *Am J Trop Med Hyg* 1986;35:1023–6.

37 Sun T, Katz S, Tanenbaum B, Schenone C. Questionable clinical significance of *Blastocystis hominis* infection. *Am J Gastroenterol* 1989;84:1543–7.

38 Johnson EH, Windsor JJ, Clark CG. Emerging from obscurity: biological, clinical, and diagnostic aspects of *Dientamoeba fragilis*. *Clin Microbiol Rev* 2004;17:553–70, table of contents.

39 Lagace-Wiens PR, VanCaeseele PG, Koschik C. *Dientamoeba fragilis*: an emerging role in intestinal disease. *CMAJ* 2006;175:468–9.

40 Stark DJ, Beebe N, Marriott D, Ellis JT, Harkness J. Dientamoebiasis: clinical importance and recent advances. *Trends Parasitol* 2006;22:92–6.

41 Stark D, Beebe N, Marriott D, Ellis J, Harkness J. *Dientamoeba fragilis* as a cause of travelers' diarrhea: report of seven cases. *J Travel Med* 2007;14:72–3.

# 31

# Intestinal Helminths: *Strongyloides stercoralis, Ascaris lumbricoides,* Hookworm, *Trichuris trichiuria, Enterobius vermicularis, Trichinella,* Intestinal Tapeworms, and Liver Flukes

Karin Leder

Royal Melbourne Hospital, University of Melbourne and Monash University, Victoria, Australia

## Introduction

This chapter focuses on intestinal helminthic infections that occur among travelers. In contrast to protozoan parasites, most helminths do not multiply in humans (*Strongyloides stercoralis* being an exception). Much of the morbidity of infection, especially in local populations, relates to worm burden. Travelers may therefore require repeated or prolonged exposure for some of the typical symptoms of infection to develop. However, some helminthic infections can be associated with a hypersensitivity reaction to the pathogen that is not dose-dependent and may therefore be seen among travelers. The most common intestinal helminthic infections will be described here, although some are not unique to travelers or alternatively are relatively unusual among traveling populations.

Helminths are multicellular organisms that often cannot complete all steps of their complex life cycles within humans. They can be divided into nematodes, cestodes, and trematodes. The classification and main treatments for the most common intestinal helminths are shown in

*Tropical Diseases in Travelers*, 1st edition. Edited by E. Schwartz.
© 2009 by Blackwell Publishing, ISBN: 978-1-4051-8441-0.

Table 31.1, and the major sites of infection are shown in Figure 31.1.

## General epidemiological and preventive measures

Of the variety of helminth infections that can affect travelers, some are transmitted only by ingestion of contaminated food or water, such as trichinellosis, taeniasis, and liver flukes. Others, such as strongyloidiasis and hookworm infections, are acquired either via the fecal–oral route or via contact with fecally contaminated soil [1]. The prevalence of infection will usually vary according to hygienic conditions. The general advice given to reduce the risk of travelers' diarrhea will decrease the risk of acquiring these pathogens (see Chapter 17). Thus, in areas where sanitation is inadequate, all raw foods (including salads, uncooked vegetables, and rare meat, fish, and shellfish) and untreated water should be avoided because they pose a high risk. Boiling water will render it safe. For strongyloidiasis and hookworm infections, prevention can also be achieved by wearing shoes in endemic areas to avoid contact with infected soil.

**Table 31.1** Classification and primary drug treatment for the most common intestinal helminths.

| Organism | Primary agent used for treatment |
|---|---|
| Nematodes [roundworms] | |
| *Ascaris lumbricoides* | Albendazole |
| *Enterobius vermicularis* | Albendazole |
| Hookworm | Albendazole |
| *Strongyloides stercoralis* | Ivermectin |
| *Toxocara* spp. (visceral larva migrans) | Albendazole |
| *Trichinella spiralis* | None or steroids ± albendazole |
| *Trichuris trichiura* | Mebendazole |
| Cestodes [flatworms] | |
| *Echinococcus* spp. | Albendazole |
| *Taenia saginata* | Praziquantel |
| *Taenia solium* | Praziquantel |
| Trematodes.[flukes] | |
| *Fasciola hepatica* | Triclabendazole |
| Other liver flukes (*Opisthorchis* spp., *Clonorchis sinensis*) | Praziquantel |
| Intestinal flukes | Praziquantel |
| *Schistosoma* species | Praziquantel |

## *Strongyloides stercoralis*

Infection with *S. stercoralis* begins when infective filariform larvae in soil penetrate human skin. They migrate hematogenously to the lungs and then ascend the tracheobronchial tree and are swallowed, reaching the gastrointestinal tract. There they mature into adult worms,

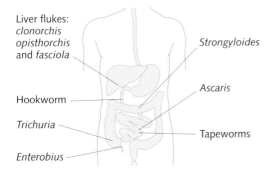

Liver flukes: *clonorchis opisthorchis* and *fasciola*

*Strongyloides*

*Ascaris*

Hookworm

Tapeworms

*Trichuria*

*Enterobius*

**Figure 31.1** Sites of helminth infections.

which live in duodenal and jejunal mucosa. Adult female worms produce eggs from which noninfectious rhabditiform larvae develop. These are generally passed in the feces; however, in contrast to other helminthic parasites, *S. stercoralis* can complete its life cycle entirely within a single human host, a process known as autoinfection. During autoinfection, the rhabditiform larvae mature into infective filariform larvae within the gastrointestinal tract. Thus, the burden of adult worms can increase in an individual even without a history of re-exposure from repeat travel. As a consequence, strongyloidiasis is unique among helminthic infections because the worm burden does not necessarily correlate with the duration of exposure, and even short-term travelers can be at risk of high worm burdens leading to symptomatic infections and complications. In addition, although each adult worm generally lives for about 5 years, the autoinfection cycle means that patients can remain infected for many decades after the initial exposure, and clinical manifestations may be delayed for many years. A case of chronic strongyloidiasis has been described in a British war veteran who served in Southeast Asia 57 years prior to diagnosis, emphasizing the need for continued diagnostic vigilance [2].

### Epidemiology in travelers

Strongyloidiasis is endemic to tropical and subtropical regions and occurs sporadically in temperate areas. High-prevalence areas include South America, South and Southeast Asia, and Sub-Saharan Africa. Infection in nonendemic settings is predominately in immigrants or expatriates rather than short-term travelers [3]. Nevertheless, strongyloidiasis associated with persistent and unexplained diarrhea has been described in international travelers [4], and even short periods of exposure may be sufficient for acquiring infection. Therefore, screening for strongyloidiasis should be considered in individuals with appropriate exposure histories, particularly those with unexplained eosinophilia or those who have lived in endemic countries, even if they are completely asymptomatic. This is particularly pertinent if they are immunocompromised and consequently at risk for complications from disseminated disease [5, 6]. A recent review highlighted that persistence of infection, increasing international travel, lack of familiarity by health care providers, and potential for iatrogenic hyperinfection all make strongyloidiasis an important infection [3].

### Clinical aspects

Manifestations of infection can range from asymptomatic eosinophilia in the immunocompetent host to disseminated disease with septic shock in the immuno-compromised host. Most symptomatic patients have mild cutaneous, pulmonary, or gastrointestinal symptoms that can persist for years. Symptoms can be divided according to the stage of the disease.

- *During penetration*: Cutaneous reactions may develop when larvae penetrate the skin, most commonly affecting the feet and causing inflammation, edema, serpiginous tracts, and pruritus. With chronic infection, intradermal migration of the filariform larvae in the skin may produce a distinctive eruption termed larva currens. Although infrequently seen, this is a pathognomonic sign of strongyloidiasis, consisting of a transient serpiginous and highly pruritic dermatitis, and is commonly seen on the buttocks.
- *During migration*: The transient migration of larvae through the lungs can produce dry cough, throat irritation, dyspnea, wheezing, and hemoptysis. A Loeffler's-like syndrome with eosinophilia is sometimes observed. Some patients with chronic strongyloidiasis experience repeated episodes of fever and mild pneumonitis, producing a picture that resembles recurrent bacterial pneumonia. Others may develop asthma that paradoxically worsens with corticosteroid use [7] or dyspnea due to restrictive pulmonary disease [8].
- *Dwelling in the gastrointestinal tract*: Gastrointestinal symptoms, including upper abdominal pain, diarrhea, anorexia, nausea, and vomiting, may develop from mucosal inflammation caused by adult worms residing in the bowel. Symptoms may mimic peptic ulcer disease. Occasionally, chronic enterocolitis and malabsorption can result from a high intestinal worm burden.

The autoinfection cycle is usually limited by an intact immune response, but in patients with depressed cell-mediated immunity (e.g., from malignancy, alcoholism, corticosteroids, cytotoxic or anti-TNF receptor therapy, transplant recipients, human T-lymphotropic virus type I [HTLV-1] infection, or HIV), potentially fatal hyperinfection and disseminated disease can develop [9, 10]. The hyperinfection syndrome is associated with a greatly increasing parasite burden. Enormous numbers of rhabditiform larvae transform into filariform larvae, which penetrate the intestinal wall to enter the bloodstream and invade organs, leading to fever, anorexia, nausea, vomiting, diarrhea, abdominal pain, shortness of breath, wheeze, hemoptysis, and cough. The massive dissemination of filariform larvae can also be associated with secondary bacterial infections and septic shock and has case-fatality rates of over 70% [5, 10]. It is therefore extremely important to detect and eradicate *S. stercoralis* infection before initiation of immunosuppressive therapy.

There are not marked characteristic differences in clinical manifestations among travelers compared to endemic populations, although eosinophilia may be more pronounced among travelers. A small Swiss study compared clinical features of imported strongyloidosis among 12 travelers and 19 immigrants and found that abdominal symptoms (75% vs 47%) and skin problems (25% vs 16%) were more common among travelers, whereas pulmonary symptoms were more common among immigrants (25% vs 8.3%) [4]. Of note, almost a quarter of the strongyloidosis cases in this series were detected by untargeted screening.

## Diagnosis

The diagnosis of uncomplicated strongyloidiasis can be made either by detecting rhabditiform larvae in concentrated stool or via serologic methods. Larvae first appear in the stool 3–4 weeks after initial dermal penetration, and this delay means that stool examination is not helpful for achieving a diagnosis during the early symptomatic phase. Additionally, examination of a single stool sample may miss 70% or more of cases owing to intermittent larval excretion [11, 12]. Specialized tests (e.g., the Baerman concentration technique or a modified agar plate method) and testing of multiple stool samples can increase the yield, but even three or more stool examinations can fail to detect up to 25% of *Strongyloides* infections. Eosinophilia may be the only clue that the patient harbors infection, but it may be suppressed or absent in disseminated disease.

A highly sensitive and specific ELISA can detect infection in both symptomatic and asymptomatic individuals and may be positive even when repeated examinations of stool samples have been unrevealing. It is considered particularly useful in travelers compared to endemic populations, as the serology may persist for months (or even years) following infection. However, it can occasionally be falsely negative in immunocompromised hosts and is not readily available in some countries.

Other methods for diagnosis include aspiration of duodenojejunal fluid and the use of a string test (Enterotest). Upper endoscopy is not usually needed to establish the diagnosis, but if it is performed in patients with gastrointestinal symptoms with unsuspected disease, larvae may be demonstrated on biopsies of the affected mucosa. Other endoscopic findings in the stomach or duodenum include edema, mucosal erosions, and subepithelial hemorrhages. In disseminated strongyloidiasis, filariform larvae can be found in stool, sputum, and other body fluids.

## Treatment

The treatment of choice for strongyloidiasis is ivermectin 200 µg/kg. Two stat doses are usually given, either on 2 consecutive days or separated by an interval of 2 weeks [13, 14]. Albendazole (400 mg twice daily for 5–7 days) is an alternative, but cure rates are lower than with ivermectin. After treatment (usually within 3 months), patients should be followed to ensure clearance of stool examinations, resolution of eosinophilia, and declining serological antibody titer. Patients with eosinophilia that persists for more than 3 months despite therapy should be evaluated for treatment failure or other causes of eosinophilia.

Immunocompromised patients, including those with disseminated disease, need prolonged or repeated therapy, although regimens used vary [15]. Occasionally, 5–7 days of ivermectin is given, or a combination of ivermectin plus albendazole, until a response is seen [16].

## Prevention

Prevention of *S. stercoralis* infection can be achieved by avoiding skin contact with contaminated soil. Prevention of complications requires increased recognition of disease by doctors and appropriate screening to ensure that those at risk are diagnosed and treated. In a recent questionnaire administered to 363 resident physicians in the USA, Brazil, Singapore, and Thailand that involved a hypothetical case scenario of strongyloidiasis in someone with respiratory symptoms, US trainees in particular had poor recognition (9%) of the need for parasite screening and frequently advocated empiric corticosteroids (23%), potentially resulting in increased iatrogenic risks [3].

## Geohelminths: ascariasis, hookworm, and trichuriasis

*Ascaris lumbricoides* (intestinal roundworm), hookworm infection caused by *Ancylostoma duodenale* and *Necator americanus*, and *Trichuris trichiuria* (whipworm) will be considered together because these are the three main geohelminths or soil-transmitted parasite infections, and many of the epidemiological aspects, clinical findings, and treatment considerations are similar.

## Epidemiology in travelers

These three nematodes are among the commonest helminth infections worldwide and cause infection through contact with parasite eggs or larvae. The highest prevalence of these infections occurs in tropical and subtropical countries, especially in warm wet climates with moist soil conditions conducive to transmission of infection, as well as in areas where suboptimal sanitation practices lead to increased fecal contamination of soil and water. Travelers who have visited highly endemic areas, including Asia, Africa, and South America, may be infected [17].

Infection with *A. lumbricoides* and *T. trichiuria* occurs mainly via ingestion of eggs in contaminated water or food (raw vegetables or fruit in particular). Children playing in contaminated soil may also acquire the parasite from their hands. In contrast, although infection via the fecal–oral route also occurs, *N. americanus* and *A. duodenale* hookworm eggs hatch in soil, and infection occurs predominantly when mature infective motile larvae penetrate human skin. Thus, skin exposure to fecally contaminated soil, such as occurs when travelers walk barefoot with open footwear or lie on the beach, can result in acquisition of hookworm. As few as three larvae are required, so even brief exposure to contaminated soil is sufficient for acquisition of infection.

Soil-transmitted helminths do not reproduce within the host, but adult worms can live for several years in the human gastrointestinal tract [18]. In endemic areas, the greatest burden of these infections occurs in children under the age of 15, but travelers of any age may be affected.

## Clinical aspects

Eggs of *T. trichiuria* are ingested, reach the intestine, and hatch to release larvae, which develop into adult whipworms in the colon. The life cycle of *Ascaris* is more complex. Following ingestion of eggs, *A. lumbricoides* larvae are released and penetrate the intestinal wall, migrate to the liver and then to the lungs, and pass up the tracheobronchial tree and are then swallowed. Once back in the intestine, they mature into adult worms. In hookworm infection, larvae pass from the skin into the blood and lymphatics and then travel to the lungs. Like the larvae of *A. lumbricoides*, they cross from the pulmonary vasculature into the airways, ascend the tracheobronchial tree to be swallowed, and then mature into adult worms in the small intestine. Adult *Necator* and *Ancylostoma* hookworms attach to the mucosa of the upper small intestine and continually consume blood and serum proteins. Adult *T. trichiuria* worms live in the large intestine (especially the cecum), whereas adult *A. lumbricoides* parasitize the entire small intestine (especially the jejunum and ileum).

The majority of infections with these parasites are asymptomatic, with clinical disease being most common in individuals with a high worm load, which is uncommon among travelers. However, symptoms related to a hypersensitivity reaction can occur in travelers even in the absence of a high infectious load. The differences in the life cycles of the worms described above are important in understanding potential clinical manifestations, as when symptoms do occur, they can relate either to the larval migration stage or to the adult worm intestinal stage.

A Early larval migration: Migrating larvae can provoke reactions in any of the tissues through which they pass.

In hookworm infection, cutaneous symptoms can result from penetration of the skin by larvae, leading to a focal pruritic maculopapular eruption at each site of larval penetration (called "ground itch"). This occurs in the area in contact with the soil, most commonly on the feet or buttocks.

In ascariasis, larvae that die during migration through the liver can induce eosinophilic granulomas.

In ascariasis and hookworm infections, larval migration through the lungs can cause intense inflammatory pneumonitis due to a hypersensitivity reaction, resulting in transient respiratory symptoms, including wheezing, dyspnea, a nonproductive cough, and fever (Loeffler's syndrome). Eosinophilic infiltrates may be seen on chest X rays. Urticaria and other symptoms related to hypersensitivity can also occur. These symptoms are allergic manifestations and occur more frequently among travelers and nonimmune populations. They are also more common and typically more severe with ascariasis than with hookworm infection [19]. Symptoms are also more severe in children.

B Gastrointestinal symptoms: Generally only moderate- and high-intensity infections produce clinical gastrointestinal manifestations, so many travelers will be asymptomatic or have only mild nonspecific complaints.

Ascariasis: *A. lumbricoides* infection can be associated with abdominal pain, anorexia, nausea, and diarrhea. Adult worms may migrate into the biliary tree, pancreatic duct, or appendix, leading to cholangitis/obstructive jaundice, pancreatitis, or appendicitis, respectively. *A. lumbricoides* are large (sometimes measuring 40 cm in length and 6 mm in diameter) and so are clearly visible to the naked eye. Travelers may therefore also present because of visualization of passage of a worm in the feces or vomitus.

Hookworm infection: Infected patients may develop nausea, diarrhea, vomiting, and upper abdominal pain (often worse after eating). Although an uncommon presentation, abrupt onset of profuse watery diarrhea due to hookworm has been reported in returned travelers [20]. The major impact of hookworm infection, however, results from intestinal blood loss secondary to invasion and attachment by the adult worm to the mucosa and submucosa of the small intestine [19]. Each adult *N. americanus* worm consumes about 0.3 mL of blood per day and each *A. duodenale* consumes about 0.5 mL of blood daily. Iron-deficiency anemia can result in endemic populations, but very rarely occurs among travelers.

Trichuriasis: Most infections with *T. trichiura* are asymptomatic. Travelers sometimes present with diarrhea, which may contain blood and/or mucus.

C Other: Travelers are commonly diagnosed with these helminthic infections during a workup for the cause of eosinophilia, which can occur with any of these parasites but is most common early in infection during the phase of larval migration, or with established hookworm infection. Other symptoms and complications of these geohelminth infections are shown in Table 31.2.

Highlighting the minimal symptomatology that is common among travelers is a retrospective study performed among expatriates returning to the United Kingdom with a diagnosis of ascariasis, trichuriasis, or hookworm that showed that almost half the patients were completely asymptomatic and even in those with symptoms, specific clinical features were no different from those in controls [21].

## Diagnosis

The diagnosis of ascariasis, trichuriasis, and hookworm is usually made via stool microscopy. Female adult worms produce thousands of eggs per day, which are excreted in feces, so characteristic eggs for each of these helminths may be seen in fecal microscopy. However, following infection, larvae must mature, migrate to the gastrointestinal tract, and mature into adult worms before eggs will be detectable in the feces. For *A. lumbricoides* this takes about 9–11 weeks, for *T. trichiura* about 12 weeks, and for hookworm about 5–9 weeks. There are no serological tests for these helminths, so the diagnosis cannot be made during the early stages of infection. Repeated stools may be needed to make the diagnosis, but in travelers with very light infections, there may be only one or a few worms of the same sex, so eggs may be absent [12].

Endoscopy may also be used to diagnose these infections. Adult hookworms can be seen by gastroscopy. Adult worms of *T. trichiura* measure approximately 4 cm in

**Table 31.2** Symptoms related to geohelminth infections in travelers and endemic populations.

| | Endemic populations | Travelers |
|---|---|---|
| Ascariasis | (a) Transient respiratory symptoms: rare, mainly occur in children<br>(b) Heavy infections can cause anorexia, nausea, and diarrhea. Complications include abdominal obstruction, intestinal perforation with peritonitis, and death<br>(c) Aberrant migration of adult worms:<br>• into biliary tree—can cause biliary colic, cholangitis, obstructive jaundice<br>• appendix—leads to appendicitis<br>• pancreatic duct—causes pancreatitis<br>• may emerge from nasopharynx or anus | (a) Respiratory symptoms due to hypersensitivity may occur<br>(b) Worm burden usually low, so gastrointestinal symptoms are mild<br><br>(c) Obstruction of appendix, biliary tree, or pancreatic duct is rare<br>Travelers may see passage of adult worm (usually in the feces) |
| Hookworm | (a) Penetration phase symptoms rarely reported<br><br>(b) Migration phase: pulmonary symptoms are rare (especially in children)<br>(c) Gastrointestinal symptoms are common (e.g., indigestion, upper abdominal pain, nausea, vomiting, diarrhea)<br>Heavy or prolonged infections: chronic blood loss/iron-deficiency anemia, chronic protein loss, hypoproteinaemia/anasarca | (a) During penetration, papular skin lesions appear ("ground itch") with intractable itching<br>(b) Migration phase: pulmonary symptoms are common<br>(c) Gastrointestinal symptoms are less common (low worm burdens)<br>Nutritional deficiency is rare |
| Trichuriasis | Heavy infections: severe diarrhea may resemble inflammatory bowel disease<br>Nocturnal stooling and anemia occur<br>Rectal prolapse with worms directly visible embedded in rectal mucosa | Infections often asymptomatic, but travelers may develop diarrhea ($\pm$ mucus and/or blood). |
| *Strongyloides* | (a) Systemic symptoms occur usually with heavy burden of worms<br><br>(b) GI complaints are common<br>(c) Skin manifestation of chronic infection: larva currens<br>(d) Hyperinfection occurs in immunosuppressed, HTLV infection, malnourished children and occasionally in immunocompetent individuals | (a) Fever, eosinophilia, and respiratory symptoms are common during acute infection<br>(b) Mild GI complaints may exist<br>(c) Larva currens rare<br><br>(d) Hyperinfection may occur in immunosuppressed<br>Important to exclude *Strongyloides* infection before treatment with immune suppression drugs |
| Ascariasis, hookworm, and trichuriasis | Chronic nutritional impacts can result: lactose intolerance, malabsorption, nutritional deficiencies, growth retardation, impaired cognitive development, especially in children | No chronic nutritional impairment (lower worm burden, greater nutritional reserves) |

length, so if proctoscopy is performed, they may be seen protruding from the bowel mucosa. Endoscopy is also useful for diagnosis of ascariasis and its complications, including intestinal obstruction and hepatobiliary or pancreatic involvement [19]. When ascariasis involving the biliary tree or pancreatic duct is suspected, endoscopic retrograde cholangiopan-creatography (ERCP) will not only establish the diagnosis but also allow direct removal of the worm. The worm may sometimes also be seen on a barium swallow.

## Treatment

For ascariasis and hookworm, a single dose of albendazole (400 mg) is effective in almost 100% of cases. Alternatives include mebendazole (500 mg as a single dose for ascariasis or 100 mg b.i.d. for 3 days for hookworm) or pyrantel pamoate (11 mg/kg up to a maximum of 1 g/day for 1 day for ascariasis or 3 days for hookworms). This latter drug is the recommended therapy during pregnancy. Ivermectin (200 µg/kg) as a single dose can also be used in ascariasis but is ineffective for hookworm [22].

For trichuriasis, the recommended treatment of choice is 3 days of mebendazole (100 mg b.i.d., achieving cure rates of 80% to >90%). Although albendazole has also been used, it has slightly lower efficacy for trichuriasis than mebendazole, and if used needs to be given for at least 3 days [23]. Ivermectin has shown variable efficacy against *T. trichiura* [24], and pyrantel is not effective.

Nitazoxanide (100 mg, age 1–3 years; 200 mg, age 4–11 years; or 500 mg, adults twice daily for 3 days) is also effective for treatment of these helminths.

Pulmonary symptoms associated with ascariasis or hookworm infection are self-limited, but symptomatic treatment with inhaled bronchodilators or occasionally systemic corticosteroids may be required. This should be followed by standard anthelminthic therapy for intestinal disease once the worms have developed to maturity.

## Prevention

Prevention of infection in endemic areas relies on adequate disposal of human feces and good sanitary conditions to interrupt transmission. Mass community therapy is also being instituted in many developing areas. However, for travelers, prevention relies on avoiding uncooked fruits and vegetables, boiling water for drinking, and wearing shoes to avoid hookworm infection. *Ascaris* eggs are resistant to chemical methods of water purification but are removed by filtration or by boiling. No vaccines are currently available against these agents.

## Enterobiasis

Infection with *Enterobius vermicularis*, also known as pinworm, occurs worldwide in both temperate and tropical climates. It is diagnosed at least as frequently in developed countries as in tropical regions. Transmission occurs via direct anus-to-mouth spread from contact with an infected person, from eating food that has been touched by soiled hands, or via eggs that are dislodged from contaminated clothing or bed linen.

Following ingestion, the eggs hatch within the intestine and release larvae. Over a period of several weeks, larvae develop into adult worms, which live in the intestine, mainly in the cecum and appendix. The female worm does not release eggs in the intestine but instead migrates out through the rectum onto the perianal skin to deposit eggs, usually at night. Larvae inside the eggs develop into an infective form over approximately 6 hours, and the eggs can then be ingested by the same host (autoinfection) or by another person. Adult females live for approximately 3 months.

Although enterobiasis is not unique to travelers, some types of budget accommodation frequented by travelers may be conducive environments for transmission.

## Clinical aspects

Most pinworm infections are asymptomatic. When symptoms occur, they are not different in travelers compared to others. Pruritis ani is most common, and is caused by an inflammatory reaction to the presence of adult worms and eggs on the perianal skin. Occasionally, high worm burden is associated with abdominal pain, nausea, and vomiting. The adult worm can also migrate from the perianal region into the genital tract of the female host, resulting in vulvovaginitis, salpingitis, oophoritis, cervical granulomas, or peritoneal inflammation.

## Diagnosis

The diagnosis of enterobiasis is best made using a "scotch tape" test, which involves patting the sticky side of scotch tape around the perianal region, and then sticking it onto a slide for examination by microscopy. A repeated test done daily for 3 days will diagnose enterobiasis over 90% of the time, with characteristic worms and/or eggs being visible by microscopy. Sometimes female adult worms, which are white, pin-shaped, and 8–13 mm long, may also be found in the perianal area. Eggs are sometimes seen in a fecal examination. Enterobiasis does not usually cause peripheral eosinophilia, because there generally is no tissue invasion.

## Treatment

Enterobiasis should be treated with either mebendazole (100-mg dose initially and repeated after 2 weeks) or albendazole (400-mg dose initially and repeated after 2 weeks). An alternative therapy is pyrantel pamoate (11 mg/kg dose to a maximum of 1 g), which is the recommended treatment during pregnancy. Ivermectin (2 doses of ivermectin, 200 µg/kg given at an interval of 10–14 days) can also be used. Although all agents achieve cure rates close to 90%, reinfection is common. When this occurs, simultaneous treatment of all household members is indicated, and all bedding and clothes should be washed.

## Trichinellosis

Trichinellosis is caused by the nematode *Trichinella*. A number of different species of *Trichinella* are known to infect humans, the commonest being *T. spiralis*.

### Epidemiology among travelers

Human infections are acquired by eating raw or undercooked meat. Consumption of inadequately cooked pork is the most commonly recognized source, but the meat of other animals, including bear, walrus, and horse meat can also result in infection.

Although trichinellosis has been reported worldwide, the prevalence of human infection is highest in China, Thailand, Mexico, Argentina, Bolivia, the former Soviet Union, and other parts of Central Europe. Clusters of cases tend to occur when groups have consumed meat from a common infected animal. Occasionally, people who have never traveled to endemic areas become infected through importation of contaminated food products.

### Clinical aspects

The clinical disease varies from an asymptomatic infection to a severe disease course, occasionally resulting in death. The severity of infection generally correlates with the number of ingested larvae and the host response. The incubation period for clinical infections is between 7 and 30 days, with shorter incubation periods being associated with more severe disease. Initial symptoms are generally intestinal, occurring between the second and seventh days after ingestion, when encysted larvae are released from the meat by gastric juices. Larvae mature

into adult worms, which burrow into the intestinal mucosa and produce additional larvae. This may be associated with abdominal pain, nausea, vomiting, and diarrhea. Following this, adult-derived larvae in the intestines enter the bloodstream and disseminate to skeletal muscle, where, depending on the species involved, they usually encyst. Common symptoms, which appear 2–8 weeks after ingestion, include sudden onset of severe muscle pain, swelling, and weakness. Other characteristic clinical findings are splinter hemorrhages, conjunctival and retinal hemorrhages, periorbital edema, disturbed vision, ocular pain, and high fever. Macular or urticarial rashes, headache, a dry nonproductive cough, and dyspnea may also develop.

Larvae encyst only in skeletal muscle, but there may be pulmonary, cardiac, or CNS involvement in serious infections, and death can occur from myocarditis, pneumonia, meningitis, or encephalitis. Symptomatic involvement of the upper airway musculature can also occur, causing hoarseness or dysphagia. Encapsulated parasites can persist for several years before dying and calcifying [25].

A number of cases of travel-associated trichinellosis have been reported [26–29]. In an American review of trichinellosis cases reported to the Centers for Disease Control from 1975 to 1989, 26 travel-associated cases (including three clusters) were identified [30]. The majority of cases (65%) occurred among patients who had traveled to Mexico or Asian countries and were associated with consumption of undercooked pork products or with unsanitary cooking practices. In this review, 73% had eosinophilia, 65% had fever, 62% reported myalgia, and 35% had periorbital edema, confirming that the clinical symptoms do not differ according to whether infection occurs among travelers or endemic hosts.

### Diagnosis

Eosinophilia is a hallmark of clinical trichinellosis. It is present at some time in every case but not before the second week of infection (during the muscle stage). The proportion of eosinophils typically rises to a maximum of 20–90% in the third or fourth week. Myositis, periorbital edema, fever, and eosinophilia in a person who has ingested undercooked meat should suggest a diagnosis of trichinellosis [30].

Other nonspecific findings include elevated serum muscle enzymes (creatine kinase and lactate dehydrogenase) and hypergammaglobulinemia. Many different serologic assays are available and are generally reliable in confirming the diagnosis. However, antibody levels do not become detectable until a minimum of 3 weeks after infection, so serology is not useful for early diagnosis. The definitive diagnosis can be made by finding larvae in a muscle biopsy.

### Treatment
Because most trichinellosis infections are self-limited, specific therapy is usually not required. Symptomatic treatment with analgesia, antipyretics, and corticosteroids may be beneficial, particularly with severe infections. If required, prednisone is generally administered at a dose of 50 mg/day for 10–15 days. Mebendazole (200–400 mg t.i.d. for 3 days, and then 400–500 mg t.i.d. for 10 days) or albendazole (400 mg twice daily for 10–15 days) is used for symptomatic infection involving the CNS, myocardium, or respiratory muscles.

### Prevention
*Trichinella* larvae in meat are rendered noninfectious by heating to a temperature of 77°C. Therefore, pretravel counseling should include information concerning the risk of eating improperly prepared meat products [30]. Freezing at −15°C for 3 weeks, as in a home freezer, will also generally kill larvae.

### Intestinal tapeworms

A number of intestinal tapeworms can inhabit the human gastrointestinal tract, including *Taenia, Diphyllobothrium* (fish tapeworms), and *Hymenolepis* (dwarf tapeworms). The best-known among these are *T. saginata*, the beef tapeworm, and *T. solium*, the pork tapeworm, so these will be reviewed here. (For neurocysticercosis, see Chapter 28.)

### Epidemiology in travelers
Humans are infected by eating undercooked meat containing larval cysts (also known as cysticerci). Following ingestion, maturation occurs in the human intestine to form adult tapeworms. Adult tapeworms consist of a head (also known as a scolex), a neck, and a segmented body (also known as proglottids). The adults of both *Taenia* species are often over 5 m long (Figure 31.2). Proglottids become progressively more developed the more distal they are along the worm, and as they mature, they contain an increasing number of eggs. In taeniasis, the distal segments can bud off from the rest of the body and these, or the eggs they contain, can be passed rectally. When fecally contaminated food or water is ingested by an intermediate host (cattle for *T. saginata* and pigs for *T. solium*), the eggs rupture in the intestine, release embryos that pass through the intestinal wall and travel to striated muscle (or other organs), and develop into cysticerci.

*T. saginata* occurs worldwide but is most common in areas such as Europe and parts of Asia, where it is customary to eat undercooked beef. *T. solium* is highly endemic in Latin America, Africa, the Middle East, and Central Asia due to both the frequency of eating undercooked pork and the poor sanitary conditions. Travelers to endemic areas have been infected [31] and should be warned not to eat undercooked meat.

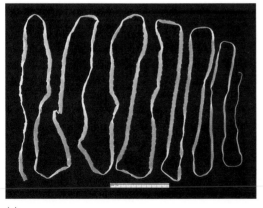
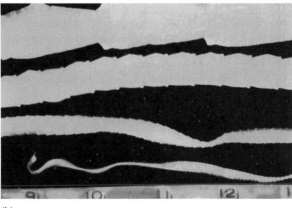

(a)                                              (b)

**Figure 31.2** *Taenia saginata* adult worms. The adult in (a) is approximately 4 meters in length. (From Centers for Disease Control and Prevention Parasite Image Library. Accessible at http://www.dpd.cdc.gov/dpdx/HTML/ImageLibrary/Taeniasis_il.htm.)

## Clinical aspects

Most humans who carry an adult tapeworm are asymptomatic. Although the conventional belief is that tapeworm infections are associated with weight loss, no clinical or experimental data support this. Patients may present because they notice intermittent passage of proglottids either with their stool (*T. solium*) or spontaneously (*T. saginata*). Sometimes patients describe finding "noodles" in their underwear. There may be other gastrointestinal symptoms including nausea, anorexia, or epigastric pain. Occasionally, segments enter the appendix, common bile duct, or pancreatic duct and cause obstruction. Headache, dizziness, and urticaria can also occur. Symptoms among travelers are not different from those in other populations.

## Diagnosis

The diagnosis of taeniasis is usually confirmed by finding characteristic eggs or proglottids in the feces. Eggs are often eliminated intermittently, so repeat stool specimens should be taken. Patients with adult tapeworm infections may have a peripheral eosinophilia.

## Treatment

Treatment is needed to precipitate complete evacuation of the worm, including the scolex. Praziquantel (5 to 10 mg/kg in a single dose) is the recommended therapy and is efficacious in >95% of cases.

## Prevention

To prevent taeniasis, travelers should be reminded not to eat undercooked meat.

## Liver flukes

The three major liver flukes that infect humans are *Clonorchis sinensis* (the Chinese liver fluke), *Opisthorchis* species, and *Fasciola hepatica*.

*C. sinensis* is common in the Far East, particularly in China, Japan, Taiwan, Vietnam, and Korea [32, 33]. The two species that most frequently cause human opisthorchiasis are *O. felineus* and *O. viverrini*. *O. felineus* occurs in Southeast Asia and in Central and Eastern Europe, particularly in Siberia and other parts of the former Soviet Union. *O. viverrini* is endemic in Thailand, Kampuchea, and Laos. *C. sinensis* and *O.* spp. both have snails as their first intermediate hosts and fish as their second in-

termediate hosts, and humans can be accidentally infected if they eat raw, pickled, or undercooked fish.

Travelers to or immigrants from endemic countries may harbor the infection and import it to nonendemic countries [34]. Contaminated frozen, dried, or pickled fish containing tiny immature larvae (metacercariae) can also be exported to nonendemic countries, so infections occasionally occur in people who have never traveled to endemic areas [35].

*F. hepatica* causes liver rot in sheep and cattle. It has a worldwide distribution but occurs mainly in sheep-rearing areas of Central and South America, Europe, China, Africa, and the Middle East [36]. Snails are the first intermediate hosts and encystation then occurs on aquatic vegetation. Humans usually acquire infection by eating contaminated freshwater plants (typically watercress, but also water lettuce, mint, alfalfa, or parsley), but can occasionally be infected by drinking unboiled contaminated water [35]. Imported infections among travelers have been reported [37, 38].

## Clinical aspects

Adult worms usually reside in the bile ducts, where they can live for many years, and produce eggs that pass out with bile into the feces.

**A** Clonorchiasis and opisthorchiasis: Most people infected with *C. sinensis* and *O.* spp. are asymptomatic and have a benign course. Symptoms are less common with light infections, so travelers often have subclinical infections. However, about 2–3 weeks after consumption of heavily infected undercooked fish, fever, anorexia, abdominal pain, myalgia, arthralgia, malaise, and urticaria can develop. Lymphadenopathy and tender hepatomegaly may be seen. High levels of circulating eosinophils are common. Liver function tests usually show normal transaminases, but in advanced disease with obstruction of the biliary tree, a raised alkaline phosphatase level may be noted.

Chronic symptoms and complications are generally associated with high worm burden and are, therefore, most common among recurrently exposed older people in endemic areas than in travelers. Prolonged fatigue, abdominal discomfort, anorexia, weight loss, dyspepsia, and diarrhea can occur. More serious complications include obstructive jaundice, recurrent cholangitis, cholangiohepatitis, and cholangiocarcinoma.

**B** Fascioliasis: When eaten by humans, *F. hepatica* larvae emerge, penetrate the small intestinal wall into the peritoneal cavity, and then penetrate the liver capsule and pass through the liver tissue into the biliary tract. They grow into mature worms within the bile ducts. Many infections in humans are mild, but morbidity can increase with heavier fluke burdens. The early phase of migration of parasites through the liver can cause liver parenchymal destruction and be associated with fever, right upper quadrant pain, and hepatomegaly beginning 6–12 weeks following ingestion. The clinical presentation may suggest a hepatic abscess. Other possible symptoms include anorexia, nausea, vomiting, myalgia, and jaundice. Marked peripheral eosinophilia is frequently present during this early stage of infection. Urticaria and other allergic symptoms, including a Loeffler's–like syndrome or right-sided pleural effusions, can develop.

Once adult flukes enter the bile ducts, obstruction can occur, leading to biliary colic, cholangitis, and obstructive jaundice. Prolonged and heavy infections can also result in sclerosing cholangitis and biliary cirrhosis [39]. Occasionally, adult worms migrate to ectopic sites such as the subcutaneous tissue of the abdominal wall, skin, lungs, heart, brain, or muscle. Pain associated with migration of the parasites can occur, and migrating, erythematous, itchy, and painful nodules may be seen.

## Diagnosis

The diagnosis is generally made via microscopy by identifying characteristic eggs in fecal samples or bile specimens. However, eggs will not appear in feces until approximately 4 weeks following infection with clonorchiasis and opisthorchiasis. In fascioliasis, egg production does not begin until approximately 3 months after infection. Multiple specimens may need to be examined, because egg excretion may be intermittent. Eggs of *C. sinensis* are difficult to distinguish from those of *O. felineus* and *O. viverrini*, and eggs of *F. hepatica* can look similar to intestinal fluke infections. Adult worms may be found by endoscopy or ERCP and will enable differentiation of species. Peripheral eosinophilia is often present, particularly during the early tissue migration phase. In advanced disease, liver function tests may show an obstructive picture.

Serology for clonorchiasis and opisthorchiasis is not generally commercially available. Serological testing for fascioliasis is available in some laboratories. In fascioliasis, serology usually becomes positive during the early phase of migration through the liver and is therefore useful in diagnosing early symptoms before the appearance of eggs in the feces.

Imaging of the liver and bile ducts with ultrasound or CT may assist with the diagnosis. In clonorchiasis and opisthorchiasis, nonspecific ultrasound findings include gall bladder enlargement or irregularities, the presence of sludge, inflammation and fibrosis of bile ducts, and liver enlargement. Sometimes ultrasound may also be able to detect aggregates of flukes as nonshadowing echogenic foci within bile ducts [40]. In early fascioliasis, CT scanning may show characteristic hypodense nodules or tunnel-like tracks up to 1 cm in diameter resulting from migration of the parasite through the liver, which may resemble hepatic abscesses. Other findings include thickening of the liver capsule, subcapsular hematoma, and parenchymal calcifications. In the later biliary stages of fasciola infection, ultrasound and ERCP may show thickening of the common bile duct wall and mobile flukes in the bile ducts and gall bladder.

## Treatment

### Clonorchiasis and opisthorchiasis

Clonorchiasis and opisthorchiasis are usually treated with praziquantel (75 mg/kg in 3 divided doses for 1 day), resulting in almost a 100% cure rate for both infections. In heavy clonorchiasis, 2 days of therapy may be required. Although clinical symptoms may take months to resolve, eggs should disappear from the stool within a week of treatment. Even asymptomatic individuals should be treated because of the risks of developing irreversible complications, such as cholangiocarcinoma following chronic infection [39, 40]. Alternative treatments include mebendazole or albendazole. For clonorchiasis, albendazole (10 mg/kg for 7 days) results in 90–100% cure [41]. For *Opisthorchis* infections, albendazole (400 mg b.i.d. for 7 days) cures approximately 60–65% of cases [42]. Although studies suggest that albendazole is not as effective as praziquantel and requires a longer course, it may be preferable because it has fewer side effects.

### Fascioliasis

Unlike most other trematode infections, *F. hepatica* is unresponsive to praziquantel, and neither mebendazole or albendazole is effective. Instead, triclabendazole (dose of 10 mg/kg for 1 or 2 days) is the drug of choice, and in most developed countries it is available on a compassionate-use basis from its manufacturer. Nitazoxanide (500 mg b.i.d. for 7 days) has also been reported to be efficacious, but experience with its use is limited [43, 44].

## Prevention

Cooking or freezing fresh water fish prevents infection with clonorchiasis and opisthorchiasis. Good hygiene measures to prevent contamination of water also decrease transmission. Prevention of fascioliasis requires avoiding consumption of raw fresh water plants in endemic areas.

# References

1 Pearson RD. An update on the geohelminths: *Ascaris lumbricoides*, Hookworms, *Trichuris trichiura*, and *Strongyloides stercoralis*. *Curr Infect Dis Rep* 2002;4:59–64.

2 Gill GV, Beeching NJ, Khoo S, et al. A British Second World War veteran with disseminated strongyloidiasis. *Trans R Soc Trop Med Hyg* 2004;98:382–6.

3 Boulware DR, Stauffer WM, Hendel-Paterson BR, et al. Maltreatment of *Strongyloides* infection: case series and worldwide physicians-in-training survey. *Am J Med* 2007;120:545 e1–8.

4 Nuesch R, Zimmerli L, Stockli R, Gyr N, Christoph Hatz FR. Imported strongyloidosis: a longitudinal analysis of 31 cases. *J Travel Med* 2005;12:80–84.

5 Lim S, Katz K, Krajden S, Fuksa M, Keystone JS, Kain KC. Complicated and fatal *Strongyloides* infection in Canadians: risk factors, diagnosis and management. *CMAJ* 2004;171:479–84.

6 Loutfy MR, Wilson M, Keystone JS, Kain KC. Serology and eosinophil count in the diagnosis and management of strongyloidiasis in a non-endemic area. *Am J Trop Med Hyg* 2002;66:749–52.

7 Sen P, Gil C, Estrellas B, Middleton JR. Corticosteroid-induced asthma: a manifestation of limited hyperinfection syndrome due to *Strongyloides stercoralis*. *South Med J* 1995;88:923–7.

8 Lin AL, Kessimian N, Benditt JO. Restrictive pulmonary disease due to interlobular septal fibrosis associated with disseminated infection by *Strongyloides stercoralis*. *Am J Respir Crit Care Med* 1995;151:205–9.

9 Marcos LA, Terashima A, Dupont HL, Gotuzzo E. *Strongyloides* hyperinfection syndrome: an emerging global infectious disease. *Trans R Soc Trop Med Hyg* 2008;102:314–18.

10 Keiser PB, Nutman TB. *Strongyloides stercoralis* in the immunocompromised population. *Clin Microbiol Rev* 2004; 17:208–17.

11 Siddiqui AA, Berk SL. Diagnosis of *Strongyloides stercoralis* infection. *Clin Infect Dis* 2001;33:1040–47.

12 Liu LX, Weller PF. Strongyloidiasis and other intestinal nematode infections. *Infect Dis Clin North Am* 1993;7:655–82.

13 Zaha O, Hirata T, Kinjo F, Saito A, Fukuhara H. Efficacy of ivermectin for chronic strongyloidiasis: two single doses given 2 weeks apart. *J Infect Chemother* 2002;8:94–8.

14 Toma H, Sato Y, Shiroma Y, Kobayashi J, Shimabukuro I, Takara M. Comparative studies on the efficacy of three anthelminthics on treatment of human strongyloidiasis in Okinawa, Japan. *Southeast Asian J Trop Med Public Health* 2000;31:147–51.

15 Segarra-Newnham M. Manifestations, diagnosis, and treatment of *Strongyloides stercoralis* infection. *Ann Pharmacother* 2007;41:1992–2001.

16 Pornsuriyasak P, Niticharoenpong K, Sakapibunnan A. Disseminated strongyloidiasis successfully treated with extended duration ivermectin combined with albendazole: a case report of intractable strongyloidiasis. *Southeast Asian J Trop Med Public Health* 2004;35:531–4.

17 Sarinas PS, Chitkara RK. Ascariasis and hookworm. *Semin Respir Infect* 1997;12:130–37.

18 Khuroo MS. Ascariasis. *Gastroenterol Clin North Am* 1996;25:553–77.

19 Bethony J, Brooker S, Albonico M, et al. Soil-transmitted helminth infections: ascariasis, trichuriasis, and hookworm. *Lancet* 2006;367:1521–32.

20 Lawn SD, Grant AD, Wright SG. Case reports: acute hookworm infection: an unusual cause of profuse watery diarrhoea in returned travellers. *Trans R Soc Trop Med Hyg* 2003;97: 414–15

21 Fryatt RJ, Teng J, Harries AD, Siorvanes L, Hall AP. Intestinal helminthiasis in ex-patriates returning to Britain from the tropics. A controlled study. *Trop Geogr Med* 1990;42:119–22.

22 Marti H, Haji HJ, Savioli L, et al. A comparative trial of a single-dose ivermectin versus three days of albendazole for treatment of *Strongyloides stercoralis* and other soil-transmitted helminth infections in children. *Am J Trop Med Hyg* 1996;55:477–81.

23 Albonico M, Smith PG, Hall A, Chwaya HM, Alawi KS, Savioli L. A randomized controlled trial comparing mebendazole and albendazole against *Ascaris*, *Trichuris* and hookworm infections. *Trans R Soc Trop Med Hyg* 1994;88:585–9.

24 Ottesen EA, Campbell WC. Ivermectin in human medicine. *J Antimicrob Chemother* 1994;34:195–203.

25 Pozio E. New patterns of *Trichinella* infection. *Vet Parasitol* 2001;98:133–48.

26 Barrett-Connor E, Davis CF, Hamburger RN, Kagan I. An epidemic of trichinosis after ingestion of wild pig in Hawaii. *J Infect Dis* 1976;133:473–7.

27 Stack PS. Trichinosis. Still a public health threat. *Postgrad Med* 1995;97:137–9, 143–4.

28 Kurup A, Yew WS, San LM, Ang B, Lim S, Tai GK. Outbreak of suspected trichinosis among travelers returning from a neighboring island. *J Travel Med* 2000;7:189–93.

29 Suwansrinon K, Wilde H, Burford B, Hanvesakul R, Sitprija V. Human trichinellosis from Laos. *J Travel Med* 2007;14:274–7.

30 McAuley JB, Michelson MK, Schantz PM. *Trichinella* infection in travelers. *J Infect Dis* 1991;164:1013–16.

31 White AC, Blum A. *Taenia saginata* tapeworm infection in a traveler to Mexico. *J Travel Med* 1994;1:168.

32 Wang KX, Zhang RB, Cui YB, Tian Y, Cai R, Li CP. Clinical and epidemiological features of patients with clonorchiasis. *World J Gastroenterol* 2004;10:446–8.

33 Rim HJ. Clonorchiasis: an update. *J Helminthol* 2005;79:269–81.

34  Lewin MR, Weinert MF. An eighty-four-year-old man with fever and painless jaundice: a case report and brief review of *Clonorchis sinensis* infection. *J Travel Med* 1999;6:207–9.

35  Chan CW, Lam SK. Diseases caused by liver flukes and cholangiocarcinoma. *Baillieres Clin Gastroenterol* 1987;1: 297–318.

36  Mas-Coma S. Epidemiology of fascioliasis in human endemic areas. *J Helminthol* 2005;79:207–16.

37  Graham CS, Brodie SB, Weller PF. Imported *Fasciola hepatica* infection in the United States and treatment with triclabendazole. *Clin Infect Dis* 2001;33:1–5.

38  Kang ML, Teo CH, Wansaicheong GK, Giron DM, Wilder-Smith A. *Fasciola hepatica* in a New Zealander traveler. *J Travel Med* 2008;15:196–9.

39  Harinasuta T, Pungpak S, and Keystone JS. Trematode infections. Opisthorchiasis, clonorchiasis, fascioliasis, and paragonimiasis. *Infect Dis Clin North Am* 1993;7:699–716.

40  Liu LX, Harinasuta KT. Liver and intestinal flukes. *Gastroenterol Clin North Am* 1996;25:627–36.

41  Liu YH, Wang XG, Gao P, Qian MX. Experimental and clinical trial of albendazole in the treatment of *Clonorchiasis sinensis*. *Chin Med J (Engl)* 1991;104:27–31.

42  Pungpark S, Bunnag D, Harinasuta T. Albendazole in the treatment of opisthorchiasis and concomitant intestinal helminthic infections. *Southeast Asian J Trop Med Public Health* 1984;15:44–50.

43  Favennec L, Jave Ortiz J, Gargala G, Lopez Chegne N, Ayoub A, Rossignol JF. Double-blind, randomized, placebo-controlled study of nitazoxanide in the treatment of fascioliasis in adults and children from northern Peru. *Aliment Pharmacol Ther* 2003;17:265–70.

44  Rossignol JF, Abaza H, Friedman H. Successful treatment of human fascioliasis with nitazoxanide. *Trans R Soc Trop Med Hyg* 1998;92:103–4.

# 32 Leishmaniasis

## Eli Schwartz

Chaim Sheba Medical Center, Tel Hashomer, Israel and Sackler School of Medicine, Tel Aviv University, Tel Aviv, Israel

## Introduction

Leishmaniasis is a vector-borne disease, seen in 88 countries, 72 of which are developing nations. Although leishmaniasis is considered a tropical disease, it is endemic in nontropical regions as well, mainly in countries of the Mediterranean basin, such as the southern European countries, Turkey, and Israel.

Leishmaniasis is an infection caused by intracellular protozoan parasites of the genus *Leishmania* and is transmitted by various species of sandflies. There are three major clinical syndromes:

- Cutaneous leishmaniasis
- Mucosal leishmaniasis
- Visceral leishmaniasis.

Based on their geographical distribution, the members of the genus can be divided into the Old World species (found in Southern Europe, the Middle East, Asia, and Africa) and New World leishmaniasis, which spreads from the southern USA through Central and South America to the highlands of Argentina. The difference between Old and New World leishmaniasis lies not only in their geographical distribution but also in the clinical spectrum of the disease. Whereas the Old World cutaneous species causes mostly benign cutaneous disease, the American species can cause diseases ranging from mild cutaneous disease to severe mucocutaneous involvement. This difference is important and requires accurate diagnosis, followed by specific treatment [1].

In returning travelers, all three syndromes, cutaneous, mucosal, and visceral leishmaniasis, have been documented; however, cutaneous leishmaniasis is the most common, particularly in the New World species. Among the New World species, *L. braziliensis* is the most severe form, with the potential for nasopharyngeal mucosal involvement (Figure 32.1). It is also the most challenging for clinicians in terms of choosing the appropriate treatment.

## Leishmaniasis in travelers—general

In returning travelers, all three syndromes have been documented. However, cutaneous leishmaniasis (CL) is the most common, especially of the New World species.

In the GeoSentinel database, CL is one of the top diagnoses among ill returned travelers with dermatological conditions, accounting for 3.3% of cases [2].

The majority of cases were acquired in Latin America (New World leishmaniasis), mainly in Bolivia [2]. Other case series from specific countries revealed similar results: in France 60% and in Germany 55% were New World CL [3, 4]. A study among German travelers estimated the relative geographical risk of *Leishmania* infection, based on the numbers of German travelers to different regions, and found that the highest risk was in Latin America, with odds ratio (OR) of 22.7 ( 95% CI 10.1–48.7), compared to the risk of infection in southern Europe. Africa and Asia had significantly less risk (Figure 32.2) [5].

Another feature shared by all previous reports is the predominance of males, who account for approximately 65–70% of all cases. Among Israeli travelers, 90% of CL is due to New World leishmaniasis, mainly caused by *L. braziliensis*, which is acquired in the Amazon region of Bolivia [6]. Male representation in leishmaniasis patients was much higher than in the general traveler population (OR 3.41). The assumption was that men have more risk-taking behavior and travel to more remote areas where the chance of acquiring the disease is greater [7].

The interval from appearance of the lesion until diagnosis and treatment initiation was studied among US travelers from 1985 to 1990 [8]. The result showed a median of 112 days (range 13–1022 days) that elapsed from when they first noticed their lesions until the CDC

*Tropical Diseases in Travelers*, 1st edition. Edited by E. Schwartz.
© 2009 by Blackwell Publishing, ISBN: 978-1-4051-8441-0.

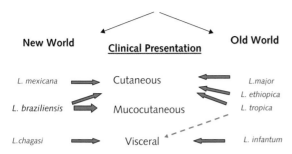

**Figure 32.1** Leishmaniasis: clinical manifestations and geographical distribution.

released sodium stibogluconate (SSG) (Figure 32.3). Although decades have elapsed since that time, and although there are an increasing number of returning travelers with leishmaniasis, the delay in diagnosis seems to be of the same magnitude. The median time for diagnosis in US military patients was 118 days [9], and in travelers from Germany 120 days [3], whereas in other reports, it was 50–60 days [3, 6]. Most of these patients had seen several doctors (some up to seven) before the diagnosis was made, and in some instances, it was the patient who proposed the diagnosis [8].

This delay between onset of symptoms and final diagnosis indicates the lack of familiarity of most physicians in nonendemic countries with leishmanial infections. In our experience with Israeli travelers in Latin America, this failure to make the diagnosis occurs even in endemic countries if medical consultation is done in major cities that are outside of the endemic areas.

It is not clear whether the increased risk to travelers going to Latin America is caused by the emergence of endemic leishmaniasis in Latin America, by frequent visits of travelers to "hot spots" of leishmaniasis transmission, or by certain risk behaviors that lead to higher exposure to the vectors, such as outdoor activities [5]. Our experience with Israeli travelers contracting the disease in a specific spot in Bolivia supports the premise that there are hot spots attractive to travelers [6].

Very few of the imported *Leishmania* infections in travelers came from the countries that account for more than 90% of leishmaniasis cases worldwide, namely: Afghanistan, Algeria, Brazil, Iran, Peru, Saudi Arabia, and Syria [10]. This observation highlights the differences in the epidemiology of leishmaniasis in travelers and native populations of endemic regions [5].

## Life cycle

The life cycles for all *Leishmania* species are similar, regardless of geographic distribution. There are three components to this cycle. The first is the pathogen, which is the Leishmania protozoon with its different species in accordance with its geographical distribution. The second component is the reservoir of the parasite, which is various vertebrate mammals, depending on the species and on the geographic area. Finally, the sandfly is the vector. Sandfly species differ according to *Leishmania* species and geographic areas and transmit the parasite to different vertebrates. In most cases, the infected vertebrates do not become ill; however, when humans become incidental victims, they do get sick with one of the clinical forms mentioned above.

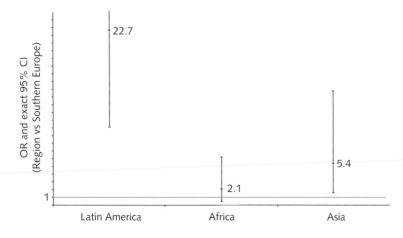

**Figure 32.2** Odds ratio (OR) of acquiring leishmania in German travelers. (With kind permission from Springer Science + Business Media: Weitzel T, Mühlberger N, Jelinek T, Schunk M, Ehrhardt S, Bogdam C, et al.; Surveillance Importierter Infektionen in Deutschland (SIMPID) Surveillance Network. Imposed leishmaniasis in Germany 2001–2004: data of the SIMPID surveillance network. *Eur J Clin Microbiol Infect Dis* 2005;24:471–6.)

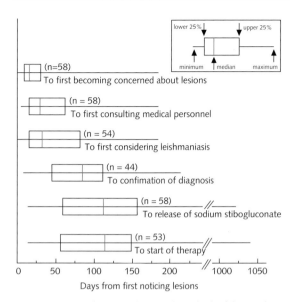

**Figure 32.3** Distributions (shown in box plots) of the numbers of days from first awareness of lesions to various events among US travelers. (Reproduced with permission of the American College of Physicians, from Herwaldt BL, Stokes SL, Juranek DD. American cutaneous leishmaniasis in U.S. travelers. *Ann Intern Med* 1993;118:779–84; permission conveyed through Copyright Clearance Center, Inc.)

The parasite, which exists in the form of promastigotes in the proboscis of a female sandfly, is introduced into the skin of a vertebrate, including a human host, during a blood meal. The promastigotes, which are in elongated, 10- to 15-μm flagellated forms, invade the reticuloendothelial cells. The tissue macrophages phagocytize the organisms, and they subsequently transform into round or oval, 2- to 3-μm, nonflagellated forms, called amastigotes. The amastigotes undergo successive asexual division until the macrophage ruptures, releasing the amastigotes, which then enter other macrophages to continue the cycle. Sandflies feeding on infected individuals ingest parasitized cells, and the amastigotes transform into promastigotes, which multiply in the gut and migrate to the proboscis, completing the cycle.

## New World leishmaniasis (NWL)

Cutaneous leishmaniasis (CL) of the New World is a zoonosis caused by parasites of the species complex *Leishmania mexicana* and the *Viannia* subgenus (*formerly L.*

**Table 32.1** New World leishmaniasis.

| Subgenus | Common species |
|---|---|
| L. Viannia | L. (V.) braziliensis |
| | L. (V.) guyanesis |
| | L. (V.) panamensis |
| | L. (V.) peruviana |
| L. mexicana | L. mexicana |
| | L. amazonensis |
| | L. venezuelensis |

*braziliensis*) (Table 32.1). They are transmitted by sandflies and cause significant ulcerative skin lesions.

Local names for New World CL include *uta* (Peru), *chiclero's ulcer* or *bay sore* (Mexico), *dicera de baurid* (Brazil), and *pian bois*, or *forest yaws* (Guyana).

In *L.* (*V.*) *braziliensis*, infected patients may develop mucocutaneous leishmaniasis, where the mucosal lesion is characterized by destructive oral, nasal, or pharyngeal lesions, locally called espundia.

The pathogens currently affecting humans are three principal organisms in the *L. mexicana* complex and four in the *L. Viannia* complex (Table 32.1). *L. chagasi*, which is the causative agent of American visceral leishmaniasis, has also been isolated on rare occasions from lesions of cutaneous leishmaniasis.

New World leishmaniasis is transmitted by sandflies of the genus *Lutzomyia*. They differ in their preference for habitat, affinity to humans, and time of feeding. In *L.* (*V.*) *braziliensis* infection, which represents the major threat, the most common vector, *Lu. wellcomei*, avidly bites humans and rodents and, unlike most sandflies, feeds during daylight hours. This means that personal protection against this vector is more difficult. In contrast, the vectors of the *L. mexicana* complex are much less anthropophilic and are usually nocturnal feeders [11].

The reservoir is usually forest rodents. Humans are incidental victims and are not the definitive hosts. In Central America, the principal reservoir is the sloth, and forest primates are secondary hosts. Thus, people who are in remote forested areas, such as military personnel training in jungles or adventure travelers, are at higher risk to contract the disease.

In the Peruvian Andes and in the highlands of Argentina, dogs are the main reservoir hosts. Thus, the human disease (uta) is contracted in and around homes, and in some villages 90% of the inhabitants are infected.

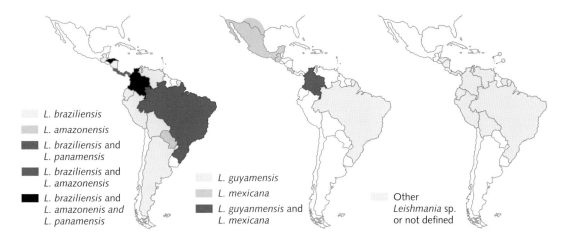

**Figure 32.4** New World *Leishmania*-infected areas. (Reprinted from Schwartz E, Hatz C, Blum J. New World Cutaneous Leishmaniasis in Travellers. *Lancet Infect Dis* 2006;6:342–9, with permission from Elsevier.)

## Epidemiology of NWL in travelers

The geographic distribution of the NWL strains is shown in Figure 32.4. As can be seen, the distribution of the disease reaches to southern Texas in the north and to Argentina in the south. Although most of the *L. mexicana* species occur in Central America and most of the *Leishmania Viannia* complex species occur in South America, there is overlap between the two complexes.

NWL is usually a disease of rural and jungle areas due to the characteristics of the hosts and the vectors, as discussed above.

The relative risk of acquiring *Leishmania* infection among German travelers was demonstrated to be highest in those who traveled to Latin America in comparison with travel to other endemic areas (Figure 32.2), with an OR of 22 compared to travelers to Southern Europe (which is also an endemic area).

The absolute risk of cutaneous leishmaniasis in travelers to Latin America is difficult to estimate because it is not notified to health authorities in most industrialized countries. It is often misdiagnosed and may also heal spontaneously. The CDC estimates an incidence between 1/1,000 (Surinam) and <1/1,000,000 (Mexico) among US travelers, based on the number of travelers and on the use of pentavalent antimonials [8].

Reports from Israel show an incidence of at least 1:360 (0.27%) in Israeli travelers to the Amazon basin (Tuichi and Beni Rivers conjunction) in Bolivia [6]. Because this region became recently a national park (Madidi National Park), which may attract more international travelers (*National Geographic*, March 2001), clinicians should be aware of this high-risk area.

## Clinical manifestations

### Cutaneous manifestation

The lesions of New World CL are generally similar at the early stage to those of Old World CL. A few weeks to several months after infection, an erythematous, often pruritic papule develops at the site of inoculation. In a group of US military personnel, cutaneous lesions were noted after a median interval of 17 days (range 2–78 days) postexposure to *L. panamensis* [12]. In French travelers, the mean interval between return and onset of lesion was 13 (1–95) days and that between return and seeking medical care was 50 (17–301) days [3]. Israeli experience with *L. (V.) braziliensis* in travelers shows that the average time that elapsed between exposure and appearance of cutaneous lesions was 1.7 months (range 1–3 months) [6].

The initial papule may become scaly or gradually enlarge, developing a raised indurated margin with central ulceration. The lesions are usually much bigger than those of the Old World disease and may reach more than 5 cm in diameter (Figure 32.5). Typically, there are 1–3 lesions, and in almost all cases they are ulcerative lesions. Other types of lesions, such as papules and nodules (which are common in Old World leishmaniasis), are rarely seen in New World CL. The ulcerative lesions are usually painless, unless secondarily infected.

### Lymphadenopathy

Enlargement of the lymph nodes draining from the bite site is a common finding in *L. (V.) braziliensis* infections. Regional lymphadenopathy was observed in two-thirds of

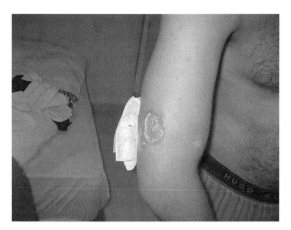

**Figure 32.5** CL due to *L. (V.) braziliensis* acquired in Bolivia; note the swollen arm (axillary lymphadenopathy was palpable).

Brazilian patients infected by *L. (V.) braziliensis*. In these patients, 62% of lymph node aspirates yielded *Leishmania* parasites in cultures [13]. Similarly, in our series of travelers infected with *L. (V.) braziliensis*, 45% had regional lymphadenopathy [6]. Lymphadenopathy may even precede the appearance of cutaneous lesions, suggesting early lymphatic spread of parasites in *L. (V.) braziliensis* infections [14]. Leishmaniasis should, therefore, be in the differential diagnosis of lymphadenopathy in travelers returning from these areas even when no skin lesion is apparent.

Multiple skin lesions due to metastatic spread along lymphatics and subcutaneous lymphatic nodules resembling sporotrichosis are often seen in *L. (V.) braziliensis* complex infections (Figure 32.6) [3, 6].

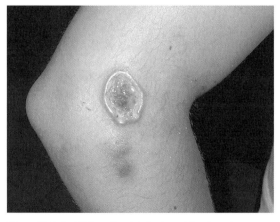

**Figure 32.6** *L. (V.) braziliensis* infection with subcutaneous nodules, sporotrichosis distribution below the lesion, and lymphangitis spread above it.

The natural history of the ulcer varies, depending on the infecting species, the location of the lesion, and host immunity. *L. mexicana* infections generally have one or a few lesions, which heal spontaneously within 6 months [9]. However, lesions on the ear, named chiclero's ulcers, occur in 40% of patients in endemic areas and are chronic, lasting for many years if not treated.

In *L. (V.) braziliensis* complex, simple cutaneous lesions generally require 6–18 months for spontaneous healing but sometimes persist much longer.

## Mucosal leishmaniasis (ML)

Mucosal leishmaniasis (espundia) is a worrisome complication of CL of the New World. It is almost exclusively a complication of *L. (V.) braziliensis* infection and, therefore, is more common in southern latitudes and much less common in northern South America and Central America.

The actual risk in endemic populations is difficult to assess. ML occurred in 2.7% of patients with CL [15] in a prospective study from Brazil, whereas it was estimated to occur in 5–20% of patients in Bolivia [16]. Interestingly, the risk of ML was 3–10 times higher in migrants than in the indigenous population [17], which may indicate that travelers could also be at higher risk to develop ML than the local population.

The mucosal lesions are more common in patients with large and multiple lesions and in those who did not receive systemic antimony treatment for the initial cutaneous lesion [15]. Additional risk factors for mucosal lesions are infection in young males, those with lesions above the waist, and those with genetic backgrounds of HLA-DR2 and HLA-DQw3 [18]. The time lag between the appearance of skin lesions and mucosal disease ranges from simultaneous appearance to as much as 35 years [19].

The metastatic spread of the infection is to the nasal, pharyngeal, and buccal mucosa. Erythema and edema of the involved mucosa are followed by ulcerations covered with a mucopurulent exudate. There is often mutilating destruction of the nasal septum, palate, lips, pharynx, and larynx. The lesions are chronic and progressive, and death can be caused by aspiration or inanition. Mucosal lesions occur rarely in *L. panamensis*, *L. guyanensis*, and *L. amazonensis* infection [20].

### ML in travelers

Reported cases of ML in travelers are extremely rare. There were only two reports of mucocutaneous lesions in the literature until 2000. However, since 2000, there have been an increasing number of reports [21]. All of these individuals contracted the disease in South

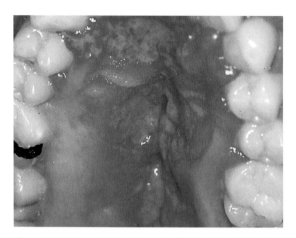

**Figure 32.7** Mucosal lesion due to *L. (V.) braziliensis* infection; note the deep ulcer in the upper palate.

America, most of them in the Amazon region of Bolivia, and none of them had systemic antimonial treatment before the appearance of mucosal lesions. For example, we encountered a case who had had 5 years of progressive mucosal ulcerations in his nose and palate after returning from the jungle areas of Bolivia [22]. The mucosal lesions appeared within 1 month of the cutaneous lesion, but they were overlooked for 5 years (Figure 32.7). Despite having multiple leishmaniasis skin lesions upon his return, he did not receive systemic treatment, but rather topical paromomycin ointment.

The risk of developing ML in travelers with *L. (V.) braziliensis* infection has never been assessed. In a series of 79 British travelers with CL from one medical center, 4 (5.1%) also had mucosal involvement [23]. In a nationwide Israeli study of CL in travelers to Latin America, out of 76 patients, 6 (7.8%) developed mucosal disease [E. Schwartz, unpublished data]. All of these cases were acquired in the Amazon region of Bolivia.

The mucosal lesions appeared within shortly after the cutaneous disease (<6 months). All the patients were HIV negative.

Clinically, patients may complain of congestion, difficulty breathing through their noses, and occasional nosebleeds as initial symptoms. Nonhealing ulcers on the palate may occur as well. Hoarseness might indicate vocal cord involvement. Therefore, our policy includes inspection of the nasopharyngeal mucosa in all patients before initiation of treatment. Hoarseness should prompt evaluation of the vocal cords for laryngeal involvement.

## Diagnostic methods

Diagnostic methods are divided into two categories. One is *genus-specific* diagnosis from which the diagnosis of a possible *Leishmania* infection can be made. The other is *species-specific* diagnosis from which the species of the *Leishmania* infection agent can be determined.

The classical method of CL diagnosis is based on direct visualization of the parasite under the microscope in Giemsa-stained smears or histological sections (for the complete method see [19]). Direct visualization of the amastigote parasite using slit skin smear is very useful, is simple, and gives rapid results (within 20 minutes) and should be the first step in establishing a diagnosis. Culturing of the aspirated material in a special medium is another method; however, this must be done in an experienced center, and it takes several weeks to obtain the final results. The sensitivity of these methods is extremely variable, from 19% to 77% for the direct demonstration of the parasite and 58% to 62% for the cultures [19, 24].

Standard serological tests are not useful for the diagnosis of CL because they are often negative. In invasive disease, such as visceral leishmaniasis or mucosal disease, they usually become positive. Serology may be helpful in monitoring the treatment response in ML [25].

The *leishmanin skin test* (Montenegro test) is another theoretical method. It is positive in almost all patients with active CL and ML, although it may take about 3 months until it becomes positive. It then remains positive for life. Thus, in endemic areas, it cannot as a rule signify active disease, and is used rather for epidemiological studies. In travelers who have not been exposed in the past to *Leishmania* infection, it could have diagnostic value; however, the test is not routinely available in most industrialized countries.

The above-mentioned methods are for genus-specific diagnosis. For species-specific diagnosis, until recently, the existing methods were isoenzyme or monoclonal antibodies analysis on cultured *Leishmania* [26]. Most laboratories do not routinely offer these tests.

PCR is now the method of choice for diagnosis in travelers. It is a rapid tool with high specificity to differentiate between Old and New World leishmaniasis and between *L. (Viannia)* and *L. mexicana* complexes in the New World forms. It is highly sensitive and requires minute amounts of DNA from dermal scrapings of cutaneous lesions. The sensitivity ranges from 89% to 100% [6, 27, 28]. Thus, beside the advantage of species-specific diagnosis, PCR has proved to be superior to the conventional methods, showing better sensitivity than the direct visualization of parasites in biopsies or smear.

Determination of the species is clinically very important because in South and Central America there is an overlap between *L. Viannia* species and the *L. mexicana* species complex, and only *L. Viannia* species cause mucosal involvement. Moreover, in travelers who may also reside in or travel through endemic areas for Old World leishmaniasis (e.g., Southern Europe and the Middle East), the causative species of skin lesions may be Old or New World *Leishmania*. It is important to make the correct diagnosis because systemic treatment is recommended for *L. Viannia* species and not required for most other cases of cutaneous leishmaniasis. Unnecessary systemic therapy may be harmful, because there is a potential for toxic side effects.

### Differential diagnosis in travelers

A typical chronic skin ulcer, together with a travel history revealing a visit to rural areas of Latin America, leads to a straightforward clinical diagnosis. However, for clinicians who are unfamiliar with the disease, common misdiagnoses include bacterial skin infections, nonspecific skin reactions to insect bites, *Mycobacterium* infections, mycosis (mainly sporotrichosis in a patient with nodular lymphangitis), and dermatologic cancers. Biopsy, which is typically done in these cases, reveals the correct leishmaniasis diagnosis.

### Treatment

The aim of treatment of CL is twofold. First is to prevent mucosal invasion by metastatic spread of the infection to the oropharyngeal site. Second is to accelerate the healing of the skin lesion(s) and to avoid disfiguring scars.

For the first, systemic treatment is needed, whereas local treatment might be sufficient for the second. The indications for systemic treatment for CL are summarized in Table 32.2.

Because *L. (V.)braziliensis* is the major culprit in mucosal involvement, treating this species is the greatest challenge and its treatment options are discussed thoroughly.

### Systemic parenteral treatment

#### Pentavalent antimony

The systemic treatment that is still considered the drug of choice by many authorities, is pentavalent antimony. This drug is available as sodium stibogluconate (SSG) (Pentostam) in most Western countries or meglumine

**Table 32.2** Indications for systemic treatment.

Lesion caused by *L. Viannia* (especially *L. (V.) braziliensis*)
Chronic ear infection (chiclero, *L. mexicana*)
Metastatic spread to lymph nodes
Localization in the face

antimoniate (Glucantime) mainly in France and Latin America countries. In the USA, SSG is available under an investigational new drug application from the CDC. The recommended dose is 20 mg /kg, without an upper limit, for 20 days [9, 19].

The drug is available only in parenteral forms (i.v. and i.m.) and the high rate of toxicity may result in hospitalization of patients for the treatment period, although in some centers with experience in this treatment, daily ambulatory treatment has been given without added complications [29].

#### *Pentavalent antimony toxicity*

Fatigue, musculoskeletal pain, and gastrointestinal symptoms are the common adverse reactions to toxicity [9].

Laboratory abnormalities include mainly elevation of liver enzymes (transaminases) and elevation of the pancreatic enzymes (amylase and lipase), both occurring frequently. The elevation in pancreatic enzymes is often without any clinical symptoms. Hematological findings include leukopenia and thrombocytopenia [9, 30, 31]. In addition, electrocardiogram disturbances with T-wave changes might occur, and life-threatening ventricular tachyarrhythmias have also been reported [32, 33].

#### *Mortality*

No deaths have been reported among travelers who have been treated with SSG. However, increased mortality is reported among patients with visceral leishmaniasis in endemic areas who were treated with antimonials rather than miltefosine [34]. In another report, 7 patients out of 553 who were improving slowly with antimony therapy died unexpectedly, which raised the suspicion that mortality in Kala-azar patients during standard antimonial therapy may be more related to the drug than the disease process [35].

#### *Management*

Our policy is to dilute the SSG in 120 ml of 5% dextrose in water and infuse intravenously over 2 hours (although others have infused it over 20–30 minutes). During drug infusion, the patients undergo ECG monitoring. Complete blood counts, basic chemistry, amylase, CPK, and ECG are analyzed during admission and biweekly during treatment.

Treatment is withheld when liver enzymes are more than 10 times normal levels or when amylase is more than 3 times normal level. Withholding treatment or decreasing the dose for a few days reverses these abnormalities, and reinstitution of treatment usually will not cause recurrence [6].

**Table 32.3** Comparison between Pentostam treatment group and AmBisome treatment group for *L. braziliensis*.

|  | AmBisome | Pentostam |
|---|---|---|
| No. of patients | 15 | 27 |
| Men:women | 11:4 | 23:4 |
| Mean age (years) | 23.1 | 24.7 |
| Infected in Bolivia | 14/15 (93%) | 25/27 (93%) |
| Mean no. of lesions | 1.4 | 2.1 |
| No. of hospitalization days | 6 | 25 |
| No. of patients with Interruption of treatment | 0 (0%) | 17/27(63%) |
| No. of patients with relapse | 0 (0%) | 10/27 (37%) |

*Source:* (Reprinted from Solomon M, Baum S, Barzilai A, Scope A, Trau H, Schwartz E. Liposomal amphotericin B in comparison to sodium stibogluconate for cutaneous infection due to *Leishmania braziliensis. J am Acad Dermatol* 2007;56:612–6, with permission from Elsevier.)

*Treatment failure*

Our past experience had been that antimonial treatment is effective in achieving clinical cure in only 75% of cases, despite the fact that this group consisted of otherwise healthy travelers who were HIV negative and without mucosal lesions. Others have reported cure rates of 85–90% in studies of cutaneous disease of the New World [9, 36]. The high failure rate observed among Israeli patients is probably related to the fact that the patient population was of *L. (V.) braziliensis* cases only, whereas in the other series reported, there were patients with other NWL complexes, such as *L. mexicana,* who had a better response to SSG.

### Liposomal amphotericin B

Amphotericin B deoxycholate and lipid-based amphotericin B products are well-established treatments for visceral leishmaniasis [37]. The latter formula is considered less nephrotoxic than nonliposomal amphotericin B because it specifically targets the macrophages in which the *Leishmania* parasites develop [38].

Amphotericin B is a well-known treatment for ML, and the liposomal form gives excellent results (~100% cure). However, because of its high cost, it is not available in the developing countries [39].

A recent study among Israeli travelers with *L. (V.) braziliensis* infection showed that among those who relapsed after SSG treatment, initiation of liposomal amphotericin B (AmBisome) treatment cured all patients, without further relapse and without any significant side effects [40]. In subsequent studies, patients with primary infection were treated with AmBisome as the first line. The

protocol used was a dose of 3 mg/kg, given for 5 consecutive days, with a 6th dose on day 10. Thus, a total dose of 18 mg/kg was given. This schedule is based on short-course treatment of visceral leishmaniasis with AmBisome [41]. All doses were given in an outpatient setting.

A comparison of the SSG treatment group to the AmBisome group is presented in Table 32.3. In this case series, there was even a high failure rate of 37% (10/27) in patients who were treated with SSG. In addition to its high failure rate, SSG treatment was associated with a very high frequency of adverse events. Consequently, the length of treatment with SSG was influenced by these significant adverse events, and frequently treatment was stopped or the dose reduced. Thus, in this study, the 20 days of SSG treatment were actually prolonged to a mean of 25 days.

AmBisome, on the other hand, was given in a short 6-day course of uninterrupted treatment. Patients achieved a complete cure in less than 1 month. Side effects were mild and could be avoided by a slow infusion rate. No laboratory abnormalities were detected during the course of treatment. This short course is very much appreciated by patients, as interference with daily activities is minimal. In addition, although the number of patients who were treated was relatively small, no case of relapse was detected for a median of a 1-year follow-up [40].

There are a number of lipid-based amphotericin B products: liposomal amphotericin B (AmBisome), amphotericin B lipid complex (Abelcet), and amphotericin B cholesteryl complex (Amphotec). In animal models, not all the compounds demonstrated similar efficacy against cutaneous leishmaniasis [42]. Thus, our success with AmBisome cannot be extrapolated to all liposomal

**Table 32.4** *Leishmania* treatment cost comparison of SSG antimony (Pentostam) vs liposomal amphotericin B (AmBisome) treatment, based on Israeli tariff.

| Regimen | Cost in US dollars | | | | |
|---|---|---|---|---|---|
| | Drug (per patient weighing 70 kg) | Hospitalization course | Extra hospitalization days (5 days due to adverse events) | Laboratory workup | Total |
| Pentostam 20 mg/kg inpatient setting (20 days) | 455 | 7,650 | 1,460 | 1,365 | 10,930 |
| Pentostam 20 mg/kg outpatient setting (20 days) | 455 | 4,200 | 800 | 1,365 | 6,820 |
| AmBisome 3 mg/kg outpatient setting (6 days) | 4,320 | 1,200 | None | 320 | 5,840 |

*Source:* (Adapted from Solomon M, Baum S, Barzilai A, Scope A, Trau H, Schwartz E. Liposomal amphotericin B in comparison to sodium stibogluconate for cutaneous infection due to *Leishmania braziliensis. J Am Acad Dermatol* 2007;56:612–6, with permission from Elsevier.)
Laboratory workup for Pentostam treatment includes CBC, electrolytes, renal function test, liver function test, amylase, lipase everyday. EKGs were analyzed during admission and biweekly during treatment.

Laboratory workup for AmBisome treatment includes CBC, electrolytes, renal function test every other day.

amphotericin products. In fact, failure of Abelcet has been reported in one case of *L. (V.) braziliensis* cutaneous leishmaniasis [43].

The major problem of using AmBisome is its high cost. However, the cost of the drug is only one component in treating patients in developed countries, where cost of hospitalization and of laboratory work-up is significant. A comparison of the total cost of the care of a patient who is treated with AmBisome versus SSG shows that despite the high cost of AmBisome, the expense for total care with AmBisome is less than with SSG: 45% less if SSG is given in an inpatient setting and 15% less if SSG is given in an outpatient setting (Table 32.4).

Thus, in the author's view, liposomal amphotericin B should be the first line of treatment of *L.(V.)braziliensis* infections, and only in case of failure should the toxic compound SSG be given.

Other therapeutic options for systemic and local treatment are listed in Table 32.5. Pentamidine might be considered as a second-line treatment [44]. In French Guiana, where *L. guyanensis* is responsible for more than 90% of the cases, it is the drug of choice [45]. Miltefosine (a phosphocholine analogue), which is the new promising oral agent for visceral leishmaniasis, shows encouraging results in treating *L. panamensis* (cure rate of 91%), but only marginal results for *L. mexicana*, and has failed in treating *L.(V.)braziliensis* [46].

For the *L. mexicana* complex treatment options, see Table 32.5.

**Local treatment**

Local treatment instead of systemic treatment is used when there is no risk of ML. Thus, it is mainly relevant in the *L. mexicana* complex. For details see below in treatment of Old World CL.

## Old World cutaneous leishmaniasis (OWCL)

Four species, *L. major*, *L. tropica*, *L. aethiopica*, and *L. infantum*, cause OWCL (see Figure 32.1). *L. infantum* is the species that may also cause visceral leishmaniasis, mainly among children; hence, its name.

The most common species in this area is *L. major*. Common names for this infection follow the associated distribution of the disease, such as Oriental sore, Baghdad sore, Rose of Jericho, or Delhi boil.

*L. aethiopica* occurs mainly in Ethiopia and Kenya, in rural mountain areas. Hyraxes, distant relatives of elephants, serve as the animal reservoir.

*L. infantum* occurs in the Mediterranean basin, China, Central Asia, and the Middle East. Adults infected with this species tend to develop a mild, self-limited cutaneous

**Table 32.5** Treatment of NWCL by species.

| Species | Drug | Dosage | Level of evidence |
|---|---|---|---|
| *L. mexicana* | Ointment: 15% Paromomycin plus 12% Methylbenzethonium chloride | Twice daily for 20 days | B |
| | Ketoconazole | 600 mg daily for 28 days | B |
| *L. panamensis* | Ketoconazole | 600 mg daily for 28 days | A |
| | Pentavalent antimonials or | 20 mg Sb/kg/day for 20 days | A |
| | Pentavalent antimonials and in addition Allopurinol | 20 mg Sb/kg/day for 15 days 20 mg/kg/day given in 4 doses for 15 days | |
| *L. guyanensis* | Pentamidine isethionate | Four injections of 3 mg/kg/day every other day | C |
| *L. braziliense* | See detailed discussion in the chapter | | |

*Source:* From [1].

Level of evidence: recommendation grade.

A = Randomized controlled trial in representative collective.

B = Randomized controlled trial in partially representative (small patient number, different species included) collective. Cohort trial or case control study in representative collective.

C = Cohort trial or case control study in partially representative collective, series of cases in representative collective.

D = Series of cases in partially representative (small patient number, different species included) collective, informal expert opinion, other information.

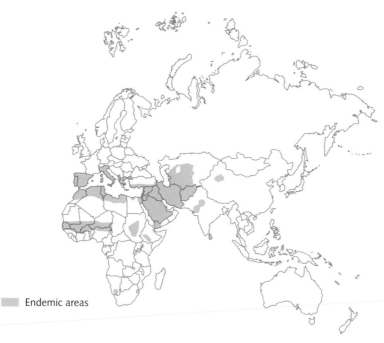

Endemic areas

**Figure 32.8** Distribution of Old World cutaneous leishmaniasis.

disease, whereas infants tend to develop a visceral disease. Animal reservoirs include domesticated and wild canines.

*L. tropica*, an emerging infection in several parts of the Middle East, and *L. major*, the common pathogen in these regions, will be discussed more thoroughly. These two pathogens have also gained lot of attention in the last decade since Western military groups participating in the conflicts in the region, such as Afghanistan, Iraq, and the Gulf, have been affected by leishmaniasis in very high numbers [47]. The distribution of OWCL is seen in Figure 32.8.

### Diagnosis of Old World CL

Methods of diagnosis are as mentioned above for NW CL. Usually, within an endemic region, each species has its own distribution area.

In these cases, *Leishmania* genus diagnosis by smear or biopsy is sufficient. In cases of co-circulation of the two species (*L. major* and *L. tropica*), species-specific diagnosis by PCR may be of value because *L. tropica* is more resistant to conventional treatment modalities. The same holds true for *travel-related* importation of *Leishmania* species from one CL-endemic area to another, or importation to nonendemic regions, where clinicians might not be familiar with local distribution of the *Leishmania* species.

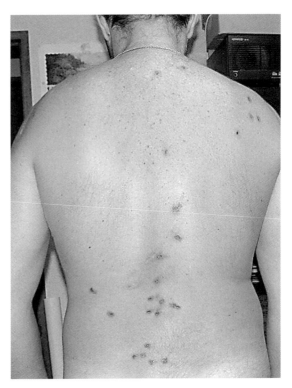

**Figure 32.9** Multiple lesions of *L. Leishmania major* infection.

### Treatment of Old World CL

Despite the fact that cutaneous leishmaniasis is a serious problem plaguing populations in more than 90 countries [10], optimal management, including indications and drugs for treatment, has yet to be clearly determined [1, 49]. Infection with CL can result in a wide spectrum of clinical manifestations from a small, benign, and self-healing condition to serious disfiguring and chronic lesions. The outcome of the disease is based on parasite and host factors.

### *Leishmania major* infection

#### Epidemiology

*L. major* is usually a disease of rural areas, because the animal reservoirs are desert rodents. It is endemic in the desert areas of northern Africa (including a wide area of the Sahel and the upper part of Sub-Saharan Africa), the Middle East, and Central Asia. In certain communities, local prevalence may approach 100% and thus travelers to desert areas in these countries may be affected.

The reservoir in Israel, Libya, and Saudi Arabia is the fat rat (*Psammomys obesus*), whereas the great gerbil (*Rhombomys opimus*) is the host in the desert areas of Central

Asia and southern Russia, throughout Iran, and in parts of Iraq and northwestern India. The vector in these areas is *Phlebotomus* spp. (mainly *P. papatasi*) [48]. The peak incidence of disease occurs in late summer and autumn.

#### Clinical features

Following inoculation by the sandfly, characteristic skin lesions generally appear within 6 weeks, but may be delayed for prolonged periods, depending on the size of the inoculum. The lesion begins as a small, pruritic, erythematous papule that slowly enlarges and breaks down to form a small ulcer or sometimes a nodular lesion. Lesions may be single or multiple and occur on exposed skin surfaces. Ulcers persist for a variable time and heal slowly, with scarring.

*L. major* often causes multiple lesions with an exudative base. Patients with 10–40 lesions are not uncommon (Figure 32.9). The infection runs a more rapid course, and the lesions may be healed in 6 months. Spread to regional lymph nodes is rare.

**Table 32.6** Treatment of OWCL by species.

| Species | Drug | Dosage | Level of evidence |
|---------|------|--------|-------------------|
| L. major | 15% paromomycin/12% methylbenzethonium chloride ointment | Twice daily for 10–20 days | A |
|  | Localized heat or cryotherapy | Two sessions with localized heat (55°C for 5 minutes) | C |
|  |  | Two to three sessions of topical application of liquid nitrogen | C |
|  | Local infiltration with antimonials | Sodium stibogluconate, meglumine antimonate Complete blanching of lesion has to be achieved See details in the chapter | A |
|  | Fluconazole | 200 mg daily for 6 weeks | A |
| L. tropica | Local infiltration with antimonials | Sodium stibogluconate, meglumine antimonate | D |
|  | 15% paromomycin/12% Methylbenzethonium chloride ointment | Twice daily for 10–20 days | D |
|  | Cryotherapy Localized heat | 2–3 sessions of topical application of liquid nitrogen 2 sessions with localized heat (55°C for 5 minutes) | C |
|  | Pentavalent antimonials | 20 mg Sb/kg/day for 10–20 days | D |
|  | Fluconazole | 200 mg daily for 6 weeks | D |

*Source:* From [1].

Level of evidence: recommendation grade.

A = Randomized controlled trial in representative collective.

B = Randomized controlled trial in partially representative (small patient number, different species included) collective. Cohort trial or case control study in representative collective.

C = Cohort trial or case control study in partially representative collective, series of cases in representative collective.

D = Series of cases in partially representative (small patient number, different species included) collective, informal expert opinion, other information.

## Treatment of *L. major*

For *L. major*, local treatment is usually sufficient, and several physical methods and topical ointments have been proposed [1, 50] (see Table 32.6). The currently employed physical methods are curettage, cryotherapy, and local heat therapy (ThermoMed, Thermosurgery Technologies).

Topical remedies are based mainly on topical paromomycin (aminosidine); it has been studied in several randomized trials of patients with CL, with variable results. The paromomycin ointments have contained different major components, including methylbenzethonium chloride, wool fat, water, white soft paraffin, and 10% urea, which might explain the different outcomes. An Israeli-made paromomycin ointment is 15% paromomycin and 12% or 5% methylbenzethonium chloride

in soft white paraffin (Leshcutan, Teva Pharmaceutical Industries, Jerusalem). Its use for the treatment of *L. major* infection in Israel was associated with a cure rate of 74% after 10–20 days [50]. Randomized clinical studies from Iran and Tunisia failed to show any clear clinical benefit of 15% paromomycin sulfate and 10% urea in Eucerin ointment [51, 52].

The usual recommended regimen is application of the ointment on the lesions twice daily for 14 days. Side effects are usually mild and include itching, erythema, edema, and tenderness, but significant local irritation may occur.

Recent study of a different ointment, S-nitroso-*N*-acetyl penicillamine (SNAP cream, Glaxo Wellcome), which generates nitric oxide, was studied by Lopez-Jaramillo et al. for treatment of new world CL in 16 patients, of whom all improved [53].

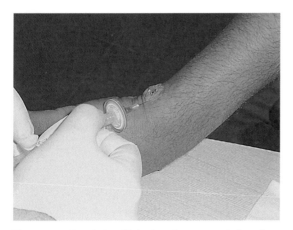

**Figure 32.10** Intralesional injection of pentostam in *L. major* lesion.

Another very effective treatment is local infiltration of the lesion with SSG. Administering SSG via the intralesional (IL) route is an attractive option, because systemic adverse events are not likely to occur and the treatment can be provided in an outpatient setting. This method is used in Europe and in Israel but has not yet been approved in the USA.

SSG is injected around the lesion (Figure 32.10) until the entire lesion has blanched, up to 0.5 cc per ulcer (50 mg). In our policy, the treatment was repeated every 2–3 weeks until the lesion had become flattened, with either complete reepithelization or reduction of the ulcer to less than 3 mm. With this schedule, 91% of our patients achieved complete cure within 3 months, with an average of 2.5 injections (range: 1–6) [54]. These results were similar to cure rate results achieved by systemic treatment with SSG. Similar results are reported by other groups [54]. Shorter intervals (< every 2 weeks) of IL SSG injection have no advantage. Thus, it seems that IL SSG treatment is highly efficacious and very convenient for the patient, as it requires infrequent visits to the outpatient clinic. Side effects are mild and consist of pain at the site of injection.

Systemic treatment should be considered in cases of failure of local treatment or in patients with multiple lesions (sometimes as many as 30–40 lesions) that cannot feasibly be treated by ointment or local infiltration. In these cases, intravenous SSG in the same dose as for NWCL (see above) is recommended, with a 10-day course usually sufficing [55].

The imidazoles, which were introduced as antifungal drugs, also have antileishmanial activity. They have the

> ### Suggested policy for treating *L. major* CL
>
> 1 Very mild disease—no treatment.
> 2 Local treatment is the preferable approach in most cases when there are only few lesions. One can try paramomycin-based ointment, or even the preferable treatment with intralesional injection of pentavalent antimony.
> 3 Failures of ointment treatment should be switched to intralesional antimony treatment.
> 4 Systemic treatment of CL ( pentavalent antimony), due to its side effects, should be provided only in the following circumstances:
>    — lesions inaccessible to local treatment (such as eyelids)
>    — failure of prior treatments
>    — multiple lesions
>    — Lesions suggest evidence of local dissemination (e.g., there are satellite papules, regional lymphadenopathy, or sporotrichoid subcutaneous nodules, which rarely occur in *L. majo*r infection).

advantage of oral administration and relatively fewer adverse effects than SSG.

*Fluconazole*, 200 mg daily for 6 weeks, was studied in Iran. Healing of lesions was complete in 79% at the 3 month follow-up compared to 34% in the placebo group. *Ketoconazole* appears to be effective as well. In studies in Turkey it had higher efficacy than topical paromomycin and intralesional injections of SSG [49]. Ketoconazole appeared to be effective in *L. major* also in Israel, with a cure rate of 70% after 200–400 mg daily for 4–6 weeks [1]. These moderate results with prolonged treatment time preclude using these drug routinely.

### *Leishmania tropical* infection

*L. tropica* usually causes urban, dry, and more often anthroponotic cutaneous leishmaniasis. Endemic areas include urban areas of the Mediterranean basin, Central Asia, and the Middle East.

It is not clear what the vertebrate reservoir of this pathogen is. Experts think that in some places (e.g., Afghanistan) humans are the primary host and may serve as a reservoir. In a recent outbreak in Israel, rock hyraxes (*Procavia capensis)* were found to be the reservoir [56].

The vectors are also *Phlebotomus* spp., although different from those of *L. major* (in Israel, mostly *P. arabicus* or *P. sergentii).*

In general, *L. tropica* has been reported to be more common in urban areas and villages than in rural areas.

In the urban setting it may be an anthroponotic, but on the outskirts of cities and villages the disease is usually contracted from animal reservoirs such as rock hyraxes [48].

## Clinical features

After an incubation period of about 3–12 weeks, CL usually appears as an erythematous papule that gradually evolves into an ulcer. Without treatment, spontaneous resolution usually occurs over a period of 6–12 months, or even longer. A scar remains at the site of the healed ulcer. It is impossible to definitively distinguish clinically between *L. tropica* and *L. major* infections. However, *L. major* has been described as an exudative, "wet" lesion that evolves and heals relatively rapidly (a few months to ~1 year). In contrast, *L. tropica* infection is usually described as a "dry" nodulo-ulcerative lesion that heals more slowly and is relatively resistant to treatment. *L. tropica* tends to affect the upper extremities and face (Figure 32.11) [57].

In addition, *L. tropica* may cause leishmania recidivans, a recrudescent infection within or at the edge of scars of previously healed *L. tropica* lesions. A systemic infection caused by *L. tropica*, characterized by fever, fatigue, diarrhea, and arthralgia, was described among US soldiers who served in Operation Desert Storm [58]. However, this viscerotropic infection seems to be exceptional.

## Treatment of *L. tropica*

There are less evidence-based recommendations for treating *L. tropica*, but it seems to be more resistant to treatment and has less of a response to paramomycin ointment [57]. In these cases, therefore, our practice is to treat with SSG, either intralesional or i.v. [57]. Recently, cases who failed i.l. SSG were treated successfully with liposomal amphotericin B (AmBisome) [E. Schwartz, unpublished data]

Large, controlled clinical trials to evaluate current treatment regimens as well as new medications for CL are urgently needed.

## Visceral leishmaniasis (VL)

Visceral leishmaniasis, or kala-azar, results from infection with protozoa such as *L. donovani* in Africa and India, *L. infantum* in the Mediterranean basin, including Southern Europe and *L. chagasi* in the New World (Figure 32.12). Like the cutaneous leishmaniases, it is transmitted by sand

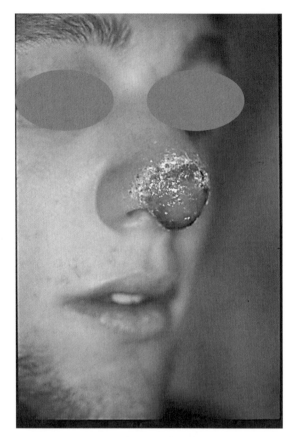

**Figure 32.11** *L. tropica* infection with erythematous–squamous type lesion.

flies, and the reservoir animals include domesticated or wild canines and various rodents, except in India, where human beings are the known reservoir.

Visceral leishmaniasis is not seen in travelers to the tropics. However, it is a re-emerging disease in developed countries, mainly in Southern Europe, where the disease often presents as *Leishmania*/HIV co-infections and intravenous drug users have been identified as a population at risk. Infrequently, organ transplant recipients have also been reported to have had VL, either acquired through the procedure or reactivated due to the immune suppression therapy.

Interestingly, in a report from Germany summarizing cases of leishmaniasis imported to Germany (2001–2004), the major group was of VL (38%) imported from Southern Europe [5] .

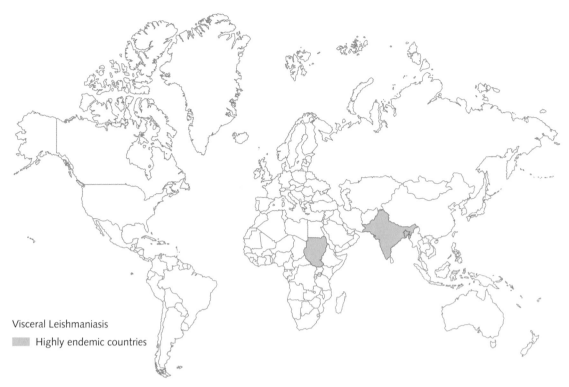

**Figure 32.12** Visceral leishmaniasis: highly endemic countries (90% of cases).

## Clinical features

VL arising in different regions may show some variations in its clinical and epidemiologic appearance. A cutaneous nodule often develops at the site of the parasitic inoculation in the African and Central Asian forms of the infection. Often this will have resolved before clinical illness develops. After an incubation period of 2–6 months, systemic manifestations develop insidiously, although the presentation may occasionally be abrupt. The earliest symptom is fever. On physical examination, the liver and spleen are large, firm, and nontender. Lymphadenopathy is more frequently reported in the Mediterranean countries, East Africa, and China.

The clinical manifestations of VL are due to the invasion of the reticuloendothelial cells of the spleen, liver, bone marrow, and skin and the subsequent multiplication of amastigotes within the cells. Untreated infections become chronic and, in addition to the above physical findings, patients typically become markedly wasted. Patients with light-colored skin may develop a grayish cast—*kala-azar* is an Indian name meaning "black fever."

Untreated visceral leishmaniasis may be complicated by concomitant infections such as pneumonia, pulmonary tuberculosis, and dysentery, and these cases often prove fatal. Some patients die from gastrointestinal hemorrhage.

The clinical presentation of VL in AIDS patients is felt to be similar to the presentation in non-HIV infected hosts. Fever, splenomegaly, and pancytopenia are common. However, involvement of the gastrointestinal tract is more common in AIDS patients where abundant parasite-laden macrophages are found in the submucosa, from the esophagus to the rectum. Management of HIV-associated leishmaniasis patients is beyond the scope of the chapter.

Among local populations, long after apparently successful treatment, some patients may develop post-kala-azar dermal leishmaniasis, a condition that resembles leprosy and features depigmented or nodular cutaneous lesions.

## Diagnosis

The diagnosis of visceral leishmaniasis should be suspected in individuals presenting with characteristic signs and symptoms and who have emigrated from or visited an area where leishmaniasis is endemic.

Laboratory studies reveal anemia, leukopenia, neutropenia, and occasionally thrombocytopenia. The eosinophil count is low. A marked hyperglobulinemia due to increased IgG is usually present.

Microscopic examination and culture of bone marrow aspirates provide the best methods for reaching a definitive diagnosis of visceral leishmaniasis, though evidence suggests that examination and culture of splenic aspirates is probably superior. In VL cases, serologic testing might be useful for diagnosis, followed by monitoring the response to treatment.

The introduction of PCR improves our diagnostic ability by testing bone marrow or splenic aspirates. Recently, it was also shown that the sensitivity of PCR of peripheral blood samples was similar to that of PCR of bone marrow aspirate (98%).

The differential diagnosis of these patients is usually of hematological malignancies due to the splenomegaly with pancytopenia observed in peripheral blood. Because of lack of awareness to the possibility of VL diagnosis in developed countries, patients may end up having a splenectomy done, and it is only the pathologist who makes the diagnosis of a medically treatable condition.

## Treatment

The traditional treatment is SSG (or meglumine antimonite), and the current regimen recommended by the CDC is 20 mg/kg/day for 28 days. Clinical resistance of *Leishmania* to antimony compounds has been noted in some countries, India in particular. An alternative regimen that has proved very effective as a shortened course is liposomal amphotericin B [41]. The response rate is close to 100%. The disadvantage of this treatment is its high cost. In Western countries, this treatment is often the first line. When cost is an issue, amphotericin B can be given at a dose of 1 mg per kilogram intravenously every other day for 30 days.

A recent study from India has shown that paramomycin (a much cheaper drug) at a dose of 11 mg/kg of body weight intramuscularly daily for 21 days was also comparable to amphotericin B treatment, with a cure rate of 95% [59].

An attractive option is the new oral anti-*Leishmania* drug miltefosine. It has been shown to be highly effective, with a 94% cure rate after 28 days of treatment (50–100 mg daily) [60]. The main adverse events associated with its use are related to gastrointestinal complaints.

## Prevention

Personal protection is the main method of protecting travelers. However, it gives only limited results. Insect repellents, long-sleeved shirts, and impregnated fine-mesh bed netting may reduce the risk of infection. However, taking into account that sandflies are much smaller than mosquitoes, standard bed nets may be useless. Although most of the sandfly vectors are nocturnal feeders, some of them, especially in South America, are day feeders. Permethrin-impregnated clothing is helpful, as was shown in a study of Colombian military personnel: soldiers wearing permethrin-impregnated uniforms in an endemic area acquired the disease significantly less often (61).

Controlling the phlebotomine population is very difficult, and a vaccine is not expected to be available in the near future. Thus, increased knowledge and increased awareness of leishmaniasis among travelers is urgently needed [62].

## References

1 Blum J, Desjeux P, Schwartz E, Beck B, Hatz C. Treatment of cutaneous leishmaniasis among travellers. *J Antimicrob Chemother* 2004;53:158–66.

2 Lederman E, Weld L, Elyazar I, Kes M, Sonnenburg F, Loutan L, Schwartz E. Keystone J. Dermatologic conditions of the ill returned traveler: an analysis from the GeoSentinel surveillance network. *Int J Infect Dis* 2008;12(6): 593–602.

3 El Hajj L, Thellier M, Carriere J, Bricaire F, Danis M, Caumes E. Localized cutaneous leishmaniasis imported into Paris: a review of 39 cases. *Int J Dermatol* 2004;43(2):120–25.

4 Harms G, Schönian G, Feldmeier H. Leishmaniasis in Germany. *Emerg Infect Dis* 2003;9:872–5.

5 Weitzel T, Mühlberger N, Jelinek T, et al.; Surveillance Importierter Infektionen in Deutschland (SIMPID) Surveillance Network. Imported leishmaniasis in Germany 2001–2004: data of the SIMPID surveillance network. *Eur J Clin Microbiol Infect Dis* 2005;24:471–6.

6 Scope A, Trau H, Anders G, Barzilai A, Confino Y, Schwartz E. Experience with New World cutaneous leishmaniasis in travelers. *J Am Acad Dermatol* 2003;49:672–8.

7 Steinlauf S, Segal G, Sidi Y, Schwartz E. Epidemiology of travel-related hospitalization. *J Travel Med* 2005;12:136–41.

8 Herwaldt BL, Stokes SL, Juranek DD. American cutaneous leishmaniasis in U.S. travelers. *Ann Intern Med* 1993;118:779–84.

9 Aronson NE, Wortmann GW, Johnson SC, et al. Safety and efficacy of intravenous sodium stibogluconate in the

treatment of leishmaniasis: recent U.S. military experience. *Clin Infect Dis* 1998;27:1457–64.

10 World Health Organization. Urbanization: an increasing risk factor for leishmaniasis. *Wkly Epidemiol Rec* 2002;77: 365–70.

11 Killick-Kendrick R. The biology and control of phlebotomine sand flies. *Clin Dermatol* 1999;17:279–89.

12 Sanchez JL, Diniega BM, Small JW, et al. Epidemiologic investigation of an outbreak of cutaneous leishmaniasis in a defined geographic focus of transmission. *Am J Trop Med Hyg* 1992;47:47–54.

13 Barral A, Barral-Netto M, Almeida R, et al. Lymphadenopathy associated with Leishmania braziliensis cutaneous infection. *Am J Trop Med Hyg* 1992;47:587–92.

14 Sousa AQ, Parise ME, Pompeu MM, et al. Bubonic leishmaniasis: a common manifestation of *Leishmania (Viannia) braziliensis* infection in Ceara, Brazil. *Am J Trop Med Hyg* 1995;53:380–5.

15 Jones TC, Johnson WD, Jr., Barretto AC, Lago E, Badaro R, Cerf B, et al. Epidemiology of American cutaneous leishmaniasis due to *Leishmania braziliensis braziliensis*. *J Infect Dis* 1987;156(1):73–83.

16 David C, Dimier-David L, Vargas F, Torrez M, Dedet JP. Fifteen years of cutaneous and mucocutaneous leishmaniasis in Bolivia: a retrospective study. *Trans R Soc Trop Med Hyg* 1993;87(1):7–9.

17 Alcais A, Abel L, David C, Torrez ME, Flandre P, Dedet JP. Risk factors for onset of cutaneous and mucocutaneous leishmaniasis in Bolivia. *Am J Trop Med Hyg* 1997;57(1): 79–84.

18 Petzl-Erler ML, Belich MP, Queiroz-Telles F. Association of mucosal leishmaniasis with HLA. *Hum Immunol* 1991;32(4):254–60.

19 Herwaldt BL. Leishmaniasis. *Lancet* 1999;354:1191–9.

20 Lucas CM, Franke ED, Cachay MI, et al. Geographic distribution and clinical description of leishmaniasis cases in Peru. *Am J Trop Med Hyg* 1998;59:312–17.

21 Schwartz E, Hatz C, Blum J. New World cutaneous leishmaniasis in travellers. *Lancet Infect Dis* 2006;6:342–9.

22 Scope A, Trau H, Bakon M, Yarom N, Nasereddin A, Schwartz E. Imported mucosal leishmaniasis in a traveler. *Clin Infect Dis* 2003;37:e83–e87.

23 Lawn SD, Whetham J, Chiodini PL, Kanagalingam J, Watson J, Behrens RH, et al. New world mucosal and cutaneous leishmaniasis: an emerging health problem among British travellers. *QJM* 2004;97(12):781–8.

24 Weigle KA, de Davalos M, Heredia P, Molineros R, Saravia NG, D'Alessandro A. Diagnosis of cutaneous and mucocutaneous leishmaniasis in Colombia: a comparison of seven methods. *Am J Trop Med Hyg* 1987;36(3):489–96.

25 OMS. *Lutte contre les leishmanioses.* Geneva: World Health Organization; 1990.

26 Desjeux P, Mollinedo S, le Pont F, Paredes A, Ugarte G. Cutaneous leishmaniasis in Bolivia. A study of 185 human cases from Alto Beni (La Paz Department). Isolation and isoenzyme characterization of 26 strains of Leishmania braziliensis braziliensis [corrected]. *Trans R Soc Trop Med Hyg* 1987;81(5):742–6.

27 Schonian G, Nasereddin A, Dinse N, Schweynoch C, Schallig HD, Presber W, et al. PCR diagnosis and characterization of Leishmania in local and imported clinical samples. *Diagn Microbiol Infect Dis* 2003;47(1):349–58.

28 Oliveira JG, Novais FO, de Oliveira CI, Cruz Junior AC, Campos LF, da Rocha AV, et al. Polymerase chain reaction (PCR) is highly sensitive for diagnosis of mucosal leishmaniasis. *Acta Trop* 2005;94(1):55–9.

29 Seaton RA, Morrison J, Man I, Watson J, Nathwani D. Out-patient parenteral antimicrobial therapy—a viable option for the management of cutaneous leishmaniasis. *QJM* 1999;92(11):659–67.

30 Hepburn NC, Siddique I, Howie AF, Beckett GJ, Hayes PC. Hepatotoxicity of sodium stibogluconate in leishmaniasis. *Lancet* 1993;342(8865):238–9.

31 Gasser RA, Jr., Magill AJ, Oster CN, Franke ED, Grogl M, Berman JD. Pancreatitis induced by pentavalent antimonial agents during treatment of leishmaniasis. *Clin Infect Dis* 1994;18(1):83–90.

32 Antezana G, Zeballos R, Mendoza C, Lyevre P, Valda L, Cardenas F, et al. Electrocardiographic alterations during treatment of mucocutaneous leishmaniasis with meglumine antimoniate and allopurinol. *Trans R Soc Trop Med Hyg* 1992;86(1):31–3.

33 Lawn SD, Armstrong M, Chilton D, Whitty CJ. Electrocardiographic and biochemical adverse effects of sodium stibogluconate during treatment of cutaneous and mucosal leishmaniasis among returned travellers. *Trans R Soc Trop Med Hyg* 2006;100(3):264–9.

34 Ritmeijer K, Dejenie A, Assefa Y, Hundie TB, Mesure J, Boots G, et al. A comparison of miltefosine and sodium stibogluconate for treatment of visceral leishmaniasis in an Ethiopian population with high prevalence of HIV infection. *Clin Infect Dis* 2006;43:357–64.

35 Ahasan HA, Chowdhury MA, Azhar MA, Rafiqueuddin AK, Azad KA. Deaths in visceral leishmaniasis (kala-azar) during treatment. *Med J Malaysia* 1996;51:29–32.

36 Herwaldt BL, Berman JD. Recommendations for treating leishmaniasis with sodium stibogluconate (Pentostam) and review of pertinent clinical studies. *Am J Trop Med Hyg* 1992;46(3):296–306.

37 Minodier P, Retornaz K, Horelt A, Garnier JM. Liposomal amphotericin B in the treatment of visceral leishmaniasis in immunocompetent patients. *Fundam Clin Pharmacol* 2003;17:183–8.

38 Musa AM, Khalil EA, Mahgoub FA, Hamad S, Elkadaru AM, El Hassan AM. Efficacy of liposomal amphotericin B (AmBisome) in the treatment of persistent post-kala-azar dermal leishmaniasis (PKDL). *Ann Trop Med Parasitol* 2005;99: 563–9.

39 Amato VS, Tuon FF, Siqueira AM, Nicodemo AC, Neto VA. Treatment of mucosal leishmaniasis in Latin America: systematic review. *Am J Trop Med Hyg* 2007 Aug;77(2):266–74.

40 Solomon M, Baum S, Barzilai A, Scope A, Trau H, Schwartz E. Liposomal amphotericin B in comparison to sodium stibogluconate for cutaneous infection due to *Leishmania braziliensis*. *J Am Acad Dermatol*. 2007;56:612–6.

41 Davidson RN, DI Martino L, Gradoni L, Giacchino R, Gaeta GB, Pempinello R, et al. Short-course treatment of visceral leishmaniasis with liposomal amphotericin B (AmBisome). *Clin Infect Dis* 1996;22:938–43.

42 Yardley V, Croft S. Activity of liposomal amphotericin B against experimental cutaneous leishmaniasis. *Antimicrob Agents Chemother* 1997;41:752–6.

43 Wortmann GW, Fraser SL, Aronson NE, Davis C, Miller RS, Jackson JD, et al. Failure of amphotericin B lipid complex in the treatment of cutaneous leishmaniasis. *Clin Infect Dis* 1998;26:1006–7.

44 Soto J, Buffet P, Grogl M, Berman J. Successful treatment of Colombian cutaneous leishmaniasis with four injections of pentamidine. *Am J Trop Med Hyg* 1994;50(1):107–11.

45 Nacher M, Carme B, Sainte MD, Couppie P, Clyti E, Guibert P, et al. Influence of clinical presentation on the efficacy of a short course of pentamidine in the treatment of cutaneous leishmaniasis in French Guiana. *Ann Trop Med Parasitol* 2001;95(4):331–6.

46 Soto J, Arana A, Toledo J, Rizzo N, Vega JC, Diaz A, et al. Miltefosine for New World cutaneous leishmaniasis. *Clin Infect Dis* 2004;38:1266–72.

47 Weina P, Neafie R, Wortmann G, Polhemus M, Aronson N. Old world leishmaniasis: an emerging infection among deployed US military and civilian workers. *Clin Infect Dis* 2004;39:1674–80.

48 Klaus S, Frankenburg S. Cutaneous leishmaniasis in the Middle East. *Clin Dermatol* 1999;17:137–41.

49 Khatami A, Firooz A, Gorouhi F, Dowlati Y. Treatment of acute Old World cutaneous leishmaniasis: a systematic review of the randomized controlled trials. *J Am Acad Dermatol* 2007;57:335.e1–335.

50 el-On J, Halevy S, Grunwald MH, Weinrauch L. Topical treatment of Old World cutaneous leishmaniasis caused by *Leishmania major*: a double-blind control study. *J Am Acad Dermatol* 1992;27:227–31.

51 Ben Salah A, Zakraoui H, Zaatour A, et al. A randomized, placebo controlled trial in Tunisia treating cutaneous leishmaniasis with paromomycin ointment. *Am J Trop Med Hyg* 1995;53:162–6.

52 Faghihi G, Tavakoli-kia R. Treatment of cutaneous leishmaniasis with either topical paromomycin or intralesional meglumine antimoniate. *Clin Exp Dermatol* 2003;28:13–16.

53 Lopez-Jaramillo P, Ruano C, Rivera J, et al. Treatment of cutaneous leishmaniasis with nitric-oxide donor. *Lancet* 1998;351:1176–7.

54 Solomon M, Baum S, Barzilai A, Pavlotzki F, Trau H, Schwartz E. Treatment of cutaneous leishmaniasis with intralesional Pentostam in Israel. In press (publication very soon).

55 Wortmann, G, Miller, RS, Oster, C, Jackson, J, Aronson, N. A randomized, double-blind study of the efficacy of a 10- or 20-day course of sodium stibogluconate for treatment of cutaneous leishmaniasis in United States military personnel. *Clin Infect Dis* 2002;35:261–7.

56 Svobodova M, Votypka J, Peckova J, Dvorak V, Nasereddin A, Baneth G, et al. Distinct transmission cycles of *Leishmania tropica* in 2 adjacent foci, Northern Israel. *Emerg Infect Dis* 2006;12:1860–68.

57 Shani-Adir A, Kamil S, Rozenman D, Schwartz E, Ramon M, Zalman L, et al. *Leishmania tropica* in northern Israel: a clinical overview of an emerging focus. *J Am Acad Dermatol* 2005;53:810–15.

58 Magill AJ, Grogl M, Gasser RA Jr, et al. Visceral infection caused by *Leishmania tropica* in veterans of Operation Desert Storm. *N Engl J Med* 1993 13;328:1383–7.

59 Sundar S, Jha TK, Thakur CP, Sinha PK, Bhattacharya SK. Injectable paromomycin for visceral leishmaniasis in India. *N Engl J Med* 2007;21;356(25):2571–81.

60 Sundar S, Jha TK, Thakur CP, Engel J, Sindermann H, Fischer C, et al. Oral miltefosine for Indian visceral leishmaniasis. *N Engl J Med* 2002;28;347(22):1739–46.

61 Soto J, Medina F, Dember N, Berman J. Efficacy of permethrin-impregnated uniforms in the prevention of malaria and leishmaniasis in Colombian soldiers. *Clin Infect Dis* 1995;21(3):599–602.

62 Bauer IL. Knowledge and behavior of tourists to Manu National Park, Peru, in relation to leishmaniasis. *J Travel Med* 2002;9(4):173–9.

# 33 Ectoparasites: Myiasis, Tungiasis, Scabies

## Eli Schwartz[1] and Eric Caumes[2]

[1]Chaim Sheba Medical Center, Tel Hashomer, Israel and Sackler School of Medicine, Tel Aviv University, Tel Aviv, Israel
[2]Hôpital Pitié-Salpêtrière, University Pierre et Marie Curie, Paris, France

## Introduction

Ectoparasites are arthropods living on the outside of the host from which they obtain their nutrients. Some of them have direct intrinsic cutaneous effects on their human hosts. They cover a large spectrum of genera and species. Many can cause dermatitis, but very few are commonly found in travelers. The three most frequent ectoparasitic skin infections in the post-travel setting are cutaneous myiasis, tungiasis, and scabies [1, 2]. Other arthropods considered as ectoparasites (according to the largest definition), such as louse, or ticks and mites (with the exception of those causing scabies), will not be covered by this review.

## Myiasis

Myiasis is an infestation of human tissue by larvae of some types of fly (Table 33.1). There are many forms of myiasis, including cutaneous (localized furuncular, creeping dermal, and wound myiasis) and body cavity myiasis [3].

In returning travelers, localized furuncular myiasis is the common form. It is 1 of the 10 leading causes of skin diseases in travelers, accounting for 2.7% of all dermatological conditions, according to the GeoSentinel network [2].

It exists in the tropics in several forms. In Africa, furuncular myiasis is mostly due to the tumbu fly (*Cordylobia anthropophaga*), whereas in Central and South America the human botfly (*Dermatobia hominis*; Diptera: Cuterebridae) is the major cause [3].

According to the results of a series of imported cases in Western countries, very few types of myiasis are observed in travelers [1, 4, 5]. The frequencies of the types of myiasis seen in returning travelers are probably a reflection of their corresponding destinations. For example, in a series of 25 imported cases seen in France, 20 were due to *C. anthropophaga*, 4 to *D. hominis*, and 1 to *Cochliomyia hominivorax* [1]. In a series of 19 imported cases in England, 9 were due to *C. anthropophaga*, 4 to *D. hominis*, 1 to *Cochl. hominivorax*, 2 to *Oestrus ovis*, and 3 to other species [5]. In a series of 13 imported cases seen in Germany, 6 were due to *C. anthropophaga*, 6 to *D. hominis*, and 1 to *Hypoderma lineatum* [4]. Of 29 myiasis cases in Israeli travelers (where Latin America is a much more frequent destination than Africa), 95% were due to *D. hominis*, whereas *C.* spp. was seen only in one case [unpublished data].

## American furuncular myiasis due to *Dermatobia hominis*

In Latin America the causative agent of furuncular myiasis is *Dermatobia hominis*. Despite its name, its main hosts are livestock mammals, although humans are accidentally infested [6]. The fly is endemic from central Mexico through Central and South America (geographical distribution: 18°S–25°N). In the Caribbean islands, it has been reported only on Trinidad. Its habitats are forest and jungle areas around rivers and streams and along coastal areas. The fly deposits its packet of eggs on the abdomen of a mosquito or other blood-feeding insect. Then, when the biting insect lands on a warm-blooded animal, the eggs hatch and the larvae enter the skin. Humans can be accidental hosts. The larva then spends 4–14 weeks in the animal skin, develops into a third-stage larva measuring 2 cm or more in length, and falls to the ground to pupate.

*Tropical Diseases in Travelers*, 1st edition. Edited by E. Schwartz.
© 2009 by Blackwell Publishing, ISBN: 978-1-4051-8441-0.

**Table 33.1** The common forms of myiasis in travelers.

| Infesting fly | Other names | Geographic distribution | Mode of transmission | Type of lesion |
| --- | --- | --- | --- | --- |
| *Dermatobium hominis* | Botfly | Latin America | Mosquitoes | Furuncular myiasis |
| *Cordylobia anthropophaga* | Tumbu fly | Sub-Saharan Africa | Contact with infested cloth | Furuncular myiasis |
| *Cordylobia rodhaini* | Lund's fly | Sub-Saharan Africa | Contact with infested soil | Furuncular myiasis |
| *Cochliomyia hominivorax* | Screwworm fly | New World | Fly directly to the wound | Wound myiasis |
| *Oestrus ovis* | Sheep nasal botfly | Cosmopolitan | Fly directly to conjunctiva | Conjunctival myiasis |

After 14–30 days, the adult fly emerges and the life cycle resumes. Each larva penetrates individually, forming the typical warble or boil in almost any exposed area of the host's surface.

The highest proportion of morbidity from this condition in travelers to Latin America was recorded in Belize, where 43% of all skin diseases are due to myiasis, in Bolivia 20%, and in Costa Rica 10%. Based on Israeli travelers' data, the highest risk area for myiasis in Bolivia was in the Amazon basin (Madidi National Park), where the estimated risk of acquiring the disease was 1:190 travelers [7].

### Clinical aspects

The common scenario is a patient who can recall several mosquito bites, most of which have already healed. One or more, however, have not healed and have grown larger, accompanied by a crawling sensation (the patient describes a feeling of movement within the lesion). The skin lesion starts as a red papule that gradually enlarges and develops into a furuncle-like lesion that has a serotic, sometimes bloody discharge. In the center of the lesion is an opening through which the larva breathes and discharges its serosanguinous feces. This hole and the crawling sensation are the important clues for diagnosis. The lesion can be painful, and sometimes a white tip proturbing out through the central hole may be seen. While the larva is alive, secondary infection does not occur due to the bactericidal nature of its secretions.

The mean time from exposure to diagnosis was 1.5 months (3–7 weeks) in 12 Israeli travelers after return from the Amazon River basin of Bolivia [7]. Similarly, the time from return to diagnosis varied from 15 to 45 days in four French travelers [1].

The number of larvae per person usually ranges from one to four, and any uncovered part of the body that has been exposed to mosquito bites, including the scalp, can be affected [1, 7].

### Diagnosis

A nonhealing nodular, furuncle-like lesion in someone who returns from an endemic area is the first clue to this condition. Careful examination of the lesion may reveal a central hole within the lesion (Figure 33.1), which is unique to this condition. After an ointment covering the

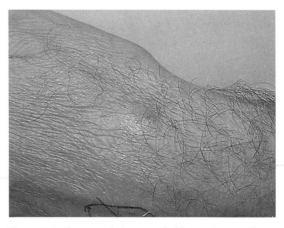

**Figure 33.1** Cutaneous lesion typical of furuncular myiasis.

lesion is applied, a white tip may bulge out, which is the tip of the larva after it has suffocated.

Blood tests are normal (unless there is a secondary bacterial infection), without eosinophilia.

For physicians who are familiar with this condition, there is no need for radiological confirmation. However, in the literature, there are reports of using ultrasound imaging for correct diagnosis [8].

The definitive diagnosis is made after the extraction and identification of the maggot (Figure 33.2).

## Treatment

Treatment can be conservative or surgical. Applying a sealing ointment (e.g., paraffin ointment) to occlude the breathing opening results in suffocation of the larva; then with manual pressure, force the larva to migrate out from the skin (Figure 33.3). Brewer et al. applied bacon to the larval apertures and caused the larva to migrate sufficiently far out of the skin to be removed with tweezers. Others injected lidocaine underneath the larva, thus producing sufficient pressure to push the larva out of the skin [9].

Our experience is that when the patient presents at an early stage, while the larva is still small and superficial, it can be removed nonsurgically without difficulty. However, as the larva matures, it grows numerous concentric rows of backward-projecting spines that lock it in place, which causes difficulty in dislodging it from the skin. In these cases, prolonged application (24 hours) of an occlusive sealing ointment is necessary to avoid surgical removal, which may finally be needed [10].

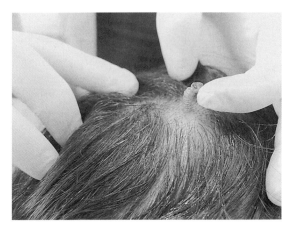

**Figure 33.3** Extraction of *D. hominis* from the scalp.

Topical ivermectin was successfully used to kill the larvae and facilitated their extraction in the particular case of an HIV-infected patient presenting with voluminous inflammatory nodules due to *D. hominis* [11].

Surgically, from our experience and supported by that of others, the best method of evacuating the larva is making a small incision through the opening, inserting a small hemostat, and pulling the larva out; the wound usually heals with no complications [10].

Disinfection of myiasis wounds, with antibiotic treatment only in cases of bacterial secondary infection, and updating tetanus vaccination should complete the treatment.

In all methods of treatment, there is typically full healing with no scarring.

## African furuncular myiasis due to *Cordylobia spp.*

*C. anthropophaga* (the tumbu fly) is the most common furuncular myiasis in Africa. The genus *Cordylobia* also contains two less common species, *C. ruandae* and *C. rodhaini* (Table 33.1).

The tumbu fly exists throughout tropical Africa and is also known as the *putsi* fly or mango fly. The gravid fly oviposits on wet clothing and also on urine-soaked soil. Rodents are the natural hosts. Humans are usually infected by wearing clothes that were hanging outdoors. The eggs usually hatch in 2–4 days and the larvae, when in contact with human skin, penetrate the skin painlessly, burrowing into the subdermal layer, causing furuncular myiasis within a few days.

The incubation period is shorter than in the case of American furuncular myiasis. The time from return to

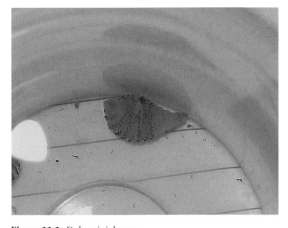

**Figure 33.2** *D. hominis* larvae.

diagnosis varied from 7 to 10 days in 20 French travelers infected with *C. anthropophaga* [1]. Cutaneous lesions are more commonly multiple than in American furuncular myiasis, the largest number of lesions ever reported being 94 in a child from Ghana [11]. Another distinctive feature is that lesions are usually located on areas of the body covered by clothing (e.g., the trunk) (11).

Infection with *C. rodhaini* (Lund's fly) appears to be very uncommon and it is transmitted differently. *C. rodhaini* is confined to tropical Africa, especially areas of rain forests in Sub-Saharan Africa (Senegal through Central Africa, to Angola and Zimbabwe) [12]. The literature reveals only seven cases of *C. rodhaini* myiasis in travelers, all acquired in the eastern and western parts of Central Africa [13]. The mode of transmission is by direct contact of the eggs with the host. Patients might be infected while sleeping on the ground in huts in rainforests. In about 3 days, the larva is activated by the warm body of the host, hatches, and invades the skin. As the larva matures, it induces a furuncular swelling. In 12–15 days, the larva reaches a length of about 23 mm, exits the skin, and falls to the ground to pupate. The adult fly emerges in 23–26 days and the life cycle resumes.

## Clinical aspects

The clinical picture of *C. anthropophaga* and *C. rodhaini* myiasis is of furuncular myiasis, that is, a 1–2-cm furuncle-like lesion with a crawling sensation within the lesion. The skin lesion starts as a red papule that gradually enlarges and develops into a furuncle. In the center of the lesion is an opening through which the larva breathes and discharges its serosanguinous feces. The lesion is associated with increasing pain until the larva exits the skin.

The disease is usually uncomplicated and lesions heal without scarring. In endemic regions, natives usually dig into the wound with sharp instruments to extract the larva. Any attempt to probe the wound with nonsterile equipment can result in bacterial infection, cellulitis, abscess formation, or even tetanus.

Systemic symptoms were described in one case of massive infestation with *C. rodhaini*. This person was infested with 150 larvae and had systemic signs of fever and lymphadenopathy [14].

The time that the larva spends in the human skin is only 12–15 days in *Cordylobia* infestation, compared to 6–14 weeks in the case of *D. hominis*. Because of the shorter cycle time in *Cordylobia* infestation, the larvae may exit the skin of the patient before the diagnosis is made.

## Treatment

Because of the round shape of the African larvae and because penetration is not as deep as in American myiasis, conservative treatment is easy. Most of the time, manual pressure to the lateral aspects of the lesion easily allows the extraction of the maggot [11]. Otherwise, applying a sealing ointment and occluding the breathing opening causes suffocation of the larva and encourages it to migrate from the skin [3]. It is important to evacuate the whole larva; otherwise, it may cause a secondary infection, as in a foreign body reaction. Surgical removal of the larva is usually not needed.

Disinfection of myiasis wounds, with antibiotics treatment if bacterial secondary infection occurs, and updating tetanus vaccination should complete the treatment.

## Prevention

It is important to educate travelers and particularly expatriates about the need to iron clothes that are hung outside. Alternatively, drying them inside a screened area or using a laundry dryer will prevent infestation. Travelers in Africa should also be aware of infestation not only by direct contact with clothes left outside, but also by direct contact with infested sand. The fly requires a special climate to reproduce; thus, the disease is confined to Sub-Saharan Africa. It is unlikely that travelers will spread the disease to their homelands.

## Other forms of myiasis of interest for travelers

Very few other clinical forms of myiasis have been described in travelers (Table 33.1). Wound myiasis due to *Cochl. hominivorax*, conjunctival myiasis due to *Oestrus ovis*, and dermal migrating myiasis due to *H. lineatum* have occasionally been reported in travelers [1, 4, 5]. In Brazil and Colombia, oral use of ivermectin has been reported as a useful surgery-associated treatment in severe orbital myiasis due to *Cochl. hominivorax* [11].

## Tungiasis

The disease is caused by a chigoe flea, which is a hematophagous insect, meaning that it procures blood by burrowing into the host tissue. The causative agent is called *Tunga penetrans*. Other synonyms are sand flea, jigger, nigua, or chigo.

Tungiasis is endemic in Central and South America, the Caribbean, the whole Sub-Saharan region of Africa, the Seychelles Islands, Pakistan, and the west coast of India [11].

The natural habitat of *T. penetrans* is the sandy, warm soil of deserts and beaches.

Reviews summarizing the reported cases in travelers showed that 39% were acquired in South America (primarily Brazil), 39% in Sub-Saharan Africa (especially Kenya and Tanzania), and 6% in Central America (mainly Mexico) and the Caribbean [15].

A study done among French travelers demonstrated that tungiasis accounted for 6% of skin disorders in travelers returning from the tropics [1]. A recent survey that was done at an airport in Brazil found that 3.2% of travelers returning from northeast Brazil had been infested with *Tunga* [16].

*T. penetrans* is the smallest known flea, reaching a length of only 1 mm. The adult female fleas feed intermittently, only on warm-blooded hosts. The fertilized females require a host to complete their life cycle, and they penetrate into the epidermis of a suitable one. The victims can be humans or other mammals. Once the parasite lies within the skin, it thrusts its head into the superficial layers of the dermis, looking for nourishment by puncturing the blood vessels. Its tail is oriented toward the surface, maintaining communication with the outside through a hole in the stratum corneum. This opening provides air for breathing and a passage for both excretions and eggs. The eggs are white and ovoid and number between 100 and 150. Once deposited on the ground, if the environmental conditions are favorable, they enter into the developmental process. They hatch in 3–4 days, liberating larvae that develop into pupae within 10–15 days. After 1–2 weeks, these pupae become adults, thus completing the cycle, which takes about 1 month.

## Clinical presentation

The incubation period is short. In a series of 17 imported cases, the median lag time between return and presentation was 12 days (range, 5–40 days) and all lesions were located on a toe, usually the tip [1]. In another study of 19 imported cases, all the lesions were also located on the feet, on a toe [17].

Infestation usually occurs under the toenails, between the toes, or on the plantar surface of the foot. Review of lesions reported in travelers documented only about 10% in ectopic sites such as fingers, backs, or breasts [15]. This is in contrast to inhabitants of endemic areas, where ectopic localizations are more common. The penetration of the flea is asymptomatic. The inflammatory process, which occurs within a few days, causes the lesion to be pruritic.

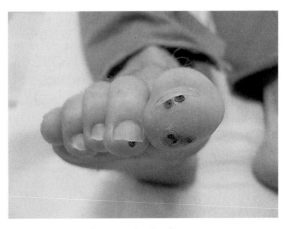

**Figure 33.4** Tunga lesion on the tip of a toe.

The flea can increase in size to a pea-sized volume while sucking the host's blood, causing increasing subungual pain. The lesion appears as a white papule, either single or multiple, with a central black depression that is the posterior portion of the flea (Figure 33.4).

Superinfections are not uncommon and are mainly caused by *Staphylococcus aureus*. In endemic countries, secondary tetanus has been reported [18].

In travelers, the symptoms of tungiasis are similar to those of people from endemic areas. However, the number of lesions is usually less and complications are less frequent, presumably because travelers have fewer lesions as a result of their higher living standards.

## Diagnosis

The diagnosis can be made clinically by taking into consideration the travel history of the patient and the description of the evolving lesion. The typical traveler has the lesion after a stay on the seashore and walking barefoot. Many travelers will notice eggs being expelled after they manipulate the lesion. The observation of eggs being expelled or eggs attached to the skin around the rear cone and the release of brownish threads of feces are pathognomonic signs. Lately, dermoscopy has been shown to be helpful in confirming the clinical diagnosis of tungiasis by showing the presence of eggs within the lesion [19] (Figure 33.5). Feces threads have a helical structure and often spread into the dermal papillae. Expulsion of eggs can be provoked by massaging the hypertrophic zone slightly.

Differential diagnoses include myiasis, warts, dermoid cysts, bites or stings of other injurious arthropods, and foreign-body reactions.

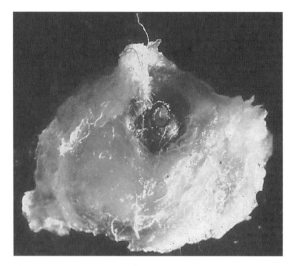

**Figure 33.5** Focus on tunga lesion.

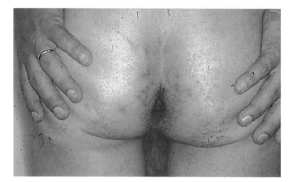

**Figure 33.6** Cutaneous lesions of the buttocks secondary to itching in a patient with scabies.

## Treatment and Prevention

Surgical extraction of the flea under sterile conditions is the appropriate treatment. The extraction should include the entire flea; otherwise, severe inflammation ensues. After extraction, the wound should be treated with antiseptics. Administration of tetanus prophylaxis and oral antibiotic therapy in case of secondary bacterial infection may be necessary.

Because the most common mode of acquiring the disease is by walking barefoot on the sand, walking with shoes is recommended. Immediate extraction of the embedded fleas protects against complications.

## Scabies

Scabies, infestation by the mite *Sarcoptes scabei*, is the most common cause of diffuse pruritic skin disease diagnosed in travelers returning from the tropics [20]. Scabies is acquired by skin-to-skin contact.

## Clinical aspects

Patients usually complain of generalized itching, worsening at night, usually sparing the face and head. It occurs within 1 month after contact in the case of primary exposure and within a few days in persons with a history of previous scabies exposure [21]. The most specific skin findings include 5–10-mm burrows, vesiculopustules, and papulonodular genital lesions. However, these specific findings are seldom found in persons with good personal hygiene. Most of the time, skin changes are limited to those induced by pruritus, including excoriation (Figure 33.6), lichenification, and impetiginization. The classic distribution of lesions is in the interdigital web spaces and on the flexor surfaces of the wrists, the elbows, the axillae, the buttocks (Figure 33.6), the genitalia in men, and the breasts in women.

## Diagnosis

A family's or a companion's travel history of pruritus is a classical clue to the diagnosis ("itching in the marital bed is scabies"). Otherwise, the diagnosis must be considered in every patient complaining of chronic and generalized pruritus. Diagnosis may be confirmed by the microscopic identification of the female mite, the eggs, or fecal pellets on skin scrapings of a cutaneous lesion. Nonetheless, the sensitivity of the parasitological examination is known to be less than 50% even in experienced hands [22]. Therefore, the diagnosis of scabies in negative patients cannot be eliminated. Dermoscopy may also be helpful [21].

## Treatment

Treatment may be topical and/or oral. Topical treatment includes permethrin cream 5%, lindane 1% (gamma-benzene hexachloride), and benzyl benzoate (available in Europe and Africa). Benzyl benzoate is applied once during a 24-hour period. Some authors recommend another application 24 hours later. However, the moderate difference in the efficacies of the two different modalities of application suggests that one application can be recommended as a standard first-line treatment of common scabies.

Oral ivermectin is a simple and well-tolerated alternative. A single 12 mg oral dose is recommended, but a second dose 10–15 days later should be added. Although the two regimens have not been compared yet, it must be kept in mind that ivermectin is active against the adults, not the eggs, and that it takes 15–21 days for the eggs to mature in adults. A recent meta-analysis concluded that there has been no argument until now establishing the superiority of oral ivermectin over topical treatments for common scabies [23]. In addition, the cost of scabies treatment must be taken into consideration, given that there is often a need to treat families. Economic considerations also favor the generic form of benzyl benzoate (approximately 0.1 euro per person).

The best treatment for scabies in countries where neither permethrin nor lindane is available is a combination of one application of benzyl benzoate and one single oral dose of ivermectin. Otherwise, the application of benzyl benzoate or the administration of oral ivermectin must be repeated, 24 hours and 10 days later, respectively.

Bedding and clothing must be laundered or removed from contact for at least 3 days. Personal and household contacts must also be treated.

## References

1 Caumes E, Carriere J, Guermonprez G, Bricaire F, Danis M, Gentilini M. Dermatoses associated with travel to tropical countries: a prospective study of the diagnosis and management of 269 patients presenting to a tropical disease unit. *Clin Infect Dis* 1995;20:542–8.

2 Lederman E, Weld L, Elyazar I, et al. Dermatologic conditions of the ill returned traveler: an analysis from the GeoSentinel surveillance network. *Int J Infect Dis* 2008;12:593–602.

3 White GB. Flies causing myiasis. In Cook GC, editor. *Manson's Tropical Diseases*. London: WB Saunders; 1996. p. 1661–3.

4 Jelinek T, Nothfurft HD, Rieder N, Loscher T. Cutaneous myiasis: review of 13 cases in travelers returning from tropical countries. *Int J Dermatol* 1995;34:624–6.

5 McGarry JW, McCall PJ, Welby S. Arthropod dermatoses acquired in the UK and overseas. *Lancet* 2001;357:2105–6.

6 Hall M, Wall R. Myiasis of humans and domestic animals. *Adv Parasitol* 1995;35:257–334.

7 Schwartz E, Gur H. *D. hominis* myiasis among Israeli travelers to South America: an emerging disease in the Amazon basin of Bolivia. *J Trav Med* 2002;9:97–9.

8 Quintanilla-Cedillo MR, León-Ureña H, Contreras-Ruiz J, Arenas R. The value of Doppler ultrasound in diagnosis in 25 cases of furunculoid myiasis. *Int J Dermatol* 2005;44:34–7.

9 Nunzi E, Rongioletti F, Rebora A. Removal of *Dermatobia hominis* larvae. *Arch Dermatol* 1986;122:140.

10 Tamir J, Haik J, Orenstein A, Schwartz E. *Dermatobia hominis* myia among travelers returning from South America. *J Am Acad Dermatol* 2003;48:630–2.

11 Hochedez P, Caumes E. Common skin infections in travelers. *J Travel Med* 2008;15:223–33.

12 Geary MJ, Hudson BJ, Russell RC, Hardy A. Exotic myiasis with Lund's fly (*Cordylobia rodhaini*). *Med J Aust* 1999;171:654–5.

13 Tamir J, Haik J, Schwartz E. Myiasis with Lund's fly (*Cordylobia rodhaini*) in travelers. *J Travel Med* 2003;10:293–5.

14 Pampiglione S, Schiavon S, Candiani G, Fioravanti ML. Clinical and parasitological observations on a case of disseminated furuncular myiasis caused by *Cordylobia rodhaini* in a man in Ethiopia. *Parassitologia* 1991;33:159–67.

15 Franck S, Feldmeier H, Heukelbach J. Tungiasis: more than an exotic nuisance. *Travel Med Infect Dis* 2003;1:159–66.

16 Heukelbach J, Gomide M, Araújo F Jr, Pinto NS, Santana RD, Brito JR, et al. Cutaneous larva migrans and tungiasis in international travelers exiting Brazil: an airport survey. *J Travel Med* 2007;14:374–80.

17 Veraldi S, Valsecchi M. Imported tungiasis: a report of 19 cases and review of the literature. *Int J Dermatol* 2007;46:1061–6.

18 Greco JB, Sacramento E, Tavares-Neto J. Chronic ulcers and myiasis as ports of entry for *Clostridium tetani*. *Braz J Infect Dis* 2001;5:319–23.

19 Cabrera R, Daza F. Tungiasis: eggs seen with dermoscopy. *Br J Dermatol* 2008;158:635–6.

20 Ansart S, Perez L, Jaureguiberry S, Danis M, Bricaire F, Caumes E. Spectrum of dermatoses in 165 travelers returning from the tropics with skin diseases. *Am J Trop Med Hyg* 2007;76:184–6.

21 Chosidow O. Clinical practices. Scabies. *N Engl J Med* 2006;354:1718–27.

22 Grossin M. Searching for sarcoptes. *Ann Dermatol Venereol* 2001;112:69–70.

23 Walker GJA, Johnston PW. Interventions for treating scabies. *Cochrane Database Syst Rev* 2000;3 CD000320.

# 34 Helminthic Skin Diseases in Travelers

Eric Caumes

Hôpital Pitié-Salpêtrière, University Pierre et Marie Curie, Paris, France

## Introduction

Helminths are microscopic worms with complex life cycles. Helminths that infect human beings and are able to produce cutaneous signs belong to three groups: nematodes, which are roundworms, and trematodes and cestodes, which are both flatworms.

The skin manifestations vary according to the helminth species and the phase of the helminth's cycle, with different clinical presentation between the penetration, invasive, and chronic phases [1, 2]. Helminths can survive for years.

During the *penetration phase* of the cycle, cutaneous signs are observed only for helminths that infect mammals by skin penetration. Signs are directly related to the presence of the larvae. In such cases, the signs last a short time for human helminths or a longer time for animal helminths, such as animal hookworms.

During the *acute (invasive) phase* of the helminthic cycle, the primary cutaneous finding is urticaria, related to the immunological response to helminth, involving Th2 cell activation with hypereosinophilia, hyper IgE, and mastocytosis. Again, the duration of the episode is short when the helminths are well adapted to humans, whereas it may last for weeks or even months when they are not, as for toxocariasis.

During the *chronic phase*, cutaneous manifestations vary according to the type of helminth and are related to the presence of the adult worm or the eggs or larvae in the subcutaneous tissue or skin. The most common clinical presentations are creeping dermatitis, panniculitis, papules, or nodules, and are more directly associated with the presence of the helminths or their eggs or larvae.

The most common helminthic infections worldwide are infections by intestinal nematodes (ascariasis, enterobiasis, hookworms, strongyloidiasis), filariasis, cysticercosis, and schistosomiasis. Apart from hookworm-related cutaneous larva migrans (HrCLM), helminthic diseases are uncommon causes of skin diseases in returning travelers [3, 4]. However, skin lesions may provide important diagnostic clues for many helminthic infections (Tables 34.1 and 34.2) [2].

Helminth infection may be accompanied by eosinophilia and hyper IgE. However, levels of eosinophils in the blood vary according to the species and to the stage of infection. In those helminths that elicit eosinophilia, the level slowly increases from baseline during the penetration phase to reach its peak during the invasive phase of the cycle. Thereafter, it often decreases slowly and may fluctuate more or less above the normal value during the chronic phase. IgE levels, which are often parallel to the presence of eosinophilia, point toward the diagnosis of a helminth infection (and to a lesser degree, allergy) in travelers with no other clues for diagnosis.

## Human nematodes

### Intestinal nematodes

Infections by intestinal human nematodes (namely ascariasis, enterobiasis, hookworm disease, and strongyloidiasis; see Chapter 31) [1, 2] share a common mode of acquisition (orally or transcutaneously), a tropical and subtropical distribution (the exception is enterobiasis, distributed worldwide), a common clinical presentation (the majority of infections being asymptomatic or mild), a lack of serological tests (e.g., in ascaris and hookworm) or lack of reliability of serologic tests (cross-reactions between various nematodes), and a common means of definitive

*Tropical Diseases in Travelers*, 1st edition. Edited by E. Schwartz.
© 2009 by Blackwell Publishing, ISBN: 978-1-4051-8441-0.

**Table 34.1** Cutaneous manifestations of infections by nematodes.

| Family | Agent | Disease | Skin manifestations |
|---|---|---|---|
| Intestinal nematodes | *Ascaris lumbricoides* | Ascariasis | Urticaria (invasive phase) |
| | *Enterobius vermicularis* | Enterobiasis | Anal pruritus |
| | *Ancylostoma duodenale, Necator americanus* | Hookworm disease | Ground itch (penetration phase), urticaria (invasive phase) |
| | *Strongyloides stercoralis* | Strongyloidiasis | Urticaria (invasive phase), larva currens (chronic phase), thumbprint sign of periumbilical purpura |
| Filariasis | *Wuchereria bancrofti, Brugia malayi,* B. timori | Lymphatic filariasis | Acute retrograde lymphangitis, adenitis, hydrocele, lymphedema, elephantiasis, lymphatic varicosities |
| | *Loa loa* | Loiasis | Pruritus, limb swelling (Calabar edema), creeping dermatitis, creeping ophthalmitis, Mazzoti averse reaction |
| | *Onchocerca volvulus* | Onchocerciasis | Pruritus, prurigo, pigmentation disorders (hypopigmentation, hyperpigmentation, leopard skin), lichenification, onchocercoma, limb swelling, Mazzoti averse reaction |
| | *Mansonella perstans* | Mansonellosis | Itching rash |
| | *Streptocerca* spp. | Streptocerciasis | Itching rash |
| Other human nematodoses | *Dracunculus medinensis* | Dracunculiasis | Skin emergence, infectious complications |
| Animal nematodes in men | *Toxocara canis, T. cati* | Toxocariasis | Urticaria, prurigo |
| | *Gnathostoma* spp. | Gnathostomiasis | Urticaria (invasive phase), eosinophilic panniculitis, creeping dermatitis, limb swelling |
| | *Anisakis simplex* | Anisakiasis | Urticaria (penetration phase) |
| | *Trichinella spiralis* | Trichinosis | Conjunctivitis, edema, urticaria, maculopapular rash, subungual hemorrhages |
| | *Ancylostoma* sp. | Hookworm-related cutaneous larva migrans | Creeping dermatitis, hookworm folliculitis |
| | *Dirofilaria repens, D. tenuis, D. ursi, D. immitis* | Dirofilariasis | Nodules, creeping eruption |

diagnosis (eggs or larvae found in anal or stool tests) and treatment (albendazole, mebendazole, ivermectin). They also have some skin manifestations in common, but differ as to where in the cycle they occur (Table 34.1).

Of these four infections, human hookworm is the only disease associated with cutaneous signs during the cutaneous penetration of the larvae. It presents as a localized erythema, edema, papule, or papulovesicular

**Table 34.2** Cutaneous manifestations of infections by trematodes and cestodes.

| Family | Agent | Disease | Cutaneous signs |
|---|---|---|---|
| Schistosomes | Nonhuman schistosomes | Cercarial dermatitis | Pruritic skin rash |
| | *Schistosoma haematobium, S. mansoni, S. intercalatum, S. japonicum, S. mekongi* | Schistosomiasis | Cercarial dermatitis (penetration phase), urticaria (invasive phase), late cutaneous schistosomiasis, perineal tumor (chronic phase) |
| Flukes | *Fasciola hepatica, F. gigantica* | Liver flukes (fascioliasis) | Urticaria (invasive phase) |
| | *Paragonimus* spp. | Lung flukes (paragonimiasis) | Nodules (ectopic localizations) |
| Echinococcosis | *Echinococcus granulosis* | Unilocular echinococcis (hydatid disease) | Urticaria, anaphylaxis (cyst opening) Nodules (ectopic localizations) |
| Taeniasis | *Taenia solium* | Cysticercosis | Nodules |
| Other cestodes | *Multiceps* spp. | Coenurosis | Nodules |
| | *Spirometra* spp. | Sparganosis | Nodules |

lesion known as "ground itch." It usually begins 1–2 days after contamination and may last up to 1 month without treatment. It is most commonly located on the feet or buttocks, which are the areas of skin penetrated by the larvae (Figure 34.1). In travelers, there is usually a history of recreational activities such as walking barefoot or lying on ground contaminated by human feces.

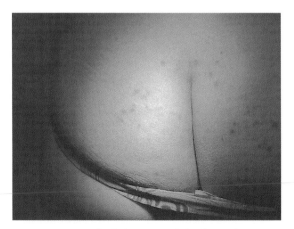

**Figure 34.1** Ground itch. (Courtesy of Eli Schwartz.)

The invasive phase of these diseases, which begins 10–14 days after the contamination, may be manifested by urticaria. It is usually associated with the pulmonary manifestations of Loeffler's syndrome (cough, wheezing, dyspnea), fever, and later vague gastrointestinal symptoms during ascariasis. Urticaria is less likely to occur during the invasive phases of hookworm disease, strongyloidiasis, and enterobiasis. Transient bilateral infiltrates on chest X ray films may be seen. There is high blood eosinophilia and elevated IgE. Eggs or larvae are not found in the stool until at least 4 weeks after acquisition. Thus, during the acute phase, a definitive diagnosis cannot be made.

During the chronic phase, cutaneous signs are only present in enterobiasis and strongyloidiasis. Enterobiasis is associated with nocturnal anal and perianal pruritus that begins 4–6 weeks after ingestion and may last for months. The skin may become impetiginized. In women, vulvovaginitis may occur.

In addition to nonspecific gastrointestinal complaints, chronic strongyloidiasis gives rise to a pathognomonic skin manifestation known as larva currens (Figure 34.2). Larva currens presents as a transient (lasting a few hours) pruritic creeping eruption that migrates fast (up to 5–10 cm/hour). It is usually located on the buttocks, groin,

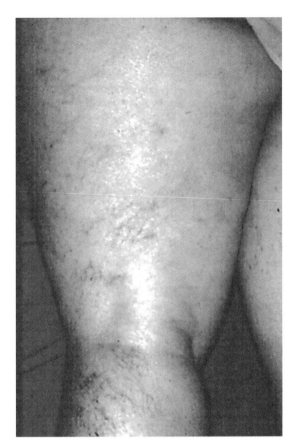

**Figure 34.2** Larva currens associated with *S. stercoralis* infection in a woman from the French West Indies.

and trunk. The eruption recurs throughout the course of the disease, lasting weeks to years, because infection can persist indefinitely due to autoinfestation.

Hyperinfection may also be discovered by cutaneous manifestations caused by massive dissemination of filariform larvae to the skin. It manifests as a rapid and progressively diffuse petechial and purpuric eruption that typically involves the trunk and proximal extremities. The phrase "thumbprint sign" has been used in disseminated strongyloidiasis to describe a unique pattern of periumbilical purpura that resembles multiple thumbprints. Peripheral eosinophilia fluctuates more or less above the normal value during the chronic phase.

The drugs with potential activity include fluromebendazole, mebendazole, thiabendazole, albendazole, pyrantel pamoate, and ivermectin. The efficacy of these drugs has been well established only during the chronic phase of the disease and varies according to the causal helminth.

For hookworm infection, there is no referral treatment for ground itch, but it is presumed that treatment of chronic hookworm infection could work (see Chapter 31). Such treatments include pyrantel pamoate, mebendazole, and albendazole. Ivermectin is not effective in human hookworm, in contrast to animal hookworm. Effective drugs for enterobiasis include fluromebendazole, albendazole, mebendazole, and pyrantel pamoate. In any case, treatment should be repeated after 2 weeks and concurrent treatment of household members may be necessary. Ivermectin (12 mg, single dose) or albendazole (400 to 800 mg/day for 3 days) is the treatment of choice for larva currens [2]. Patients with HTLV-1 infection or immunosuppression who have disseminated infections must receive more prolonged initial therapy as well as repeated courses of ivermectin as long as the immunosuppression lasts, to avoid relapse.

For prevention in travelers, see Chapter 31.

### Filariasis (see Chapter 25)

The spectrum of filariasis in travelers has recently been updated. Of the 43,722 medical conditions reported to the GeoSentinel network by December 2004, 271 (0.62%) were related to filariasis [5]. Of these 271 patients, 37% were diagnosed with onchocerciasis, 25% with loiasis, and 25% were found to be infected with *Wuchereria bancrofti*, the main agent of lymphatic filariasis. The majority of cases (62%) occurred among immigrants or refugees native to endemic countries. The main reasons for travel were immigration (44%), visiting friends and relatives (19%), and missionary service (16%), but tourists accounted for 9% of the cases. Most of the infections were acquired in Sub-Saharan Africa (75%). Almost one-third (30%) of patients native to nonendemic regions acquired their infections during trips of less than 1 month duration. Filariasis can thus be acquired with relatively short-term exposure, and a risk of acquisition does exist among tourists.

From a clinical point of view, infected patients with lifelong exposure to filariae are more commonly asymptomatic (or subclinical) than those from nonendemic regions (5).

Patients with filariasis have peripheral eosinophilia, which may be high grade, and elevated IgE. The diagnosis relies on demonstration of microfilariae, usually in blood or in the skin. The usefulness of serological tests is limited by cross-reactions with other nematodes. Newer tests with better specificity, such as PCR and antigen detection, are becoming available.

Patients with filariasis may be referred for treatment in specialized units. The treatment, which usually combines different drugs, is potentially associated with severe adverse events, called the Mazzoti reaction, which consists of exacerbation of the skin manifestations. Thus, the Mazzoti reaction, in addition to being an adverse event related to treatment, has a high diagnostic value. Drugs with antifilarial activity include diethylcarbamazine (DEC), ivermectin, and albendazole. However, they must also be used with doxycycline, except in loiasis.

## Onchocerciasis

Onchocerciasis is caused by the filarial nematode *Onchocerca volvulus* and is transmitted by the bite of blackflies of the genus *Simulium*. Onchocerciasis affects primarily immigrants living near fast-flowing rivers in Africa and the Arabian Peninsula [6]. But it can also be observed in travelers with short-term exposure. Among travelers from nonendemic regions and diagnosed with imported filariasis, onchocerciasis was the most common, and 77% acquired it during trips of less than 1 month duration [5].

The incubation period is usually 1–2 years (several months to several years), but 67% of the travelers with onchocerciasis in the GeoSentinel study presented within 1 month after return [5]. The skin and the eyes are the two most commonly involved organ systems. The symptoms last for years.

The skin manifestations of onchocerciasis are the consequences of itching, which is chronic and severe. Skin manifestations include papules, nodules, lichenified dermatitis, atrophy, and hyperpigmented and hypopigmented lesions. Ocular findings include chorioretinitis, iritis, optic atrophy, punctate keratitis, and sclerosing keratitis. Blindness is a potential outcome. Other clinical manifestations include "hanging groin," lymphadenopathy, and lymphedema of external genitalia or limbs. These chronic manifestations of the disease are not seen in travelers.

Onchocerciasis-associated limb swelling is a particular clinical and epidemiological form of the disease that may be seen in travelers and expatriates. In contrast to other clinical forms of onchocerciasis, limb swelling is not a disease of the savanna but of forested areas [7]. Patients present with acute pruritic and erythematous swelling of a limb known as onchocerciasis-associated limb swelling, as first described in 1974 [8].

The low prevalence of severe adverse reactions in the treatment of onchocerciasis in indigenous adult patients (the prevalence of minor to moderate side effects varies from 15% to 30%) contrasts with the higher frequency (up to 61%) of mild to moderate adverse reactions in expatriates with onchocerciasis [9]. These side effects include itching, urticarial rash, localized edema, and fever,

which usually occur 6–36 hours after the dose and may continue for 1–14 days. In contrast with adult indigenous patients, in whom the incidence of reactions is related to high microfilarial load, expatriates had very low microfilarial loads. Apparently, reactions to ivermectin occur much more frequently in expatriates and children, with recent infections and no immune tolerance, compared to indigenous adults, with lifelong exposure and a degree of immune tolerance [9].

## Loiasis

Loiasis is due to the filarial nematode, *Loa loa*, and transmitted by the bite of *Chrysops* in forested areas of Central Africa. It is more commonly reported in autochthonous populations, migrants, and expatriates than in travelers with short-term exposure, but it is still the second most common filarial infection in travelers [5].

Symptoms begin a mean of 24 months after exposure (4 months to 20 years). Loiasis is manifested by pruritus, migration of the worm under the skin or across the eye, and Calabar swellings (10). Calabar swelling, the characteristic manifestation of loiasis, is a subcutaneous localized edema, from 5 to 20 cm in diameter, which lasts a few days but may recur for years. It occurs predominantly on the upper extremities (more commonly than the lower), especially around joints, such as the wrist.

A migrating adult worm may be seen crossing the conjunctivae or the bridge of the nose or migrating under the skin, causing a creeping eruption (Figure 34.3). It presents as a serpiginous or linear erythematous cutaneous trail that is less than 10 cm long and advances very fast (1 cm/minute). It lasts no more than a few hours.

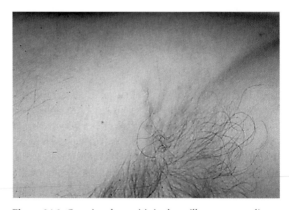

**Figure 34.3** Creeping dermatitis in the axillary area revealing loiasis in a French expatriate working in the forest industry in Gabon.

Serious life-threatening complications, such as encephalopathy, may occur as a complication of treatment with DEC [10] or ivermectin [11].

## Lymphatic filariasis

Lymphatic filariasis is caused by three filarial nematodes: *W. bancrofti* and to a lesser extent *Brugia malay* and *B. timori*. They are found in the tropical and subtropical areas of Africa, Asia, Pacific islands, Central and South America, and the Caribbean [1, 2].

Lymphatic filariasis is acquired by the bite of an infective mosquito. Symptoms can begin as early as 1–3 months after exposure and last for years. Sequelae can persist after the death of all parasites, and the treatment does not reverse the consequences of lymphatic obstruction.

Manifestations may be acute and recurrent and then become chronic. In endemic areas, the clinical course ranges from asymptomatic manifestations to severely disabling manifestations that affect less than 1% of those infected. Initial lymphatic damages may give rise to retrograde and recurrent lymphangitis, lymphadenitis, less commonly, orchitis, or epididymitis. It takes years for the characteristic clinical features of chronic filariasis to appear. The chronic disease is a consequence of lymphatic obstruction and includes lymphedema, elephantiasis, hydrocele, and chyluria. Lymphedema is usually located at the lower extremities, scrotum, and penis.

For treatment and prevention of filarial infection, see Chapter 25.

## Mansonellosis and streptocerciasis

Mansonelliasis is an infection caused by the filarial nematodes, *Mansonella perstans*, *M. streptocerca*, and *M. ozzardi* (considered as nonpathogenic to humans). Both are transmitted by mosquito bites. Both are found in remote geographic areas, mainly in Africa. They have not been reported in travelers.

The skin rash of *M. streptocerca* and *M. perstans* looks like that seen in onchocerciasis with itching, papules, lichenification, and hypopigmented and/or hyperpigmented macules [1, 2]. Peripheral eosinophilia is usually present and low grade. The diagnosis can be made by finding microfilariae in skin snips (streptocerciasis) and blood (mansonelliasis). Ivermectin is the drug of choice.

## Dracunculiasis

Dracunculiasis is now confined to 13 countries in Africa and remains a serious health problem only in Sudan. Therefore, imported cases are now unlikely in Western countries. Humans acquire dracunculiasis by drinking infected water, usually taken from step wells and other surface water. The incubation period has been well evaluated in migrants returning from travel in endemic countries where the infection was common in the past [12]. The adult worm emerges about 1 year (range, 10–18 months) after the larvae are ingested [12]. The characteristic clinical findings of dracunculiasis include a bulla, 2–7 cm in size, that progresses within a week to an ulcer. At this stage, the adult worm may be palpated, and sometimes seen (as a cutaneous trail 55–80 cm long) under the skin. But the eruption is usually masked by localized swelling.

Visual inspection of the parasite as it emerges from the skin and identification of the discharged larvae from the ulcer confirm the diagnosis. The treatment of dracunculiasis includes extracting the worms by slowly winding them around a stick.

There is no efficient treatment. Prevention consists of avoiding drinking infested water.

## Animal nematodes in human beings

### Toxocariasis

Toxocariasis is caused by the dog roundworm, *Toxocara canis*, and the cat roundworm, *T. catis*. It is transmitted by ingesting infective eggs from contaminated soil on fingers, fruits, vegetables, and other foods. It is found worldwide.

Most infections are asymptomatic. Otherwise, the clinical spectrum of the disease comprises major forms, namely visceral larva migrans and ocular or neurological toxocariasis, and minor forms, recognized more recently, namely common and covert toxocariasis [2] (see Table 34.1).

Skin manifestations include prurigo and chronic urticaria [13, 14]. They may be associated with fever, cough, wheezing, abdominal pain, anorexia, arthralgia, myalgia, fatigue, and hepatomegaly. Signs and symptoms usually resolve over time. In heavy infections, the heart and CNS may be affected.

The level of eosinophilia is highest at the beginning of the disease. Then it decreases slowly and fluctuates more or less above the normal value. The diagnosis relies on the results of serological testing. ELISA testing has a sensitivity of up to 90% but lacks specificity. Diagnosis must therefore be confirmed with a Western blot.

The treatments that have been assessed include diethylcarbamazine (DEC) (3–4 mg/kg/day for 21 days),

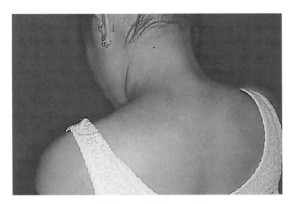

**Figure 34.4** Eosinophilic panniculitis revealing cutaneous gnathostomiasis in a woman from Southeast Asia.

mebendazole (20–25 mg/kg/day for 7–21 days), and albendazole (10 mg/kg/day for 5–15 days). Mazzoti-like reactions are observed in 10% of patients treated with DEC, calling for a progressive increase of the daily dose. The cure rate varies from 47% to 70% according to the clinical form and the treatment. Mebendazole and DEC seem to be more efficient than albendazole; longer duration of treatment is better. Ivermectin is not efficient. Corticosteroids (1 mg/kg/day for 1 month) are necessary to decrease the inflammatory response caused by the production of antigens by the larvae in associated nervous system or eye involvement. But they should not be given with diethylcarbamazine because of strong antagonism.

Prevention consists of washing the hands after contact with the ground and cleaning raw vegetables before eating them.

## Gnathostomiasis

Gnathostomiasis is caused by ingestion of uncooked food infected with the nematode larvae of *Gnathostoma* spp. (mainly *G. spinigerum*) [15] (Table 34.1). Gnathostomiasis is endemic in Southeast Asia (particularly Thailand) and Latin America (particularly Mexico). Cases of cutaneous gnathostomiasis have also been reported in travelers returning from these areas [16].

The most common clinical presentation of gnathostomiasis is cutaneous gnathostomiasis. Typical cutaneous manifestations are recurrent subcutaneous swelling (Figure 34.4), creeping eruption, and edema of the extremities, all more or less pruritic. In travelers, cutaneous lesions appear within a mean period of 62 days (range 10–150 days) after return [16]. Symptoms last 1–4 weeks each, but recurrence occurs in a different area. Severe neurological

complications have been reported. Thus, the diagnosis of cutaneous gnathostomiasis calls for early treatment before the onset of neurological involvement.

Diagnosis of cutaneous gnathostomiasis usually relies on the association of recurrent dermatological manifestations, a history of ingestion of uncooked meat of animal hosts in endemic areas, hypereosinophilia (common but not constant), and results of serological tests, which should be repeated if negative [15, 16]. Some authors report definitive confirmation by the isolation of the nematode's larva in a biopsy specimen. However, because biopsy is frequently unsuccessful, it is not usually recommended [16].

The effective treatments are albendazole (400–800 mg/day for 21 days) and ivermectin (0.2 mg/kg for 1 or 2 days). Cure rates in Thailand are 78–94% with albendazole, 76–95% with a single dose of ivermectin, and 100% with two doses of ivermectin. However, in imported cases treated in Western countries, a single course of albendazole cured 81% of a series of British patients and 40% of a series of French patients with cutaneous gnathostomiasis [16]. Because relapses may occur up to 24 months after apparent cure, a prolonged period of follow-up is necessary before cure.

*Prevention* consists of avoiding eating raw or insufficiently cooked freshwater fish or flesh from other mammal hosts.

## Trichinosis

Trichinosis is caused by *Trichinella spiralis* (see Table 34.1). Humans are incidental dead-end hosts. They ingest raw meat containing the infective larvae, mainly pork, and become infected. Many times trichinosis appears as a small outbreak in hunters who shared undercooked flesh. Trichinosis is present in most countries.

The usual incubation period is 10–30 days. Gastrointestinal symptoms (abdominal pain, diarrhea, and vomiting) may begin as early as 1–2 days after eating infected meat and continue during the first week of infection.

Symptoms of trichinosis occur later during larval migration, before encystment. Ten days after the ingestion of larvae, the cutaneous signs appear in association with fever (90% of cases), fatigue, and severe myalgia.

Cutaneous manifestations are varied and are seen in about 75% of cases of symptomatic trichinosis [17]. The most frequent dermatological manifestations are periorbital and facial edema (75–95% of the cases), conjunctivitis (50%), and a macular or papular (sometimes urticarial) rash (15%). Hand swelling and volar surface erythema followed by desquamation have been also reported [2].

Subconjunctival and splinter hemorrhages are less common [17]. The severity of trichinosis ranges from asymptomatic to fatal, fatalities usually being related to CNS or cardiac involvement.

Peripheral eosinophilia may be marked and may persist for months. Muscular enzymes (creatine phosphokinase) are increased. Serological tests become positive about 20 days after ingestion. Otherwise, definitive diagnosis is possible after the 17th day and relies on identification of the parasite in a muscle biopsy.

For treatment and prevention, see Chapter 31.

## Hookworm-related cutaneous larva migrans

Hookworm-related cutaneous larva migrans (HrCLM) is one of the most frequent travel-associated skin diseases of tropical origin [3, 4]. HrCLM is usually caused by the penetration of the human skin by infective larvae of animal hookworms, usually cat or dog hookworm larvae (*Ancylostoma braziliense*, *A. caninum*, and *Uncinaria stenocephala*), while lying or walking on beaches (or any ground contaminated with animal feces) in hot seaside areas of tropical and subtropical countries worldwide (Table 34.1).

The incubation period of HrCLM is rarely more than 1 month. In series of HrCLM diagnosed in returning travelers, the cutaneous lesions appeared in approximately half of the patients upon their return, whereas in the remaining patients the mean time of onset after return was usually less than 1 month [18]. However, some extremely long incubation periods have been reported.

The striking symptom of HrCLM is pruritus localized at the site of the eruption and reported in 100% of patients [18]. The most frequent and characteristic sign of HrCLM is "creeping dermatitis," an erythematous, subcutaneous linear or serpiginous track that is approximately 3 mm wide and may be up to 15–20 cm long, which may extend a few millimeters to a few centimeters daily [19] (Figure 34.5). The mean number of lesions per person commonly varies from one to three. Other clinical signs are local swelling, reported in 6–17%, and vesiculobullous lesions, reported in 4–40% of returning travelers [18]. The most frequent location of HrCLM lesions is the feet, followed by the buttocks and thighs. Without any treatment, the eruption usually lasts between 2 and 8 weeks, but they may continue for as long as 2 years.

Hookworm folliculitis is a particular form of HrCLM, related to other species of animal nematodes, consisting of pruritic folliculitis-like lesions associated with numerous relatively short tracks, generally arising from follicular

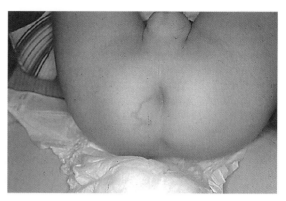

**Figure 34.5** Hookworm-related cutaneous larva migrans revealed by creeping dermatitis in a child coming back from the Caribbean.

lesions and located on the buttocks [19]. The term "hookworm folliculitis" was first used in 1991, and *A. caninum* was the identified hookworm.

Diagnosis of HrCLM is usually based on the typical clinical presentation in the context of recent travel to a tropical country and beach exposure [18]. The differential diagnoses include the other dermatoses that give rise to creeping eruptions and the other causes of the cutaneous larva migrans syndrome [19].

### Treatment

Topical application of a 15% tiabendazole ointment to the affected areas (2–3 times per day for 5–10 days) has been shown to be efficacious for decades, with cure rates of more than 95%. Nonetheless, ivermectin and albendazole are more convenient and more widely available. Ivermectin, taken in a single 12-mg oral dose, is well tolerated and highly efficacious, with cure rates of 94–100% in all but one of the largest series of imported HrCLM in travelers [18]. Oral albendazole (400–800 mg/day) gives similar cure rates but has to be administered for 3 days. In hookworm folliculitis, treatment necessitates repeated courses of ivermectin [18]. For low-weight children or when oral ivermectin and albendazole are contraindicated, the application of a 10% albendazole ointment twice a day for 10 days is a safe and effective alternative treatment.

### Prevention

The best way to prevent HrCLM is to wear protective footwear, use mattresses, and prefer sand washed by the tide when walking or lying on tropical beaches frequented by dogs and cats [18].

## Dirofilariasis

The organisms responsible for dirofilariasis include the nematodes of several species of the genus *Dirofilaria*, most importantly *D. immitis* (the dog heartworm). It has been reported from all continents (see Table 34.1). Humans acquire the disease from mosquito bites. The interval between exposure and development of symptoms is usually at least 2–3 months. Cutaneous dirofilariasis is characterized by well-defined firm subcutaneous nodules 1–5 cm in diameter that are usually single [20]. Occasionally, lesions may be migratory [2]. Definitive diagnosis relies on identification of the worm after surgical excision of the nodule.

## Trematodes

### Schistosomes

#### Cercarial dermatitis

Cercarial dermatitis results from the penetration of the skin by cercariae of nonhuman schistosomes during bathing in fresh water or coastal water (Table 34.2). The usual hosts of these schistosomes are birds and small mammals. The cercariae penetrate intact skin of swimmers in endemic areas on all continents. Identified risk factors in the USA (Lake Michigan) and Switzerland (Lake Leman) are bathing in shallow water and in areas with onshore winds, greater number of days of lake use, previous history of cercarial dermatitis, time spent in the water, time of day, and climatic conditions [21, 22].

A significant outbreak, which occurred in Lake Annecy in France, provides a good description of the disease because the exposure during a swimming race was unique [23]. The time from exposure to onset of symptoms varies from a few minutes to a maximum of 24 hours after exposure. A prickling sensation during or shortly after exposure to infested water may be reported. Typically, approximately 1 hour later, the eruption begins with numerous pruritic macular erythematous cutaneous lesions that progress to papular, papulovesicular, or urticarial eruptions. The eruptions peak in 1–3 days and last 1–3 weeks [23]. They usually involve exposed parts of the skin, but involve the parts covered by the bathing costume in approximately 20% of cases [22, 23]. The diagnosis is made by history of water exposure, other cases in exposed bathers, and the characteristic dermatological findings.

Cercarial dermatitis is self-limited and treatment with corticosteroid ointment is only symptomatic.

Prevention consists of avoiding swimming in infested water. No topical barrier method has shown preventive efficacy, except DEET application, but this needs to be confirmed.

### Human schistosomiasis

Human schistosomiasis is the only helminthic infection associated with skin manifestations during the three phases of its cycle (see Table 34.2).

A cercarial dermatitis-like reaction may occur during the penetration phase but is transient (a few hours).

Acute urticaria is a typical skin manifestation of acute schistosomiasis (or invasive schistosomiasis). It can be observed 2–6 weeks after exposure to infested fresh water in endemic areas (see Figure 24.6, Chapter 24). As an example, among 28 nonimmune travelers who acquired schistosomiasis after having swum once (unique exposure) in freshwater pools in Mali, 10 (36%) complained of pruritic cercarial like dermatitis just after swimming and 15 (54%) further presented with signs of invasive schistosomiasis (fever, urticaria, cough, headaches) [24].

Diagnosis should thus be systematically considered for any febrile traveler with acute urticaria and a history of exposure to fresh water in an endemic area. The diagnosis relies on serology and eosinophilia, which both might be within normal limits at the beginning of the invasive phase (usually < 2 weeks after exposure) and, therefore, must be repeated. Praziquantel, which kills only adult worms and is associated with worsening acute schistosomiasis in 40% of cases, should not be given during the acute phase [24].

Late cutaneous schistosomiasis and perineal tumors may be observed during the chronic phase. These conditions present as papulonodular skin lesions located in the perineal area, including the genitalia in women (perineal tumor), or with a zosteriform distribution (late cutaneous schistosomiasis). The diagnosis relies on histopathology as well as stool test or urinalysis [2].

Treatment and prevention are discussed in Chapter 24.

### Flukes other than schistosomes

Flukes other than schistosomes include liver flukes (*Fasciola hepatica* and, less commonly, *F. gigantica*), which cause fascioliasis, and lung flukes (*Paragonimus westermani* and more than 10 species of *Paragonimus*), which cause paragonimiasis. Both diseases are acquired orally, by ingestion of watercress and other plants (fascioliasis) or raw or undercooked freshwater crayfish, crab or shrimp (paragonimiasis). Fascioliasis and paragonimiasis have common skin manifestations.

Urticaria and other allergic manifestations (wheezing, angioedema, fever) may be associated with hepatic manifestations in fascioliasis and pulmonary manifestations in paragonimiasis. Marked leukocytosis and eosinophilia characterize acute infection.

In later stages, ectopic cutaneous manifestations may include firm, slightly mobile subcutaneous nodules containing immature flukes [25]. These occur more frequently in paragonimiasis than in fascioliasis. Fascioliasis may also present as eosinophilic panniculitis [2]. One case of creeping eruption due to the subcutaneous migration of the immature form of *F. gigantica* has been described in Vietnam [2]. Eosinophilia may be low grade or absent when the parasites are encysted.

The identification of eggs confirms the diagnosis. An immunoblot serological test that has high sensitivity and specificity is available for both infections.

Treatment and prevention are discussed in Chapter 31.

## Cestodes

### Echinococcosis

Echinococcal diseases (see Chapter 27) include hydatid cyst disease caused by *Echinococcus granulosus* and alveolar cyst disease caused by *E. multilocularis* (see Table 34.2). These diseases are not currently observed in travelers but are particularly common in endemic countries and in immigrants from those countries.

Acute urticaria, like other manifestations of anaphylaxis, may be seen during accidental rupture of a hydatid cyst and is related to allergic reaction to foreign antigens released from cyst fluid. Otherwise, skin and soft tissue manifestations are rare. Ectopic echinococcal cysts can appear as firm subcutaneous nodules. Infection with *E. multilocularis* may cause cutaneous localizations but result from the extension of an underlying visceral localization [2]. Peripheral eosinophilia is present in only a small percentage of patients with cysts. In contrast, leakage of cyst fluid causes eosinophilia in nearly all patients.

Diagnosis relies on serological testing and was formerly made by examination of the contents of the cyst after surgery.

### Taeniasis

### Cysticercosis

The larval stage of the pork tapeworm, *Taenia solium*, causes cysticercosis (see Chapter 28). *T. solium* is a common parasite in Central and South America, Africa, parts of Asia, and Eastern Europe (Table 34.2). In Western countries, this disease appears primarily in immigrants but has been described in travelers [2]. Cysticercosis is the most common helminthic infection of the CNS, but skin manifestations are uncommon. The skin findings are single or multiple firm, mobile, round, well-circumscribed (a few mm to 2-cm diameter) subcutaneous nodules. The prognosis of subcutaneous cysticercosis is related to the involvement of other organ systems (mainly the eyes and nervous system). The presence on thigh X rays of calcified larvae of cysticercae in the muscles is of high diagnostic value, but is more likely to be seen in migrants with past exposure than in travelers with recent exposure.

Peripheral eosinophilia is absent. Definitive diagnosis relies on identification of the parasite after surgical excision of a cutaneous nodule. Serological tests are also available.

### Other cestodes: coenurosis and sparganosis

Coenurosis and sparganosis are uncommon infections even in autochthonous populations. Cutaneous coenurosis and sparganosis may present as firm, well-delimited subcutaneous nodules that are solitary cysts. Size varies from 1 to 6 cm in diameter. The lesion is often painless. Definitive diagnosis is made by identification of the parasite in the surgically excised nodule.

## Conclusion

Skin manifestations provide important diagnostic clues for many helminthic infections. They can be seen during the three phases of the helminth life cycle within human hosts.

Hookworms are the main cause of cutaneous lesions during the penetration phase. Human hookworms give rise to a relatively short-lasting ground itch, whereas infective larvae of animal hookworms give rise to a characteristic chronic creeping dermatitis (HrCLM). This is the most common helminthic skin disease to be seen in travelers. Urticaria is the most common sign seen during the invasive phase of the cycle, and its most common cause in travelers is acute schistosomiasis. During the chronic phase, skin manifestations are rare, especially in travelers. However, they may be seen in a spectrum of helminthic diseases, where they offer a unique opportunity for easy diagnosis by skin lesion biopsy or surgical excision.

# References

1 Canizares O, et al. Helminthic diseases I, II, III. In: Canizares O, Harman R, editors. *Clinical Tropical Dermatology*, 2nd ed. Oxford: Blackwell Sciences; 1992. p. 324–71.

2 Caumes E, Wilson ME. Helminthic infections. In: Freedberg IM, Eisen AZ, Wolff K, Austen KF, Goldsmith LA, Katz SI, editors. *Fitzpatrick's Dermatology in General Medicine*, 7th ed. New York: McGraw-Hill; 2007. p. 2011–29.

3 Lederman ER, Weld LH, Elyazar IR, et al. Dermatologic conditions of the ill returned traveler: an analysis from the GeoSentinel Surveillance Network. *Int J Infect Dis* 2008;12:593–602.

4 Caumes E, Carriere J, Guermonprez G, Danis M, Bricaire F, Gentilini M. Dermatoses associated with travel to tropical countries: a prospective study of the diagnosis and management of 269 patients presenting to a tropical disease unit. *Clin Infect Dis* 1995;20:542–8.

5 Lipner EM, Law MA, Barnett E, et al. Filariasis in travelers presenting to the GeoSentinel surveillance network. *PLoS Negl Trop Dis* 2007;1(3):e88.

6 Borup LH, Peters SS, Sartori CR. Onchocerciasis (river blindness). *Cutis* 2003;72:297–302.

7 Nozais JP, Caumes E, Datry A, Bricaire F, Danis M, Gentilini M. A propos de cinq nouveaux cas d'oedème onchocerquien. *Bull Soc Pathol Exot* 1997;90:335–8.

8 Wolfe MS, Petersen JL, Neafie RC, Connor DH, Purtilo DT. Onchocerciasis presenting with swelling of limb. *Am J Trop Med Hyg* 1974;23:361–8.

9 Davidson RN, Godfrey-Fausset P, Bryceson AD. Adverse reactions in expatriates treated with ivermectin. *Lancet* 1990;336:1005.

10 Carme B, Namboueni JP, Copin N, Noireau F. Clinical and biological study of *Loa loa* filariasis in Congolese. *Am J Trop Med Hyg* 1989;41:331–7.

11 Gardon J, Gardon-Wendel N, Demanga-Ngangue J, Kamqno J, Chippaux JP, Boussinesq M. Serious reactions after mass treatment of onchocerciasis with ivermectin in an area endemic for *Loa loa* infection. *Lancet* 1997;350: 18–22.

12 Carme B, Duda M, Datry A, Gentilini M. *Dracunculus medinensis* infestation following holidays in West Africa.

Epidemiological implications. *Nouv Presse Med* 1981;10: 2711–13.

13 Humbert P, Niezbola M, Salembier R, et al. Skin manifestations associated with toxocariasis: a case-control study. *Dermatology* 2000;201:230–4.

14 Wolfrom E, Chene G, Lejoly-Boisseau H, Beylot C, Geniaux M, Taieb A. Chronic urticaria and *Toxocara canis* infection. A case-control study. *Ann Dermatol Venereol* 1996;123:240–6.

15 Rusnak JM, Lucey DR. Clinical gnathostomiasis: Case report and review of the English-language literature. *Clin Infect Dis* 1993;16:33–50.

16 Ménard A, Dos Santos G, Dekumyoy P, et al. Imported cutaneous gnathostomiasis: report of five cases. *Trans R Soc Trop Med Hyg* 2003;97:200–2.

17 Bournerias I, Danis M, Nozais JP, et al. Cutaneous signs of trichinosis. A propos of the 1985 outbreak. *Ann Dermatol Venereol* 1986;113:1139–44.

18 Hochedez P, Caumes E. Hookworm-related cutaneous larva migrans. *J Travel Med* 2007;14:339–46.

19 Caumes E, Danis M. From creeping eruption to hookworm-related cutaneous larva migrans. *Lancet Infect Dis* 2004;4:359–60.

20 Pampiglione S, Rivasi S, Angeli G, et al. Dirofilariasis due to *Dirofilaria repens* in Italy, an emergent zoonosis: report of 60 new cases. *Histopathology* 2001;38:344–54.

21 Hoeffer DF. Swimmer's itch (cercarial dermatitis). *Cutis* 1977;19:461–5.

22 Chamot E, Toscani L, Rougemont A. Public health importance and risk factors for cercarial dermatitis associated with swimming in Lake Leman, Geneva, Switzerland. *Epidemiol Infect* 1998;120:305–14.

23 Caumes E, Felder-Moinet S, Couzigou C, Darras-Joly C, Latour P, Leger N. Failure of an ointment based on IR3535 (ethyl butylacetylaminopropionate) to prevent an outbreak of cercarial dermatitis during swimming races across Lake Annecy, France. *Ann Trop Med Parasitol* 2003;97:157–63.

24 Grandière-Perez L, Ansart S, Paris L, et al. Efficacy of praziquantel during the incubation and invasive phase of S. *haematobium* schistosomiasis in 18 travellers. *Am J Trop Med Hyg* 2006;74:814–18.

25 Arjona R, et al. Fascioliasis in developed countries: a review of classic and aberrant forms of the disease. *Medicine (Baltimore)* 1995;74:13–23.

# 35 Delusional Parasitosis

Eli Schwartz,[1] Jay Keystone,[2] and Henry Abramovitch[3]

[1] Chaim Sheba Medical Center, Tel Hashomer, Israel and Sackler School of Medicine, Tel Aviv University, Tel Aviv, Israel
[2] Toronto General Hospital, University of Toronto, Toronto, ON, Canada
[3] Sackler School of Medicine, Tel Aviv University, Tel Aviv, Israel

## Introduction

The clinical presentation of delusional parasitosis (DP) was first described in 1894 when a French dermatologist introduced the term *acarophobia* to describe patients who were convinced that they had been infested with mites. In the following decades numerous reports appeared in the literature describing similar phenomena with different names (Table 35.1). In 1946, Wilson and Miller published their case series in a dermatology journal [1] and introduced the term "delusional parasitosis" or "delusion of parasitosis," which became the most widely accepted term.

Patients with DP believe they are infested with parasites or other microorganisms, and this idea is a fixed, unshakeable belief held in the absence of any medical finding. The complaints are mostly of the skin, and less commonly involve the gastrointestinal tract. The majority of patients are female. Delusional parasitosis is very distressing to the patient, causing him or her to visit medical centers for advice from family practitioners, dermatologists, infectious disease specialists, and travel and tropical medicine practitioners. Despite the fact that technically it is a psychiatric disease, psychiatrists rarely encounter the condition. Most patients refuse psychiatric help because they firmly believe they are suffering from a serious medical condition. In the words of one patient, "I am not crazy, why would I want to go to a headshrinker?" Paradoxically, psychiatrists who have a great interest in such patients only seldom see them. On the other hand, family physicians, dermatologists, and infectious disease specialists, who do see them, are often at a loss as to how to treat them. The majority of case reports and treatment approaches are found in the dermatological literature.

Conceptually, DP may be understood in terms of what medical anthropologists call the disease–illness dichotomy [2]. DP is a special case of illness/no disease, in which the patient is sure he or she suffers from a specific disease. The doctor finds no medical evidence to support the patient's interpretation of the illness as a disease. Instead, the physician interprets the intensity of the patient's fixed belief as indicative of a delusional disorder, somatic subtype (DSM IV-TR). At this point, the physician and patient are at loggerheads because they fundamentally disagree concerning the nature of the illness and the disease. In the ensuing mismeeting [3], the patient continues to suffer and implicitly accuses the doctor of incompetence and withholding treatment, while the physician thinks that he or she is not the appropriate physician to be treating this patient.

In their frustration in trying to find cures for their problem patients with DP then turn to those who specialize in exotic diseases, that is, travel/tropical medicine practitioners. These patients do so for a number of reasons. A few have returned from travel that might be the trigger for the appearance of the DP. The majority, however, have not traveled but are convinced that they have a parasite that only a specialist in exotic diseases can treat. Thus, travel/tropical medicine physicians must be acquainted with this unique disorder, its symptomatology, its impact on the doctor-patient relationship, and its treatment modalities.

## Epidemiology

Delusional parasitosis (DP) reporting is mostly anecdotal and, therefore, little is known about its epidemiology, nosological classification, therapy, and course. Trabert,

*Tropical Diseases in Travelers*, 1st edition. Edited by E. Schwartz.
© 2009 by Blackwell Publishing, ISBN: 978-1-4051-8441-0.

**Table 35.1** Reports in the literature describing delusional parasitosis with different names.

| Description | Authors | Year |
| --- | --- | --- |
| Acarophobia | Thibierge | 1894 |
| Parasitophobic neurodermatitis | Perrin | 1896 |
| Presenile parasthesias | Ekbon | 1938 |
| Delusion of parasitosis | Wilson and Miller | 1946 |
| Chronic tactile hallucination | Bers and Conrad | 1954 |
| Delusion of infestation | Hopkinson | 1970 |
| Monosymptomatic hypochondrial psychosis (which includes delusional parasitosis as a subtype) | Riding and Munro | 1975 |

*Source:* Adapted from [4, 5].

who reviewed 1223 cases [4], found that DP may occur at any point in the human life cycle but is most commonly found in women in their fifties, with a mean age of $57\pm14$ years. The ratio of female to male patients was 1.4:1 for persons aged <50 years and 2.5:1 for those aged 50 years or more. Most DP cases have no previous psychiatric history and are middle class. Psychiatric symptoms are limited to this single delusion.

The prevalence of these delusions is unknown. Baker estimated their prevalence as 7 cases per 10,000 psychiatric admissions, which is clearly an underestimate, because psychiatrists do not encounter the majority of patients [5]. Trabert [4] estimated that the annual incidence in Germany was 16 cases per million people and its prevalence is 83 per million. When Reilly and Batchelor surveyed 386 British and English dermatologists, 66% of the replies indicated that they had seen at least one such patient in the previous 5 years [6].

It is important to note that most cases of DP have no history of psychiatric illness. The precipitating factor for delusional parasitosis may not be identifiable. However, it has been reported that the death of a family member, flooding in the patient's home, injury, contact with people infested with parasites, and travel are possible psychosocial triggers associated with the onset of DP [7]. Even without a history of travel, patients may claim to have been infected with a variety of exotic parasites.

Shared delusion—*folie a deux*—is a known phenomenon in delusional parasitosis [8, 9]. One or more members of the same family suffer from a monosymptomatic psychosis, the characteristic delusional state being identical. The secondary victims are often family members, who are dominated by their spouses, show filial devotion, or are trying to keep family harmony. The outbreak may occur at intervals of several months. The moving spirit in most of the cases is the mother. This phenomenon was reported in approximately 5–15% of the reported cases.

There are reports of DP from Japan and India and it is likely that it is to be found in many non-Western and nonindustrialized countries [9, 10].

## Epidemiology in travelers

Travel as a precipitating factor for delusional parasitosis, either for the traveler himself or for relatives and friends, has been described [11–13].

The GeoSentinel database, which accumulates information from ill returned travelers in more than 40 clinics worldwide, includes 103 cases of DP out of approximately 60,000 travelers with reported various illnesses post-travel. At the Centre for Travel and Tropical Medicine, Toronto, Canada, a 5-year review of 4100 referrals to the center showed that 62 patients were diagnosed with DP. Three of these cases were associated with travel. Similarly, in the Center for Travel and Tropical Medicine, Tel Hashomer, Israel, among a cohort of 2500 returned travelers, 2 cases were due to DP with a possible association with the travel. The 10 other cases were unrelated to travel [unpublished data].

Thus, as mentioned above, travel clinic/tropical medicine practitioners who see returned travelers may encounter patients who have no history of travel but complain of being infested with exotic parasites, believing that only a specialist in "exotic diseases" can treat them.

## Clinical aspects

Patient complaints of infection by parasites usually concern the skin. The patient may describe parasites coming out of the skin, or burrowing under the skin, causing terrible itching, crawling, biting, and the like. Usually, the skin will be damaged because of scratching or attempts to extract the organism. Often, patients will present in the clinic with containers containing the "parasites," which are collections of hair, scabs, and flakes of skin (called the "matchbox sign" in older publications and the "Ziploc bag sign" in the modern literature). Usually, repeated samples of these materials have been sent to different laboratories that have not identified any microorganisms. The patient may attribute these negative findings to the lack of expertise of the local laboratories.

In some cases, the patient may point to a trigger (as in the case described below), but most often there is no clear precipitating factor. The typical patient is middle-aged, with no psychiatric history, and belongs to the middle class economically. Usually, the patient has seen several doctors, including family physicians and dermatologists, and several nonphysicians, such as entomologists and parasitologists. She or he has tried several remedies, including a variety of anti-scabies medications and other conventional and alternative medicine approaches (pharmacological and nonpharmacological compounds).

In addition to the ritual of cleaning themselves, patients will focus on the cleansing of their surroundings (the bed, the house, the pet). Fumigators may be called in to debug the home. "To rid themselves of the 'bugs,' patients with DP may become desperate and quit their jobs, use pesticides dangerously and repeatedly" [14]. In severe cases, patients will sell their furniture or move to new premises in an attempt to eliminate the infestation.

Recently, patients have focused on an entity that was first reported in the 1600s, Morgellons syndrome, described as a condition in which fine fibers are found to extrude from the skin [15].

In some cases, the delusion will be directed to the gastrointestinal system. In these cases, the patient will complain of having a worm inside the body, which cannot be eliminated. It may cause abdominal discomfort, or irritation around the anus. In an era where electronic information is readily available, the patient may be convinced that he or she has a specific parasite, without any plausible explanation for it (e.g., having schistosomiasis without any travel history, or with all tests being negative). In such cases, patients may have tried conventional antiparasitic agents and/or alternative methods such as herbal preparations or enemas (e.g., garlic enema).

It is important to emphasize that patient distress and suffering from DP are intense; it may result in financial losses due to absence from work, cleaning costs, and visits to specialists. Those with DP often consider themselves contagious and, therefore, isolate themselves from family members or friends, leading to secondary agoraphobia.

### An illustrative case

A 56-year-old female biologist came to the Travel and Tropical Medicine Clinic after having been treated by

at least 20 physicians [12]. She suffered from generalized pruritus; her symptoms started about 1 week after her 25-year-old daughter returned from a trip to Southeast Asia and brought as presents yak-wool sweaters from Nepal. Believing that the sweaters were infested with fleas, the mother sealed them in plastic bags and cleaned the house thoroughly several times. She underwent treatment for scabies and with antihistamines and even went for a vacation overseas. None of these measures provided permanent relief. She then began to suffer from diarrhea, reduced appetite, and weakness and as a result was absent from work for several days. Direct examination of the skin for bites, stings, and scabies burrows were negative, as were examination of dust samples collected from her immediate surroundings. Stool samples were examined three times for helminths and protozoa and were also negative. Treatment with metronidazole and mebendazole provided no relief.

After 2–3 months, other members of the family began to complain of being infected by parasites. Altogether, four other members were affected, but the daughter who came back from Nepal was not affected. They, too, had visited several physicians and brought samples from their homes, as well as skin and stool samples for examination. All laboratory tests were negative for pathogens. In this case, DP may have resulted from pathological family dynamics and appeared to cause a high level of family stress.

### Diagnosis

Typically, the diagnosis of delusions of parasitosis is made on the basis of a thorough history alone, but it is important to do a careful physical examination and to examine the samples brought in by the patient. In addition, one must ensure that the patient does not have an organic skin disorder and that the delusion is not secondary to another mental or physical illness. Several systemic diseases have been associated with DP, such as diabetes mellitus, renal disease, and vitamin deficiencies, such as pellagra and vitamin B12 deficiency [16]. Cerebral disorders such as brain tumors, dementia, syphilis, HIV, cerebral infarction, and head injury have all been associated with DP [16].

In addition, medications and substance abuse such as corticosteroids, phenelzine, amphetamines, and cocaine abuse may cause secondary DP. Recently, ciprofloxacin was reported to induce a psychosis in a 45-year-old man without a previous history of mental disorder, who developed DP after administration of the antibiotic. After discontinuation of the drug, complete remission occurred within a few days without the use of psychopharmacologic medication [17].

Laboratory tests to evaluate causes of unexplained pruritus may include a complete blood count and differential, especially looking for eosinophilia (which might point to a parasitic infection), electrolytes, urea, creatinine, liver function tests, fasting blood sugar, thyroid stimulating hormone level, B12 and folate levels, calcium, and magnesium. Based on the individual's risk factors, additional tests such as serology for HIV infection, rapid plasma reagin test, or radiological imaging (e.g., chest X rays, CT, or MRI of the brain) may be indicated but in most cases are unnecessary.

## Approach to the patient and treatment

The diagnosis of primary DP is made when there is no objective evidence for a parasitic infection, and the condition is not secondary, or associated with underlying medical illness or medications/toxins. Although a psychiatric opinion is invaluable in assessing these patients, they typically refuse psychiatric assessment.

The key to treating patients with DP is the confirmation of the patient's experience of suffering as well as the provision of empathy for how difficult it is to live with such a chronic condition. Many patients express dissatisfaction with previous physicians who they believe are incompetent and uncaring. As a result, patients often fail to attend follow-up appointments and receive inadequate therapy or no therapy at all. Thus, a nonjudgmental approach, acknowledgment that the patient's symptoms are real, and empathetic exploration into the effects the symptoms have had on his or her daily life can instill a sense of trust. Patients who bring specimens should be reassured that these will be sent to a proper laboratory and/or entomologist for examination.

Repeated follow-up visits provide the opportunity for serial examination of the skin and allow the patient to develop trust in the physician. Repeated assessments are helpful in determining whether the patient has a shakable belief rather than a true delusion. One question that may be useful in trying to determine whether a belief is shakable is to ask, "If we come up with an alternative diagnosis other than a parasitic infection, how would you feel about it?" Patients with DP invariably reply that the cause of their symptoms *is* parasites.

During the clinical encounter, it is important not to contradict the patient's heath beliefs. Indeed, a trial of an antiparasitic drug may be warranted in some cases.

Because many of these patients have used several kinds of antiparasitic drugs previously, a different, difficult-to-obtain medication, used for "very exotic parasites," with a very low profile of adverse events (as are most of the antiparasitic drugs) may be prescribed. In our experience in Israel, a significant number of patients will respond to this approach. The effect may be due to the better doctor-patient relationship combined with the placebo effect of the drug, and it seems to work in the subset of DP patients who approached us early during the course of the disease. Some patients will have temporary relief with this approach, and repeated courses of these medications may help. This approach, we feel, may pave the way to offer an antipsychotic drug at the second stage, although some may argue that this approach might be problematic because the patient may desire not to stop the antiparasitic drug.

In most cases of DP that have persisted for several months, antipsychotic medication is warranted. As mentioned above, these patients refuse psychiatric consultation, and especially antipsychotic medication when it is prescribed as such.

One approach that has been used successfully is the "chemical imbalance theory" (J. S. Keystone, personal communication, 2008): "You may have been infected with a parasite (which even might be true in his past) and this has led to a 'chemical imbalance' which persists long after the infection has resolved." The patient may be given a similar example of drug-induced urticaria that continues for many weeks or months after the reaction had occurred. The role of antipsychotic drugs in these cases could be explained as antipruritic drugs or as restoring the patient's "chemical balance." It must be made very clear to the patient that the drug being prescribed *is* an antipsychotic; if one does not clarify its nature, the pharmacist or the World Wide Web will. One can say honestly that the drug was originally indicated for schizophrenia, "but you do not have schizophrenia!" It can be further explained that many drugs that were designed for one purpose may be used for another, including psychiatric drugs such as amitriptyline for depression and for neurological pain, or chlorpromazine, an antipsychotic that is used for the treatment of emesis, insomnia, and itching.

For those who ask why they are not being treated for parasites although they still *see* parasites, one may invoke the phenomenon of the "phantom limb," in which amputees still feel the presence of the amputated limb. It is very important to remember that the chemical imbalance theory should not be discussed until patients have had every opportunity to have one or more specimens examined to their satisfaction and all test results are negative.

## Treatment with antipsychotic drugs

The use of psychopharmacological medication, according to Trabert, increased the rate of full remissions from 33.9% to 51.9% [4]. Until recently, pimozide was the drug of choice, with a reported efficacy of up to 90% [18].

However, given the resistance to psychiatric referrals, the recommendation of a treatment of choice is largely based on case reports and not on systematic control studies.

Recently, the newer atypical antipsychotics, such as risperidone, olanzapine, and seroquel have been utilized as first-line agents because of the lower incidence of the extrapyramidal side effects associated with pimozide and other older agents [19].

These medications are not without problems that patients often find unacceptable. Significant weight gain is common, as is the occasional risk of diabetes with olanzapine, and drowsiness and "fogginess" with all of these drugs. Our practical approach is to start at a very low dose and build up to maintenance therapy over several weeks. It is interesting to note that most patients require relatively low doses to improve, between one-third and one-fourth of the maximum dose for maintenance.

The question is how long responders should remain on their drug. Trabert in his review mentioned that for a number of patients, DP will resolve, but others may require lifetime therapy [20]. Thus, the approach is to keep the patient on the minimum effective dose, determined by trial and error. Symptoms may recur while the medications are tapering off. A recurrence of symptoms would necessitate a more prolonged trial of therapy.

Despite these explanations, many patients will refuse the medication because of the stigma associated with mental illness and antipsychotic medication, but mostly because they believe that they do not have a mental illness.

DP is considered a delusional disorder, somatic subtype, and treated with antipsychotic medication, with poor compliance and mixed outcomes. DP may also be understood as a chronic somatoform disorder, in which some underlying emotional disturbance is expressed via physical symptoms. Treatment involves brief, but regularly scheduled clinic visits, stress reduction, and self-help techniques, as well as a family assessment (as in the case example presented earlier).

Treatment is care-oriented and not cure-oriented and focuses on a return to normal daily functioning.

## Outcome

Our knowledge of outcomes of this disorder is minimal, because patients tend to switch from one physician to another. Accurate follow-up data, prospective studies, and longitudinal studies are rare. Many reports consider DP a chronic condition [20], although Trabert claimed otherwise. In one study, about half the patients experienced a remission during the observation period. Other observations are that the use of psychopharmacological medication increased the rate of full remission. Response, however, is in part related to duration of symptoms, with full remission less likely in patients with longer-term symptoms.

Relapses are common, although relapse rates have not been reported. Relapses often respond to reinstitution of therapy, regardless of the neuroleptic agent used.

The literature includes one report of suicide in a 40-year-old man with DP [21] and another of attempted homicide [22].

## Conclusions

DP is a chronic delusional and somatoform disorder with mixed outcomes. With the ever-growing number of people traveling to exotic countries, we anticipate that more patients with these disorders will attend travel/tropical medicine clinics, which specialize in post-travel problems. It is, therefore, important to be aware of this unique and rare disorder. Although travel and tropical medicine clinicians may feel uncomfortable with the diagnosis and management of patients with DP, they need to understand that psychiatric evaluation is usually not an option. However, consultation with a psychiatric colleague and having him or her observe one's interaction with the patient in a discreet manner may be helpful. In any case, the management of DP takes considerable empathy, time, and patience. On the other hand, the rewards of successful therapy and of the effort it takes to achieve it are enormous, not only for the patient and his or her family but also for the physician personally.

# References

1 Wilson JW, Miller HE. Delusions of parasitosis. *Arch Derm Syphilol* 1946;54:39–56.

2 Kleinman A, Eisenberg L, Good B. Culture, illness, and care: clinical lessons from anthropologic and cross-cultural research. *Ann Intern Med* 1978;88:251–8.

3 Abramovitch H, Schwartz E. The Three Stages of Medical Dialogue. *Theor Med* 1996;17:175–87.

4 Trabert W. 100 years of delusional parasitosis. Meta-analysis of 1,223 case reports. *Psychopathology* 1995;28(5):238–46.

5 Baker PB, Cook BL, Winokur G. Delusional infestation. The interface of delusions and hallucinations. *Psychiatr Clin North Am* 1995;18:345–61.

6 Reilly TM, Batchelor DH. The presentation and treatment of delusional parasitosis: a dermatological perspective. *Int Clin Psychopharmacol* 1986;1:340–53.

7 Alexander JO'D. *Arthropods and Human Skin.* Berlin: Springer; 1984. p. 391–8.

8 Gieler U, Knoll M. Delusional parasitosis as "folie a trois." *Dermatologica* 1990;181:122–5.

9 Ohtaki N. Delusions of parasitosis—report of 94 cases. *Jap J Dermatol* 1991;101:439–46.

10 Srinivasan TN, Suresh TR, Jayaram V, Fernandez MP. Nature and treatment of delusional parasitosis: a different experience in India. *Int J Dermatol* 1994;33:851–5.

11 Prociv P. Trans-Pacific delusional parasitosis: the suitcase sign. *J Travel Med* 1997;4(3):154–5.

12 Schwartz E, Witztum E, Mumcuoglu KY. Travel as a trigger for shared delusional parasitosis. *J Travel Med* 2001;8(1):26–8.

13 Gill CJ, Hamer DH. "Doc, there's a worm in my stool": Munchausen parasitosis in a returning traveler. *J Travel Med* 2002;9(6):330–2.

14 Goddard, J. Analysis of 11 cases of delusions of parasitosis reported to the Mississippi Department of Health. *South Med J* 1995;88:837–9.

15 Murase JE, Wu JJ, Koo J. Morgellons disease: a rapport-enhancing term for delusions of parasitosis. *J Am Acad Dermatol* 2006;55:913–14.

16 Lyell A. Delusions of parasitosis. *Br J Dermatol* 1983:108:485–99.

17 Steinert T, Studemund H. Acute delusional parasitosis under treatment with ciprofloxacin. *Pharmacopsychiatry* 2006 1;39(4):159–60.

18 Lorenzo CR, Koo J. Pimozide in dermatologic practice. *Am J Clin Dermatol* 2004;5:339–49.

19 Lee CS. Delusions of parasitosis. *Dermatol Ther* 2008;21:2–7.

20 Editorial: Delusions of parasitosis. *Br Med J* 1977;84:790–1.

21 Monk BE, Rao YJ. Delusions of parasitosis with fatal outcome. *Clin Exp Dermatol* 1994;19(4):341–2.

22 Bourgeois ML, Duhamel P, Verdoux H. Delusional parasitosis: folie à deux and attempted murder of a family doctor. *Br J Psychiatry* 1992;161:709–11.

# Syndromic Approach

# 36 Approach to Patients with Post-Travel Diarrhea

Eli Schwartz[1] and Bradley A. Connor[2]

[1]Chaim Sheba Medical Center, Tel Hashomer, Israel and Sackler School of Medicine, Tel Aviv University, Tel Aviv, Israel
[2]Weill Medical College of Cornell University, New York, USA

## Introduction

Gastrointestinal illnesses are the most common disorders in travelers, with up to 70% of travelers affected by travelers' diarrhea (TD) during travel [1, 2]. Gastrointestinal (GI) complaints are also the most common cause for seeking medical advice post-travel, accounting for about 40% of all referrals [3]. However, there are differences between the "during" and "post-travel" presentations. Whereas bacterial diarrhea is reported as the main cause of TD, in post-travel referrals chronic diarrhea and chronic GI complaints become the major reasons for seeking medical care. The explanation for this discrepancy is the relatively short incubation period and the usually mild and self-limited nature of the bacterial diarrhea group, which usually resolves during the trip. The chronic GI complaints may be due to parasitic infections, which have longer incubation periods and tend to be more chronic, or alternatively to noninfectious conditions. Because in most cases stool tests are negative in these patients, the clinician who cares for post-travel patients faces a greater challenge.

## Clinical definition

Most studies define TD as the passing of three or more unformed stools per day in association with at least one other enteric symptom, such as nausea, vomiting, cramps, bloating, fecal urgency, tenesmus, or the passage of bloody, mucoid stool.

However, because travel-related diarrhea is not a single disease but rather a multietiologic syndrome, symptoms may differ according to the different pathogens (mainly bacterial vs parasitic), and on many occasions GI complaints may be disturbing enough for patients to seek medical care but without having the criteria of >3 unformed stools. Parenthetically, patients may complain of constipation with other enteric symptoms.

Symptoms may also be divided according to their duration from onset. Those who are seen within 2 weeks of onset of symptoms are said to have *acute diarrhea*, and those who are seen with more than 2 weeks of symptoms are defined as having *persistent or chronic diarrhea*.

## Acute diarrhea

Acute post-travel diarrhea may be due to viral, bacterial, or parasitic infection.

### Bacterial diarrheas

The bacterial diarrheas are usually characterized by the sudden onset of uncomfortable diarrhea, usually as very frequent watery diarrhea, associated with additional enteric symptoms, such as nausea, vomiting, and abdominal cramping. Fever may be present, in many cases preceding or at the onset of the enteric complaints.

The most common pathogen is enterotoxigenic *Escherichia coli*, followed by *Campylobacter jejuni*, *Shigella* spp., and *Salmonella* spp. Enteroadherent and other *E. coli* species have been found to be common pathogens in bacterial diarrhea.

In post-travel bacterial diarrhea, the most commonly isolated pathogens reported are *Campylobacter* species, followed by *Shigella* and nontyphoidal *Salmonella* [3].

*Tropical Diseases in Travelers*, 1st edition. Edited by E. Schwartz.
© 2009 by Blackwell Publishing, ISBN: 978-1-4051-8441-0.

Although less common in the post-travel setting, diarrhea may lead to hospitalization. Between 3% and 14% of adult hospital admissions after travel are reported to be due to febrile gastroenteritis.

The incubation period of bacterial diarrhea is short, about 1–3 days. Thus, patients will present shortly after their arrival, unless they were infected back home with similar pathogens.

## Diagnosis

The diagnosis of bacterial diarrhea is based on a positive stool culture. However, this method has several limitations. The chance to recover a pathogen even in the best laboratory is no more than 50%. The most common pathogens causing bacterial diarrhea are pathogenic *E. coli*, which in most laboratories are not routinely tested for. In addition, results of stool culture are relatively slow, with results usually taking up to 3 days. Thus, stool culture in general is not a useful tool for clinicians.

Direct stool examination that reveals excess white blood cells is highly suggestive of bacterial infection. This test is simple and rapid, but it is not available in every clinic and is generally underused.

Thus, decisions on treatment should be based on the clinical symptoms and their severity.

## Treatment

The principles that guide treatment of the returned traveler with acute travelers' diarrhea apply as well to enlightened self-treatment by the traveler acutely ill with travelers' diarrhea in the field. As bacterial causes of travelers' diarrhea far outnumber other microbial etiologies, empirical treatment with an antibiotic directed at enteric bacterial pathogens remains the most definitive therapy for travelers' diarrhea. Adjunctive agents, such as loperamide, may be used for symptom control. The benefits of antibiotic treatment of travelers' diarrhea are clear, with treated travelers experiencing both faster resolution and less severe diarrhea. A recent Cochrane analysis demonstrated that travelers receiving antibiotics were almost six times more likely to have rapid resolution of diarrhea than untreated travelers [4]. This may ultimately translate to a lower likelihood of developing persistent diarrhea and postinfectious sequelae of diarrhea, such as Guillain–Barré syndrome, reactive arthritis, and more commonly and importantly, postinfectious irritable bowel syndrome (PI-IBS) (see Chapter 17).

The history of antibiotic treatment for travelers' diarrhea has been marked by the almost universal development of resistance amongst bacterial enteropathogens to commonly used antibiotics, beginning in the 1970s and early 1980s with trimethoprim/sulfamethoxazole and doxycycline and in the early 1990s and early 2000s initially with quinolone-resistant *Campylobacter* and now other quinolone-resistant enteric bacterial pathogens [5]. With a growing recognition of resistance patterns, the choice of empirical antibiotic treatment needs to be matched as well as possible to the destination. Unfortunately, there is no clear threshold as to when antibiotic resistance mandates a change in empirical treatment. Thus, quinolones are still recommended by many authorities. Azithromycin has now become the treatment of choice for bacterial diarrhea in travelers returning from Thailand, where the highest rate of *Campylobacter* resistance is reported, and in febrile gastroenteritis in most regions (Figure 36.1).

## Viral diarrheas

Viral gastroenteritis often cannot be distinguished clinically from bacterial diarrhea at the outset, but studies show that viruses account for a maximum of 10% of cases of travelers' diarrhea for most common travel destinations. Vomiting is usually a more predominant feature of viral gastroenteritis. Viral diarrhea can be caused by a number of viral pathogens, including noroviruses, rotaviruses, and astroviruses.

Toxic gastroenteritis, which is caused by the ingestion of preformed toxins and not by a bacterial enteric infection, does not appear to be a common cause of travelers' diarrhea, and it is self-limited in its course.

## Protozoan diarrheas

A major difference between diarrhea during travel and post-travel is that whereas bacterial pathogens are the main cause of travelers' diarrhea, in post-travel diarrhea, even shortly after travel, parasitic diseases are more common, with *Giardia* being the leading identifiable cause.

Protozoan diarrhea is often characterized by gradual onset and less severe diarrhea. Often, weeks of symptoms elapse before medical care is sought. In many cases, it is not the diarrhea but rather the other intestinal symptoms that bring the patient to medical care. These symptoms may include alternating diarrhea and constipation, increased gas and bloating, foul-smelling burps, and increased fatigue. In some cases, low-grade fever may accompany them.

Protozoan diarrhea usually has a minimum incubation period of 7–10 days.

**Approach to the patient with acute diarrhea (< 2 weeks duration)**

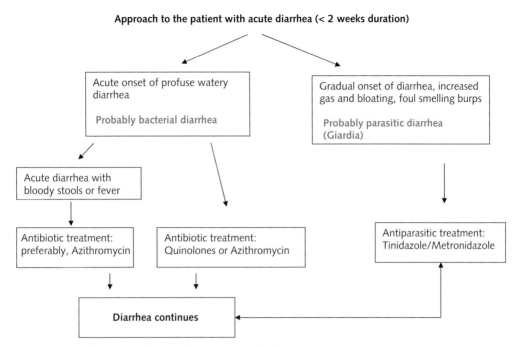

**Figure 36.1** Approach to the patient with acute diarrhea (<2 weeks duration).

*Giardia* is the main protozoal pathogen found in travelers. *Entamoeba histolytica* is relatively uncommon in travelers. *Cryptosporidium parvum* is also relatively uncommon. The risk of *Cyclospora* is highly geographic and seasonal, with the best-known risks in Nepal, Peru, Haiti, and Guatemala. *Dientamoeba fragilis* is occasionally diagnosed in travelers and its role as a causative diarrheal agent is controversial.

### Diagnosis and treatment

The diagnosis of protozoan infection theoretically should be based on direct stool examination with recovery of the protozoa. However, the sensitivity of this test is low. Providing three stool samples may increase the yield of recovery, but it is time-consuming and the sensitivity is still low. Using ELISA tests for antigen detection of *Giardia* and *E. hystolitica* may increase sensitivity, but these are not available in every center, and negative results do not preclude protozoan infection (see Chapter 30).

Thus, a practical approach is to treat the patient according to clinical symptoms, and when symptoms fit protozoan infection, to treat empirically with metronidazole (500 mg × 3/day for 5–7 days) or more conveniently with tinidazole (2 g/day for 3 days), which will cover both giardiasis and amebiasis (Figure 36.1).

### Chronic (persistent) diarrhea and GI complaints

Although travelers' diarrhea is typically a self-limiting illness, some patients may experience a more prolonged clinical course. Diarrhea lasting more than 2 weeks is considered persistent travelers' diarrhea, although other gastrointestinal symptoms such as bloating, cramping, flatulence, nausea, and rectal urgency may predominate. Symptoms such as headache, joint pains, and extreme fatigue may also be present. A "post-travel diarrhea and fatigue syndrome" has been described [6].

### Epidemiology of post-travel diarrhea

In post-travel referrals, chronic diarrhea is the major reason for seeking medical care, with a rate of 10–17% of all referrals [3]. Persistent diarrhea was ranked second in causing inability to work among returning travelers [2].

Several published studies suggest that a certain percentage of individuals with travelers' diarrhea will experience persistent symptoms. One of these studies evaluated the health problems that occurred among 7886 Swiss international tourists after travel to developing countries for ≤3 months [7]. Approximately 1% of patients reported chronic diarrhea, which was defined as persisting illness with at least three unformed stools per day that resulted in at least five medical consultations, hospitalization of at least 5 days, inability to work for at least 15 days, or no cure by 4–7 months after return. A second study estimated the incidence of chronic diarrhea among 4607 US Peace Corps volunteers stationed in 43 countries [8]. During the previous 2 years, an estimated 78 volunteers (1.7%) experienced chronic diarrhea, which was defined as the presence of ≥3 loose stools per day that usually persisted for ≥3 months, marked fecal urgency, the absence of systemic symptoms, and no known etiology. In a third study, persistent diarrhea (i.e., persisting for ≥2 weeks) occurred in 1 of 35 students (2.9%) who had traveled to Latin America [9]. Collectively, these three studies demonstrate that persistent diarrheal illnesses in travelers are not uncommon, with up to 3% of individuals experiencing symptoms for at least 2 weeks and up to several months.

## Etiology

The etiology of prolonged symptoms may be assigned to several categories: persistent infection, co-infection, temporary postinfectious phenomena, malabsorptive syndromes, or underlying GI disease. Recently, postinfectious irritable bowel syndrome (PI-IBS) has gained increased recognition as another potential cause of persistent gastrointestinal symptoms in returned travelers (Table 36.1).

Even though chronic diarrhea is highly prevalent among returning travelers who seek medical care, little information on this condition exists in the published literature. There are numerous reviews with only scanty good systematic studies.

A study that summarized the stool results obtained from travelers who returned from developing countries with post-travel chronic diarrhea and presented to referral centers situated in Israel and in Germany revealed similar results [E. Schwartz, T. Jelinek, unpublished data]. In the two centers, the positive stool finding in each group was present in only 29% of cases (Table 36.2). *G. lamblia* and *E. histolytica* combine to account for 80% of the positive results. Other pathogens such as *Cyclospora cayetanesis*, *Cryptosporidium parvum*, and *Microsporidia*, although thoroughly investigated, were found to consist of only a very few positive results.

The stool specimens were examined in referral centers. This might cause a sample bias in which all who were diagnosed or successfully treated by primary care physicians were unrepresented.

**Table 36.1** Possible etiologies of prolonged travelers' diarrhea.

| Conditions | Considerations |
| --- | --- |
| Persistent infection | Protozoal infection<br>Helminthic infection<br>Persistent bacterial infection (rare) |
| Co-infection | Undocumented additional pathogen<br>*Clostridium difficile* after antibiotic therapy |
| Temporary postinfectious phenomena | Intestinal disaccharidase deficiency<br>Small intestinal bacterial overgrowth |
| Malabsorption | Celiac sprue<br>Tropical sprue |
| Underlying GI disease | Inflammatory bowel disease<br>Colon cancer |
| Postinfectious irritable bowel syndrome | |

As can be seen, most travelers with chronic symptoms have negative stool findings, and it is this majority of patients who become the challenge for the clinician. In addition to those who had initial negative findings, there are some patients with positive stool findings, either those with nonpathogenic protozoa (Table 36.3) or those who will continue to have symptoms despite the fact that pathogen is not recovered after treatment.

Discussion on possible etiologies follow.

**Table 36.2** Stool findings among returning travelers in Israel and Germany.

| | Israel<br>$n = 81$ | Germany<br>$n = 139$ |
| --- | --- | --- |
| Positive findings, total | 24 (29.6%) | 41 (29.5%) |
| *E. histolytica* | 14 (17.2%) | 12 (8.6%) |
| *G. lamblia* | 5 (6.1%) | 21 (15.1%) |
| *B. hominis* | 1 (1.2%) | 8 (5.7%) |
| *Schistosoma* | 1 (1.2%) | 0 |
| Hookworm | 1 (1.2%) | 1 (0.7%) |
| *Entamoeba coli* | 2 (2.4%) | 6 (4.3%) |
| *Cryptosporidium* | 0 | 0 |
| *Cyclospora/Microsporidium* | 0 | 2 (1.4%) |
| Others | 0 | 0 |

**Table 36.3** Nonpathogenic protozoa.

*Entamoeba* spp. (non-*histolytica*)
   *E. hartmani*
   *E. moshkovskii*
   *E. coli*
   *E. dispar* (morphologically similar to *E. histolytica*)
*Endolimax nana*
*Iodameba bütschlii*
*Chilomastix mesnii*
*Enteromonas hominis*
*Blastocystitis hominis* (questionable role as a pathogen)

### Persistent infection

The infecting pathogen should be considered in the evaluation of individuals with persistent travelers' diarrhea. In general, the usual approach is to rule out a persistent bacterial or protozoan infection.

Although bacteria such as *Salmonella* may persist, bacterial pathogens are rarely associated with persistent symptoms. Conversely, parasites (protozoa and helminths) are more likely to cause protracted illness in travelers, particularly in patients who describe an insidious onset of symptoms. Parasitic infections probably represent the most common cause of persistent diarrhea in returning travelers. With symptoms continuing for more than 14 days, parasitic causes are more likely. In travelers to Nepal, protozoans were detected in 10% of travelers with symptoms for less than 14 days and in 27% of those with symptoms for more than 14 days [10, 11]. The most common protozoan pathogen isolated in travelers with persistent diarrheal symptoms is *G. lamblia*. Other protozoan pathogens that cause prolonged illness include *Cyclospora* and *Cryptosporidium*, which are much less common in travelers. For some patients with persistent diarrhea, a stool analysis by microscopy may only identify "nonpathogenic" protozoa such as *E. coli*, *Endolimax nana*, *Iodamoeba büetschlii*, and the questionable pathogen *Blastocystitis hominis*, which most authorities consider nonpathogenic (Table 36.3; see Chapter 30).

As mentioned above, in many travelers with chronic diarrhea, stool findings are negative. A negative stool test does not preclude occult infection.

There are several possible explanations for the high negative detection rate reported. One possible explanation is that the current methods for the detection of known infectious pathogens have low sensitivity. The sensitivity of laboratory detection of intestinal protozoa depends on several factors, including the number and types of specimens collected, the processing methods employed, and the experience and training of laboratory staff involved in the identification of these organisms. In addition, the shed of protozoa in the stool might be intermittent, necessitating repeated stool tests.

Another possibility that should not be ignored is that some enteric pathogens have yet to be discovered. Thus, symptomatic patients may have unrecognized pathogens in their GI tracts. The fact that *Cryptosporidium* and *Cyclospora* were only discovered in the last two decades supports this hypothesis.

### Co-infection

Persistent diarrhea may be due to co-infection with an untreated second infection (e.g., *Giardia*) in patients effectively treated for a different pathogen.

*Clostridium difficile* infections may be a cause of persistent diarrhea in returned travelers, because many travelers have had a history of prior treatment of diarrheal episodes or other infection with antibiotics. *C. difficile* may also result from the use of doxycycline as an antimalarial chemoprophylactic agent [12].

Even though fluoroquinolones are still recommended as a first-line treatment and prophylaxis option for traveler's diarrhea, and *C. difficile* associated disease has been shown to be associated with fluroquinolone use [13], *C. difficile* infections are uncommonly reported in travelers [14]. A careful history of prior antibiotic used during travel is important in suggesting this diagnosis. An examination of stool for *C. difficile* toxin should be included as part of the workup.

Another phenomenon that may lead to persistent symptoms is small intestinal *bacterial overgrowth*. An acute enteric infection can cause changes in small bowel motility and lead to stasis and secondary bacterial overgrowth, although this condition is rarely found in returning travelers.

Noninfectious causes for the syndrome that should be considered are as follow:

### Temporary postinfectious phenomena

Temporary postinfectious phenomena may cause persistent symptoms in returned travelers as a result of gastrointestinal damage or compromise. For example, an attack of acute infectious diarrhea may precipitate intestinal disaccharidase deficiency (e.g., lactase or sucrase deficiency). Patients typically report symptoms of chronic diarrhea, abdominal pain, and gaseous distention. These symptoms usually resolve within a few weeks, although certain individuals with a genetic predisposition may have permanent lactose intolerance unmasked by an acute episode of infectious diarrhea. Thus, a nonpharmacological recommendation for patients with chronic diarrhea is a trial of a lactose-free diet.

## Malabsorption

Persistent diarrhea, especially when accompanied by weight loss, may be related to malabsorption. *Tropical sprue* is a clinical entity of unknown etiology that is associated with chronic diarrheal illness and malabsorption, mainly in long-term travelers and expatriates in developing countries [15]. Tropical sprue, however, is very uncommon in returning travelers [16].

More common is celiac sprue, which may be unmasked by an acute episode of infectious diarrhea and present as persistent travelers' diarrhea. *Celiac sprue*, an autoimmune inflammatory condition of the bowel, has become more easily diagnosed by serological tests. Thus, part of the evaluation of persistent diarrhea in the patient should be serologies for endomysial and tissue transglutaminase antibodies. Celiac disease is generally responsive to a gluten-free diet.

## Underlying gastrointestinal disease

Travelers' diarrhea may also uncover an underlying chronic GI disease. A review of the case notes for 129 returned travelers with *bloody diarrhea* admitted to the Hospital for Tropical Diseases in London from 1978 to 1984 found that a quarter of the patients (32/129) had inflammatory bowel disease (IBD), and an additional two patients (2%) had colon cancer [17]. Other clinicians have described the detection of colon cancer in a patient who developed diarrhea during international travel. Therefore, the clinician should be alert to alarming symptoms and signs of fever, bloody diarrhea, nocturnal diarrhea, and weight loss that are not typical for post-travel chronic diarrhea. In addition, blood tests are typically normal in post-travel chronic diarrhea. Thus, inflammatory signs such as high sedimentation rate, C-reactive protein, and thrombocytosis are all alarming signs. Appearance of anemia should also prompt further evaluation.

Elderly travelers, especially when there is a family history of GI malignancy, should have GI screening.

## Postinfectious irritable bowel syndrome (PI-IBS)

A diagnosis of PI-IBS should be considered in returned travelers with chronic symptoms for which no specific etiology is identified. PI-IBS is associated with an onset of IBS symptoms after an acute episode of enteric infection in patients with previously normal bowel function. In-

creasing evidence supports PI-IBS as a specific diagnosis [18]. Acknowledgment of PI-IBS represents a paradigm shift in assuming that a peripheral event (infection) leads to prolonged, permanent changes in GI function.

In the context of travelers' diarrhea, PI-IBS has been defined as new IBS symptoms by Rome III criteria:
- At least 3 months of symptoms (need not be consecutive)
- Onset of at least 6 months previously of recurrent abdominal pain or discomfort associated with two or more of the following features: improvement with defecation, onset associated with a change in the frequency of stool, or onset associated with a change in form (appearance) of stool
- Following an episode of gastroenteritis or travelers' diarrhea
- Workup for microbial pathogens and underlying GI disease is negative [18].

Although not conclusive, epidemiological studies suggest that PI-IBS may be a relatively common complication of travelers' diarrhea. Increasing etiological and pathological data highlight the importance of effective prevention and treatment of acute bacterial illness as a strategy to reduce the risk of PI-IBS. Quantitative histology data indicating persistent low-grade inflammation following an acute enteric infection support additional studies to investigate the potential benefits of anti-inflammatory agents and antibiotics in the treatment of PI-IBS [19].

One of the important criteria for PI-IBS is that the workup for enteric microbial pathogens is negative. When physical examination and laboratory workup are normal, the main differential diagnosis is usually between persistent parasitic infection and postinfectious IBS. However, because stool tests for ova and parasites are relatively insensitive, broad-spectrum antiparasitic treatment might be warranted to exclude an infectious etiology. Clinical experience suggests that travelers may respond to antiparasitic therapy even when repeated stool tests are negative.

## The approach to the patient

A detailed medical history should be taken, which will both help in the assessment of the patient and allow a more comprehensive follow-up of the patient's condition, particularly in tracking any improvement subsequent to medical intervention.

Common symptoms of parasitic infections, as described above, may include alternating diarrhea and constipation, increased gas and bloating, foul-smelling burps, and increased fatigue. Many patients will describe a cyclic pattern of symptoms, with several days of suffering from gastrointestinal complaints accompanied by significant fatigue (often affecting their daily activities), alternating with periods of well-being. In contrast to patients with chronic fatigue syndrome, in most cases, there is no depression or other overt psychological disturbance.

Physical examination as a rule is normal. Typically, despite the prolonged GI symptoms, there is no weight loss.

Unusual symptoms or abnormal physical findings such as bloody diarrhea, nocturnal diarrhea, and fever should prompt a full systemic and GI evaluation. These symptoms, however, as stated earlier, are only found in a minority of patients.

## Laboratory workup

Stool tests should be ordered, preferably three times for ova and parasites, as this will increase sensitivity by 10–30%, depending on the pathogen [20]. ELISA antigen detection assays for *G. lamblia* and *E. histolytica* also increase sensitivity of the stool test. Acid fast staining of stool specimens is required for the detection of *Cyclospora*, *Cryptosporidia*, and *Isospora* spp. This test is not done routinely in most laboratories; however, these pathogens are uncommon in travelers (see Table 36.2). *C. difficile* toxin should be checked when the history suggests antibiotic-associated diarrhea.

When stool tests are positive for pathogenic parasites, treatment should be given accordingly.

Blood tests may help in several aspects. A complete blood count in some cases may reveal eosinophilia, which together with GI complaints may point to a helminthic infection (protozoa such as *G. lamblia* or *E. histolytica*, as a rule, do not cause eosinophilia). In these cases, anthelminthic treatment is recommended , and albendazole, a broad spectrum anthelminthic, covers most pathogens (see also Chapter 39).

B12 may occasionally be low, even without any dietary restriction of the patient.

Other blood tests should be performed to exclude any systemic disease.

Anemia is not part of the common parasitic infection presentation and therefore should be evaluated if found.

Laboratory evidence of active inflammation, such as high sedimentation rate, high C-reactive protein, thrombocytosis, and abnormal liver function tests, should prompt systemic evaluation (including IBD and colon cancer).

**Table 36.4** Intestinal protozoa associated with chronic diarrhea and irritable bowel syndrome-like symptoms.

| Species | Global distribution | Stool diagnosis |
|---|---|---|
| *G. intestinalis* | Worldwide | Permanent stain, antigen detection assay |
| *E. histolytica* | Developing countries | Permanent stain, antigen detection assay |
| *D. fragilis* | Worldwide | Permanent stain fixation of fecal material |
| *Cr. parvum* | Worldwide | Modified acid fast stain |
| *C. cayetanensis* | Developing countries | Modified acid fast stain |
| *Bl. hominis* | Worldwide | Wet preparation |
| *Isospora belli* | Tropical, developing countries | Wet preparation |
| *B. coli* | Developing countries, particularly warm and temperate climates | Wet preparations |

*Source:* Reprinted from Stark D, van Hal S, Marriott D, Ellis J, Harkness J. Irritable bowel syndrome: a review on the role of intestinal protozoa and the importance of their detection and diagnosis. *Int J Parasitol* 2007;37:11–20, with permission from Elsevier.

TSH should also be evaluated, because abnormal function may affect the GI system.

Because infection may unmask celiac disease, celiac serologies should be checked.

HIV should be excluded because positive cases necessitate further evaluation, which is beyond the scope of the chapter.

If all of these tests are normal, including the stool test, which is the situation in most cases, the main differential diagnoses are unrecognized persistent parasitic infection and PI-IBS.

## Treatment

Infectious diarrhea may cause temporary lactase deficiency and, therefore, a trial of a lactose-free diet is recommended. In fact, many patients may report that their

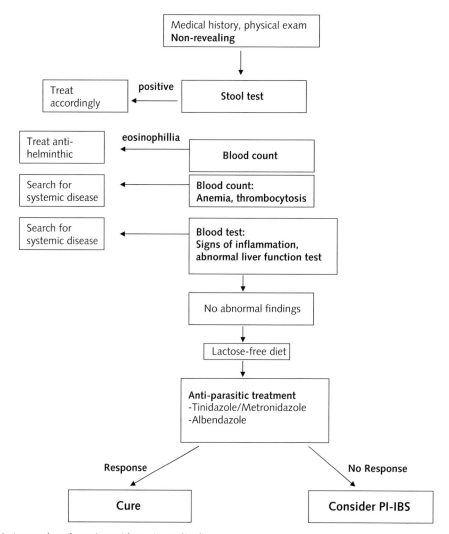

**Figure 36.2** Approach to the patient with persistent diarrhea.

symptoms are aggravated after dairy meals. Additionally, low-volume meals may be helpful.

Because several protozoa may cause IBS-like symptoms (Table 36.4), and sensitivity of stool tests is far from being optimal, we recommend a trial of broad-spectrum antiparasitic treatment.

The treatment recommended is tinidazole 2g/day for 2–3 days (preferable to metronidazole), and if there is no response, followed by albendazole 400 mg b.i.d. for 5–7 days. This regimen will cover a broad spectrum of protozoa, helminths, and *C. difficile* as well. It should be remembered that albendazole, in addition to its broad anthelmintic activity, is valuable for metronidazole-resistant giardia-

sis. When there is no response to treatment, a diagnosis of PI-IBS is probably established and further evaluation and treatment by a gastroenterologist may be warranted (Figure 36.2).

## Lesson from travel medicine for the developed world

Diarrheal diseases are very common in travelers and often are due to infectious agents. However, diarrheal diseases exist as well in industrialized countries in those without a history of travel to developing countries. Clinicians in industrialized countries may fail to consider infectious diseases in the differential diagnosis of patients with diarrhea.

Although the contribution of viruses is higher in Western countries, with seasonal outbreaks of norovirus occurring annually, acute diarrhea may be caused by pathogens similar to those seen in travelers, even without a travel history. As mentioned above, stool culture has several limitations for clinical decisions, so it may not be unreasonable to consider a course of empirical antibiotic treatment. Short-course antibiotics may quickly alleviate suffering, and may prevent unnecessary hospitalization even in the Western setting.

Chronic diarrhea is not an uncommon complaint in industrialized countries and may be due to parasitic infection even without a travel history, as some protozoa have worldwide distribution (Table 36.4). Fecal–oral transmission may occur in restaurants in the West where large populations of persons from endemic countries are working, in homes with housekeepers from endemic countries, after camping in the countryside, and in other circumstances.

In cases acquired in the Western countries, clinicians may neglect to order stool for ova and parasites. Because antiparasitic treatment is safe and short, it should be considered also in these cases without a travel history and with negative stool microscopy, as it may prevent prolonged suffering and save the costs associated with lengthy and invasive medical evaluations.

# References

1 DuPont HL, Ericsson CD. Prevention and treatment of traveler's diarrhea. *N Engl J Med* 1993;328:1821–37.

2 Steffen R, Rickenbach M, Wilhelm U, Helminger A, Schär M. Health problems after travel to developing countries. *J Infect Dis* 1987;156:84–91.

3 Freedman DO, Weld LH, Kozarsky PE, Fisk T, Robins R, von Sonnenburg F, et al. Spectrum of disease and relation to place of exposure among ill returned travelers. *N Engl J Med* 2006;354:119–30.

4 Al-Abri SS, Beeching NJ, Nye FJ. Traveller's diarrhea. *Lancet Infect Dis* 2005;5:349–60.

5 Hoge CW, Gambel JM, Srijan A, Pitarangsi C, Echeverria P. Trends in antimicrobial resistance among diarrheal

pathogens isolated in Thailand over 15 years. *Clin Infect Dis* 1998;26:341–5.

6 Schwartz E, Connor B. Chronic post-travel fatigue (CPTF) syndrome. 5th Conference of the International Society of Travel Medicine. Geneva: Switzerland; March 1997.

7 Steffen R. Epidemiology of travellers' diarrhoea. *Scand J Gastroenterol Suppl* 1983;84:5–17.

8 Addiss DG, Tauxe RV, Bernard KW. Chronic diarrhoeal illness in US Peace Corps volunteers. *Int J Epidemiol.* 1990;19:217–18.

9 Merson MH, Morris GK, Sack DA. Travelers' diarrhea in Mexico: a prospective study of physicians and family members attending a congress. *N Engl J Med* 1976;294:1299.

10 Hoge CW, Shlim DR, Echeverria P., et al. Epidemiology of diarrhea among expatriate residents living in a highly endemic environment. *JAMA* 1996;275:533–8.

11 Taylor DN, Houston R, Shlim DR, Bhaibulaya M, Ungar BLP, Echeverria P. Etiology of diarrhea among travelers and foreign residents in Nepal. *JAMA* 1988;260:1245–8.

12 Golledge CL, Riley TV. *Clostridium difficile*-associated diarrhoea after doxycycline malaria prophylaxis. *Lancet* 1995;345:1377–8.

13 Loo VG, Poirier L, Miller MA, et al. A predominantly clonal multi-institutional outbreak of *Clostridium difficile*-associated diarrhea with high morbidity and mortality. *N Engl J Med* 2005;353:2442–9.

14 Norman FF, Pérez-Molina J, Pérez de Ayala A, Jiménez BC, Navarro M, López-Vélez R. *Clostridium difficile*-associated diarrhea after antibiotic treatment for traveler's diarrhea. *Clin Infect Dis* 2008;46:1060–63.

15 Walker MM. What is tropical sprue? *J Gastroenterol Hepatol* 2003;18:887–90.

16 Klipstein FA. Tropical sprue in travelers and expatriates living abroad. *Gastro* 1981;80:590–600.

17 Harries AD, Myers B, Cook GC. Inflammatory bowel disease: a common cause of bloody diarrhoea in visitors to the tropics. *Br Med J (Clin Res Ed)* 1985;291:1686–7.

18 Connor BA. Sequelae of traveler's diarrhea: focus on postinfectious irritable bowel syndrome. *Clin Infect Dis* 2005;41(suppl 8):S577–S586.

19 Spiller RC. Postinfectious irritable bowel syndrome. *Gastroenterology* 2003;124:1662–71.

20 Hiatt RA, Markell EK, Ng E. How many stool examinations are necessary to detect pathogenic intestinal protozoa? *Am J Trop Med Hyg* 1995;53:36–9.

21 Stark D, van Hal S, Marriott D, Ellis J, Harkness J. Irritable bowel syndrome: a review on the role of intestinal protozoa and the importance of their detection and diagnosis. *Int J Parasitol* 2007;37:11–20.

# 37 Approach to Patients with Fever

Eli Schwartz

Chaim Sheba Medical Center, Tel Hashomer, Israel and Sackler School of Medicine, Tel Aviv University, Tel Aviv, Israel

## Introduction

Fever in the returned traveler is one of the most challenging conditions to treat because it may be the manifestation of a self-limited, trivial infection, but it can also presage an infection that could be rapidly progressive and lethal. International travel expands the list of infections that must be considered but does not eliminate common, worldwide (cosmopolitan) infections. Initial attention should focus most urgently on infections that are treatable and transmissible and that cause serious sequelae or death.

The art of taking a medical history is essential in these cases, and in addition to this skill, which is taught in medical schools, getting a detailed travel history is mandatory. The characteristics of the places visited, types of exposure, and time frame of the travel are highly valuable in evaluating the patient.

This chapter will focus on the pertinent issues that help to identify the cause of fever in a returned traveler.

## Epidemiology of fever in returning travelers

Fever, in the absence of other prominent findings, has been reported in 2–3% of European and American travelers to developing countries. Among 784 American travelers who traveled for 3 months or less to developing countries, 3% reported fever that was not associated with other illnesses [1]. These results are similar to those reported in classic studies by Steffen et al., in which about 2% of 7886 Swiss travelers reported "high fevers over several days" on questionnaires completed several

months after return from short visits to developing countries. Of those with fever, 39% reported fever only while abroad, 37% had fevers while abroad and at home, and 24% had fevers at home only [2].

In the GeoSentinel database, among 17,353 ill returned travelers, fever was the second most common complaint (after gastrointestinal complaints), accounting for about 25% of the cases, including outpatients and hospitalized patients [3] (see Chapter 3, Figure 3.2). Among inpatients, this rate is expected to be higher, as was shown in an Israeli study in which 77% of hospitalized travelers had been admitted for fever evaluation [4]. Among the outpatient Israeli population, fever was still a major reason to seek medical care, but accounted for only 29% of those seeking post-travel care.

## Causes of fever in returned travelers

Several studies have examined the causes of fever after tropical travel. Malaria poses by far the most frequent cause in hospitalized patients, with a prevalence ranging between 13% and 48% (see Chapter 3, Table 3.2).

Dengue fever is the second most common cause of fever in most studies. Whereas malaria is mainly seen in travelers returned from Sub-Saharan Africa, dengue is more common than malaria in all other tropical and subtropic areas [3].

The largest published case series in travelers, that of GeoSentinel, which examined the causes of fever seen in both hospitalized and outpatient settings, demonstrated the major groups of febrile illnesses, as shown in Table 37.1 [5]. These findings show that systemic febrile illnesses constituted the largest group, followed by diarrheal and respiratory febrile illnesses. Vaccine-preventable diseases, such as hepatitis and typhoid fever, still account for a number of cases.

*Tropical Diseases in Travelers*, 1st edition. Edited by E. Schwartz.
© 2009 by Blackwell Publishing, ISBN: 978-1-4051-8441-0.

**Table 37.1** Summary of diagnosis group and selected specific diagnosis in febrile patients after travel (6957 febrile patients out of 24,920 ill returned travelers in the GeoSentinel database).

| | |
|---|---|
| Systemic febrile illness (35%) | Malaria 21% |
| | Dengue 6% |
| | Enteric fever 2% |
| | Rickettsia 2% |
| Unspecified febrile illness (22%) | |
| Acute diarrhea (15%) | Travelers' diarrhea |
| | Acute gastroenteritis |
| Respiratory illness (14%) | Pneumonia |
| | Bronchitis |
| | Tonsilitis |
| | Sinusitis |
| Vaccine preventable (3%) | Hepatitis A, B |
| | Enteric fever |

*Source:* Reprinted from Wilson ME, Weld LH, Boggild A, et al. Fever in returned travelers: results from the GeoSentinel Surveillance Network. *Clin Infect Dis* 2007;44:1560–8, with permission from University of Chicago Press.

Among the systemic febrile illnesses, malaria, dengue, enteric fever, and rickettsial diseases were the most common (Table 37.1). Also, in these large case series, malaria was the most common specific agent identified [5].

It is interesting to note that the cause of fever remained undefined in about one-fourth of cases in the GeoSentinel study, and similar results were reported even in case series of hospitalized patients in referral medical institutions (Table 37.1 and Table 3.2). However, these cases are usually associated with favorable outcomes [6].

## Differences between travelers and local populations

Important differences exist between travelers to developing countries and local residents in terms of types of infections commonly seen and their clinical manifestations. These differences reflect variations in both likelihood of exposure to infections and intensity of exposure, which is higher in local populations, as well as differences in background immunity. For example, melioidosis (caused by the gram-negative soil- and water-associated bacterium *Burkholderia pseudomallei*) is a common cause of community-acquired sepsis in northern Thailand, yet is rarely seen in travelers (see Table 41.1). The same holds true for sleeping sickness, filarial infection, and cholera,

which are rarely seen in travelers. On the other hand, due to background immunity, malaria in adult populations of endemic countries may not cause a life-threatening disease and is normally not expressed as a febrile illness, whereas in travelers, even low-grade parasitemia may cause a severe and life-threatening condition.

Another example is acute schistosomiasis (Katayama syndrome), which is an immune-complex-mediated disease and is commonly seen in travelers and persons newly infected with schistosomiasis, but not in residents of endemic areas who have been repeatedly exposed to the parasite (see details in Chapter 24).

## Approach to the patient with fever

In addition to the patient's signs and symptoms, pertinent information concerning the travel history needs to be taken into consideration. These aspects can be summarized in the acronym S.I.T.E. and will be discussed in detail.

Signs and symptoms
Incubation
Travel—where
Exposed—to what

### Incubation period

Incubation time is an extremely valuable clue in evaluating the febrile patient. In many instances, the exact day of exposure cannot be determined (e.g., in food-borne or mosquitoe-borne diseases, where the exact day of exposure during the trip is unknown). However, the time interval from departure from the endemic area to onset of fever is known, and that should be considered the minimal incubation period (assuming a possibility of exposure on the last day in the endemic area). The time interval from the beginning of the trip to the onset of fever should be considered the "maximal incubation time" [ Figure 37.1]. Understanding these incubation periods can enable the exclusion of infections that are not biologically plausible. For example, dengue fever typically has an incubation time of 3–14 days. Thus, fever that begins more than 2 weeks after return from endemic areas is not likely to be related to dengue fever. On the other hand, in cases of fever that begin immediately after a short stay (e.g., < a week), the maximum incubation time (Figure 37.1) is less than 1 week, which excludes all diseases with longer incubation periods, such as malaria (usually 10–14 days), viral hepatitis, and so on.

In cases where fever begins shortly after return from a long travel, the differential diagnosis is very wide, because

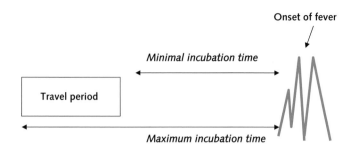

**Figure 37.1** Estimation of incubation period.

it may include all the diseases with short incubation periods and also diseases with prolonged incubation periods.

In contrast, the list of infections that may occur more than 3 months after return is very limited and includes non-falciparum malaria, amebic liver abscess, and hepatitis B. Visceral leishmaniasis is another possibility, but is rarely seen in travelers (Table 37.2).

In a GeoSentinel study, the majority of ill returned travelers with systemic febrile illnesses present fairly soon after their return, with the majority being admitted to hospital within 1–2 weeks [5]. However, a substantial number may present later, with *Plasmodium vivax* being a dominant pathogen, especially in those who took malaria chemoprophylaxis [7].

Approximately 30% of patients with vivax malaria in the USA had their onset of symptoms more than 6 months after return. In 2–4% of cases of malaria, symptoms began a year or more after return [8, 9,]. It is important to note that falciparum malaria is rarely seen in travelers as a late infection (>3 months after return ); however, among

immigrants, late falciparum infection is well documented [10]. This fact highlights the importance of travel history in all cases, because remote travel that may lead to fever may easily be overlooked by the patient and by the physician.

Table 37.2 lists many of the common febrile infections seen in travelers according to their incubation times. As mentioned, in assessing potential incubation periods, one must take into account the duration of the trip (and points of potential exposure during travel) and time from return to onset of fever.

## Geographic area of exposure

The most common systemic febrile illnesses are listed in Table 37.3. However, as shown, they are not evenly distributed within the tropics. Falciparum malaria is the most common pathogen seen in Sub-Saharan Africa, whereas dengue is the most common febrile disease outside of Africa, with the highest attack rate in Southeast Asia and the India subcontinent [11].

**Table 37.2** Causes of fever by usual incubation periods.

| Incubation time | Viral | Bacterial | Parasites |
|---|---|---|---|
| Short<br>< 14 days | Dengue fever<br>Chikungunia<br>West Nile fever<br>Acute HIV fever<br>Viral<br>hemorrhagic fever | Bacterial diarrhea<br>Typhoid fever<br>Leptospirosis<br>Rickettsiosis<br>Relapsing fever<br>Meningococcemia | Malaria (all species)<br>Acute histoplasmosis |
| Medium<br>14–60 days | Hepatitis A, E<br>Acute HIV | Typhoid fever<br>Brucellosis<br>Q fever | Acute schistosomiasis<br><br>Malaria (all species) |
| Long<br>> 60 days | Hepatitis B<br>Rabies | Tuberculosis | Malaria<br>(non-falciparum)<br>Amebic liver abscess<br>Visceral leishmaniasis |

**Table 37.3** Main etiologies of fever according to region visited.

|  | Sub-Saharan Africa (N = 1401) | Southeast Asia (N = 381) | Latin America (N = 146) | North Africa and Middle East (N = 103) |
|---|---|---|---|---|
| Falciparum malaria | 30% | 2% | 0 | 1% |
| Non-falciparum malaria | 5% | 9% | 4% | 4% |
| Rickettsia | 5% | 2% | 0 | 1% |
| Dengue | 0.1% | 13% | 8% | 0% |
| Acute schistosomiasis | 2% | 0 | 0 | 0 |
| Enteric fever | 0.2% | 3.4 % | 0 | 0 |
| Cosmopolitan causes | 30% | 41% | 45% | 41% |
| Unknown | 24% | 21% | 33% | 39% |

*Source*: From [5].

Enteric fever is most commonly seen in travelers returning from the Indian subcontinent.

The common type of rickettsiosis seen in travelers is *Rickettsia africae*, which is usually seen after travel to the southern part of Africa.

Acute schistosomiasis, which often presents as a febrile disease, is mostly seen in Africa, although recently it has been seen more often in travelers with exposure to the Mekong River in Laos (see Chapter 24).

It is important to know that some diseases that are associated with a specific system, such as the respiratory system, have endemic distributions. For example, histoplasmosis, which is the most common endemic mycosis seen in travelers, is almost invariably restricted to Latin America (see Chapter 29). Meliodosis, which is a bacterial infection, is confined to Southeast Asia, mainly Thailand (see Chapter 41).

## Mode of exposure

Specific types of exposures are associated with specific infections, and therefore getting exposure details from the traveler is important. The common modes of exposure are as follow:

Person-to-person contact
Arthropod-borne
Contaminated food and water
Fresh water exposure

Person-to-person exposure may include air-borne, blood-borne, and sexually transmitted infections. These infections exist in the tropics as well as in the developed countries and will not be discussed here.

Infections that can be acquired by a single bite of an infective arthropod include viruses such as the flaviviruses

(dengue, West Nile) and parasitic infections, with the most important being malaria. However, most patients with mosquito-borne diseases cannot recall specific mosquito bites, and many travelers with a history of mosquito bites will present with unrelated febrile illnesses. More exact information is a history of tick bites, which is less common in travelers but is a mode for the transmission of several specific illnesses such as *R. africae* (tick-bite African fever) and *Borrelia* infection (relapsing fever, Lyme disease).

The same holds true for the ingestion of contaminated food or beverages. On one hand, it is a very common mode for transmitting infections, but on the other hand, it is not specific enough, in that almost all travelers have been exposed to suspect food or beverages. More specific information includes ingestion of raw shellfish (*Clonorchis, Paragonimus*), raw meat (*Trichinella*), or unpasturized milk products (*Brucella*).

Exposure to fresh water by swimming, rafting, and so on is a very important and specific mode of exposure. The two most common diseases seen from this mode of exposure are schistosomiasis and leptospirosis. Whereas schistosmiasis has a very defined geographic distribution, leptospirosis is a worldwide zoonosis (see Chapter 20). Another feature that might be associated with both of these pathogens is the high attack rates among members of the same groups of travelers who had identical exposure. In the case of schistosomiasis, this rate of infection may reach as high as 90% [12].

## Impact of pretravel vaccination

The history should include a review of pretravel vaccines, including dates of vaccination, types of vaccines received, and numbers of doses in the case of multidose vaccines. Vaccines vary greatly in efficacy, and knowledge of vaccination status can influence the probability that certain infections are present. For example, hepatitis A and yellow fever vaccines have high efficacy and only rare instances of infection have been reported in vaccinated travelers. In contrast, the typhoid fever vaccines (oral and parenteral) give incomplete protection for *S. typhi* (estimated to be 60–72%), and do not protect against *S. paratyphi* [13].

## Symptoms and signs

### Clinical presentation

Many febrile infections are associated with focal signs or symptoms, which may help to limit the differential diagnosis. The other chapters provide more detailed discussions of diarrheal, skin, respiratory, and CNS infections. Undifferentiated fever in returning travelers is a more challenging situation.

It is highly important for the physician to remember that focal signs and symptoms might be part of systemic illnesses. For example, in malaria, respiratory symptoms occur in up to half the patients and are not limited to cases of severe malaria with pulmonary edema and ARDS [14]. Similarly, cough is not rare in enteric fever [15] or leptospirosis [16], which are sometimes initially mistaken for a respiratory infection.

*Hemorrhagic fever* usually refers to a group of viral diseases in which the worrisome aspect of their clinical manifestation is hemorrhage (see Chapter 13). These infections usually carry a high mortality rate for the patient, and in addition may carry risk for the caretakers; therefore, vigilance and prompt diagnosis and treatment are essential.

Several systemic infections, in addition to those exotic infections (e.g., Ebola and Marburg), can cause fever and hemorrhage in travelers, and many are treatable. Leptospirosis, meningococcemia, and other bacterial infections can cause hemorrhage. Rickettsial infections can produce a petechial rash or purpura, and severe malaria may be associated with disseminated intravascular coagulation. In the diseases mentioned above, a specific treatment exists and therefore early recognition may save lives.

### Undifferentiated fever

The patient with undifferentiated fever usually presents with high fever and nonspecific symptoms such as headache, asthenia, mild joint pain, and mild gastrointestinal upset (it is often difficult to interpret whether the gastrointestinal complaints are part of the specific febrile illness or acquired separately along the trip).

### Pattern of fever

The pattern of fever received lot of attention and detailed description in the old medical literature. However, in this day and age, with the liberal use of antipyretic medications, it has become much less important.

In spite of this, there are a few patterns of fever to be emphasized.

#### Gradual onset versus acute onset

Several diseases are characterized by an acute onset of spiking fever, sometimes with chills. A good example is dengue. Typhoid fever, on the other hand, is described classically as having a gradual onset of fever with incremental increases in fever until it reaches its maximum (sometime accompanied by relative bradycardia). Malaria also may have a prodromal phase of 1–2 days of an unwell feeling with low-grade fever culminating with spiking fever and rigors.

#### Intermittent fever

In most febrile cases, fever occurs daily. Intermittent fever means an episode of fever separated by days of normal temperature. According to textbooks, tertian malaria, which means a spike in fever every 48 hours (fever on the first day separated by normal temperature and spiking fever again on the third day), may occur with *P. falciparum* and with *P. vivax* infection. In reality, it almost never occurs with falciparum malaria, but this synchronization is quite often seen with vivax malaria. However, the patient usually does not offer this information spontaneously and it should be part of the detailed medical history taken by the clinician.

#### Relapsing fever

In cases of relapsing fever, bouts of several days of fever are separated by several days of normal temperature. This is described in African *Tryponasoma* infection, which is hardly ever seen in travelers. It is, however, a common pattern of untreated *Borrelia* infection (non-Lyme), in which bouts of about 4–5 days of fever are separated by 5–7 days of normal temperature.

### Other physical signs

A careful, complete physical examination should be carried out, looking with special care for rashes or skin lesions, lymphadenopathy, retinal or conjunctival changes, enlargement of the liver or spleen, genital lesions, and neurological findings.

Mild hepatosplenomegaly or lymphadenopathy may be found in several infectious diseases and usually does not help to limit the differential diagnosis. A rash is commonly found in dengue, but in most cases toward the end of the febrile period (4–5 days from onset of fever); thus, rash that appears at the onset of the fever raises the likelihood of some other cosmopolitan viral infection (such as measles).

A skin ulcer (eschar) in a febrile patient who has returned from Africa is highly suggestive of tick-bite African fever (due to *R. africae*) (see Chapter 18).

## Laboratory clues

Results of routine laboratory findings may provide clues to diagnosis in febrile travelers.

### Blood count

An elevated white blood cell count may suggest a typical bacterial infection, but a number of infections that are seen in travelers, such as the bacterial infections of typhoid fever (uncomplicated), leptospirosis, rickettsial infections, and brucellosis, are associated with a normal or low white blood cell count. In addition, malaria is characterized by a low to normal white count, and viral infections are associated with low white counts. Dengue is usually characterized by a very low count ($<3,000/mm^3$) and has the lowest count among the common tropical diseases in travelers [17]. Thus, as a general rule, most of the systemic febrile infections seen in travelers will present with low to normal white counts, usually accompanied by a low level of platelets ($<150,000 \times 10^9$/L). An exception is amebic liver abscesses, which usually present with high white counts.

The hemoglobin level in most of these infections, including malaria, is usually normal (in contrast to local populations, where anemia is the hallmark of malaria). Typhoid fever often presents with mild anemia.

The C reactive protein (CRP) in most of the systemic febrile illnesses will be normal or near normal [17].

### Elevated liver enzymes

Mild elevation of the liver function tests (LFT), mainly of the transaminases, is often seen in many febrile infections, either travel-related or cosmopolitan. Frank hepatitis, in which LFTs are more than 20 times normal (transaminase in thousands), is seen in viral hepatitis. In the past, hepatitis A virus was the most common cause of travel-related hepatitis, but with increasing awareness of this risk and the use of hepatitis A vaccine, acute hepatitis A

now is seen primarily in persons who failed to receive the vaccine. Hepatitis B is much less common in travelers and remains a risk for unvaccinated persons. Hepatitis E, which is transmitted via fecally contaminated water or food and clinically resembles acute hepatitis A, is seen in travelers and should be suspected in cases of acute hepatitis in hepatitis A vaccinated travelers. Cases have been reported in travelers [18].

Cases of amebic liver abscesses (and liver flukes) often cause right upper quadrant pain, tender liver, and elevated alkaline phosphatase.

A unique pattern is often seen in leptospirosis, where significant elevation of direct bilirubinemia may be associated with normal or near-normal transaminases.

In malaria, where hemolysis occurs, elevated indirect bilirubin may seen. In falciparum malaria, direct hyperbilirubinemia may also be seen, usually accompanied by significant elevation of transaminases as a sign of direct liver damage by the parasite.

Table 37.4 provides a summary of findings on routine laboratory studies for infections commonly seen in febrile travelers.

### Fever and eosinophilia

Eosinophilia is not uncommon in returning travelers and usually is due to helminthic infection (see Chapter 39). However, the combination of fever and eosinophilia is quite uncommon. In travelers, the most common cause for it is acute schistosomiasis (Katayama syndrome). Several other helminths (ascaris, hookworm), during their migration through the lungs, may cause fever, pulmonary symptoms, and significant eosinophilia (Loeffler's syndrome). Examples of such conditions also include trichinosis, fascioliasis, gnathostomiasis, lymphatic filariasis, tropical pulmonary eosinophilia, toxocariasis, and loiasis. Many of these helminth infections are seen primarily in local populations or in persons who have made prolonged stays in tropical or developing countries. The protozoan infections, such as malaria, amebiasis, giardiasis, and leishmaniasis, are not associated with eosinophilia. Acute coccidioidomycosis, an endemic fungal infection, and a few other nonhelminthic infections may also be associated with eosinophilia [19].

## Initial diagnostic workup

The initial laboratory evaluation in a febrile patient with a history of tropical exposures should generally include

**Table 37.4** Usual laboratory findings and diagnostic tests for infections common in febrile travelers.

| | WBC total | Eosinophils | Platelets | Liver enzymes | Main diagnostic tests |
|---|---|---|---|---|---|
| **Viral infections** | | | | | |
| Dengue fever | Very low | Low | Very low | Mild elevation | Serology;PCR |
| Chikungunya | Normal/low | Normal/low | Normal/low | Mild elevation | Serology;PCR |
| West Nile fever | High/normal/low | Normal/low | Normal/low | Mild elevation | Serology; |
| Viral hepatitis (A, B, E) | Normal/low | Normal/low | Normal/low | Very high | Serology; PCR for Hep E |
| **Bacterial infections** | | | | | |
| Typhoid fever | Normal/low | Very low | Normal/low | Mild elevation | Isolate bacteria (blood, feces) |
| Rickettsial infections | Normal/low | Normal/low | Normal/low | Mild elevation | Serology; PCR |
| Leptospirosis | Low/normal/high | Normal/low | Normal/low | Mild to high | Serology; |
| Relapsing fever | Normal/low | Normal/low | Normal/low | Mild elevation | Blood smear; PCR |
| **Protozoa** | | | | | |
| Malaria | Normal/low | Low | Low | Mild elevation | Identify parasites on blood smear; detect antigen in blood |
| Visceral leishmaniasis | Low | Normal/low | Low | | Identify parasite in tissue culture; PCR |
| Amebic liver abscess | Normal/high | Normal/low | Normal | Elevated (mainly alkaline phosphatase) | Serology; identify trophozoites in tissue/aspirate |
| **Helminths** | | | | | |
| Acute schistosomiasis (Katayama fever) | Normal/high | Very high | Normal | Mild elevation | Serology; identify eggs (may be absent at time of symptom onset) |

all or most of the following:

    Complete blood count with the differential count
    Liver enzymes
    Blood smears for malaria
    Blood cultures
    Urinalysis
    Chest radiography.

If malaria is suspected, it is essential not only to request the appropriate tests for malaria, but also to make certain that tests are done expeditiously and by experienced technicians. A rapid test for malaria can be done as a first malaria assesment, especially where technicians are not experienced with malaria smear.

Serology tests for various pathogens should be sent after the initial evaluation.

In a patient with persistent fever, a repeat physical examination will sometimes uncover new findings (e.g., new rash, splenomegaly) that can provide useful clues to the diagnosis.

Table 37.4 lists tests used to diagnose common infections in febrile returned travelers.

Travel itself may lead to medical problems. Immobility associated with travel may predispose individuals to deep vein thrombosis; sinusitis may flare up during or after travel, related to changes in pressure during ascent and descent. Fever with a noninfectious etiology, such as drug fever and pulmonary emboli, or fever unrelated to travel should also be considered if initial studies do not confirm the presence of an infection.

## Look for malaria

Malaria remains the most important infection to consider in anyone with fever after visiting or living in malarious areas. In nonimmune travelers, falciparum malaria can be fatal if not diagnosed and treated promptly. Although most patients with malaria will report fever, 40% or more may not have fever at the time of initial medical evaluation [20]. Risk of malaria varies greatly from one endemic region to another, but in general is highest in parts of Sub-Saharan Africa; the most severe cases in travelers and the most fatalities follow exposure in this region. Tests to look for malaria should be done urgently (same day). Negative smear (and rapid malaria test) might be due to a low level of parasitemia, which still may cause severe disease in travelers. (In *P. falciparum* infection, the infected erythrocytes may be sequestered in the deep vasculature and therefore may not be seen on a blood smear, even in a severely ill patient). Therefore, a repeated malaria smear about 24 hours after the initial blood smear is mandatory.

No chemoprophylactic agent is 100% effective, so malaria tests should be done even in persons who report taking chemoprophylaxis. Prompt evaluation is most critical in persons who have visited areas with falciparum malaria in recent weeks. About 90% of reported patients with acute falciparum malaria had an onset of symptoms within a month of return [10]. Use of chemoprophylaxis may ameliorate symptoms or delay their onset. Similarly, several antimicrobials (e.g., TMP-SMX, azithromycin, doxycycline, clindamycin) have some activity against plasmodia. Taking these drugs for reasons unrelated to malaria may delay the onset of symptoms of malaria or modify the clinical course. Immigrants from endemic countries may also present with late infection.

Although fever and headache are commonly reported in malaria, gastrointestinal and pulmonary symptoms may be prominent and may misdirect initial attention toward other infections. Thrombocytopenia and absence of leukocytosis are common laboratory findings and serve as good predictors of malaria infection [17].

## Management

A traveler returning with fever poses an urgent challenge to any clinician, and it is essential that a diagnosis be made and treatment be initiated without delay. In cases such as falciparum malaria, this timing may be life-saving. In addition to the traveler's well-being, clinicians need to consider the potential impact of an unknown infection on public health. The task of rapid diagnosis is often a daunting one and clinicians should be aware of outside resources, such as the Center for Disease Control and Prevention (CDC) or other reference laboratories with special expertise, to help in making these timely diagnoses and offering other clinical support (see Appendix B).

Geographical diversity also brings with it multidrug-resistant organisms, even in infections that are cosmopolitan, such as pneumococcal pneumonia or gonorrhea, or in infections, such as *Salmonella*, *Campylobacter*, and, of course, malaria, that are more often associated with travel to developing countries. In cases such as malaria or multidrug-resistant typhoid fever, these infections are potentially lethal. A patient who does not respond to seemingly appropriate treatment needs to be reassessed for the following conditions:

    Drug-resistant infection
    Misdiagnosis
    Co-infection.

The presence of two infections is not uncommon in the tropics, mainly due to several gastrointestinal pathogens. Dual pathogens causing febrile illnesses are less common. However, a number of case reports document the simultaneous presence of dual febrile infections, such as malaria and typhoid fever or amebic liver abscess and hepatitis A [21–23].

It is certainly helpful for clinicians to be familiar with the epidemiology of infectious diseases worldwide. However, it is often very difficult to ascertain up-to-date information about infections from specific locations.

The advent of the Internet and e-mail and their widespread adoption in the last decade allow a constant flow and interchange of clinical observations in close to real time. This has led to the establishment of several international communication networks, such as ProMED-mail, which is an Internet-based reporting system dedicated to rapid global dissemination of information on outbreaks of infectious diseases and acute exposures to toxins that affect human health. It provides up-to-date and reliable news to a worldwide audience from which every clinician may benefit.

## References

1 Hill D. Health problems in a large cohort of Americans traveling to developing countries. *J Travel Med* 2000;7:259–66.

2 Steffen R, Rickenbach M, Willhelm U, et al. Health problems after travel to developing countries. *J Infect Dis* 1987;156:84–91.

3 Freedman DO, Weld LH, Phyllis E, Kozarsky PE, et al. Spectrum of disease and relation to place of exposure among ill returned travelers. *N Engl J Med* 2006;354 (2):119–30.

4 Steinlauf S, Segal G, Sidi Y, Schwartz E. Epidemiology of travel-related hospitalization. *J Travel Med* 2005;12:136–41.

5 Wilson ME, Weld LH, Boggild A, et al. Fever in returned travelers: results from the GeoSentinel surveillance network. *Clin Infect Dis* 2007;44:1560–68.

6 Bottieau E, Clerinx J, Schrooten W, Van den Enden E, Wouters R, Van Esbroeck M, et al. Etiology and outcome of fever after a stay in the tropics. *Arch Intern Med* 2006;166:1642–8.

7 Schwartz E, Parise M, Kozarsky P, Cetron M. Delayed onset of malaria—implication for chemoprophylaxis in travellers. *N Engl J Med* 2003;349:1510–16.

8 Centers for Disease Control and Prevention. CDC surveillance summaries. Malaria surveillance: United States, 1997. *MMWR Morb Mortal Wkly Rep* 2001;50(SS-1):25–44.

9 Centers for Disease Control and Prevention. CDC surveillance summaries. Malaria surveillance–United States, 1998. *MMWR Morb Mortal Wkly Rep* 2001;7:1–18.

10 D'Ortenzio E, Godineau N, Fontanet A, Houze S, Bouchaud O, Matheron S, et al. Prolonged *Plasmodium falciparum* infection in immigrants, Paris. *Emerg Infect Dis* 2008;14: 323–6.

11 Schwartz E, Weld LH, Wilder-Smith A, von Sonnenburg F, Keystone JS, Kain KC, et al.; GeoSentinel Surveillance Network. Seasonality, annual trends, and characteristics of dengue among ill returned travelers, 1997–2006. *Emerg Infect Dis* 2008;14:1081–8.

12 Schwartz E, Kozarsky P, Wilson M, Cetron M. Schistosome infection among river rafters on Omo River, Ethiopia. *J Travel Med* 2005;12:3–8.

13 Schwartz E, Shlim DR, Eaton M, et al. The effect of oral and parenteral typhoid vaccination on the rate of infection with *Salmonella typhi* and *Salmonella paratyphi* among foreigners in Nepal. *Arch Intern Med* 1990;150:349–51.

14 Anstey NM, Jacups SP, Cain T, Pearson T, Ziesing PJ, Fisher DA, et al. Pulmonary manifestations of uncomplicated falciparum and vivax malaria: cough small airways obstruction, impaired gas transfer, and increased pulmonary phagocytic activity. *J Infect Dis* 2002 1;185:1326–34.

15 Su CP, Chen YC, Chang SC. Changing characteristics of typhoid fever in Taiwan. *J Microbiol Immunol Infect* 2004;37:109–14.

16 Tattevin P, Léveiller G, Flicoteaux R, Jauréguiberry S, Le Tulzo Y, Dupont M, et al. Respiratory manifestations of leptospirosis: a retrospective study. *Lung* 2005;183:283–9.

17 Bottieau E, Clerinx J, Van den Enden E, Van Esbroeck M, Colebunders R, Van Gompel A, et al. Fever after a stay in the tropics: diagnostic predictors of the leading tropical conditions. *Medicine (Baltimore)* 2007;86:18–25.

18 Piper-Jenks N, Horowitz HW, Schwartz E. Risk of hepatitis E to travelers. *J Travel Med* 2000;7:194–9.

19 Meltzer E, Percik R, Shatzkes J, Sidi Y, Schwartz E. Eosinophilia among returning travelers: a practical approach. *Am J Trop Med Hyg* 2008;78(5):702–9.

20 Dorsey G, Gandhi M, Oyugi JH, Rosenthal PJ. Difficulties in the prevention, diagnosis, and treatment of imported malaria. *Arch Intern Med* 2000;160:2505–10.

21 Gopinath R, Keystone JS, Kain KC. Concurrent falciparum malaria and salmonella bacteremia in travelers: report of two cases. *Clin Infect Dis* 1995;20:706–8.

22 Schwartz E, Piper-Jenks. Simultaneous amebic liver abscess and hepatitis A infection. *J Trav Med* 1998;5:95–6.

23 Badiaga S, Imbert G, La Scola B, Jean P, Delmont J, Brouqui P. Imported brucellosis associated with *Plasmodium falciparum* malaria in a traveler returning from the tropics. *J Travel Med* 2005;12:282–4.

# 38 Approach to Returning Travelers with Skin Lesions

Eric Caumes

Hôpital Pitié-Salpêtrière, University Pierre et Marie Curie, Paris, France

## Introduction

Dermatoses are a leading cause of health problems in travelers. According to various studies, they are the third to sixth cause of consultation in returning travelers. They cover a large spectrum of diseases that includes infectious skin diseases of exotic or cosmopolitan origin as well as environmental skin diseases [1].

## Epidemiological data

Three studies have focused on skin diseases diagnosed in returning travelers. In an international study concerning 17,353 returning travelers, dermatological disorders (reported in 18% of the patients) were the third most common cause of health problems after systemic febrile illness and acute diarrhea. The most common causes of dermatological problems in these 4594 patients were hookworm-related cutaneous larva migrans (HrCLM) (9.8%), insect bites (8.2%), skin abscesses (7.7%), superinfected insect bites (6.8%), allergic rashes (5.5%), rashes of unknown etiology (5.5%), dog bites (4.3%), superficial fungal infections (4%), dengue (3.4%), and leishmaniasis (3.3%) [2]. The percentage of imported skin diseases was 24%. In contrast, in a prospective study of 269 travelers (tourists, business persons) who presented in the early 1990s to a clinic in Paris that specializes in tropical and skin diseases, there were 137 (53%) patients with imported tropical skin diseases [3]. In a prospective study done 10 years later in the same hospital unit among a broader spectrum of travelers (immigrants returning from visiting their home

countries, expatriates, business travelers, and tourists), the percentage of imported dermatoses declined to 33% [4]. A total of 165 skin diseases were diagnosed, the main dermatoses being cellulitis, scabies, pruritus of unknown origin, pyoderma, myiasis, dermatophytic infection, filariasis, hookworm-related cutaneous larva migrans, and urticaria [4].

All together, these three studies show that the leading causes of skin diseases are bacterial skin infections, hookworm-related cutaneous larva migrans, and insect bites (with or without secondary infection). The percentage of tropical, exotic skin diseases averaged 30%; however, these were more common in the past and are more often seen in specialized units.

## Clinical approach

The patient's history should include all of the events related to travel: the geographic area visited, the duration of stay, the means of transportation, activities, housing, risky behavior (food and water hygiene, clothing and shoes worn, exposures to sand, fresh or salt water, insects, plants and animals, and personal contacts), a history of similar signs and symptoms in fellow travelers, and use of preventive measures (insect repellent, mosquito netting). Physicians should be aware of any known recent outbreaks and of diseases endemic to the geographic areas visited. The history should also include a review of all medications that the patient may have taken.

The dermatological history should focus on the initial presentation, the progression of lesions, their duration, and the time of onset relative to potential exposures and return. Any underlying skin disease should be taken into account. Clinical examination should focus on the morphological characteristics of cutaneous lesions

*Tropical Diseases in Travelers*, 1st edition. Edited by E. Schwartz.
© 2009 by Blackwell Publishing, ISBN: 978-1-4051-8441-0.

**Table 38.1** Causes of localized skin diseases in travelers according to the primary cutaneous lesion.

Papules and nodules

Noninfectious causes: arthropod bites,* sea urchin granuloma, tick granuloma, acne exacerbation

Bacterial infection: pyodermas,* mycobacterial infection (leprosy, tuberculosis, etc.)

Parasitic infection: scabies,* leishmaniasis,* tungiasis,* myiasis,* onchocerciasis, gnathostomiasis, cysticercosis, late cutaneous schistosomiasis, dirofilariasis, paragonimiasis, sparganosis, trypanosomiasis

Fungal infection: lobomycosis, mycetoma, paracoccidioidomycosis, chromomycosis, sporotrichosis, West African histoplasmosis

Viral infection: Orf, milker's nodules

Erythematous plaque

Noninfectious causes: cellulite-like reactions to arthropods*

Bacterial infection: cellulitis,* Lyme disease

Parasitic infection: African trypanosomiasis, leishmaniasis

Fungal infection: dermatophytosis*

Vesicles and bullae

Noninfectious causes: sunburn,* blister beetle dermatitis, contact dermatitis,* irritant dermatitis, phytophotodermatitis, arthropod bites,* fixed drug eruption

Bacterial infection: bullous impetigo*

Parasitic infection : hookworm-related cutaneous larva migrans*

Viral infection: herpes simplex infection,* herpes zoster, varicella, pox virus

*Source*: Adapted from [1].

*More common in travelers.

(e.g., nodules, ulcers) together with their anatomical distribution (localized, generalized, or limited to a specific anatomical location). Any associated local and systemic signs and symptoms should be noted.

Further diagnostic procedures such as blood tests, serologies, skin biopsies, PCR, cultures, and imaging studies may be warranted, according to the results of clinical examination.

Skin diseases and diseases with dermatological manifestations that are encountered most frequently by travelers will now be reviewed according to their dermatological presentation. The presenting cutaneous signs or symptoms in travelers are papules and nodules, vesicles and bullae, plaque (Table 38.1), creeping dermatitis, ulcers, localized pruritus, febrile exanthema, acute urticaria, disseminated pruritus with or without rash, nodular lymphangitis, and localized edema.

## Skin diseases

### Pyoderma and common bacterial skin infections

Bacterial skin infections are one of the most common dermatoses in travelers. The clinical spectrum ranges from impetigo and abscesses (Fig. 38.1) to erysipelas and necro-tizing cellulites. Lesions usually appear while the patient is still abroad, but are also a leading cause of consultation in returning travelers [2–4]. In a prospective study of 48 returning travelers with pyoderma, 75% were diagnosed with impetigo, erysipelas, or ecthyma. Among the 19 patients with impetigo, *Staphylococcus aureus* and *Streptococcus* species were identified in 80% of the 15 available swab samples and 63% were secondary to insect bites

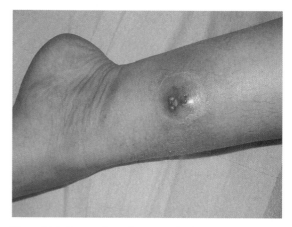

**Figure 38.1** Abscess due to Panton–Valentine positive methicillin *S. aureus* in a traveler returning from Ivory Coast.

[3]. In another prospective series of 165 returning travelers, bacterial skin infections were the leading cause of dermatoses (21%) and were secondary to insect bites in 28.6% [3]. Insect bites with superinfection were also the fourth etiological diagnosis in 2947 travelers with dermatological disorders in the GeoSentinel skin study [2]. Hence, insect bites are often complicated by superinfection because bites may either act as a portal of entry or become superinfected secondary to itching.

Most of these infections, such as folliculitis, carbuncles, and abscesses, are due to *S. aureus*, either methicillin-resistant (MRSA) or methicillin-sensitive (MSSA). Both can carry the gene of Panton–Valentine leukocidin (PVL), a cytotoxin that confers higher morbidity. Recently, cases have been reported of PVL-positive *S. aureus* infections acquired abroad with subsequent transmission of the infection upon return home [5, 6]. Moreover, an Irish study showed that one-third of PVL-positive MRSA infections were observed in patients of non-Irish ethnic origin, reflecting the importation of diverse genotypes of PVL-positive MRSA into Ireland [7]. Foreign importation of particular strains of MRSA through travelers could be one of the reasons for this diversity. Some of these staphylococcal skin infections can lead to chronic or recurrent furunculosis in previously healthy travelers. Therefore, in cases of recurrence, returning travelers should be screened as carriers for *S. aureus* and be decontaminated in case of positive results.

## Creeping dermatitis

Creeping eruption, a cutaneous sign, is defined as a linear or serpiginous cutaneous track that is slightly elevated, erythematous, and mobile [8] (Table 38.2).

The main causes of creeping dermatitis are found among the causes of cutaneous larva migrans (CLM), a syndrome defined clinically and parasitologically by the subcutaneous migration of a nonhuman nematode larva, such as hookworm (hookworm-related cutaneous larva migrans), *Gnathostoma* spp. (gnathostomiasis), *Pelodera strongyloides*, various zoonotic *Strongyloides* spp., and *Spirurina* spp. [8], making the infected human a dead-end host. The most frequent cause of CLM in travelers is hookworm-related cutaneous larva migrans (HrCLM) due to nonhuman hookworms and caused by the penetration of the skin by nonhuman (cat, dog) nematodes larvae (see Figure 34.5).

Creeping eruptions may also be seen in diseases involving larvae such as fly maggots (migratory myiasis), adult nematodes (*Loa loa, Dracunculus medinensis, Dirofilaria* spp.), trematode larva (*Fasciola gigantica*), mites

**Table 38.2** Causes of creeping eruption in travelers.

| Nematode larvae |
|---|
| Animal hookworms (HrCLM),* *Pelodera strongyloides*, zoonotic *Strongyloides* spp. |
| Gnathostomiasis (*Gnathostoma* spp.) |
| *Spirurina* spp. |
| Larva currens (*Strongyloides stercoralis*) |
| Adult nematodes |
| Loiasis (*Loa loa*) |
| Dracunculiasis (*Dracunculus medinensis*) |
| Dirofilariasis (*Dirofilaria immitis*, etc.) |
| Trematode larvae |
| Fascioliasis (*Fasciola gigantica*) |
| Fly maggots |
| Migratory myiasis (*Gasterophilus* spp.) |
| Arthropods |
| Scabies (*Sarcoptes scabiei*) |

*Source*: Adapted from [1].
*More common in travelers.

(*Sarcoptes scabiei*), and human nematode larvae (*Strongyloides stercoralis*) [9].

## Cutaneous ulcer

The main cause of cutaneous ulcers (Table 38.3) in this setting is localized cutaneous leishmaniasis (LCL). The clinical forms of LCL also include papules, nodules, plaques, and nodular lymphangitis. The average number of

**Table 38.3** Causes of cutaneous ulcer in travelers.

| |
|---|
| Noninfectious causes: spider bites, cupping |
| Bacterial infections: ecthyma,* rickettsial tick eschar, syphilis, anthrax, mycobacterial infection (*M. ulcerans*), melioidosis, glanders, tularemia, cutaneous diphtheria, plague |
| Parasitic infections: leishmaniasis,* sporotrichosis, cutaneous amebiasis, dracunculiasis |
| Fungal infection: mycetomas, West African histoplasmosis, North American blastomycosis, paracoccidioidomycosis, chromomycosis |
| Viral infection: herpes simplex infection |

*Source*: Adapted from [1].
*More common in travelers.

cutaneous lesions varies from 1 to 3 and the number rarely exceeds 10 per patient. Usual features of LCL include return from endemic countries in the New or the Old World, anatomical location on exposed skin (face, arms, legs), absence of pain, chronicity (more than 15 days duration), and failure of antibiotics (which are often prescribed, given that it often looks like pyoderma) [1] (see Chapter 32).

A few cases of African trypanosomiasis (also known as sleeping sickness) have been reported in travelers returning from endemic areas and presenting with a trypanosomal chancre, which is the early stage of the disease and occurs at the inoculation site of the tsetse bite [10]. Trypanosomal chancres occur more frequently in infections due to *Trypanosoma brucei rhodesiense* than in those due to *T. b. gambiense*, with a frequency up to 70% [1]. Onset of infection usually occurs 1–10 days after the infective bite. The lesion, which may ulcerate, consists of a circumscribed, indurated, red or violaceous inflammatory plaque, or nodule measuring 2–5 cm in diameter (see Figure 26.2, Chapter 26). The primary lesion usually resolves in 3 weeks.

Only two cases of cutaneous anthrax have been reported in travelers, whereas up to 100,000 cases of anthrax have been estimated to occur worldwide annually [11]. Cutaneous anthrax is acquired from contact with infected animals or contaminated animal products. Skin manifestations typically appear 1–7 days after infectious contact, beginning with a pruritic papule, which becomes vesiculous with a surrounding edema and, finally, becomes a necrotic ulcer presenting as a black eschar.

Cases of Buruli ulcer have been reported extremely rarely in travelers [1]. In contrast, *Mycobacterium ulcerans* infection is considered an emerging disease in endemic countries, with hundreds of cases reported yearly. The typical cutaneous manifestation of *M. ulcerans* infection is a progressive ulcer appearing after journeys to endemic areas (mainly Africa).

### Localized pruritic eruptions

Table 38.4 lists major causes of localized pruritic eruptions.

### Arthropod-related dermatitis

Arthropod-related dermatitis is one of the main reasons for consultation in returning travelers [2, 3]. Identification of the implicated arthropod is always difficult because arthropods of different species may give rise to similar dermatological manifestations, or a given arthropod may provoke multiple dermatological manifestations.

**Table 38.4** Causes of localized pruritus in travelers.

Noninfectious causes: contact dermatitis,* irritant dermatitis,* phytophotodermatitis

Arthropods: arthropod bites,* lice

Parasitic infection: hookworm-related cutaneous larva migrans* and other causes of creeping dermatitis (see Table 38.2), enterobiasis (perianal)

*Source*: Adapted from [1].
*More common in travelers.

However, this has no significant consequence, as the treatment is the same. Local treatment with a corticoid-based ointment is indicated in mild to moderate cases, whereas systemic corticosteroids should be considered in more severe cases. Oral antihistamines may improve the symptoms. In addition, for irritant contact dermatitis, the irritant should be removed by washing the implicated area, and antibiotics may be indicated if secondarily infected [1].

Apart from the bacterial superinfection previously described, another predominant feature of the arthropod reaction is prurigo (Figure 38.2), an eruption of intensely pruritic erythematous and excoriated papules [3]. This reaction is considered to be an evolutive stage of papular urticaria related to a hypersensitivity reaction to the bites of insects such as fleas, bedbugs, and less commonly mosquitoes, chiggers, and mites [12]. Arthropod bites may also result in vesiculobullous lesions.

### Contact dermatitis

Allergic contact dermatitis after contact with plants in the family *Anacardiaceae*, which includes cashew nut trees, poison ivy/oak (poison ivy dermatitis), mango, and pistachio [13] has been widely reported. Poison ivy dermatitis clears by itself in absence of renewed exposure to the allergen.

*Paederus* dermatitis (blister beetle dermatitis) occurs when nocturnal beetles of the genus *Paederus* (rove beetles) are crushed on the skin, releasing the vesicant pederin and resulting in geographic, linear, erythematous plaques with the presence of vesicles or pustules, 1 or 2 days after contact with the insect (Figure 38.3). An outbreak where staphylinid (rove) beetles were implicated has been recently reported among 191 US personnel deployed in Pakistan [14].

Dermatitis related to contact with moths has been reported in travelers returning from Mexico [15]. It presents

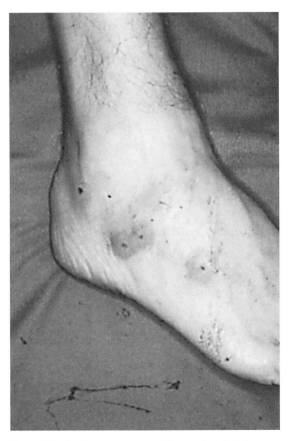

**Figure 38.2** Acute prurigo after walking accidentally into an anthill in Niger.

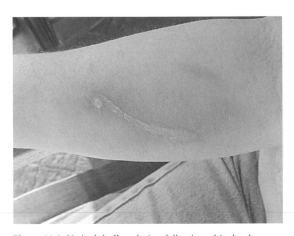

**Figure 38.3** Vesiculobullous lesion following a bite by the Nairobi fly, a poisonous beetle of the species *Paederus crebinpunctatis* or *Paederus sabaeus* in an Israeli traveler. (Courtesy of Eli Schwartz.)

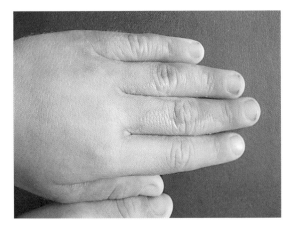

**Figure 38.4** Phytophotodermatitis associating postbullous lesions and hyperpigmented well-delimited hyperpigmented plaques in a child returning from the French West Indies (Guadeloupe).

as a highly pruritic papular eruption localized on uncovered areas targeted by the spines released by the moths.

Phytophotodermatitis is a cutaneous phototoxic reaction that occurs after contact with a variety of plant substances (e.g., limes, lemons) followed by sunlight exposure. The acute presentation is similar to sunburn but with well delimited and circumcised erythema and vesiculation. Secondarily, the involved skin has marked hyperpigmentation [16] (Figure 38.4).

### Dermatophytosis

Dermatophytosis is a worldwide cutaneous infection but its incidence is higher in the tropics. It ranks among the most common skin diseases observed during travel abroad [2–4]. It may present as tinea corporis (infection of the nonhairy glabrous skin), tinea cruris and axillaris (infection of the groins and axillae), and tinea of the feet (the most common dermatophytic infection to be encountered in travelers). In contrast, tinea capitis is more likely to be seen in children coming back from visiting friends and relatives or in children adopted from Africa [17].

## Disseminated diseases with skin involvement

### Febrile exanthema

Febrile exanthema (Table 38.5) deserves particular attention because it may reveal potentially life-threatening

**Table 38.5** Causes of febrile widespread rash in travelers.

Noninfectious causes: adverse drug reactions*

Viral infections: dengue,* chikungunya,* other arboviral infections,* measles,* rubella, HIV, EBV and cytomegalovirus primary infection, viral hemorrhagic fever

Bacterial infections: rickettsial infections,* typhoid fever,meningococcemia (purpura), syphilis, rat-bite fever, leptospirosis, trench fever, brucellosis

Parasitic infections: African trypanosomiasis, trichinellosis, toxoplasmosis

*Source*: Adapted from [1].
*More common in travelers.

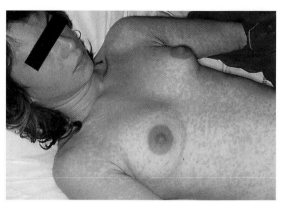

**Figure 38.5** Exanthema associated with measles in a patient returning from Southeast Asia.

disease. In a prospective study of 62 returning travelers presenting with fever and exanthema, a specific etiology was found in 57 cases (92%), whereas 5 cases remained of undetermined origin [18]. The three main etiologies were chikungunya (35%), dengue (26%), and African tick-bite fever (ATBF) (10%). Travel to the Indian Ocean was significantly associated with the diagnosis of chikungunya, whereas travel to South Africa was significantly associated with the diagnosis of ATBF. Two life-threatening diseases were diagnosed in this study: an adverse drug reaction (DRESS) and a streptococcus-associated exanthema similar to that seen in streptococcal toxic shock syndrome [18]. Other life-threatening bacterial infections that may be revealed by febrile exanthema in a traveler include meningococcal disease, toxic staphylococcal syndrome, measles (Figure 38.5), and leptospirosis, in addition to other rickettsioses [1]. Some of these infections deserve particular attention given their ability to be transmitted to others (e.g., measles, rubella, varicella, viral hemorrhagic fever).

### Arboviroses

The two main arboviroses giving rise to febrile exanthema in travelers are dengue (Chapter 7) and chikungunya (Chapter 11) [18, 19]. Chikungunya and dengue skin manifestations are difficult to differentiate. Each has a diffuse (potentially pruritic) macular or maculopapular exanthema in which small islands of normal skin are spared. Clinical and biological presentations of chikungunya and dengue infections were compared in one study performed more than 40 years ago among children in Thailand [20]. In chikungunya, the onset of symptoms was more abrupt, the febrile course was shorter, and mac-

ulopapular rashes, conjunctival injection, and arthralgia were more common than in dengue. Shock and gastrointestinal hemorrhage occurred only in dengue patients. Recently, the manifestations of chikungunya and dengue among returning, mostly adult travelers have been compared [18, 19]. Arthralgia and lymphopenia were more frequently observed in chikungunya, whereas leukopenia, neutropenia, and thrombopenia were more frequently observed in dengue fever [18].

Regarding the subset of patients with rashes of undetermined origin, other less frequent arboviral diseases presenting with fever and rash could be implicated. In a study conducted with sera from 86 travelers to Britain from tropical Africa, evidence of infections with dengue and chikungunya were found, but also with O'nyong-nyong, Ntaya, and Zinga virus [21]. In this setting, physicians should be aware that some rashes of undetermined origin could be related to unusual arboviroses. Therefore, travelers should be screened according to the area visited for the Ross River and Barmah Forest viruses in the South Pacific, O'nyong-nyong and Sindbis viruses in tropical Africa, and Mayaro virus in South America [1].

### Viral hemorrhagic fever

Although extremely rare, viral hemorrhagic fevers (VHFs; see Chapter 13) such as rift valley fever, Crimean–Congo hemorrhagic fever, Marburg virus disease, and Ebola hemorrhagic fever have been reported in travelers [1, 22]. Yellow fever should also be suspected in any nonvaccinated traveler returning from areas of endemicity. VHFs should be systematically ruled out in facing travelers with fever and exanthema because they are part of the clinical manifestations for several of them, especially in Africa.

Effective protective measures must be activated as soon as a diagnosis of VHF is suspected because most of them are associated with a high case fatality rate and risk of nosocomial transmission [1].

### Rickettsioses and scrub typhus

African tick bite fever (ATBF) is considered the most commonly encountered rickettsiosis in travelers, mostly those returning from rural Sub-Saharan Africa and the eastern Caribbean [23]. Other rickettsioses that may be observed in travelers are Rocky Mountain spotted fever (caused by *Rickettsia rickettsii*, transmitted by ticks, and endemic in the Americas); Mediterranean spotted fever (caused by *R. conorii*, transmitted by dog ticks, and endemic in Mediterranean Europe, Africa, and Asia); scrub typhus (caused by *Orientia tsutsugamushi*, transmitted by the bite of larval trombiculid mites, and endemic in rural south and southeastern Asia and the western Pacific); and murine typhus (caused by *R. typhi*, transmitted by fleas, and widely distributed in tropical and subtropical regions) [24]. (See Chapter 18 for more information on these conditions.)

Typical presentation includes recent (< 1 week) travel in an endemic area and clinical features such as fever, flu-like symptoms, a generalized maculopapular cutaneous rash, and an inoculation eschar at the site of the tick bite (for conditions transmitted by ticks). Although these rickettsioses are usually self-limiting, multiorgan failure and fatal cases have been reported [1]. Therefore, presumptive therapy with doxycycline is recommended whenever a case of rickettsiosis is suspected, allowing rapid recovery and prevention of complications [24].

### Parasitic diseases

Three parasitic diseases may present with a febrile disseminated rash.

Although rarely observed, severe acute disseminated toxoplasmosis has been reported among immunocompetent patients in French Guiana. It presents as fever, myalgias, arthralgias, fatigue, generalized lymphadenopathy, hepatosplenomegaly, and a maculopapular rash [25].

The hemolymphatic stage of African trypanosomiasis is classically associated with fever, lymphadenopathies, and disseminated cutaneous lesions known as trypanides. Trypanides are characteristic but reported in less than 10% of cases [1]. The eruption is an evanescent macular erythematous rash with polycyclic plaques and centrally pale, occurring on the trunk or the proximal side of the limbs [10]. A diffuse and severe pruritus is also reported. Involvement of the CNS has to be systematically ruled out by lumbar puncture and CSF examination.

Trichinosis may also be associated with a febrile rash but more classically with typical acute urticaria (see Chapter 34).

### Hypersensitivity reaction to drugs

Hypersensitivity reaction to drugs must always be considered in the diagnosis of fever and exanthema. They are classically a leading cause of febrile exanthema, usually considered as the second etiological group of febrile exanthema after viral infections. However, in travelers, they may be less common, having been observed only once in a series of 67 travelers presenting with febrile exanthema [18]. However, in travelers, cutaneous reactions among users of malaria prophylaxis have been reported [26].

### Acute urticaria

Table 38.6 lists causes of acute urticaria.

### Acute schistosomiasis

Acute schistosomiasis is probably the leading cause of urticaria in travelers. Among 14 nonimmune travelers who bathed once in the Dogon region of Mali, acute schistosomiasis was accompanied by fever in 93% and by acute urticaria in 57%. Urticarial rash was observed a mean of 1 month after exposure to infested fresh water, whereas the mean intervals from exposure to hypereosinophilia and from exposure to seropositivity were 47 and 46 days, respectively. Serology and eosinophilia should thus be repeated if negative at the beginning of the invasive phase (see Chapter 34).

**Table 38.6** Causes of urticaria in travelers.

Noninfectious causes: adverse drug reaction*

Viral infection: hepatitis A infection

Parasitic infections: invasive phase of helminthic diseases (ascariasis, hookworm, strongyloidiasis, anisakiasis, gnathostomiasis, schistosomiasis, fascioliasis),* chronic helminthic infections where humans are dead-end hosts (trichinellosis, toxocariasis), and rupture of cysts during hydatid disease

Unknown*

*Source*: Adapted from [1].
*More common in travelers.

## Other helminthic diseases

Other helminthic diseases can present with urticaria during the invasive or chronic phases of their cycles. Examples are ascariasis, toxocariasis, gnathostomiasis, trichinosis, fascioliasis, and to a lesser extent, other helminthic diseases (see Chapter 34).

## Other diseases

Hypersensitivity reaction to drugs and viral hepatitis A should also be considered in the differential diagnosis of urticaria in travelers [1, 26].

## Disseminated pruritus with or without rash

Table 38.7 lists causes of disseminated pruritus.

## Scabies

Scabies is the most common cause of diffuse pruritic skin disease diagnosed in travelers returning from the tropics (see Chapter 33).

## Ciguatera

Ciguatera is a significant cause of pruritus that can last for months after the initial event. This form of fish poisoning is acquired by the ingestion of fish containing the toxins produced by the dinoflagellate *Gambierdiscus toxicus*, which is frequently found in damaged coral reef systems in tropical and subtropical regions.

In a series of 13 Italian travelers returning from the Caribbean, the incubation period varied between 2 and 9 hours. Nearly all patients had initial gastrointestinal symptoms. Itching occurred in 8 patients and cold-to-hot reversal of temperature sensation occurred in 2 patients [27]. The duration of symptoms varied from 1 to 16 months.

**Table 38.7** Causes of disseminated pruritus in travelers.

Noninfectious causes: adverse drug reactions, ciguatera fish poisoning,* atopic dermatitis exacerbation, seabather's eruption

Viral infections: varicella (in adults), dengue, chikungunya

Parasitic infections: scabies,* loiasis, onchocerciasis, African trypanosomiasis, cercarial dermatitis, and in association with urticarial rash during the invasive phase of some helminthic diseases (see Table 38.6)

*Source*: Adapted from [1].
*More common in travelers.

In a series of 18 cases seen between 1997 and 2002 in Marseille, patients returned to France and suffered from arthralgias, myalgias, or pruritis for 2 to 18 months (28).

The diagnosis relies on history of fish consumption, other cases among exposed persons, a short incubation period (2–30 hours), and the association of gastrointestinal symptoms (nausea, vomiting, diarrhea, and abdominal cramps) and neurological signs such as fatigue, myalgias (particularly of the lower extremities), pruritus, and neurosensory manifestations (peri-oral and distal extremity paresthesias). Patients experience tingling, burning, "dry ice-like," smarting, and "electric" sensations, and the paradoxical reversal of temperature perception (i.e., cold beverages and objects are described as feeling hot) is unique to ciguatera. Gastrointestinal symptoms resolve within a few hours; myalgias, pruritus, and neurosensory symptoms last longer. There is no etiological treatment. Gabapentine given orally can attenuate the neurological symptoms.

## Cercarial dermatitis

Cercarial dermatitis results from penetration of the skin by nonhuman schistosomal cercariae in fresh water (swimmer's itch) or coastal water (clam digger's itch; see Chapter 34).

## Seabather's eruption

Seabather's eruption (also called sea lice) is a highly pruritic eruption generally confined to the skin under swimwear and occurs after bathing in the ocean. It is caused by larval forms of sea anemones (e.g., *Edwardsiella lineata*) and jellyfish (e.g., *Linuche unguiculata*) that become trapped under swimwear [29]. Seabather's eruption has been widely reported on the Atlantic coast of the USA and in the Caribbean, Central and South America, and Southeast Asia. A prospective cohort study conducted in Palm Beach County, Florida concluded that children, people with a history of seabather's eruption, and surfers were at the greatest risk for seabather's eruption [30].

The time from exposure to onset of symptoms is usually a few minutes to a few hours. Individuals with a history of previous exposure may develop a prickling or stinging sensation while in the water. The clinical features include pruritic, erythematous macules that progress to papules, vesicles, and urticarial lesions. The anatomical distribution typically includes skin surfaces covered by swimwear and uncovered skin surfaces where there is friction (e.g., axillae, medial thighs, surfer's chest). The eruption can last from 3 days to 3 weeks. The average duration of the eruption and pruritus was 12.5 days in 70 patients in southeast Florida [29]. Topical use of corticosteroids may be indicated in case of severe itching.

### Pruritus of unknown origin

Some travelers present with pruritus without a rash except for the skin changes secondary to pruritus (i.e., excoriation, lichenification, impetiginization). In cases of localized or limited pruritus, the main cause of pruritus is acclimatization-related xerosis, a phenomenon usually limited to the legs and more commonly observed in aged travelers and those of African origin returning from their countries of origin [4]. Miliaria rubra is usually associated with particular climatic conditions and gives rise to vesicular lesions located on the trunk. In cases of disseminated pruritus, exacerbation of chronic pruritic diseases, such as atopic dermatitis, may occur. If eosinophilia is present, helminthic infections must be ruled out (see preceding discussion).

### Other dermatological syndromes

The most classical cause of nodular lymphangitis (defined by the presence of nodular and/or ulcerative lesions distributed along the line of lymphatic drainage) is sporotrichosis, but in travelers, cutaneous leishmaniasis due to *L. braziliensis* is the major cause (Table 38.8).

The most common cause of localized edema is a cellulitis-like reaction to insect bites, but infectious cellulitis must be kept in mind (Table 38.9).

### Conclusions

In conclusion, dermatoses are common health problems in returning travelers. The array of dermatoses ranges from benign to serious infections, some cosmopolitan and some exotic, but many can be distressing to the patient. It is

**Table 38.8** Causes of nodular lymphangitis in travelers.

Parasitic infection: New World cutaneous leishmaniasis*

Mycosis: sporotrichosis

Bacterial infection: tularemia, cat-scratch disease, pyogenic or mycobacterial infection (*M. marinum*)

Adapted from [1].
*More common in travelers.

**Table 38.9** Causes of localized edema in travelers.

Noninfectious causes: cellulitis-like reaction to arthropods*

Bacterial infection: infectious cellulitis*

Parasitic infections: acute lymphatic filariasis, lymphedema of onchocerciasis, Calabar swelling of loiasis, gnathostomiasis, American trypanosomiasis, or trichinellosis (located on the face)

*Source*: Adapted from [1].
* More common in travelers.

imperative to obtain a detailed travel history, including the specific nature of exposure, and to examine skin lesions carefully in order to provide needed clues for diagnosis. Identifying the etiology of a traveler's skin infection is essential to offer timely and appropriate treatment, avoid unnecessary testing, alleviate the traveler's suffering, and prevent further transmission in the community.

### References

1 Hochedez P, Caumes E. Common skin infections in travelers. *J Travel Med* 2008;15:223–33.

2 Lederman ER, Weld LH, Elyazar IR, et al. Dermatologic conditions of the ill returned traveler: an analysis from the GeoSentinel surveillance network. *Int J Infect Dis* 2008;12:593–602.

3 Caumes E, Carriere J, Guermonprez G, et al. Dermatoses associated with travel to tropical countries: a prospective study of the diagnosis and management of 269 patients presenting to a tropical disease unit. *Clin Infect Dis* 1995;20:542–8.

4 Ansart S, Perez L, Jaureguiberry S, et al. Spectrum of dermatoses in 165 travelers returning from the tropics with skin diseases. *Am J Trop Med Hyg* 2007;76:184–6.

5 Schleucher RD, Gaessler M, Knobloch J. Panton–Valentine leukocidin-producing methicillin-sensitive *Staphylococcus aureus* as a cause for recurrent, contagious skin infections in young, healthy travelers returned from a tropical country: a new worldwide public health problem? *J Travel Med* 2008;15:137–9.

6 Helgason KO, Jones ME, Edwards G. Panton–Valentine leukocidin-positive *Staphylococcus aureus* and foreign travel. *J Clin Microbiol* 2008;46:832–3.

7 Rossney AS, Shore AC, Morgan PM, et al. The emergence and importation of diverse genotypes of methicillin-resistant *Staphylococcus aureus* (MRSA) harboring the Panton–Valentine leukocidin gene (pvl) reveal that pvl is a poor marker for community-acquired MRSA strains in Ireland. *J Clin Microbiol* 2007;45:2554–63.

8 Caumes E. It's time to distinguish the sign 'creeping eruption' from the syndrome 'cutaneous larva migrans'. *Dermatology* 2006;213:179–81.

9 Hochedez P, Caumes E. Hookworm-related cutaneous larva migrans. *J Travel Med* 2007;14:339–46.

10 Ezzedine K, Darie H, Le Bras M, Malvy D. Skin features accompanying imported human African trypanosomiasis: hemolymphatic *Trypanosoma gambiense* infection among two French expatriates with dermatologic manifestations. *J Travel Med* 2007;14:192–6.

11 Van den Enden E, Van Gompel A, Van Esbroeck M. Cutaneous anthrax in a Belgian traveler. *Emerg Infect Dis* 2006;12: 523–5.

12 Steen CJ, Carbonaro PA, Schwartz RA. Arthropods in dermatology. *J Am Acad Dermatol* 2004;50:819–42.

13 Maje HA, Freedman DO. Cashew nut dermatitis in a returned traveler. *J Travel Med* 2001;8: 213–15.

14 Dursteler BB, Nyquist RA. Outbreak of rove beetle (staphylinid) pustular contact dermatitis in Pakistan among deployed U.S. personnel. *Mil Med* 2004;169:57–60.

15 Jamieson F, Keystone JS, From L, Rosen C. Moth-associated dermatitis in Canadian travellers returning from Mexico. *CMAJ* 1991;145:1119–21.

16 Weber IC, Davis CP, Greeson DM. Phytophotodermatitis: the other "lime" disease. *J Emerg Med* 1999;17:235–7.

17 Markey RJ, Staat MA, Gerrety MJ, Lucky AW. Tinea capitis due to *Trichophyton soudanense* in Cincinnati, Ohio, in internationally adopted children from Liberia. *Pediatr Dermatol* 2003;20:408–10.

18 Hochedez P, Canestri A, Guihot A, Brichler S, Bricaire F, Caumes E. Management of travelers with fever and exanthema notably dengue and chikungunya infections. *Am J Trop Med Hyg* 2008;78:710–13.

19 Nicoletti L, Ciccozzi M, Marchi A, et al. Chikungunya and dengue viruses in travelers. *Emerg Infect Dis* 2008;14:177–8.

20 Nimmannitya S, Halstead SB, Cohen SN, Margiotta MR. Dengue and chikungunya virus infection in man in Thailand, 1962–1964. I. Observations on hospitalized patients with hemorrhagic fever. *Am J Trop Med Hyg* 1969;18:954–71.

21 Woodruff AW, Bowen ET, Platt GS. Viral infections in travellers from tropical Africa. *Br Med J* 1978;1:956–8.

22 Isaacson M. Viral hemorrhagic fever hazards for travelers in Africa. *Clin Infect Dis* 2001;33:1707–12.

23 Raoult D, Fournier PE, Fenollar F, et al. *Rickettsia africae*, a tick-borne pathogen in travelers to Sub-Saharan Africa. *N Engl J Med* 2001;344:1504–10.

24 Jensenius M, Fournier PE, Raoult D. Rickettsioses and the international traveler. *Clin Infect Dis* 2004;39:1493–9.

25 Bossi P, Paris L, Caumes E, Katlama C, Danis M, Bricaire F. Severe acute disseminated toxoplasmosis acquired by an immunocompetent patient in French Guiana. *Scand J Infect Dis* 2002;34:311–14.

26 Schlagenhauf P, Tschopp A, Johnson R, et al. Tolerability of malaria chemoprophylaxis in nonimmune travellers to sub-Saharan Africa: multicentre, randomised, double blind, four arm study. *BMJ* 2003;327:1078–84.

27 Bavastrelli M, Bertucci P, Midulla M, Giardini O, Sanguigni S. Ciguatera fish poisoning: an emerging syndrome in Italian travelers. *J Travel Med* 2001;8:139–42.

28 de Haro L, Pommier P, Valli M. Emergence of imported ciguatera in Europe: report of 18 cases at the Poison Control Centre of Marseille. *J Toxicol Clin Toxicol* 2003;41:927–30.

29 Wong DE, Meinking TL, Rosen LB, Taplin D, Hogan DJ, Burnett JW. Seabather's eruption. Clinical, histologic, and immunologic features. *J Am Acad Dermatol* 1994;30:399–406.

30 Kumar S, Hlady WG, Malecki JM. Risk factors for seabather's eruption: a prospective cohort study. *Public Health Rep* 1997;112:59–62.

31 Kostman JR, DiNubile MJ. Nodular lymphangitis: a distinctive but often unrecognized syndrome. *Ann Intern Med* 1993;118:883–8.

# 39 | Approach to Travel-Related Eosinophilia

Eyal Meltzer and Eli Schwartz

Chaim Sheba Medical Center, Tel Hashomer, Israel
Sackler School of Medicine, Tel Aviv University, Tel Aviv, Israel

## Introduction

Eosinophils constitute a small percentage of peripheral blood leukocytes in healthy adults, and although different cutoffs are used by different authors [1–3], they usually fall below $0.4 \times 10^9$/L or 5%.

Eosinophil cells were described (with the other leukocyte populations) by Paul Ehrlich in 1878. The association of eosinophilia with helminthic diseases was soon discovered, and eventually a large number of different diseases were found to cause eosinophilia.

Although eosinophilia is relatively infrequent, a great number of possible causes exist, and evaluation of a patient with eosinophilia can be extensive, protracted, and inconclusive. In developing countries, helminths are the main cause, whereas in developed countries, helminths are infrequent even in patients with eosinophilia. Travelers are a unique population in this respect because they stand at a midpoint between the developed and developing world. The approach to eosinophilia in travelers should therefore be unique as well. In this chapter, the etiologies of eosinophilia in general and in travelers will be discussed, together with a rational approach to post-travel eosinophilia.

## Mechanism of eosinophil recruitment

Eosinophils develop from myeloid precursors in the bone marrow. The half-life of eosinophils in the peripheral circulation of normal individuals is approximately 18 hours, with an average blood transit time of about 26 hours,

similar to that of neutrophils [4]. However, although their blood transit time is short, they survive much longer in tissues. Therefore, the majority of eosinophils actually reside inside various organs, and eosinophilic organ infiltration can occur prior to or completely without peripheral blood eosinophilia.

Eosinophil production is usually dependent on cytokine activation. Granulocyte–monocyte colony stimulating factor (GM-CSF) and interleukin-2 (IL-2) are both inducers of eosinophilia. Most of their effect is mediated through the release of IL-5 from activated $T_H$-2 CD4 lymphocytes (Figure 39.1). Cytokine secretion leading to eosinophilia can be the result of either a reactive inflammatory process or clonal/neoplastic disease, leading to $T_H$-2 lymphocytic activation. Several disease groups are associated with a predominantly $T_H$-2 response and, therefore, are frequently associated with eosinophilia. These include tissue-invasive helminthic diseases and much less frequently some other infections, atopic diseases and allergic reactions (including drug reactions), and immune-complex-mediated diseases. In addition, cytokine release induced by clones of malignant cells, especially of lymphatic or hematopoietic origin, gives rise to the eosinophilia sometimes seen in lymphoma, leukemia, myeloproliferative, or myelodysplastic disorders.

Glucocorticosteroids are potent inhibitors of eosinophilia, and most conditions associated with acute stress, including infections (e.g., malaria or typhoid fever), are typified by eosinopenia. The decrease in glucocorticosteroid levels, as in the recovery phase of such infections, causes relative or absolute eosinophilia.

The hypereosinophilic syndrome constitutes a collection of rare conditions in which chronic (usually high-level) idiopathic eosinophilia exists. In many of these cases, idiopathic high levels of IL-5 are the driving force

*Tropical Diseases in Travelers*, 1st edition. Edited by E. Schwartz.
© 2009 by Blackwell Publishing, ISBN: 978-1-4051-8441-0.

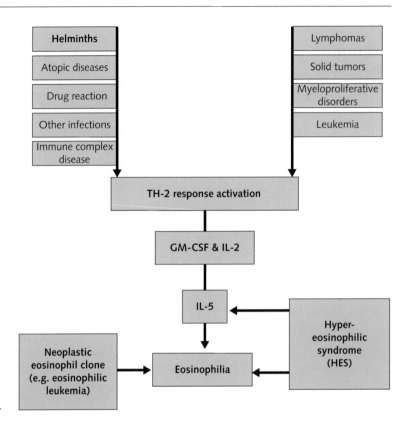

**Figure 39.1** Mechanisms of eosinophilia.

behind eosinophilia, whereas in others, mutations such as Fip1-like 1–platelet-derived growth factor receptor fusion gene [FIP1L1–PDGFRA] are the cause of a unique myeloproliferative disorder, chronic eosinophilic leukemia. Despite its rarity, HES has been the focus of much research, and specific therapies, including imatinib, a tyrosine kinase inhibitor for the clonal variants, and mepolizumab, a monoclonal anti-IL-5 antibody for other cases, have been found to be effective [3, 5].

The degree of eosinophilia is probably associated with its etiology. Eosinophilia has been classified as mild (<1.5 × 10⁹/L), moderate (<5 × 10⁹/L), and severe (>5 × 10⁹/L) [3]. Atopic conditions are usually associated with mild eosinophilia, whereas lymphoproliferative and neoplastic diseases often present with moderate to severe eosinophilia. This is recognized by the inclusion of an eosinophil count >1.5 × 10⁹/L in the diagnostic criteria for HES (the other criteria are a duration of more than 6 months, evidence of target organ damage, and the ruling out of secondary causes). Although these definitions are arbitrary, there are data to suggest that different etiologies for eosinophilia segregate according to numbers. Kobayashi et al. have established a cutoff of 2 × 10⁹/L

as differentiating between asthma and other allergic conditions and conditions explaining HES [6]. The degree of eosinophilia with helminthic infections is highly variable, with some enteric helminths (e.g., *Taenia*) causing little or no eosinophilia. Invasive helminths tend to cause marked eosinophilia, but this is also associated with the phase of infection (migration phase in hookworm or *Ascaris* infection) and most importantly with chronicity: for example, heavily helminth-infested patients in developing countries can present with a normal eosinophil count [7].

## Causes of eosinophilia in the general population

Only a few studies exist concerning the prevalence and causes of eosinophilia in developed countries. Although many conditions can be associated with eosinophilia (Table 39.1), allergic/atopic conditions consistently predominate overall. The eosinophil count is quite variable even in the apparently healthy population, with values of 0.15–0.65 × 10⁹/L found, for example, in healthy

**Table 39.1** Major etiologies of eosinophilia.

| Etiology | Major group | Examples/comments |
|---|---|---|
| Infections—helminthic | Trematodes<br>Nematodes<br>Cestodes | Schistosomiasis<br>Geohelminths, filaria<br>Occasional eosinophilia |
| Infections—ectoparasites | Miasis<br>Scabies | Eosinophilia uncommon |
| Infections—protozoan | *Sarcocystis*<br>*Dientamoeba* | Association with<br>eosinophilia questionable |
| Infections—fungal | Coccidioidiomycosis<br>Paracoccidiomycosis<br>Allergic bronchopulmonary<br>aspergillosis (ABPA) | |
| Atopic diseases | Asthma<br>Allergic rhinitis<br>Eczema/atopic dermatitis | |
| Bullous dermatoses | Bullous pemphigoid | |
| Medications | Antimicrobials<br><br>Anti-inflammatory<br>Metabolic<br>Antihypertensive<br>Gastric acid–lowering agents<br>Antidepressants and<br>antipsychotics | Beta lactams, sulfonamides,<br>nitrofurantoin, tetracyclines<br>Nonsteroidals, gold salts<br>Allopurinol<br>Hydralazine<br>Ranitidine, omeprazole |
| Collagen vascular diseases | Rheumatoid vasculitis<br>Churg–Strauss syndrome | Other associations are<br>anecdotal |
| Hematological neoplastic<br>diseases | Myeloproliferative diseases<br>Leukemia<br>Lymphoma<br>Systemic mastocytosis | |
| Hypereosinophilic syndrome | Idiopathic | Some cases associated with<br>FIP1L1/PDGFRA fusion<br>tyrosine kinase |

medical students [8]. Even within this "normal" range, the prevalence of allergic/atopic diseases tends to increase from $0.275 \times 10^9$/L upward [9]. Brigden and Graydon [10] have evaluated the causes of eosinophilia from a large cohort of ambulatory patients in Canada and found eosinophilia (defined as an eosinophil count above 5% or $0.7 \times 10^9$/L) in 0.1% out of 195,300 patients. In the majority of cases, eosinophilia was an incidental finding. Atopic diseases were the leading cause established, with 52% of patients reporting asthma/allergic rhinitis/eczema or atopic dermatitis. It should be noted, however, that

nearly one-third of the patients did not have a repeat clinical evaluation, and only 20% had a stool sample performed for ova and parasites [10].

In another report, Kivity and co-workers studied the causes of eosinophilia among 100 hospitalized patients from a tertiary center in Israel [11]. Despite the inherent bias of studying such a population, allergic conditions were still predominant at 15%, and another 6% were caused by medications, whereas neoplasms represented only 10% of cases. A definitive diagnosis of helminthic disease was made in only 1%. It should be noted that even in this hospital-based series and despite an extensive evaluation, about one-third of the patients remained without a specific diagnosis.

A third study evaluated 1862 outpatients with eosinophilia who had been referred to an allergy clinic in northern Italy. Of these cases, 79.7% were attributed to atopic conditions, 5% were associated with either solid or hematological malignancies, and 8.2% were caused by helminths, although no data were offered on disease stage, immigrant status, or travel history [12].

Conditions other than allergy may contribute greatly to the concerns of physicians in evaluating patients with eosinophilia. These include neoplastic diseases, especially carcinomas, lymphomas, and leukemia, and also vasculitis and collagen vascular diseases. It is important to note that for most patients found to have cancer-associated eosinophilia, the tumor had already been diagnosed and usually was in an advanced stage [13]. Eosinophilia is therefore unlikely to indicate an otherwise occult cancer. Similarly, eosinophilia is unlikely to be the initial finding of an otherwise silent rheumatic condition [10]. Eosinophilia is an infrequent finding for most autoimmune diseases. In a survey of 1000 patients referred to rheumatological evaluation, only 7.7% had eosinophilia, which was largely due to drug therapy [14].

To summarize, in a developed country eosinophilia in the general population is usually due to atopic disease, medications, and skin disorders. It may infrequently be associated with advanced malignant neoplasms and with collagen vascular diseases, but not usually as a presenting finding. Helminths appear to be a relatively infrequent cause for eosinophilia in developed countries, although a thorough diagnostic effort to rule them out has not usually been performed, and a large proportion of cases remain without a specific diagnosis.

## Causes of eosinophilia in immigrants and refugees

It is of the utmost importance to understand that for the majority of the human population, helminthic diseases remain a commonplace, everyday occurrence. Geohelminths, filaria, and schistosomiasis probably affect more than 2 billion persons worldwide [15]. In many parts of the world, helminths infect the majority of the population. This can be attested by data from deworming studies in both schoolchildren and adults, in which 62–91% have been shown to carry hookworms [16]. Migrant workers and immigrants from developing nations also frequently harbor helminths, and a high prevalence is reported from refugee camps. It is only to be expected, therefore, that the prevalence of eosinophilia is higher in such populations. Seybolt et al., for example, found eosinophilia in 12% of cases [17]. Similarly, Ugandans perceived as healthy have a mean eosinophil count of about $1.0 \times 10^9$/L, reflecting the ubiquity of helminthic infection in Africa [18].

Several studies have evaluated the incidence and the etiology of eosinophilia in refugees and immigrants, with helminthic diseases causing the majority of cases, whereas atopic diseases are rare and neoplasms are not reported at all [17, 19]. Two types of helminths form the bulk of diagnoses made in refugees and immigrants: geo-helminth nematodes (*Ascaris*, hookworms, *Strongyloides*, and *Trichuris*) are the most frequent and have a global distribution; schistosomiasis and filariasis are also frequent, but largely in immigrants or refugees from Africa, and are infrequent in Asian or South American refugees [12, 19, 20]. Furthermore, in immigrants with eosinophilia, even after screening did not find a specific diagnosis, most patients with unexplained eosinophilia were still found to be infected with hookworms or *Strongyloides* when further evaluated [20]. Other helminths, including tissue trematodes (e.g., *Clonorchis, Opistorchis, Fasciola*, and *Paragonymus*) and cestodes, are also reported, but much less frequently.

## Causes of eosinophilia in travelers

Eosinophilia usually accounts for 4–12% of all referrals for post-travel medical care [21–25], which approaches the prevalence of eosinophilia in immigrants. However, different travel characteristics may result in markedly increased risk of eosinophilia. In British military personnel, for example, 50% had eosinophilia after deployment in West Africa [26].

Several studies have reported on the etiology of eosinophilia in returning travelers [22–26]. The results show differences that are understandable, because the populations studied were somewhat different in each study, sometimes including immigrants or those visiting friends and relatives (VFRs), and sometimes including only recreational tourists native to a developed country. However, several features are common to all reports: first, in many cases no definite diagnosis is established (22–64%); second, among the established diagnoses, helminthic diseases were the most common.

**Table 39.2** Epidemiological and diagnostic features of post-travel eosinophilia.

| Feature | Meltzer et al. [24] (N = 38) | Whetham et al. [21] (N = 175) | Schulte et al. [22] (N = 648) | Harries et al. [25] (N = 114) |
|---|---|---|---|---|
| **Demographic and epidemiological features** | | | | |
| % of all post-travel referrals | 4.3 | 4.5 | 2.6 | NR |
| Symptomatic eosinophilia (%) | 94.7 | 79 | 67 | NR |
| Age (years) | 30.8 | 31 | 34.3 | 33 |
| Immigrants (%) | 0 | NR | 26.4 | NR |
| Expatriates (%) | 0 | NR | NR | NR |
| Destination (%) | | | | |
|    Africa | 7.9 | 47.7 | 50.2 | 64 |
|    Asia | 62.8 | 52.3 | 36.6 | 29 |
|    America | 26.3 | | 16.5 | 7 |
|    Other | 7.9 | | 7.5 | 0 |
| **Diagnosis** | | | | |
| A final cause of eosinophilia established (%) | 36.8 | 78 | 36 | 44.5 |
| Helminth-associated eosinophilia (%) | 31.6 | 63.8 | 32.7 | 40.3 |
| Atopy-associated eosinophilia (%) | 2.6 | 13.4 | 3.2 | 4.2 |
| Other noninfectious diagnoses (%) | 2.6 | 0.8 | 0.1 | 0 |

NR = not reported.

Allergies were diagnosed in some travelers as a cause of eosinophilia, but other diagnostic groups such as autoimmune diseases and malignancies were very rare or nonexistent (Table 39.2).

Whereas reports of eosinophilia in the general population find that eosinophilia, especially mild eosinophilia, is often an incidental finding, among travelers the bulk of referrals are due to symptoms. Among Israeli travelers, for example, nearly 80% of patients were symptomatic (with most of the asymptomatic cases being cases of schistosomiasis, diagnosed through active screening) [24].

The most frequently diagnosed helminth in travelers is *Schistosoma* [21–24]. Patients with *Schistosoma*-associated eosinophilia acquired the disease mostly through freshwater exposure in Africa, with a small minority being diagnosed after exposures elsewhere. There are probably several reasons for the prominence of schistosomiasis among the helminthic diagnoses. Schistosomiasis necessitates freshwater exposure, which is reliably elucidated through a travel history, and the areas of endemic schistosomiasis are well delineated. The reliability and availability of specific diagnostic tests, including serology, make it relatively easy to confirm a clinical suspicion. Also, schistosomiasis is highly infectious and tends to oc-

cur in outbreaks or clusters among groups of travelers. Once an index case is diagnosed, it is easy to screen other members of the group and diagnose many more cases.

The diagnosis next in frequency was geohelminth nematodes, which figured more prominently in travelers returning from Asia [21, 24], with hookworms and *Strongyloides* predominating. Other helminths are reported only occasionally and include a variety of species. Filaria were largely reported from immigrant VFRs from Africa [27] and are very rare in other travelers, as are tissue trematodes and cestodes (Table 39.3).

## Symptoms associated with helminthic infection

Because eosinophilia in travelers is mostly due to helminthic infection, physicians should be acquainted with associated symptoms. During helminth migration and maturation within humans, symptoms are varied and transient. Patients should be specifically asked about these; otherwise, they may not report them, as they seem to be irrelevant to the current situation.

**Table 39.3** Helminthic infections causing eosinophilia in travelers [24].

| Name | Mode of transmission | World distribution | Diagnosis | | | Treatment |
|------|---------------------|--------------------|-----------|--|--|-----------|
| | | | Time to patency[a] | Stool[b] | Serology[b] | |
| *Frequently described travel-associated pathogens with frequent eosinophilia* | | | | | | |
| *Ascaris lumbricoides* | Geohelminth | Cosmopolitan, mostly tropical, subtropical | 8 weeks | + | − | Albendazole Mebendazole Ivermectin |
| Human hookworm spp. | Geohelminth | Cosmopolitan, mostly tropical, subtropical | 5–6 weeks | + | − | Albendazole Mebendazole |
| *Strongyloides stercoralis* | Geohelminth | Cosmopolitan, mostly tropical, subtropical | 4 weeks | ± | + | Albendazole Ivermectin |
| *Schistosoma* spp. | Aquatic | Africa ≫ South America, Asia | 4–6 weeks | +(urine) | + | Praziquantel |
| *Frequently described travel-associated pathogens with infrequent eosinophilia* | | | | | | |
| *Trichuris trichiura* | Geohelminth | Cosmopolitan, mostly tropical, subtropical | 12 weeks | + | − | Albendazole Mebendazole |
| Zoonotic hookworms (cutaneous larva migrans) | Geohelminth | Cosmopolitan, mostly tropical, subtropical | Never | − | − | Albendazole Mebendazole |
| *Rarely described travel-associated pathogens with frequent eosinophilia* | | | | | | |
| Lymphatic filariasis | Mosquito bite | Africa ≫ Asia, South America | 12–32 weeks | − | + | Ivermectin Albendazole Doxycycline DEC |
| *Loa loa* | *Chrysops* flies | West/Central Africa | 20 weeks | − | + | Ivermectin DEC |
| *Onchocerca volvulus* | Blackfly bite | Africa | 26–52 weeks | − | + | Ivermectin |
| *Trichinella* spp. | Food-borne | Cosmopolitan | Never | − | + | Albendazole (if early) |
| *Capillaria philippinensis* | Food-borne | Philippines, Thailand | 4 weeks | + | − | Albendazole |
| *Ancylostoma caninum* Eosinophilic gastroenteritis | Geohelminth Fecal–oral | Cosmopolitan, mostly tropical, subtropical | Never | − | Experimental | Albendazole Mebendazole |
| *Taenia solium/saginata* (taeniasis) | Food-borne | Cosmopolitan | 8 weeks | + | ± | Praziquantel |

*(Continued)*

**Table 39.3** (*Continued*)

| Name | Mode of transmission | World distribution | Diagnosis | | | Treatment |
|------|----------------------|--------------------|-----------|---|---|-----------|
| | | | Time to patency[a] | Stool[b] | Serology[b] | |
| *Taenia solium* (cysticercosis) | Food-borne | Cosmopolitan | 8 weeks | ± | + | Albendazole |
| *Fasciola* (liver flukes) | Food-borne | Cosmopolitan | 16 weeks | + | + | Triclabendazole |
| *Paragonimus* (lung flukes) | Food-borne | Asia, Latin America | 10–12 weeks | + (sputum) | + | Praziquantel |
| *Gnathostoma spinigerum* | Food-borne | Southeast Asia, Latin America | Never | − | + | Albendazole |

[a]Patency = the time from exposure to the first detection of ova/larvae in clinical samples (stool/urine/blood).
[b](+) = available, (−) = not available, (±) = available, but infrequently positive, DEC = diethylcarbamazine.

The main stages of helminth migration are associated with different symptoms. *Penetration* into the body can cause symptoms such as transient abdominal pain when hatched larva penetrate the gut, or transient rash when larva penetrate the skin, such as hookworm and *Strongyloides* (ground itch) and *Schistosoma* cercariae (swimmer's itch). Such symptoms may be fleeting and may therefore not be recalled (swimmer's itch is in fact recalled only by a minority of cases of acute schistosomiasis [28]), or may be prolonged and dominate the patients' concerns (as is often the case with hookworm-associated ground itch, where the intensely pruritic rash may take several weeks to resolve).

The second phase is *migration* through the body. This is often associated with blood-borne transit through the lungs (as occurs in *Schistosoma* and most geohelminths). In some cases, the migration occurs via body cavities (e.g., the peritoneum in *Fasciola* and the pleura in *Paragonymus*, as occurs with tissue trematodes). The result is often a combination of respiratory symptoms and concomitant systemic symptoms of fever, arthralgia, and myalgia. Respiratory symptoms are less recognized in the literature but can dominate the clinical presentation. These include prolonged cough, usually a dry and often nocturnal cough, occasionally with accompanying wheezes, and sometimes associated with pulmonary infiltrates. The acute eosinophilia that often appears during this phase can result in nonspecific symptoms that are caused by the effects of systemic eosinophil activation and include transient urticarial rashes and facial or limb edema. Occasionally, these larvae lose their way, causing variations on the more common manifestations.

The third phase, *maturation and oviposition*, occurs when the worm settles in at the target organ, with symptoms pertaining to that organ. Thus, genitourinary symptoms occur with *Schistosoma hematobium*, gastrointestinal symptoms with geohelminths, pedal edema with lymphatic filariasis, and so forth.

The late symptoms of chronic infection are the main findings in endemic populations and are therefore very well known through descriptions of large cohorts. The acute symptoms are rarely seen in developing countries. In fact, acute phenomena are mostly known through studies on travelers and from a few volunteer studies. It is, therefore, reasonable to assume that knowledge of the extent of acute symptoms and their variability is incomplete, and physicians need to be aware of this.

The majority of travelers who presented to our clinic with eosinophilia were symptomatic. There is a difference in the presentation of travelers with schistosomiasis-associated eosinophilia and with non-*Schistosoma* eosinophilia. As seen in Figure 39.2, fever, rash/itch, and respiratory complaints predominate in acute schistosomiasis, whereas abdominal complaints predominate in non-*Schistosoma* eosinophilia, and fever is rare.

To summarize, in travelers, eosinophilia in helminthic infection is likely to present itself in the early, acute phase. Although each symptom or sign at this stage is rarely diagnostic, a pattern of changing, additive, or sequential symptoms is often a clue to the diagnosis. The physical findings most likely to contribute to the diagnosis are

(a)

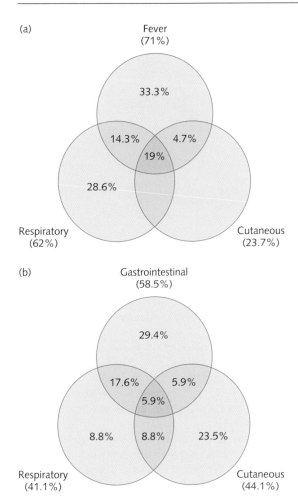

Fever
(71%)

33.3%

14.3%    4.7%

19%

28.6%

Respiratory
(62%)

Cutaneous
(23.7%)

(b)

Gastrointestinal
(58.5%)

29.4%

17.6%    5.9%

5.9%

8.8%    8.8%    23.5%

Respiratory
(41.1%)

Cutaneous
(44.1%)

**Figure 39.2** Distribution of major symptoms in acute schistosomiasis ($N = 21$) (a) and post-travel non-schistosoma eosinophilia ($N = 34$) (b). (From [24]).

cutaneous, including nonspecific urticarial rash and a fixed papular rash, which is typical for hookworm penetration (Figure 39.3).

## Clinical hints for the diagnosis of post-travel eosinophilia

The clinical approach to the returning traveler with eosinophilia should begin with a thorough travel history and physical examination. Analysis of the "where, what, and when" of the travel itinerary, combined with the symptom complex presented, should enable the physician to create a plausible differential diagnosis.

The issue of "where" is paramount. Several helminthic diseases reported in travelers are geographically distinct,

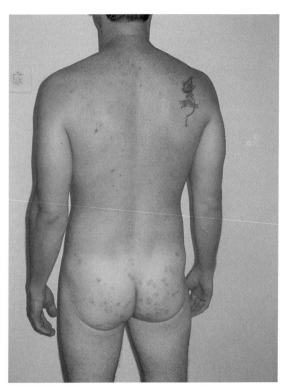

**Figure 39.3** Acute hookworm infection. A fixed papullar pruritic rash, after exposure to a sandy beach in Thailand—typical of acute hookworm dermatitis.

especially schistosomiasis and filariasis. Schistosomiasis, which is an emerging infection among travelers, is seen mostly in travelers returning from Africa, where the greatest burden of schistosomiasis exists [28]. A few travelers also acquire schistosomiasis through travel elsewhere, for example, the Mekong region in Southeast Asia (mainly Laos) and the northeastern region of Brazil [29, 30]. Filariasis is geographically more widespread, existing in Sub-Saharan Africa, the Indian subcontinent, East Asia, the Pacific region, and South America. However, most cases reported in travelers were acquired in Africa [27] . Unlike schistosomiasis, filariasis is rarely seen in travelers, probably because of the need for prolonged exposure to establish the infection.

The distribution of most other helminths is global, and the question of "where" in these cases is unlikely to aid in narrowing the differential diagnosis.

The question of "what" refers to the kind of activities or forms of exposure during travel. The most pertinent data that can be obtained relate to freshwater exposure through bathing, diving, or swimming. This information is usually well retained, and when such exposures are definitely excluded, this virtually rules out schistosomiasis.

Another important piece of information is a history of bodily contact with potentially contaminated soil. Very frequently, this takes the form of walking barefoot, or of reclining or playing on sandy beaches. In developing countries, the ground is often littered with either animal or human excreta and is therefore a frequent source of inoculation with geohelminths. This mode of exposure may lead to cutaneous larva migrans syndromes (due to zoonotic geohelminths—a rare cause of systemic eosinophilia) or to ground itch due to human hookworm and *Strongyloides* infections—which are an important cause of eosinophilia.

Information regarding food and water consumption is usually of limited value (as in travelers' diarrhea). However, recalling some more memorable foodstuffs can sometimes assist in forming a differential diagnosis. For example, a traveler may recall eating uncooked freshwater crabs, which can harbor *Paragonimus*, or a recent snail dinner, which can point to *Angiostrongylus*. Several of these hints are summarized in Table 39.4.

The issue of when the exposure occurred, and when symptoms began, is highly important in travel medicine, as it may reflect the incubation time for the illness. It is often complicated by the fact that the time of exposure is not always well demarcated. Furthermore, due to the complex life cycle of the helminth inside the human host, symptoms may appear and change over long periods of time. Eosinophilia may present as early as 1–2 weeks after exposure and may last for months or years.

## Diagnosis and diagnostic pitfalls

Helminthic diseases are classically proven by showing the pathogen or its ova or larvae in clinical samples. Serology is another diagnostic method, which is largely irrelevant for diagnosis in endemic populations but can be very important in travelers.

## Stool (and blood) microscopy

This classical diagnostic test often fails to establish a parasitological diagnosis in travelers, for several reasons.

The most important shortcoming of microscopy is the time required for oviposition to begin. Helminths are complex multicellular organisms, which undergo sexual development and pass through several stages. The period during which infection exists but no ova/larvae can be detected, called the prepatent period, is usually measured in weeks or months (Table 39.3). It is important to note that symptoms begin during the prepatent period, and because it is these symptoms that bring the traveler to the travel clinic, a direct parasitological diagnosis at this time is unlikely.

The sensitivity of stool/urine microscopy is markedly dependent on the inoculum. A low burden of infection (often with a very low egg count in the stool) is usually encountered in travelers, even when marked symptoms and vigorous eosinophilia are present. Furthermore, some helminths exhibit intermittent release of progeny (e.g., a diurnal variation in microfilaremia and in the presence of schistosomal ova in excreta). Some helminthic infections never result in the production of eggs in the stool. Strongyloidiasis is probably the most important of these, where only larvae, which are notoriously difficult to visualize, are present in stool.

## Serological tests

These are also used for the diagnosis of helminthic infections in travelers, but present with several problems, and are sometimes difficult to interpret. In many helminthic serological tests, the antigens used are not well standardized. Cross-reactivity between helminths is an important limitation.

Current helminth serologies are not able to differentiate between acute and past infections; a serological test can remain positive for many years or may be lifelong. Therefore, when patients report a history of past travel or immigration, a positive serological test cannot be used to establish the presence of active infection. Theoretically, avidity studies can differentiate between recent and past exposures, but such tests have only been reported in a few diseases (e.g., for toxocariasis [31]) and are not clinically available.

Furthermore, the best serological tests can be negative in patients with very early infection, even when severe symptoms are present. Such has been our experience, for example, with schistosomiasis, where repeated sera are sometimes needed before the diagnosis is established. Many helminths undergo a complex life cycle within the host, which entails a dramatic shift in expressed antigens. It may be that because many serological tests utilize adult worm antigens, they may initially be falsely negative in early infection, which is the main problem encountered among travelers.

Finally, for some of the most important helminthic diseases, no serological tests are commercially available at all. This is most evident in hookworm, one of the most prevalent helminthic diseases.

**Table 39.4** Helminths: association with specific foodstuffs/exposures.

| | Helminth | Details of food/exposure | Main symptoms |
|---|---|---|---|
| Soil | Hookworm (human)* | Soil contaminated by sewage (e.g., walking barefoot on a beach) | Rash, pneumonitis, anemia |
| | Hookworm (zoonotic) | Soil contaminated by animal excreta | Cutaneous larva migrans |
| | *Strongyloides stercoralis** | Soil contaminated by sewage | Rash, respiratory symptoms |
| Freshwater | *Schistosoma* spp.* | Freshwater exposure (bathing, diving) | Swimmers' itch, fever, respiratory symptoms, urticaria, GI/GU symptoms |
| Food | *Ascaris lumbricoides** | Food contaminated by sewage/night soil | Pneumonitis, abdominal pain |
| | *Trichuris trichura* | Food contaminated by sewage/night soil | Tenesmus, rectal pain |
| | Hookworm (zoonotic) | Food contaminated by animal excreta | Eosinophilic gastroenteritis |
| | *Gnathostoma* spp. | Saltwater fish | Larva migrans |
| | *Angiostrongylus* spp. | Freshwater snails | Eosinophilic meningitis |
| | *Clonorchis* spp. *Opistorchis* spp. | Freshwater fish | Abdominal pain, biliary colic |
| | *Capillaria* spp. | Freshwater fish | Abdominal pain, diarrhea |
| | *Fasciola/Fasciolopsis* | Leafy vegetables (watercress, lettuce, alfalfa, etc.) | "Hepatitis"/migrating "hepatic abscess," biliary colic |
| | *Taenia saginatta* | Uncooked beef | Abdominal discomfort, excretion of proglottides |
| | *Taenia solium* | Uncooked pork | Abdominal discomfort, excretion of proglottides |
| | | Fecal contamination of food (infected food handlers) | Cysticercosis |
| | *Difilobotrium latum* | Saltwater fish | Abdominal discomfort, excretion of moving proglottides |
| | *Trichinella spiralis* | Uncooked meat (mostly game) | Fever, myositis, edema, urticaria |
| Contact with animals/animal excreta | *Toxocara* spp. *Himenolepis* spp. | Contact with cats/dogs Rodents? | Fever, abdominal pain, organomegaly Abdominal discomfort, excretion of proglottides |

* = Frequent cause of post-travel eosinophilia.
GI/GU = gastrointestinal/genitourinary.

Despite these limitations, some serological tests are of proven value in evaluating eosinophilia in travelers. *Schistosoma* serology is diagnostic in a traveler without prior exposure to endemic areas. This test is useful for diagnosis, but is of little use for follow-up after therapy, because antibodies persist for years [32]. *Strongyloides* serology, on the other hand, may be used not only for diagnosis, but for follow-up as well. Ascertaining the eradication of this infection is very important because it is one of only a few helminths that can reproduce inside the host and perpetuate infection, sometimes causing hyperinfection. Data suggest that after successful treatment, the anti-*Strongyloides* antibody titer decreases [33].

Overall, most groups studying post-travel eosinophilia have reported that a specific diagnosis was absent in most or many cases. In our experience, a specific parasitological diagnosis could be established in only about 20% of cases.

## A suggested algorithm for the approach to post-travel eosinophilia

How should physicians approach eosinophilia in the returning traveler? Clearly, with the limitations inherent in the currently available diagnostic tools and the nonspecific nature of many of the symptoms associated with early helminthic diseases, a specific diagnosis is not easily made. With these limitations in mind, we propose an algorithmic approach, which apparently leads to a cure in most cases [24] (Figure 39.4).

If the patient is an acutely ill febrile traveler, we believe that the initial clinical focus should be the ruling out of possible co-infection with potentially life-threatening conditions, such as malaria. Malaria and bacterial diseases such as typhoid are typically associated with marked eosinopenia. Because there is a significant overlap in the distribution of schistosomiasis (the main cause of fever and eosinophilia in travelers) and malaria, active exclusion of the latter with rapid tests and repeated blood smears is essential. Taking a blood culture in this scenario is always warranted as well, helping to exclude concomitant bacterial infection, such as typhoid fever.

After a life-threatening co-infection is ruled out, schistosomiasis should be excluded through history and specific tests, if exposure to potentially infected fresh water has occurred. Schistosomiasis is a frequent diagnosis in travelers with eosinophilia, and the therapeutic approach is established, with limitations [28].

In some cases of nonschistosomal eosinophilia, the physical findings, especially the dermatological findings, may suffice to establish a specific diagnosis (e.g., the papular, intensely pruritic, nonmigratory rash of human hookworm infection, especially if a history of exposure to soil or contaminated beaches is elicited). However, the bulk of cases will remain without a specific diagnosis even after a thorough history, physical examination, and routine tests such as a chemistry panel, stool exams, and even imaging studies. We believe that empirical therapy should take precedence over extensive diagnostic efforts. Our experience shows that if after the exclusion of schistosomiasis, no specific diagnosis is made through physical examination and a twice-repeated stool examination, a course of albendazole 400 mg b.i.d. for 5–7 days should be used. We have shown that among Israeli travelers with nonschistosomal eosinophilia, albendazole was very effective in improving both symptoms and eosinophil count [24]. Symptomatic relief is usually evident within a few days, and eosinophilia will usually decrease within a month, although the time to eosinophil normalization is sometimes much longer.

Albendazole is a broad-spectrum anthelminthic, with activity against human (and zoonotic) hookworms, many other intestinal helminths such as *Ascaris lumbricoides* and *Trichuris trichura*, and other common helminthic infections that travelers are likely to encounter (Table 39.3). Although albendazole is less effective than ivermectin for *Str. stercoralis*, a cure rate of 45–78% is achieved even in endemic populations [34, 35]. Its safety record is excellent, its cost is low, and it, therefore, figures prominently on the WHO Essential Drugs List. Ivermectin is not readily available in many developed countries, but can also be used empirically with albendazole. In fact, empirical anthelminthic therapy has been shown both in the USA and in Israel to be highly cost-effective and beneficial in immigrants [36–38].

Several helminthic infections that may not be addressed by this approach are tissue trematodes and (to some extent) filariasis. Filariasis has only rarely been described in travelers who are not expatriates or returning immigrants. The major area of risk for acquiring these infections is Africa. When filariasis cannot be clearly ruled out on epidemiological grounds, its presence should be pursued with specific laboratory studies. These include nocturnal blood smears and serology. Tissue trematodes have also been infrequently reported even among travelers with eosinophilia; these include the lung fluke *Paragonimus* spp. [39] and the liver flukes *Fasciola hepatica* and *Fasciolopsis buski* [40]. There are few data about the acute manifestations following infection with these agents. Both can result in a migratory rash. The rash in paragonimiasis is accompanied by cough, chest pain, and hemoptysis, and may mimic tuberculosis; in fascioliasis, abdominal pain and "hepatitis" may occur. Although the classical diagnosis is through finding the ova in stool (and in sputum in paragonimiasis), this is highly unlikely in the acutely ill traveler (Table 39.3). A tentative diagnosis often rests on imaging of the lungs and liver, respectively, although serological tests for *Fasciola* and *Paragonimus* are available in some countries.

Additional tests, including other serologies, imaging studies, and invasive procedures, should be reserved for the minority of cases with no symptomatic relief and laboratory improvement within 1 month after treatment when

no diagnosis was achieved. These patients should be evaluated for the causes of eosinophilia in the general population, including allergies, medications, and rarer conditions such as neoplasms and rheumatic diseases.

A specific population of travelers with eosinophilia consists of patients who are asymptomatic. They are sometimes discovered by screening, for example, after a co-traveler is diagnosed with a helminthic disease, such as schistosomiasis. In our experience, such cases constitute the majority of asymptomatic eosinophilia [24]; in other reports, asymptomatic eosinophilia was typically found in expatriates after a long stay, especially in Africa

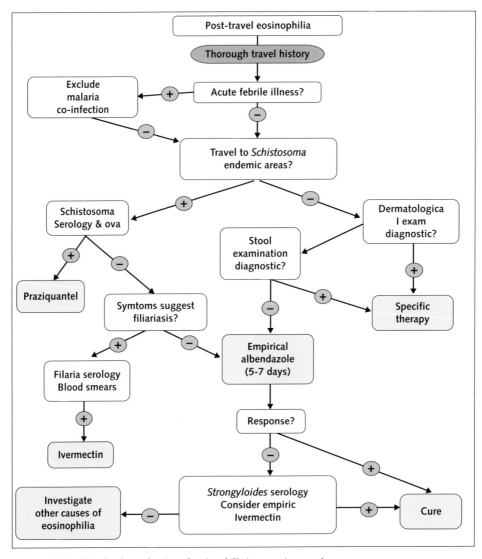

**Figure 39.4** Suggested algorithm for the evaluation of eosinophilia in returning travelers.

[41]. We believe that cases of asymptomatic post-travel eosinophilia will benefit from the same algorithmic approach suggested above. We have shown that among the initially asymptomatic schistosomiasis patients, a significant proportion eventually developed symptoms of chronic schistosomiasis [29]. Similarly, a timely diagnosis of strongyloidiasis may prevent late, fatal hyperinfection, developing decades after exposure, that may be misdiagnosed because the travel history was not considered [42, 43].

## Conclusions

Eosinophilia in returning travelers is not rare and is often accompanied by symptoms. Careful history-taking may reveal an additive or migratory pattern of symptoms (dermatological, respiratory, and gastrointestinal), which is highly suggestive of helminthic disease. Travelers usually present during the acute phase of the infection, so a parasitological diagnosis by ova detection is unlikely. The helminths most often diagnosed in travelers include *Schistosoma* and geohelminths. Using a simple algorithmic approach, with empirical albendazole therapy in cases of nonschistosomal eosinophilia, most cases will demonstrate resolution of symptoms and eosinophilia. Noninfectious causes of eosinophilia, especially malignant and rheumatological diseases, are less frequent in travelers. Therefore, additional diagnostic measures should probably be reserved for patients who have not responded to empirical albendazole.

## References

1 Rothenberg ME. Eosinophilia. *N Engl J Med* 1998;338:1592–1600.

2 Brito-Babapulle F. The eosinophilias, including the idiopathic hypereosinophilic syndrome. *Br J Haematol* 2003;121(2):203–23.

3 Tefferi A, Patnaik MM, Pardanani A. Eosinophilia: secondary, clonal and idiopathic. *Br J Haematol* 2006;133(5):468–92.

4 Ackerman SJ, Butterfield JH. Eosinophilia, eosinophil associated diseases, chronic eosinophil leukemia, and the hypereosinophilic syndromes. In: Hoffman R, Benz E, Shattil S, Furie B, Cohen H, editors. *Hoffman: Hematology: Basic Principles and Practice*, 4th ed. Philadelphia: Elsevier; 2005.

5 Rothenberg ME, Klion AD, Roufosse FE, Kahn JE, Weller PF, Simon HU, et al.; Mepolizumab HES Study Group. Treatment of patients with the hypereosinophilic syndrome with mepolizumab. *N Engl J Med* 2008;358(12):1215–28.

6 Kobayashi S, Inokuma S, Setoguchi K, Kono H, Abe K. Incidence of peripheral blood eosinophilia and the threshold eosinophile count for indicating hypereosinophilia-associated diseases. *Allergy* 2002;57(10):950–6.

7 Carranza-Rodriguez C, Pardo-Lledias J, Muro-Alvarez A, Pérez-Arellano JL. Cryptic parasite infection in recent West African immigrants with relative eosinophilia. *Clin Infect Dis* 2008;46(6):e48–50.

8 Krause JR, Boggs DR. Search for eosinopenia in hospitalized patients with normal blood leukocyte concentration. *Am J Hematol* 1987;24:55.

9 Mensinga TT, Schouten JP, Rijcken B, Weiss ST, Speizer FE, van der Lende R. The relationship of eosinophilia and positive skin test reactivity to respiratory symptom prevalence in a community-based population study. *J Allergy Clin Immunol* 1990;86(1):99–107.

10 Brigden M, Graydon C. Eosinophilia detected by automated blood cell counting in ambulatory North American outpatients. Incidence and clinical significance. *Arch Pathol Lab Med* 1997;121:963–7.

11 Sade K, Mysels A, Levo Y, Kivity S. Eosinophilia: a study of 100 hospitalized patients. *Eur J Intern Med* 2007;18(3):196–201.

12 Lombardi C, Passalacqua G. Eosinophilia and diseases: clinical revision of 1862 cases. *Arch Intern Med* 2003;163(11):1371–3.

13 Lowe D, Jorizzo J, Hutt MS. Tumour-associated eosinophilia: a review. *J Clin Pathol* 1981;34(12):1343–8.

14 Kargili A, Bavbek N, Kaya A, Koşar A, Karaaslan Y. Eosinophilia in rheumatologic diseases: a prospective study of 1000 cases. *Rheumatol Int* 2004;24(6):321–4.

15 Nutman TB. Asymptomatic peripheral blood eosinophilia redux: common parasitic infections presenting frequently in refugees and immigrants. *Clin Infect Dis* 2006;42(3):368–9.

16 Flohr C, Tuyen LN, Lewis S, Minh TT, Campbell J, Britton J, et al. Low efficacy of mebendazole against hookworm in Vietnam: two randomized controlled trials. *Am J Trop Med Hyg* 2007;76(4):732–6.

17 Seybolt LM, Christiansen D, Barnett ED. Diagnostic evaluation of newly arrived asymptomatic refugees with eosinophilia. *Clin Infect Dis* 2006;42:363–7.

18 Lugada ES, Mermin J, Kaharuza F, Ulvestad E, Were W, Langeland N, et al. Population-based hematologic and immunologic reference values for a healthy Ugandan population. *Clin Diagn Lab Immunol* 2004;11(1):29–34.

19 López-Vélez R, Huerga H, Turrientes MC. Infectious diseases in immigrants from the perspective of a tropical medicine referral unit. *Am J Trop Med Hyg* 2003;69(1):115–21.

20 Nutman TB, Ottesen EA, Ieng S, Samuels J, Kimball E, Lutkoski M, et al. Eosinophilia in Southeast Asian refugees: evaluation at a referral center. *J Infect Dis* 1987;155(2):309–13.

21 Whetham J, Day JN, Armstrong M, et al. Investigation of tropical eosinophilia; assessing a strategy based on geographical area. *J Infect* 2003;46:180–5.

22 Schulte C, Krebs B, Jelinek T, et al. Diagnostic significance of blood eosinophilia in returning travelers. *Clin Infect Dis* 2002;34:407–11.

23 Whitty CJ, Carroll B, Armstrong M, et al. Utility of history, examination and laboratory tests in screening those returning to Europe from the tropics for parasitic infection. *Trop Med Int Health* 2000;5:818–23.

24 Meltzer E, Percik R, Shatzkes J, Sidi Y, Schwartz E. Eosinophilia among returning travelers: a practical approach. *Am J Trop Med Hyg* 2008;78(5):702–9.

25 Harries AD, Myers B, Bhattacharrya D. Eosinophilia in Caucasians returning from the tropics. *Trans R Soc Trop Med Hyg* 1986;80:327–8.

26 Bailey MS, Thomas R, Green AD, Bailey JW, Beeching NJ. Helminth infections in British troops following an operation in Sierra Leone. *Trans R Soc Trop Med Hyg* 2006;100(9):842–6.

27 Lipner EM, Law MA, Barnett E, Keystone JS, von Sonnenburg F, Loutan L, et al.; for the GeoSentinel Surveillance Network. Filariasis in travelers presenting to the GeoSentinel surveillance network. *PLoS Negl Trop Dis* 2007;1(3):e88.

28 Meltzer E, Artom G, Marva E, Assous MV, Rahav G, Schwartz E. Schistosomiasis among travelers: new aspects of an old disease. *Emerg Infect Dis* 2006;12(11):1696–700.

29 Jelinek T, Nothdurft HD, Löscher T. Schistosomiasis in travelers and expatriates. *J Travel Med* 1996;3(3):160–164.

30 Grobusch MP, Mühlberger N, Jelinek T, Bisoffi Z, Corachán M, Harms G, et al. Imported schistosomiasis in Europe: sentinel surveillance data from TropNetEurop. *J Travel Med* 2003;10(3):164–9.

31 Dziemian E, Zarnowska H, Kolodziej-Sobocińska M, Machnicka B. Determination of the relative avidity of the specific IgG antibodies in human toxocariasis. *Parasite Immunol* 2008;30(3):187–90.

32 Tsang VC, Wilkins PP. Immunodiagnosis of schistosomiasis. Screen with FAST-ELISA and confirm with immunoblot. *Clin Lab Med* 1991;11(4):1029–39.

33 Boscolo M, Gobbo M, Mantovani W, Degani M, Anselmi M, Monteiro GB, et al. Evaluation of an indirect immunofluorescence assay for strongyloidiasis as a tool for diagnosis and follow-up. *Clin Vaccine Immunol* 2007;14(2):129–33.

34 Nontasut P, Muennoo C, Sanguankiat S, et al. Prevalence of strongyloides in Northern Thailand and treatment with ivermectin vs. albendazole. *Southeast Asian J Trop Med Public Health* 2005;36:442–4.

35 Marti H, Haji HJ, Savioli L, et al. A comparative trial of a single-dose ivermectin versus three days of albendazole for treatment of *Strongyloides stercoralis* and other soil-transmitted helminth infections in children. *Am J Trop Med Hyg* 1996;55:477–81.

36 Nahmias J, Greenberg Z, Djerrasi L, et al. Mass treatment of intestinal parasites among Ethiopian immigrants. *Isr J Med Sci* 1991;27:278–83.

37 Geltman PL, Cochran J, Hedgecock C. Intestinal parasites among African refugees resettled in Massachusetts and the impact of an overseas pre-departure treatment program. *Am J Trop Med Hyg* 2003;69:657–62.

38 Muennig P, Pallin D, Sell RL, Chan MS. The cost effectiveness of strategies for the treatment of intestinal parasites in immigrants. *N Engl J Med* 1999;340:773–9.

39 Malvy D, Ezzedine KH, Receveur MC, Pistone T, Mercié P, Longy-Boursier M. Extra-pulmonary paragonimiasis with unusual arthritis and cutaneous features among a tourist returning from Gabon. *Travel Med Infect Dis* 2006;4(6):340–42.

40 Metter K, Glöser H, von Gaisberg U. Fascioliasis after a stay in Turkey. *Dtsch Med Wochenschr* 2000;125(39):1160–63.

41 Libman MD, MacLean JD, Gyorkos TW. Screening for schistosomiasis, filariasis, and strongyloidiasis among expatriates returning from the tropics. *Clin Infect Dis* 1993;17:353–9.

42 Gill GV, Beeching NJ, Khoo S, et al. A British Second World War veteran with disseminated strongyloidiasis. *Trans R Soc Trop Med Hyg* 2004;98:382–6.

43 Williams BT, Guerry-Force ML. Disseminated strongyloidiasis in a World War II veteran with metastatic undifferentiated carcinoma of neuroendocrine type. *South Med J* 1992;85:1023–6.

# 40 Approach to Patients with Protracted Rheumatological Manifestations

Eli Schwartz[1] and Michael Ehrenfeld[2]

[1]Chaim Sheba Medical Center, Tel Hashomer, Israel and Sackler School of Medicine, Tel Aviv University, Tel Aviv, Israel
[2]Chaim Sheba Medical Center, Tel Hashomer and Tel Aviv University Faculty of Medicine, Tel Aviv, Israel

## Introduction

Arthralgia is a common manifestation in many acute infectious diseases. The symptoms usually subside within few days, in parallel to recovery from the febrile illness. However, several infectious diseases may cause a long and protracted course of rheumatic symptoms. Thus, patients may seek medical advice for the rheumatic pain without any febrile condition.

It should be noted that a recent onset of arthritis poses a diagnostic and prognostic challenge to primary care physicians and rheumatologists. Because the medical encounter may take place long after the travel, the association between the disease and the travel might not be considered, either by the patient or by the physician. It is estimated that in 30–40% of patients presenting with early arthritis, the disease remains unclassified [1]. Without knowing the underlying etiology, it is difficult to distinguish benign forms of arthritis, which follow a self-limiting course, from forms that proceed to an aggressive, erosive disease, requiring intensive immunosuppressive therapy. Having a travel history may help to reveal the etiology.

Rheumatological manifestations may occur in association with viral, bacterial, and fungal infections and can also occur in the course of some parasitic infections. The aim of this chapter is to call attention to the possibility of travel-associated arthritis, which usually has an infectious disease etiology. Noninfectious causes will be discussed as well.

## Viral infections

### Alphaviruses

The most common causative agents of joint manifestations among travelers are the alphaviruses. The alphaviruses are a separate genus in the family of Togaviridae and are unique because nearly all symptomatic infections in adults lead to joint symptoms (febrile polyarthritis). The alphaviruses are a group of RNA viruses, reservoir of which consists of vertebrates (mammals and birds), and which are transmitted by various mosquitoes (arboviruses).

### Epidemiology

The geographical distribution of the alphaviruses is wide-ranging, as listed in Table 40.1. A special feature of these viruses is that there are often long intervals between outbreaks.

The *Sindbis* virus is the most widely distributed virus among the arboviruses. When isolated in Egypt in 1952, it was considered "a virus without a disease"; however, the disease was found subsequently to be characterized by fever, rash, arthralgia, or arthritis and paresthesias. It occurs mainly in Africa, Australia, and Asia, but also in Europe. In Northern Europe, there are three closely related Sindbis-like viral strains, Ockelbo virus in Sweden, Karelian fever virus in Russia (Karelia), and Pogosta virus in Finland. All three are spread by mosquitoes (for the

**Table 40.1** Alphavirus infections causing persistent arthritis.

| Pathogen | Vector | Main exposure time | Distribution |
|---|---|---|---|
| Ross River | *Aedes* (rarely *Culex*) | Daytime | Australia and Pacific |
| Barmah Forest | *Aedes* | Daytime | Australia |
| Chikungunya | *Aedes aegypti, Aedes albopictus, Culex (in Asia)* | Daytime | Africa, Indian subcontinent, recent outbreak in Italy |
| Mayaro | *Aedes, Hemagogus* mosquitoes (vector of yellow fever) | Daytime | South America |
| *Sindbis* | *Culex* (mainly) | Night-time | Africa, Asia, and Australia |
| *Sindbis*-like viruses (including Ockelbo, Pogosta, and Karelian fever) | *Culex* (mainly) | Night-time | Northern Europe |
| O'Nyong-Nyong | *Anopheles* | Night-time | Africa |

specific vectors see Table 40.1) and have a similar clinical picture, namely fever, rash, and arthralgia or arthritis, which may be quite incapacitating and persist for months, or even years [2].

The *Sindbis*-like virus in Finland has been described as having 7 year intervals between outbreaks [2].

Ross River and Barmah Forest viruses (see Chapter 12) cause significant disease in Australia, where they are responsible for about 5000 to 8000 cases of epidemic polyarthritis annually. Barmah Forest virus is responsible for only about 10% of cases. Ross River virus (RRV) is found throughout Australia, in the Solomon Islands, and in Papua New Guinea, whereas Barmah Forest virus occurs only in mainland Australia [3].

Mayaro virus is endemic in South America, usually near tropical rain forests. The first epidemics were described in Brazil and Bolivia. Cases were afterward reported from other countries in South America, mostly in visitors around forests [2].

O'Nyong-Nyong caused an outbreak in Africa in 1959, disappeared for 35 years, and was again seen in Uganda in 1996.

Chikungunya (CHIK) virus (see Chapter 11) is the most recent emergent arbovirus infection. Its epidemiological behavior is similar to that of the O'Nyong-Nyong virus, to which it is related. It was isolated for the first time in Congo in 1958, disappeared for over 30 years, and then reappeared in Congo in 1999 and 2000 after heavy rain-

falls, infecting an estimated 50,000 persons. In Southeast Asia, it was the cause of sporadic outbreaks in the late twentieth century and then, after not having been isolated for about 20 years, reappeared in Indonesia in 2000 and 2001. A recent epidemic took place in 2005–2006 in the Indian Ocean islands, spread out to India, and ended up affecting over 1.5 million persons. On Réunion Island, up to 35% of the inhabitants were affected and, more alarmingly, 237 deaths were recorded, all from a disease that had been considered not to be fatal [4].

During this period of millions of cases in endemic areas, there was a corresponding increase in the number of cases that were diagnosed among travelers returning to Europe and the USA. Further, because the efficient vector of this virus, *Aedes albopictus*, is present in many parts of Europe and the USA, there is a potential for autochthonous spread. This in fact took place in northern Italy in September 2007, when a local outbreak was reported, with almost 200 people being affected [5]. Among the whole range of arthritogenic viruses, CHIK virus is undoubtedly the most significant, with a potential for more widespread occurrence.

Taking into account that virtually all clinical cases have rheumatic manifestations, and that chronic symptoms continue for more then 6 months in about half of the patients, these patients could easily be referred for rheumatological evaluation long after their acute febrile illness, when only an alert clinician taking the appropriate epidemiological history of high-risk travel might possibly make the correct diagnosis.

## Clinical manifestations of alphaviruses

The recent large outbreak of chikungunya affected large numbers of international travelers, and detailed clinical studies show a picture similar to that which has been reported in natives of endemic countries [6].

The clinical pictures of the alphaviruses are quite similar, with an incubation period of about 2–7 days, virtually always less than 10 days. High-grade fever for several days is typical, although in RRV infection about half of the patients are afebrile. An erythematous rash, often with maculopapules, is an important clue, particularly in the absence of a known epidemic. Headaches and myalgia are usually present. Severe asthenia is common. The Australians coined the term "epidemic polyarthritis" to highlight the significant rheumatological manifestations of RRV infection, a clinical pictures that was subsequently described in other alphaviruses as well.

The rheumatological manifestations involve small and medium-sized joints, with the main targets being the wrists, ankles, fingers, knees, and metacarpophalangeal joints; however, the knees and, more rarely, the shoulders may be involved. A symmetric distribution is the rule. The severity of joint involvement ranges from isolated arthralgia to arthritis, synovitis, and tenosynovitis. The joint manifestations usually make up the predominant clinical picture, and the joint pain is typically incapacitating.

A tendency toward a chronic course is a distinctive feature of alphavirus-induced arthritis, and patients more than 40 years old are at increased risk for chronic disease. Depending on the study, 5–50% of the patients experienced temporary incapacitation, usually of less than 1 year duration. Prolonged absence from work and high healthcare costs result from this chronic course.

Recently, in a large study of 88 adult patients with persistent arthralgia associated with chikungunya virus, it was shown that polyarticular persistent arthralgia was present in up to 63% of patients up to 18 months after the infection [7]. The factors predicting persistent or relapses of arthralgia were studied among the chikungunya patients, and both interestingly and paradoxically, it was demonstrated that the more severe the acute disease (lower platelet count, higher liver enzymes), the more favorable the outcome, with less chronicity [7]. Pre-existing joint pain was associated more often with persistent arthralgia in chikungunya and Ross River infections [7–8].

Rheumatoid factor may be detected in low titer in patients with prolonged symptoms, and the symmetric chronic arthritis of the distal joints may simulate rheumatoid arthritis, inviting diagnostic errors. However, there is no convincing proof that alphavirus infection can lead to joint destruction [9].

## Cosmopolitan viruses

Some globally distributed viruses may also have a prolonged course of arthritis or arthralgia, affecting the general population as well as international travelers. However, in contrast to alphaviruses, arthritis is usually a rare manifestation of these diseases.

Approximately 5% of patients with HIV infection (in the nonacute HIV phase) suffer from diffuse arthralgias or arthritis. Other features include HIV-reactive arthritis, atypical mycobacterial and fungal joint infections, vasculitis, undifferentiated spondylarthritis, myalgias, myositis, and fibromyalgia. The scope of this chapter does not allow us to elaborate extensively on the various clinical presentations of HIV-associated rheumatic symptoms [10].

Rubella virus typically manifests as a self-limited polyarthritis, following the natural infection or vaccination, although occasionally patients will develop a chronic course of the disease. Arthritis or arthralgias, although uncommon in males and in prepubescent girls, occurs in up to 50% of adult females with rubella virus infection.

Parvovirus joint disease typically presents as a rheumatoid arthritis-like disease, lasting days to weeks or even months after the infection. Some 50% of adults and 10% of children will develop joint manifestations.

Hepatitis B virus joint disease presents with an acute symmetrical polyarthritis in the prodromal phase of the disease. The arthritis may thus precede the jaundice by days or weeks, but it usually subsides following the onset of jaundice. In patients who develop chronic active hepatitis, recurrent polyarthralgia or polyarthritis may develop.

Similarly, in Hepatitis C virus joint disease, articular manifestations tend also to be chronic with polyarthralgias or polyarthritis, which occasionally mimic rheumatoid arthritis.

## Clinical presentations

As noted previously, early viral arthritis, as seen in Parvovirus B19 infection and in other viral infections, may at times mimic rheumatoid arthritis, with a typical small joint polyarticular symmetric arthritis [11]. Arthralgias or arthritis tend to have a rather sudden onset, and usually tend to be of short duration. Joint symptoms may be accompanied by a rash, and in most cases tend not to recur. However, there have been reports of either persistence or recurrence of the joint symptoms in rubella parvovirus, as mentioned for alphavirus infections [11, 12]. In these instances, the arthritis is generally of a nondestructive nature.

## Pathogenesis

The pattern of acute viral infection followed by protracted arthralgias or arthritis led to the search for a mechanism of possible pathogenesis to explain it. Several pathogenic mechanisms have been implicated in these presentations. One of these is direct invasion of the virus into the synovium, as has been suggested in the case of Ross River infection. It is assumed that productive viral infections in synovial macrophages, which persist despite neutralizing antibodies and antiviral cytokine responses, are responsible for the polyarthritis [13, 14].

Indeed, virus particles were detected in the synovium in few cases of parvovirus, enterovirus, rubella, and RRV infection [12, 15, 16]. Little is known about the pathogenesis of chikungunya arthritis. The synovitis, when present, probably results from direct viral invasion and infection of the synovium. In a recently published mouse model of chikungunya virus infection, the authors were able to show hind limb weakness, muscle wasting, weight loss, and mononuclear cell infiltrates into skeletal muscle [17]. These findings were comparable to previous reports on animal models of RRV infection and may thus provide a useful model for determining the pathogenesis of the clinical features of these viral diseases.

The second major mechanism implicated in the clinical features is the formation of immune complexes. In this case it has been suggested that viral antigens or whole virons lead to immune complexes being formed via the humoral response to the viral infection. These immune complexes, which are deposited in the skin or the joint, lead to the clinical features of many of these diseases, including rashes, arthralgias, or even frank arthritis [14]. This type of synovitis may be demonstrated by local complement consumption, immunoglobulin deposition by immunofluorescence, or immune complex deposition by electron microscopy. This would be the case in hepatitis B and C (via the formation of cryoglobulins in many instances) [18]. Antibodies that are directed against viral antigens cross-react with tissue antigens, typically known as molecular mimicry [19]. This process of viral cross-reactivity may lead to autoimmunity with immune recognition of either self antigens or neoantigens in the joints. It has been recently shown that macrophage-derived prod-

ucts play an important role in the development of arthritis and myositis triggered by alphavirus infection [20].

## Diagnosis

Acute febrile infection with rheumatological manifestations may raise the suspicion of a viral etiology. However, in the prolonged rheumatic manifestations due to pathogens mentioned above, the patient in most cases will be afebrile when seeking medical care. Thus, the most important clue in these cases is the travel history and the history of acute onset, usually with a febrile episode lasting a few days. However, some infections may give rise to joint manifestations without the febrile stage, such as RRV infection (see Chapter 12).

A diagnosis of viral arthritis should be taken into account in patients with acute arthritis and a positive antibody titer against a distinct virus, especially of the IgM class. Because acute phase serology (IgM) in many infections remains positive for ∼3 months, in some cases it can still be detected even when the patient presents several months after the onset of symptoms. In other cases, when the infection was remote, IgG will be positive. Because many of the etiological pathogens are endemic in specific areas of the world, the presence of positive serology provides strong support for the diagnosis. For example, the presence of antibodies to RRV in a non-Australian patient with a travel history to Australia prior to disease onset supports the diagnosis of RRV as the etiology.

The diagnosis of acute arthritis as viral arthritis is rarely confirmed by viral isolation because this can be done only in specific medical centers, and also because patients usually do not present early enough in the course of the disease. Even serological diagnosis of the alphaviruses may be limited due to unavailability of these tests as routine diagnostic tests in many instances.

Detection of antiviral antibodies in the synovial fluid of an affected joint, or detection of viral particles or gene products in an affected joint, obviously strengthens the diagnosis. However, this is rarely available.

In most patients with viral arthropathy, the rheumatoid factor (RF) is not present in the patient's serum. However, occasionally one may note a positive RF and antinuclear antibody, as well as anti-DNA and other autoantibodies. These positive laboratory tests, which are occasionally seen in parvovirus infection or post-Epstein–Barr virus infection, are obviously nonspecific and may lead to a delay of the actual diagnosis. Similarly, hepatitis C virus-infected individuals have a high prevalence of RF activity (50–60%), probably related to the high prevalence of cryoglobulins among these patients. Other laboratory serological autoimmune tests may also be positive in this group of patients, including antiphospholipid antibody and antineutrophil cytoplasmic antibody.

Thus, sorting out the differential diagnosis and coming up with the correct diagnosis in this whole group of patients depends on the travel history of these patients, as well as on the clinical presentation, which may reveal a history of an acute febrile illness with or without a rash.

## Treatment of viral arthralgia/arthritis

Given the benign self-limited course of this type of joint symptoms, treatment is usually symptomatic and geared toward maintenance of function. Thus, simple analgesics and nonsteroidal anti-inflammatory drugs, as used in any other inflammatory arthropathy, are the hallmark of the therapy. In rare instances of acute severe inflammatory arthritis not responsive to nonsteroidal anti-inflammatory drugs (NSAIDs), a short course of glucocorticosteroids may be used. Long-term treatment with corticosteroids has been suggested but is probably not generally justified, given the potential side effects. However, in a small cohort of serologically confirmed RRV-infected patients, corticosteroid therapy did not lead to an exacerbation of the disease [21].

Uncontrolled reports suggest beneficial effects of antimalarial therapy in patients with Lyme arthritis. This attempt may also be made in protracted forms of chronic viral arthritis, but there is no good data in the literature to support this approach. Occupational therapy may be initiated in order to maintain joint function and range of movement.

## Bacterial infection

Acute bacterial infection may invade the joints and cause septic arthritis. These cases are rarely associated with travel, and they are not associated with chronic pain, because of the rapid intervention needed.

However, reactive arthritis (ReA) may also develop following a bacterial infection. This is most common following bacterial diarrhea, a genitourinary infection, or a sexually transmitted disease (STD). The pathogens commonly associated with ReA are *Chlamydia*, *Salmonella*, *Shigella*, *Yersinia*, and *Campylobacter* species [22, 23].

Although traveler's diarrhea is the most common illness that affects travelers to developing countries, reactive arthritis is relatively uncommon.

The rheumatological manifestations of a ReA appear usually 2–3 weeks after the infection. The clinical manifestations usually include a lower extremity asymmetric oligoarthritis, which may mimic septic arthritis, and thus warrant a joint aspiration. Other characteristic features include enthesitis (inflammation of the insertion sites of tendons, ligaments, and fascia to bone) and lower back pain. Extra-articular features of ReA include urethritis (in cases of genitourinary infection), conjunctivitis or anterior uveitis, oral ulcers, circinate balanitis, and various other skin lesions. The rheumatological manifestations of ReA are similar whether the preceding infection is genitourinary, an STD, or a gastrointestinal infection.

ReA is considered one of the spondyloarthropathies, a group of diseases that also includes psoriatic arthritis, ankylosing spondylitis, and enteropathic arthritis associated with inflammatory bowel disease.

Factors associated with the development of postinfection ReA are not clear. Despite the strong association with the HLA-B27 antigen, the mechanism whereby this HLA gene might confer disease susceptibility to ReA remains unknown. One of the existing alternative theories is molecular mimicry, whereby an autoimmune response develops after the infection because of cross-reactivity of host and microbial antigens. Alternatively, in an altered cellular immune response to the pathogen, unique determinants in the antigen-binding groove of the HLA-B27 molecule may specifically present arthritogenic peptides to the responding CD8+T-cell population. The third possibility is an altered microbial–host cell interaction by which certain HLA alleles modulate the host response to arthritogenic organisms. Whichever mechanism is true, it is likely that the synovitis that develops is related to local deposition and persistence of microbial antigens, although there is no definitive proof of this so far.

In some other bacterial infections, such as Lyme disease, *Bartonella*, and rickettsial diseases, joint manifestations may appear as well.

The majority of Lyme disease cases are localized to endemic foci in the USA, Europe, and Asia. Upon infecting humans, *Borrelia burgdorferi* replicates in the skin and then disseminates via the bloodstream to other organs, leading to extracutaneous disease manifestations. Fever, malaise, myalgias, and arthralgias generally accompany this dissemination. Late manifestations of Lyme disease may occur in the joints, nervous system, and skin. The joint manifestation of this stage would usually be an intermittent, oligoarticular arthritis, with the knee being the most common site [24].

In cat scratch disease (CSD), caused principally by *Bartonella henselae* infection, musculoskeletal manifestations are not uncommon. In a large Israeli cohort, 20% of the patients developed chronic disease persisting 16–53 months after the onset of arthropathy. The arthropathy was characterized by large and medium joint involvement and severe joint pain that was often incapacitating. Fatigue, nocturnal joint pain, morning stiffness, tendinitis, and erythema nodosum were part of the CSD-associated arthropathy syndrome. In contrast to ReA, the arthropathy appears concurrent with the onset of the disease, and not weeks after resolution of the triggering infection. Thus, *Bartonella* infection, similarly to Lyme-associated arthropathy, should be classified as part of the direct infection-related arthropathy group [25].

Rheumatic manifestations of *Brucellosis* are the most common features of the disease, and up to 30% of the patients exhibit some form of these manifestations. Among the rheumatic manifestations, sacroiliitis (40–55%), peripheral arthritis (30–40%), spondylitis (20–30%), and osteomyelitis (5–10%) are the most common. A mixture of these features with peripheral arthritis and spondylitis is quite common. The diagnosis of the disease requires a high index of suspicion and is based on a history of consumption of raw milk products or direct contact with tissues of infected animals. Diagnosis is based on isolation of the bacterium from tissue or blood and a rising titer of specific antibodies.

Long-term antibiotic treatment (6 weeks) is recommended.

Mycobacterial tuberculosis (TB) infections of the musculoskeletal system account for up to 5% of cases of TB. The main clinical presentations include spondylitis (Pott disease), arthritis, osteomyelitis, tenosynovitis, bursitis, and pyomyositis. Musculoskeletal TB remains a major cause of morbidity and mortality in developing countries. Population migration from these countries is still a major source of TB in the modern Western world.

The scope of this chapter does not allow an extensive review of this subject. Among travelers, recreational tourists are at a very low risk for acquiring TB. Among long-term residents in developing countries, relief workers, and volunteers in refugee camps, some risk exists. In these latter groups, positive PPD conversion is more common, active pulmonary TB has occasionally been reported, and extrapulmonary manifestations are extremely rare.

### Treatment

NSAIDs form the cornerstone of treatment of ReA. Occasional use of intra-articular injections of glucocorticoids may provide relief of inflammatory arthritis. Oral steroids have been also used, but there are no good studies to support this approach. The long-term use of antibiotics is probably also of no value in treating the joint symptoms. However, the use of second-line drugs, of the disease-modifying agent group, such as sulfasalazine, methotrexate, and the recently introduced tumor necrosis factor inhibitors, may provide some benefit in cases refractory to NSAIDs with a rather chronic course of active inflammation, although this approach is also not based on large-scale clinical studies.

Uncontrolled single reports suggest initiation of anti-malarial therapy in patients who suffer a protracted course of Lyme arthritis. Occupational therapy may be initiated in order to maintain joint function and range of movement.

## Parasitic infections

Parasitic infections are common among travelers. They may include protozoa, helminths, arthropods, and much less commonly, fungal infections. The most common are the food-borne protozoa and geohelminths (e.g., *Giardia lamblia*, *Entamoeba hystolitica*, *Ascaris*, hookworms, and *Strongyloides*). Although gastrointestinal complaints are the dominant ones, extraintestinal manifestations may occur, including musculoskeletal manifestations, hypersensitivity reactions, and immune complex deposition. Arthralgia is the most common symptom, but the frequency of joint involvement is not clearly known. These manifestations are usually benign and often resolve with treatment of the underlying infection. They have been reviewed extensively by Peng [26], and thus will not be discussed here. Several infections with prolonged rheumatological manifestations that may be seen in travelers will be discussed.

Trichinosis is infection with *Trichinella* species (see Chapter 31). Human infections are acquired by eating raw or undercooked meat, usually pork. Following this, the larvae in the intestines enter the bloodstream and disseminate to skeletal muscle. In these cases, the hallmark of the disease is invasion of muscles, causing severe myalgias and elevated muscle enzymes (creatine kinase). The presentation of myalgias with severe proximal muscle weakness may be confused with polymyositis [27].

Symptoms appear 2–8 weeks after ingestion and include a sudden onset of severe muscle pain, swelling, and weakness. The pain may be so severe as to limit function of the arms and legs and inhibit walking, speaking, moving the tongue, breathing, and swallowing. Weakness is also a consequence of muscle involvement.

The severity of the clinical course depends on host factors and on the species involved.

After the acute period, convalescence follows (lasting from months to years), usually with complete recovery. However, some investigators report "persisting sequelae," meaning the persistence of myalgia, early fatigability, ocular signs, and headache for up to 10 years after clinical recovery [28].

Eosinophilia is a hallmark of trichinellosis and is present at some time in every case. The level of eosinophils rises to a range of 20–90% (for methods of diagnosis see Chapter 31).

Symptomatic treatment with analgesics, antipyretics, and corticosteroids may be beneficial, particularly with severe infections. Prednisone is generally administered at a dose of 50 mg/day for 10–15 days. In addition, the antiparasitic drugs mebendazole and albendazole are warranted.

Schistosomiasis is a water-borne helminth that resides within the blood vessels of the urinary system in the case of *Schistosoma hematobium*, and within the mesenteric blood vessels in the cases of *S. mansoni* and *S. japonicum* (see Chapter 24). The mature worms lay eggs that are expelled via the urine or gastrointestinal system. However, ectopic migration of eggs via the blood stream may result, with unusual manifestations, such as cerebral schistosomiasis (mainly in cases of *S. japonicum*). Rarely, this ectopic migration can terminate in the blood vessels of a joint, causing severe monoarthritic pain, with reactive fluid in the joint [29]. In populations of endemic areas, large proportions of patients with *S. mansoni* infection reported rheumatological manifestations [30]. The most common syndromes resemble classical ReA or other seronegative spondyloarthropathies, with varying combinations of peripheral enthesitis, large joint asymmetric oligoarthritis (typically of the knee), and sacroiliitis; other studies report a relatively high percentage of rheumatoid arthritis-like presentations involving the MCP and PIP joints, wrists, ankles, and knees. Some of these manifestations might be the result of circulating immune complexes, which are known to exist in this infection.

Briefly, the treatment is directed against the parasite, and it is a course of 40–60 mg/kg of praziquantel. Fungal infection by endemic mycoses is relatively rare among travelers (Chapter 29). Among fungal infections, histoplasmosis is the most common and, in almost all cases, in travelers the infection was acquired in Latin America (visiting bat caves is a risk factor). The major symptoms associated with this infection are flu-like and respiratory symptoms, including granulomas in the lung. There are reported cases where prolonged rheumatological manifestations occurred [31]. The rheumatological manifestations during histoplasmosis infection are thought to represent a systemic inflammatory reaction to the primary pulmonary infection. Typically, these patients have rapidly additive arthritis or arthralgia, which tends to be symmetric in 50% of cases [32]. Knees, ankles, wrists, and small joints of the hand are the most common sites affected. About 40% may have monoarticular disease. Nearly half of patients with rheumatological manifestations exhibit erythema nodosum and/or erythema multiforme [32].

For diagnosis, see Chapter 29.

Pulmonary histoplasmosis in immune-competent patients is considered to be a self-limited disease without need for antifungal treatment. The rheumatological manifestations do not change this policy [33]. Thus, only therapy with NSAIDs for 2–12 weeks, depending on the resolution of the symptoms and of erythema nodosum, is recommended. Relapse may occur after anti-inflammatory therapy is stopped, requiring reinstitution of the same therapy [33].

## Prognosis

The prognosis of the postinfectious rheumatic manifestations is generally good, although few cases of viral infection, such as in chikungunya, or bacterial infection, such as in Lyme disease, may develop a protracted chronic course, which is, however, nondestructive in nature. It should be noted that patients who bear HLA-B27 antigen, and have developed ReA, are prone to a much more severe course of their disease.

The generally favorable prognosis of the postinfectious rheumatic diseases highlights the need for an accurate diagnosis in these cases.

## Noninfectious causes

Noninfectious etiologies, including various toxins, have been reported as causing prolonged rheumatological manifestations.

A large epidemic appeared in Spain in 1981, following the consumption of adulterated rapeseed oil. A new systemic disease was described and the name *toxic-oil syndrome* (TOS) was coined [34]. The musculoskeletal manifestations of the new syndrome were characterized by the presence of arthralgias, sometimes arthritis, extensive muscle atrophy, severe neuropathy, and scleroderma-like skin involvement. Other scleroderma-like features were the Raynaud phenomenon, pulmonary hypertension, sicca syndrome, and liver disease [34]. This epidemic affected more than 20,000 persons in Spain, including international travelers to Spain [35].

## Eosinophilia–myalgia syndrome

In 1989, a new syndrome appeared in the USA following the consumption of L-tryptophan containing products. This syndrome was termed *eosinophilia–myalgia syndrome* (EMS), and symptoms and laboratory findings were similar to those of the epidemic of TOS. The chronic phase of EMS was characterized by long-term disability, sclerodermatous skin thickening, sensorimotor polyneuropathy, and severe episodic myalgias [36].

Due to their clinical similarities, researchers tried to link both epidemics to the same altered metabolism of L-tryptophan [37].

From a tropical medicine perspective, it is important to note that these two syndromes were associated with significant peripheral eosinophilia, in addition to the rheumatological manifestations. This combination is unusual, and among the helminthic diseases (which are usually associated with eosinophilia), trichinosis is the disease in which rheumatological manifestations are accompanied by significant eosinophilia.

## Ciguatera

Ciguatera is a disease caused by the ingestion of fish containing the toxins of *Gambierdiscus toxicus*. Ciguatera toxin, also known as ciguatoxin, is a class of polyether toxins that act on the sodium channels of cells, causing changes in their electrical potential and permeability. This dinoflagellate is frequently found in damaged coral reef systems in several parts of the tropics: the Pacific Ocean, Red Sea, Indian Ocean, and Caribbean. It is estimated that at least 25,000 cases occur each year worldwide. The disease is now seen in tourists returning from tropical countries. Eighteen French patients who were examined between 1997 and 2002 acquired the disease on Atlantic Ocean islands, Pacific Ocean islands, and one on the Egyptian Red Sea coast [38]. A series of 13 Italian travelers were reported with ciguatera poisoning after returning from the Caribbean [39]. Patients suffered initially from gastrointestinal complaints and sensory disturbances. In addition,

patients suffered for 2–18 months from arthralgias, myalgias, or pruritis [38].

No specific effective treatment for ciguatera fish poisoning has been proven; supportive treatment is based on symptomatic treatment. It is important to note that cases of fish poisoning might have happened in travelers returning from tropical countries after having ingested fish imported from the Caribbean and Pacific.

## Plant thorn synovitis

Plant thorn synovitis is an uncommon cause of monoarthritis. Pathologically, thorn synovitis represents a foreign body reaction to retained plant material and is mostly aseptic. The presentation is delayed (mean time to diagnosis was 10 weeks with a range of 2 weeks to 9 months in one study), with a history of antecedent injury, often forgotten. Thus, diagnosis relies on careful elicitation of the history. Symptoms include joint pain, swelling, and stiffness. Synovitis is usually present on examination, along with decreased range of motion of the affected joint [40]. Imaging may be helpful in localizing the plant material when the history is not clear. Initial conservative treatment with nonsteroidal anti-inflammatory NSAIDs, antibiotics, or splinting is usually unsuccessful, and many of the patients need an arthrotomy, removal of the foreign body, and partial or total synovectomy, which generally leads to complete resolution without any sequelae. Plant thorn synovitis must be therefore included in the differential diagnosis of monoarthritis. Histologically, it can mimic sarcoidosis, tuberculosis, or a fungal infection.

## Conclusions

Protracted rheumatological manifestations, especially polyarthritis/arthralgia, may occur as a consequence of a wide range of pathogens, including viral, bacterial, and parasitic agents. Although the pathogenesis varies, the prognosis overall is good, with full recovery, without sequelae, albeit sometime very drawn out. Treatment is symptomatic in most cases. Diagnosis of infectious-related arthritis/arthralgia leads to a better prognosis, and can relieve anxiety among patients who are afraid of chronic rheumatic disease.

Because many patients will seek medical advice with these chronic complaints long after travel, physicians should be aware of the possible association between these complaints and remote travel. Travel history is mandatory, even in a rheumatological setting.

# References

1 El-Gabalawy, HS, Duray P, Goldbach-Mansky R. Evaluating patients with arthritis of recent onset: studies in pathogenesis and prognosis. *JAMA* 2000;284:2368.

2 Toivanen A. Alphaviruses: an emerging cause of arthritis? *Curr Opin Rheumatol* 2008;20:486–90.

3 Suhrbier A, La Linn M. Clinical and pathologic aspects of arthritis due to Ross River virus and other alphaviruses. *Curr Opin Rheumatol* 2004;16:374.

4 Enserink M. Infectious diseases. Chikungunya: no longer a Third World disease. *Science* 2007;318:1860–1.

5 Bonilauri P, Bellini R, Calzolari M, Angelini R, Venturi L, Fallacara F, et al. Chikungunya virus in *Aedes albopictus*, Italy. *Emerg Infect Dis* 2008;14:852–4.

6 Simon F, Parola P, Grandadam M, Fourcade S, Oliver M, Brouqui P, et al. Chikungunya infection: an emerging rheumatism among travelers returned from Indian Ocean islands. Report of 47 cases. *Medicine (Baltimore)* 2007;86: 123–37.

7 Borgherini G, Poubeau P, Jossaume A, et al. Persistent arthralgia associated with chikungunya virus: a study of 88 adult patients on Reunion Island. *Clin Infect Dis* 2008;47:469–75.

8 Mylonas AD, Brown AM, Carthew TL, McGrath B, Purdie DM, Pandeya N, et al. Natural history of Ross River virus-induced epidemic polyarthritis. *Med J Aust* 2002;177:356–60.

9 Colin de Verdière N, Molina JM. Rheumatic manifestations caused by tropical viruses. *Joint Bone Spine* 2007;74: 410–13.

10 Louthrenoo W. Rheumatic manifestations of human immunodeficiency virus infection. *Curr Opin Rheumatol* 2008; 20:92–9.

11 Naides SJ. Rheumatic manifestations of parvovirus B19 infection. *Rheum Dis Clin North Am* 1998;24:375.

12 Chantler JK, Tingle AJ, Petty RE. Persistent rubella virus infection associated with chronic arthritis in children. *N Engl J Med* 1985;313:117–23.

13 Fraser JR, Ratnamohan VM, Dowling JP, et al. The xanthema of Ross virus infection: histology, location of virus antigen and nature of inflammatory infiltrate. *J Clin Pathol* 1983;36:1256–63.

14 Morrison TE, Whitmore AC, Shabman RS, et al. Characterization of Ross River virus tropism and virus-induced inflammation in a mouse model of viral arthritis and myositis. *J Virol* 2006;80:737–49.

15 Moore TL. Parvovirus associated arthritis. *Curr Opin Rheumatol* 2000;12:289–94.

16 Soden M, Vasudevan H, Roberts B, et al. Detection of viral ribonucleic acid and histologic analysis of inflamed synovium in Ross River virus infection. *Arthritis Rheum* 2000; 43:365–9.

17 Ziegler SA, Lu L, Travassos da Rosa APA, et al. An animal model for studying the pathogenesis of chikungunya virus infection. *Am J Trop Med Hyg* 2008;79:133–9.

18 Lai CL, Ratziu V, Yuen MF, et al. Viral hepatitis B. *Lancet* 2003;362: 2089–94.

19 Albert LJ, Inman RD. Molecular mimicry and autoimmunity. *N Engl J Med* 1999;341:2068–74.

20 Lidbury BA, Rulli NE, Suhrbier A, et al. Macrophage-derived proinflammatory factors contribute to the development of arthritis and myositis after infection with an arthrogenic alphavirus. *J Infect Dis* 2008;197:1585–93.

21 Mylonas AD, Harley D, Purdie DM, Pandeya N, Vecchio PC, Farmer JF, et al. Corticosteroid therapy in an Alphaviral arthritis. *J Clin Rheumatol* 2004;10:326–30.

22 Sieper J, Rudwaleit M, Braun J, et al. Diagnosing reactive arthritis: role of clinical setting in the value of serologic and microbiologic assays. *Arthritis Rheum* 2002;46:319–29.

23 Rihl M, Klos A, Kohler L, et al. Infection and musculoskeletal conditions: Reactive arthritis. *Best Pract Res Clin Rheumatol* 2006;20:1119–37.

24 Steere AC, Cobourn J, Glickstein L. The emergence of Lyme disease. *J Clin Invest* 2004;113:1093–1101.

25 Giladi M, Maman E, Paran D, et al. Cat-scratch disease-associated arthropathy. *Arthritis Rheum.* 2005;52:3611–17.

26 Peng SL. Rheumatic manifestations of parasitic diseases. *Semin Arthritis Rheum* 2002;31:228–47.

27 Santos Durán-Ortiz J, García-de la Torre I, Orozco-Barocio G, Martínez-Bonilla G, Rodríguez-Toledo A, Herrera-Zárate L. Trichinosis with severe myopathic involvement mimicking polymyositis. Report of a family outbreak. *J Rheumatol* 1992;19:310–12.

28 Bruschi F, Murrell KD. New aspects of human trichinellosis: the impact of new *Trichinella* species. *Postgrad Med J* 2002;78:15–22.

29 Bassiouni M, Kamel M. Bilharzial arthropathy. *Ann Rheum Dis* 1984;43:806–9.

30 Atkin SL, Kamel M, el-Hady AM, el-Badawy SA, el-Ghobary A, Dick WC. Schistosomiasis and inflammatory polyarthritis: a clinical, radiological and laboratory study of 96 patients infected by *S. mansoni* with particular reference to the diarthrodial joint. *Q J Med* 1986;59:479–87.

31 Alonso D, Munoz J, Letang E, Salvado E, Cuenca-Estrella M, Buitrago MJ, et al. Imported acute histoplasmosis with rheumatologic manifestations in Spanish travelers. *J Travel Med* 2007;14:338–42.

32 Rosenthal J, Brandt KD, Wheat LJ, Slama TG. Rheumatologic manifestations of histoplasmosis in the recent Indianapolis epidemic. *Arthritis Rheum* 1983;26:1065–70.

33 Wheat J, Sarosi G, McKinsey D, et al. Practice guidelines for the management of patients with histoplasmosis. *Clin Infect Dis* 2000;30:688–95.

34 Sánchez-Porro Valadés P, Posada de la Paz M, de Andrés Copa P, et al. Toxic oil syndrome: survival in the whole cohort between 1981 and 1995. *J Clin Epidemiol* 2003;56: 701–8.

35 Araoz D, Fabre J. Poisoning by adulterated edible oil. *Schweiz Med Wochenschr* 1981;111:1818–22.

36 Sullivan EA, Kamb ML, Jones JL, Meyer P, Philen RM, Falk H, et al. The natural history of eosinophilia-myalgia syndrome in a tryptophan-exposed cohort in South Carolina. *Arch Intern Med* 1996;156:973–9.

37 Silver RM, Sutherland SE, Carreira P, Heyes MP. Alterations in tryptophan metabolism in the toxic oil syndrome and in the eosinophilia–myalgia syndrome. *J Rheumatol* 1992;19:69–73.

38 de Haro L, Pommier P, Valli M. Emergence of imported ciguatera in Europe: report of 18 cases at the Poison Control Centre of Marseille. *J Toxicol Clin Toxicol* 2003;41:927–30.

39 Bavastrelli M, Bertucci P, Midulla M, et al. Ciguatera fish poisoning: an emerging syndrome in Italian travelers. *J Travel Med* 2001;8:139–42.

40 Carandell M, Roig D, Benasco C. Plant thorn synovitis. *J Rheumatol* 1980;7:567–79.

# 41 Travel-Related Respiratory Infections

Eyal Meltzer and Eli Schwartz

Chaim Sheba Medical Center, Tel Hashomer, Israel
Sackler School of Medicine, Tel Aviv University, Tel Aviv, Israel

## Introduction

Respiratory tract infections are ubiquitous in developed and developing countries. Seasonal outbreaks of the common cold, pharyngitis, and influenza form a part of the medical landscape of everyday life, and pneumonia is one of the most frequent community-acquired infections in most countries. The importance of respiratory infections in travelers stems from their high frequency, pathogens that occur out of season, the possibility of less known but life-threatening pathogens, and other clinical pitfalls. The aim of this chapter is to consider the epidemiology of travel-related respiratory tract infections, to review certain less frequent pathogens, and to suggest a clinical approach to diagnosis.

## Epidemiology of travel-related respiratory infections

Respiratory tract infections (RTIs) are the most prevalent infectious disease in humans. Surveys in the USA have established that RTIs affect more than 70% of the population yearly, with adults suffering at least two yearly episodes [1]. The incidence of respiratory disease in the UK usually peaks at about 600/100,000 or 0.6% during winter months, but may reach 1% of the population in some years [2]. Whether travel per se increases the risk for RTIs is unknown. The incidence of RTIs changes markedly throughout the year in all temperate countries; it may differ markedly from year to year, between regions, and among different age groups. It is certain, however, that RTIs appear to be very frequent among travelers. In the USA, a prospective study has found that among internal air travelers during the winter season, 20% developed RTIs (3).

Several studies have reported on the occurrence of RTIs in travelers to developing countries using different methodologies. Only a few prospective studies have addressed this issue: Rack et al. have found among German travelers an RTI incidence of 13.8% [4], whereas among Israeli and American travelers, as many as 25–26% reported post-travel RTIs ([5, 6]. Several retrospective surveys on very large numbers of returning travelers have reported similar findings: in a seminal article 30 years ago, Steffen et al. reported that the incidence of respiratory symptoms was 12% among more than 10,000 travelers to developing countries [7]. Among nearly 5,000 Scottish travelers, 16.8% reported an RTI during travel [8]. In all these surveys, RTIs were second only to diarrhea as the most prevalent health event during travel.

Another set of data can be found in registries of ill returning travelers presenting at travel clinics or hospitals. These reports have an inherent selection bias toward more severe illnesses. Despite this, RTIs still figure high among travel-related infectious diseases. The most comprehensive registry of ill returning travelers is the multinational GeoSentinel registry. In this report, RTIs accounted for 77/1000 travelers, and were again second only to diarrhea in prevalence [9]. Other reports have focused on febrile illness in returning travelers. In another GeoSentinel study of febrile patients, RTIs accounted for 14% of all cases [10]. RTIs assume even greater importance among HIV-infected travelers, whereas among febrile patients, they were the leading diagnosis [11]. Hospital-based series from different countries show RTIs to be the diagnosis

*Tropical Diseases in Travelers*, 1st edition. Edited by E. Schwartz.
© 2009 by Blackwell Publishing, ISBN: 978-1-4051-8441-0.

in 2.6–46% of febrile hospitalized patients [12]. These marked differences probably reflect local differences in hospitalization practices, rather than local differences in RTI incidence.

To summarize, although it is not known whether travelers to developing countries are more or less prone to RTIs, these conditions are highly prevalent among them, causing significant travel disruption and a significant number of post-travel hospital admissions.

## Upper respiratory tract infections in travelers

Upper respiratory tract infection (URTI) is usually defined as an acute illness causing cough, with or without coryza, sore throat, and systemic symptoms such as fever and malaise [13]. As discussed previously, the true incidence of URTI in travelers is not really known, but is in all likelihood very high, second only to diarrhea in prevalence. Most cases are mild and therefore unreported. However, the burden of short-term morbidity, travel disruption, and cost is probably very considerable. The mode of transmission for most of the common viruses causing URTI is probably similar in travelers and the general population, with droplet infection and close contact accounting for most cases. Several viruses that cause RTIs can be transmitted orally, such as enteroviruses and adenoviruses, and may, therefore, be transmitted via food and water [14]. However, this mode of transmission is probably not important.

The spectrum of viral agents causing travel-related URTIs is similar to that seen in the general population. Camps et al. have diagnosed at least one virus from 56% of travelers with fever and respiratory symptoms [15]. The most frequent viruses detected were influenza virus (38%), rhinovirus (23%), adenovirus (9%), and respiratory syncytial virus (9%). Similar results were reported in German travelers, where again influenza was the most frequent isolate [16].

Most data regarding respiratory viruses among travelers relate to influenza. Large outbreaks of influenza have been reported among travelers, and the global fear of pandemic influenza and the spread of avian influenza have focused research on this field. Already during the pandemic of 1889–1890, the advance of pandemic influenza along lines of travel was well established [17]. Today, air travel is of great importance in influenza dissemination [18].

Influenza is not rare among travelers. The Hajj is probably the largest annual transit of persons in the world

and has presented an excellent opportunity to study influenza. In a large survey among Hajj pilgrims in 2003, RTIs accounted for 40% of all illnesses reported, and influenza virus accounted for half the respiratory viruses isolated [19]. In 2006, a detailed laboratory analysis for viral causes of URTIs in Hajj pilgrims found influenza to be second only to rhinovirus (11% and 15%, respectively) [20]. Apart from Hajj pilgrims, additional studies on Western travelers attest to the high incidence of influenza. Mutsch et al. have established in Swiss travelers an incidence rate of 1 case/100 travel months, with 2.8% overall incidence and 12.8% among travelers with a history of febrile illness. An important feature was that most cases occurred outside the usual North European influenza season [21]. Large outbreaks of influenza were also reported in cruise ships because the confined onboard conditions promote outbreaks [22].

## Lower respiratory tract infections in travelers

Pneumonia is not a rare condition among returning ill travelers. Although it is significantly less prevalent than URTI in most series, it still accounts for many hospital admissions due to post-travel respiratory illness [12, 23]. Pneumonia is also an important cause of infectious mortality post-travel [9] and, in fact, was the only cause of mortality among 1106 ill Australian travelers over a 6 year period [24]. Due to its potential severity and associated mortality, post-travel pneumonia is a major medical concern in returning travelers. These concerns were accentuated after the SARS outbreak due to the fears of global spread of the disease and the attendant risks to healthcare personnel.

Most of the major causes of pneumonia have a global distribution. *Streptococcus pneumoniae, Hemophilus influenza,* and *Staphylococcus aureus* are the dominant pneumonia isolates in developing countries [25–27]. Some agents of travel-related pneumonia have a global distribution, but are reported infrequently. Q fever, for example, is only rarely diagnosed in travelers, and in fact has more often been associated with a nonspecific febrile illness than with RTI, sometimes diagnosed only as part of an outbreak investigation [28, 29]. The majority of travel-related Q fever is reported from Africa. Whether African travel is indeed a risk factor for *Coxiella* infection or the disease is underreported from other locales (e.g., Southern Europe, where Q fever is quite prevalent [30]) is not known.

Some agents of travel-related pneumonia are rare in most developed countries and may, therefore, be missed by practitioners if the travel itinerary is not taken into account. These include most helminthic and some bacterial and fungal respiratory infections, which will be discussed below.

The etiology of travel-related pneumonia has in fact received scant attention. In a small study by Ansart et al., most cases of pneumonia were bacterial, with *Streptococcus pneumoniae*, *Mycoplasma*, and *Legionella* diagnosed in 38% of cases [31]. Three cases were caused by organisms not included in the "core organisms" covered by guidelines for the treatment of pneumonia, including one case each of Q fever, histoplasmosis, and schistosomiasis, and two cases were diagnosed with systemic infectious agents: dengue and leptospirosis.

In the following sections, several of these travel-specific agents of pneumonia are described in detail. However, one should keep in mind that even for mundane pneumococcal pneumonia, major differences in bacterial resistance patterns are encountered in different countries. For example, pneumococcal penicillin and multidrug resistance are very frequent in South Africa, the Far East, and even Spain, but very rare in the Netherlands [32]. These issues should all be addressed in the clinical approach to the patient with post-travel pneumonia and to empirical antimicrobial therapy.

## A clinical approach to the returning traveler with respiratory symptoms

Acute and chronic respiratory symptoms are two common complaints, with the first being the most common presentation in general medical practice and the second being reported by up to 20% of the general population [33]. Clearly, therefore, in evaluating returning travelers, the first issue is to establish by a thorough medical history whether respiratory complaints are indeed temporally associated with travel. The majority of patients presenting with post-travel respiratory symptoms fall into one of two major categories: an acute febrile disease with respiratory symptoms or protracted respiratory symptoms post-travel, mainly cough.

## Acute post-travel fever and respiratory symptoms

It is of primary importance for the physician to remember at the outset that respiratory symptoms are not rare in systemic febrile illnesses that are not commonly associated with the respiratory tract. In malaria, respiratory symptoms occur in up to half the patients and are not limited to cases of severe malaria with pulmonary edema/acute respiratory distress syndrome (ARDS) [34]. Similarly, cough is not rare in enteric fever [35] and leptospirosis [36], which are sometimes initially mistaken for URTI/pneumonia. Thus, if a thorough travel history reveals a stay in malaria-endemic areas, malaria must always be actively ruled out by repeated blood smears.

The acutely ill returning traveler with fever and respiratory symptoms may be suffering from either URTI or pneumonia. As recommended in practice guidelines in the general population, a chest radiograph (CXR) is needed to exclude pneumonia [37]. Radiological findings may include not only infiltrates of "usual" pneumonia, but other findings such as the infiltrates of acute respiratory distress/pulmonary edema in *vivax/falciparum* malaria or pulmonary nodules in acute histoplasmosis.

Among patients with URTI, an immediate issue is influenza: fever and cough with an acute onset are the definition of "influenza-like-illness" (ILI). Attention to influenza is heightened due to current concerns about avian influenza and pandemics because travelers are assumed to be the main force of pandemic spread [38]. Since early identification of influenza can provide benefits for the traveler (by instituting antiviral therapy) and the community (by limiting spread), travelers should be tested for influenza virus. The patterns of influenza seasonality in travel medicine reflect the transmission pattern in the destination countries. It should be remembered that in many tropical countries influenza transmission is continuous rather than seasonal [39].

### Pneumonia
Guidelines for the assessment, triage, and treatment of pneumonia are well established [37]. We believe it is useful to consider three scenarios post-travel: usual pneumonia, severe pneumonia, and pneumonia with eosinophilia. The majority of travelers with pneumonia will not differ from routine cases of community-acquired pneumonia (CAP). Still, increased exposure to hotels requires heightened alertness to the possibility of legionellosis. Providing coverage for *Legionella* even in non-severe cases is probably merited (see discussion on legionellosis later in this chapter).

Among patients with severe CAP (SCAP), general CAP guidelines already address legionellosis. However, travelers to East and Southeast Asia may be exposed to *Burkholderia pseudomallei*—the causative agent of melioidosis. This disease can manifest as a severe necrotizing pneumonia and is not covered by usual treatment recommendations (see discussion on melioidosis later in this chapter).

Severe pneumonia can also be associated with viral infections. The most common worldwide is influenza. Primary influenza pneumonia is in fact underreported, but during pandemic years has accounted for 18% of all influenza-associated pneumonia [40]. Other rarely reported viral pneumonias in travelers include SARS and hantavirus pulmonary syndrome (HPS). No SARS activity has been recorded since the end of the 2003 epidemic. However, this situation may change, and for travelers from East and Southeast Asia with severe pneumonia, tests for possible SARS may be required. HPS, which is part of the viral hemorrhagic fever group, has been reported very rarely in travelers to South America (see Chapter 13).

### Pneumonia with eosinophilia

Acute bacterial infections, including pneumonia, are usually accompanied by eosinopenia, and, therefore, even a high normal eosinophil count should be closely followed. Pneumonia with eosinophilia can be attributed to several causes; in developed countries exposure to various drugs or toxic substances is the more frequently established cause, but many cases remain idiopathic [41]. Among returning travelers, several unusual causes should be considered initially, mainly helminthic infections.

Schistosomiasis manifests acutely as a combination of fever and respiratory symptoms, either with or without pulmonary infiltrates [42]. Other symptoms of acute schistosomiasis may include an urticarial rash, fatigue, and myalgia (see Chapter 24). Respiratory symptoms are at times the dominant symptom and may last for several weeks. Similarly, geohelminths—*Ascaris*, hookworms, and *Strongyloides*—can cause an acute febrile episode with cough, again with or without lung infiltrates. The presence of lung infiltrates in acute ascariasis defines the original Löffler syndrome.

Several dimorphic fungi may cause respiratory symptoms with pulmonary infiltrates. Among these, coccidioidomycosis in the western USA and paracoccidioidomycosis in Latin America are often associated with eosinophilia. The more frequent endemic fungal pneumonitis seen in travelers is histoplasmosis, which does not cause eosinophilia (see discussion later in this chapter and Chapter 29).

A simple algorithmic approach may be used to guide the diagnosis and therapy of acutely ill returning travelers with fever and respiratory symptoms (Figure 41.1). Clinicians are encouraged to make use of available international reporting systems (e.g., ProMed, available from http://www.promedmail.org) because these may present the earliest opportunity of recognizing an international common source outbreak (e.g., legionellosis).

### Protracted post-travel respiratory symptoms

Unlike the data on the prevalence of chronic diarrhea among travelers and its etiology, there are few data on the prevalence and etiology of protracted post-travel respiratory symptoms—mainly prolonged cough. In the majority of cases of acute respiratory infections, respiratory symptoms persist well after fever has resolved, but will usually disappear or be greatly improved after 2–3 weeks [33]. In the general population, protracted cough is frequently ascribed to a few causes, including asthma, postnasal drip, and gastroesophageal reflux. Among travelers, we have to consider several travel-related infections that may cause prolonged cough before applying the usual Western guidelines. Our approach is summarized in Figure 41.2.

A thorough medical history and physical examination are essential. An exact travel itinerary should be determined, as well as the types of exposures that have occurred (e.g., bathing in freshwater, exposure to contaminated soil, and types of raw food consumed). The geographical distribution of the major travel-related RTIs is described in Figure 41.3. Symptoms and signs that developed prior to the respiratory symptoms may suggest a specific diagnosis (e.g., ground itch, urticarial rashes, or gastrointestinal manifestations) [43]. In addition to history and physical examination, all patients with post-travel respiratory symptoms should undergo chest radiography and a complete blood count (CBC).

### Persistent cough with eosinophilia

Helminth-associated respiratory symptoms can follow a protracted course, usually associated with marked eosinophilia. We have shown, for example, that among Israeli travelers with schistosomiasis, protracted cough was not rare, with the median duration of respiratory symptoms being 6 weeks (mean ± SD 15.4 ± 22.7 weeks) [44]. Therefore, regardless of the results of the CXR (in some patients granulomatous pneumonitis was not seen at all, or was discernible only after high-resolution CT), schistosomiasis needs to be actively excluded if exposure to infected waters may have occurred. Geohelminths can cause cough and eosinophilia [45]. Infiltrates can be fleeting, and, therefore, the diagnosis should be assessed in all patients, even when the CXR is normal.

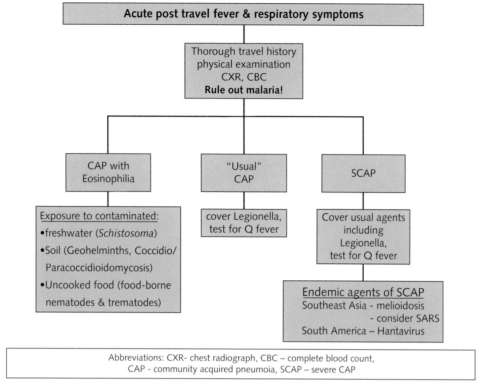

**Acute post travel fever & respiratory symptoms**

Thorough travel history
physical examination
CXR, CBC
**Rule out malaria!**

CAP with
Eosinophilia

"Usual"
CAP

SCAP

Exposure to contaminated:
- freshwater (*Schistosoma*)
- Soil (Geohelminths, Coccidio/
  Paracoccidioidomycosis)
- Uncooked food (food-borne
  nematodes & trematodes)

cover Legionella,
test for Q fever

Cover usual agents
including
Legionella,
test for Q fever

Endemic agents of SCAP
Southeast Asia - melioidosis
                    - consider SARS
South America – Hantavirus

Abbreviations: CXR- chest radiograph, CBC – complete blood count,
CAP - community acquired pneumoia, SCAP – severe CAP

**Figure 41.1** The clinical approach to the acutely ill returning traveler with fever and cough.

An additional pathogen that may present with protracted cough and eosinophilia is *Paragonimus*, which is rarely described in travelers. Paragonimiasis results from the ingestion by humans of the intermediary host of the helminth—usually by eating uncooked freshwater crabs. After an initial migratory phase, a chronic cavitary lung lesion develops, with productive cough, occasionally with hemoptysis and chest pain. The clinical–radiological picture closely mimics that of tuberculosis, for which it is often mistaken in developing countries. A careful history can sometimes reveal possible exposure. Also, some patients may recall a larva migrans like rash early in the disease course. The infection can be proven by demonstrating the ova in sputum and stool. Serological tests exist, but are not often available (see Appendix). Therapy, on the other hand is simple: a 2-day course of praziquantel. Paragonimiasis has mainly been reported from Southeast Asia and South America, but may occur in additional regions, including Africa.

A final issue in the patient with persistent cough and eosinophilia is infection with coccidioidomycosis and paracoccidioidomycosis. Travelers to North and Latin America may be exposed to these agents, but reports of infections mostly involve long-term expatriates rather than tourists. The diagnosis requires demonstrating the typical yeast in the sputum, but occasionally bronchoalveolar lavage and even lung biopsy are required. Serological tests are also available (see Chapter 29).

In the patient with persistent cough, lung infiltrates, and a normal leukocyte count, histoplasmosis should be considered. Chest CT may have a highly suggestive radiological pattern, which may direct clinicians to order specific diagnostic tests. Similarly, any traveler with a protracted cough and infiltrate should be evaluated for tuberculosis.

In a patient with a normal physical examination, a normal CXR, and without eosinophilia, pertussis should be considered. Even in developed countries, the level of immunity for *Bordetella pertussis* is inadequate in many adults [46], and travelers are not different in having little awareness of and little protection against the disease. Little is known about travel-related pertussis, but among Hajj pilgrims clinical pertussis occurred in 7.5% of travelers without immunity [47]. The disease is so underreported

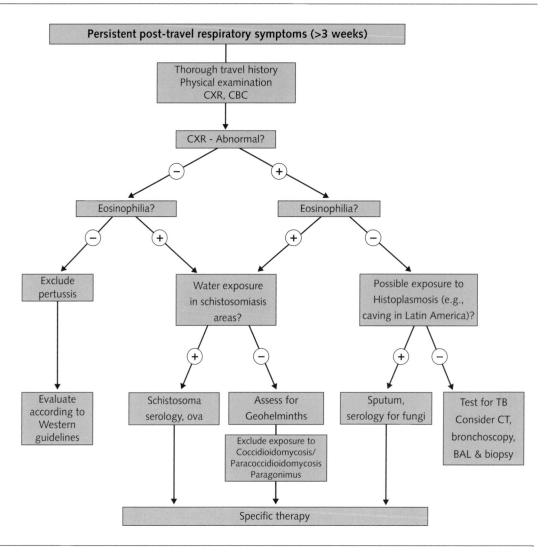

**Figure 41.2** The clinical approach to the returning traveler with protracted respiratory symptoms.

and unrecognized that testing the traveler with protracted cough is merited. Marked lymphocytosis on the CBC, an infrequent finding in the general population, is often a diagnostic clue.

In cases in which the diagnoses mentioned earlier are considered and excluded, the evaluation should generally follow established Western guidelines [33].

Following is a more detailed discussion of several pathogens that bear significant importance in post-travel pneumonia, including *Legionella*, melioidosis, fungal respiratory infection, and tuberculosis.

## Specific agents of pneumonia in travelers

### Legionella

Legionellae are a group of bacterial pathogens, whose usual habitat is aquatic environments, usually in close association with environmental amoebas. Colonization of air-conditioning systems, cooling towers, and water systems in hotels can result in aerosolization of the bacteria and outbreaks of severe pneumonia. Ever since the original

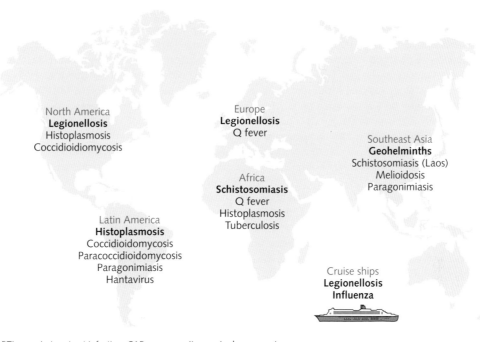

North America
**Legionellosis**
Histoplasmosis
Coccidioidiomycosis

Europe
**Legionellosis**
Q fever

Southeast Asia
**Geohelminths**
Schistosomiasis (Laos)
Melioidosis
Paragonimiasis

Africa
**Schistosomiasis**
Q fever
Histoplasmosis
Tuberculosis

Latin America
**Histoplasmosis**
Coccidioidomycosis
Paracoccidioidomycosis
Paragonimiasis
Hantavirus

Cruise ships
**Legionellosis**
**Influenza**

RTI = respiratory tract infection, CAP = community acquired pneumonia
Agents in bold = often reported in travelers with RTI from these regions

**Figure 41.3** Local distribution of travel-related agents of lower respiratory tract infections.

description of Legionnaires' disease among attendants of an American Legion conference in 1977, a connection between legionellosis and travel has been well recognized. The European Working Group for *Legionella* Infections (EWGLI) has reported on the incidence of legionellosis in the European Union. In this report, 12.1% of all cases were due to international travel, with a similar number caused by internal travel [48].

Legionellosis typically affects luxury tourism. Most cases are reported after travel to developed countries in Europe—most frequently Spain, France, and Italy—or North America. However, 10.5% had traveled to other destinations, with the resorts of southern Turkey being the most frequent, but with occasional clusters reported from the Caribbean region, Africa (both North and Sub-Saharan), and Southeast Asia [49]. In the USA, the CDC *Legionella* reporting system found that nearly a quarter of all diagnosed cases were travel-related, with between 5% and 10% being associated with international travel [50]. A specific form of travel that is frequently associated with legionellosis outbreaks is cruise ships. Many such clusters have been reported in recent decades from both the USA and Europe [51, 52].

*Legionella* pneumonia cannot be diagnosed through any combination of clinical and radiological findings. Although diarrhea, other gastrointestinal symptoms, or liver test abnormalities are sometimes deemed suggestive, all occur with other bacterial pneumonias. The only clinical finding that may increase the likelihood of legionellosis is pneumonia severity—severe and fatal pneumonia is more frequent with *Legionella*. Thus, in the European Union, the case fatality rate in travel-related legionellosis ranges between 3.8% and 5.6% [49].

To diagnose *Legionella*, clinicians need to perform additional tests. Legionellae are rarely isolated in culture, and most diagnoses are based on serology and urine antigen tests. Serology often requires paired serum samples, so that the diagnosis is often made after the event. Urine tests provide an accurate and timely diagnosis, and this probably accounts for an increasing reliance on these tests in recent years, both in Europe and in the USA [48, 51]. However, urine tests are targeted against the most frequent domestic isolate in developed countries, *L. pneumophila* serogroup 1, and their sensitivity for other *Legionella* infections is much lower [53]. The relative importance of other *L. pneumophila* serogroups and other *Legionella* species is undetermined in many locales, especially in developing countries. An example of the complexity of this issue can be seen in data from Thailand [54]. Surveys of CAP in Thailand using urinary antigen have revealed a small number of cases (0.4%) of legionella [55]. However, when a more thorough methodology was used, legionellosis was found to be quite common (at least as common as *Mycoplasma* or *Chlamidophyla* pneumonia), but was due exclusively to *L. longbeacheae*, whereas *L. pneumophila* was not diagnosed at all [56]. It is quite possible that cases of post-travel *Legionella* CAP are missed for the same reasons.

Thus, although proven post-travel legionellosis is rare, it may in fact be significantly underdiagnosed. This should certainly be assessed empirically, in light of the risk of severe or fatal disease. Tertiary health centers should be encouraged to employ serology, culture, or nucleic acid tests to further our knowledge about *Legionella* in developing countries.

## Melioidosis

Melioidosis is a bacterial infection caused by *Burkholderia pseudomallei*, a gram-negative motile rod, which is frequently found in soil and surface water. It is mostly found in South, Southeast, and East Asia and in northern Australia, although rare cases are reported from Latin America as well [57]. Within its endemic range, melioidosis is a frequent cause of bacteremia and pneumonia; in Khon Kaen, Thailand, and in Darwin, Australia, melioidosis is second only to *Pneumococcus* as a cause of CAP [58, 59]. The case density is probably highest in northeast Thailand, where isolates of *B. pseudomallei* represent 20% of all positive blood cultures [60], and the seropositivity rate reaches 60–70% [61].

By far the largest group of people from nonendemic countries ever exposed to melioidosis is army veterans. Serological surveys have suggested that up to 7% of soldiers during the Vietnam War were exposed to the disease [62]; even among aircrews stationed in Vietnam, the seroprevalence was 0.3% [63]. Similarly, among Commonwealth soldiers serving in Malaysia, the seroprevalence was found to be nearly 2%. Soldiers who tested seropositive were more likely to have engaged in recreational activities or had other surface water exposure [64]. They were also more likely to have suffered a transient, unexplained febrile illness after their deployment. Although the total number of infected US Army personnel in Southeast Asia may have numbered 200,000, only a few dozen cases of clinically diagnosed melioidosis were reported in returning GIs.

In travelers, melioidosis has been reported more frequently in its cutaneous form, but cases of severe pneumonia and sepsis have also been described [65–72]. As can be seen from the data presented in Table 41.1, many of these cases occurred in diabetic travelers, with a predilection toward middle-age males. In this respect, the data in travelers reflect the same pattern as seen in cases from endemic regions.

Several features in the pathogenesis and clinical picture make melioidosis an important pathogen to consider in a traveler returning from an endemic region. Although inhalation of bacteria, leading to the development of primary pneumonia, has long been considered to be the main source of infection, it is quite likely that primary inoculation is cutaneous, through contact with infected soil or water. Skin infection sometimes presents as an infected wound or as cutaneous abscesses, with some patients going on to develop sepsis and a secondary or hematogenous pneumonia.

Melioidosis, as is seen in other intracellular infections such as tuberculosis, can remain dormant for a protracted period of time and then reactivate in the skin or the lungs (or occasionally other organs). Indeed, extreme cases have been reported, including a reactivated cutaneous disease, 62 years after inoculation, in a World War II veteran [73]. A chronic, subacute course is often described, with a predilection to the upper lobes, and causing cavitary lesions suggestive of tuberculosis.

Another feature that makes melioidosis an important disease in travelers is that the frequently recommended regimens for CAP and even for SCAP do not cover this pathogen. *B. pseudomallei* is closely affiliated to other nonfermenting environmental species such as *Pseudomonas* and is intrinsically resistant to many antibiotics, including many beta lactams and aminoglycosides. Although it is often sensitive to trimethoprim sulfamethoxazole, tetracyclines, and quinolones, optimal therapy requires the use of an antipseudomonal cephalosporin, such as ceftazidime or a carbapenem, in combination with one of the above-mentioned agents. Furthermore, even after the resolution of the acute phase, suppressive antimicrobial therapy needs to be continued for 3–6 additional months, due to the intracellular niche of the pathogen and its predilection to cause relapse.

## Tuberculosis

Tuberculosis (TB) was the major cause of mortality in industrialized countries, right up to the early twentieth century. The question of importation of TB from other regions began to arise after the decline of endemic TB in

**Table 41.1** Clinical and epidemiological features of respiratory melioidosis in returning travelers ($N = 8$).

| Ref. | Sex/age | Diabetes | Destination | Travel duration | Radiological features | Clinical features | Outcome |
|------|---------|----------|-------------|-----------------|-----------------------|-------------------|---------|
| 65 | 42/M | + | Thailand | 6 months | Cavitation | Skin lesions, splenic abscesses | Recovered |
| 66 | 29/M | + | Thailand | NR | NR | Sepsis | Death |
| 67 | 53/M | + | Thailand | 4 weeks | Lt. lung infiltrates | Sepsis, hypoxemia | Death |
| 68 | 25/F | − | Thailand | 3 weeks | Upper lobe infiltrates | One-year latency cystic fibrosis patient | Recovered |
| 69 | 65/M | + | Thailand | NR | Bilateral nodules, infiltrates | Sepsis, abscesses, arthritis osteomyelitis | Recovered |
| 70 | NR | NR | Thailand India | 3 years | Upper lobe infiltrates | Recurrent pustules > subacute pneumonia | Recovered |
| 71 | 47/M | − | Thailand | <1 month | Cavitation, upper lobe infiltrates | Acute pneumonia | Recovered |
| 72 | 39/M | + | Thailand | 4 years | Cavitation | Initial pneumonia sepsis after >2 year latency | Recovered |

the developed world. In fact, until then, a portion of the travel industry was dedicated to the *exportation* of active TB patients to warmer climates, in the hope of inducing a remission. Today, however, TB is actively imported to most developed countries through immigration and a migrant work force. The ease with which mycobacterium TB is transmitted via aerosolized droplets has made it a real concern in the crowded environments of aircrafts and airports, although outbreak investigations have found that the true infection rate under these conditions is quite low.

## Epidemiology of post-travel tuberculosis

Clearly, not all travelers share similar risks. Former immigrants returning to visit friends and relatives (VFRs), long-term residents in developing countries, relief workers and volunteers in refugee camps, and recreational tourists are not at the same level of risk.

American Peace Corps volunteers are a well-studied group of travelers, who may represent the high end of risk for post-travel TB. Volunteers typically stay for 2 years in developing countries, usually living in close proximity to the local population. A surveillance system has established that among Peace Corps volunteers; the overall

incidence rates for positive PPD conversions and active TB cases are 1.283 and 0.057 per 1000 patient-months. This rate is far higher than that seen in the USA, which is about 4.8/100,000 or 0.004/1000 resident-months [74]. A study of Dutch travelers found a similarly high incidence of 3.5 and 2.8 per 1000 person-months of positive PPD conversions and active TB, a rate that is suggestive of that found in local populations in endemic countries [75]. Again, these were long-term travelers, often to Africa, and a significant proportion were health care professionals, a high-risk group for TB transmission. In both of these studies, the risk of TB acquisition was unevenly distributed, with travel to Africa associated with higher risk.

The risk of TB in tourists, especially in short-term travel, is not clearly established. Such cases were rarely reported to the GeoSentinel system, for example, and indeed the odds ratio for TB was 67 in favor of immigrants and VFRs as opposed to other tourists [76]. Similar results are reported from France and Italy, where TB is essentially restricted to immigrants and VFRs, mostly from Africa [77, 78]. This pattern is repeated even among HIV-infected travelers—a group highly susceptible to TB. Bottieau et al. have found that TB in HIV-infected travelers is overwhelmingly a disease among immigrants (and ex-patriates) traveling from Sub-Saharan Africa, and presents in its chronic (often extrapulmonary) stage [11].

In our experience, active tuberculosis is rarely if ever seen in returning travelers. Thus, when a traveler presents with fever and respiratory symptoms in the immediate post-travel period, he is very unlikely to be diagnosed with pulmonary TB.

## Clinical aspects of primary tuberculosis

The incubation time for TB pneumonitis (when tuber-culin sensitivity develops) is 3–8 weeks. Clinically, there is little to distinguish primary TB from other causes of CAP. It should be noted that there is a surprising dearth of clin-ical data on primary TB. Most of the literature is based on pediatric series and is 40–60 years old [79, 80]. The physical examination is usually unremarkable, as are lab-oratory studies. Occasionally, the pneumonitis may be ac-companied by other hypersensitivity reactions, erythema nodosum and keratoconjunctivitis (which is phlyctenular, i.e., involving the corneal limbus). Whereas the latter was described almost always in children, Thomas et al. have de-scribed erythema nodosum in 40% of adults with primary TB [79]. However, even these conditions are not specific to tuberculosis and can be seen, for example, in histoplas-mosis, coccidioidomycosis, and paracoccidioidomycosis.

The classical chest radiographic findings of reactiva-tion TB—apical lesion ± cavitation—are not likely to be present in primary TB. In fact, infiltrates in the lower lung fields are more common. A radiographic pattern that should heighten suspicion of primary TB is the pres-ence of a dense/nodular peripheral infiltrate coupled with ipsilateral hilar adenopathy (which eventually results in Ghon–Ranke complexes after healing and calcification) [81].

Primary TB is mostly asymptomatic in healthy adults. Even when it is symptomatic, it is mostly a self-limited process and may therefore be easily missed. Symptoms and radiographic patterns of chronic reactivation of TB will usually appear many months or several years post-travel. Here it is important to note that an illness clinically and radiographically highly suggestive of chronic TB may be due to other agents, including endemic fungal infections, paragonimiasis, and melioidosis.

## Fungal infections

Fungal pneumonia is not a frequent occurrence and is often a result of profound immune compromise in de-veloped countries. However, a group of dimorphic fungi, sometimes referred to as "endemic mycosis," is an excep-tion to this rule, and affects immunocompetent patients as well as immunocompromised patients. These dimor-phic fungi are of special interest to the travel physician because their distribution is regional, and they are, there-fore, recognized as travel-related infections. In this re-gard, histoplasmosis is the most frequent travel-related respiratory mycosis. Other endemic mycosis, including coccidioidomycosis, paracoccidioidomycosis, and blasto-mycosis, are only occasionally described in travelers (see Chapter 29).

Histoplasmosis is a disease caused by *Histoplasma cap-sulatum*. This dimorphic fungus is not really an endemic mycosis, because it can be found at low levels on all conti-nents. But autochthonous cases are rarely seen in Europe and Asia; the bulk of the disease occurs in the Ameri-cas. It is highly endemic in the Ohio and Mississippi river valleys in the USA and in Central and South America. Correspondingly, the disease is seen in travelers returning from Latin America (but it is not reported in travelers to the USA). Specific activities in endemic regions that are more likely to result in heavy exposure and infection are construction work, working near chicken coops, and agricultural work. A specific leisure activity that is an im-portant risk factor in travelers is caving. In caves housing bat colonies, the soil is highly contaminated. In fact, even staying at cave entrances can result in infection [82].

The clinical aspects of histoplasmosis are described thoroughly in Chapter 29. Briefly, after an incubation period of 1–3 weeks, pneumonitis and mediastinal lym-phadenitis develop. Symptoms include fever, malaise, headache, weakness, substernal chest discomfort, and dry cough. These are often mistaken for influenza or acute pneumonia. Physical findings are usually minimal, and atypical pneumonia agents such as *Mycoplasma* are some-times considered. Most symptoms resolve within 10 days, but a more protracted course might occur after heavy ex-posure, and histoplasmosis therefore should be part of the differential diagnosis of prolonged cough.

CXR shows patchy pneumonia in one or more lobes. Enlarged hilar and mediastinal lymph nodes are fre-quently noted, a pattern that is again similar to other granulomatous pneumonias, including primary TB and sarcoidosis.

## Prevention of travel-related RTI

RTIs are almost as prevalent as diarrhea among travelers, but there have been few reports on general measures for prevention of RTI. Only a few of the agents that cause

RTIs are spread by aerosol (measles, *Coxiella*, and tuberculosis), and these agents cause only a minority of cases. Because droplet infection and direct contact are the main modes of RTI transmission, strict hand washing and avoidance of common towels and crowding seem reasonable recommendations, but may not always be feasible in developing countries. Unfortunately, unlike traveler's diarrhea, for most cases of RTI the only treatment available is symptomatic. Travelers should be encouraged to have analgesics/antipyretics and nasal decongestants as part of their traveling kits.

The high prevalence of influenza in travelers makes it probably the most important vaccine-preventable disease among travelers. This has led to recommendations for the use of influenza vaccine in travelers. Influenza vaccine has not been prospectively addressed in travelers. However, healthy adults are expected to benefit from the vaccine regardless of travel and are included in the vaccine recommendations of the American Advisory Committee on Immunization Practices (ACIP) [83]. Furthermore, there are data to suggest vaccine efficacy among travelers. Among Malaysian Hajj pilgrims, vaccination has led to a 77% decrease in ILI [84], whereas among Pakistani pilgrims vaccination decreased ILI incidence by half [85]. Influenza vaccine is recommended to all travelers, especially those traveling during the influenza season of the destination country and to the tropics. Influenza vaccine is recommended (although not required) for all Hajj travelers [86]. Another population for whom vaccination is deemed necessary is cruise ship personnel and travelers [87].

The issue of H5N1 avian influenza remains a theoretical concern for travelers. With the ever-increasing spread of the strain (currently throughout the Old World, but with most cases still reported from East and Southeast Asia), larger cohorts of travelers are theoretically at risk. A recent study by the American CDC has concluded that the risk for travelers is extremely low. On the other hand, in the cases considered suspicious for H5N1 avian influenza, the majority were in fact infected with influenza A, again highlighting the importance of influenza vaccine for travelers [88]. Recommendations for reducing exposure to possibly infected poultry have been published by the American CDC [87].

Pneumococcal pneumonia is also a vaccine-preventable disease. No studies have specifically addressed vaccine efficacy in travelers, and the very large numbers needed for such trials to reach statistical significance make such trials unlikely. However, pneumococcal vaccines—both the polysaccharide and the conjugated vaccines—have been incorporated into childhood vaccination programs in many countries, and vaccinating the elderly and adults with many chronic illnesses is also recommended. International travel may serve as an opportunity to ascertain vaccine status and provide catch-up vaccination as required [89].

## Conclusions

Travel-related respiratory complaints are very common, usually as an acute post-travel cough, and occasionally as a chronic cough. The differential diagnosis is exhaustive, but a rational stepwise approach may aid in establishing a diagnosis and providing specific therapy. Recognition of the geographical association of some agents of pneumonia can prevent diagnostic delays. For most causative agents, only general hygienic measures serve to prevent disease, but influenza vaccination should be recommended.

## References

1 Fendrick AM, Monto AS, Nightengale B, Sarnes M. The economic burden of non-influenza-related viral respiratory tract infection in the United States. *Arch Intern Med* 2003;163(4):487–94.

2 United Kingdom Health Protection Agency (HPA) HPA national influenza graphs 2008/2009. Available from http://www.hpa.org.uk/web/HPAweb&HPAwebStandard/HPAweb_C/1201767912921. Accessed 2008 July 31 .

3 Zitter JN, Mazonson PD, Miller DP, Hulley SB, Balmes JR. Aircraft cabin air recirculation and symptoms of the common cold. *JAMA* 2002;288(4):483–6.

4 Rack J, Wichmann O, Kamara B, Günther M, Cramer J, Schönfeld C, et al. Risk and spectrum of diseases in travelers to popular tourist destinations. *J Travel Med* 2005;12(5):248–53.

5 Winer L, Alkan M. Incidence and precipitating factors of morbidity among Israeli travelers abroad. *J Travel Med* 2002;9(5):227–32.

6 Hill DR. Health problems in a large cohort of Americans traveling to developing countries. *J Travel Med* 2000;7(5):259–66.

7 Steffen R, van der Linde F, Meyer HE. Risk of disease in 10,500 travelers to tropical countries and 1,300 tourists to North America. *Schweiz Med Wochenschr* 1978;108(39):1485–95.

8 Redman CA, Maclennan A, Wilson E, Walker E. Diarrhea and respiratory symptoms among travelers to Asia, Africa, and South and Central America from Scotland. *J Travel Med* 2006;13(4):203–11.

9 Freedman DO, Weld LH, Kozarsky PE, Fisk T, Robins R, von Sonnenburg F, et al.; GeoSentinel Surveillance Network. Spectrum of disease and relation to place of exposure among ill returned travelers. *N Engl J Med* 2006;354(2):119–30.

10 Wilson ME, Weld LH, Boggild A, Keystone JS, Kain KC, von Sonnenburg F, et al.; GeoSentinel Surveillance Network. Fever in returned travelers: results from the GeoSentinel surveillance network. *Clin Infect Dis* 2007;44(12):1560–8.

11 Bottieau E, Florence E, Clerinx J, Vlieghe E, Vekemans M, Moerman F, et al. Fever after a stay in the tropics: clinical spectrum and outcome in HIV-infected travelers and migrants. *J Acquir Immune Defic Syndr* 2008;48(5):547–52.

12 Stienlauf S, Segal G, Sidi Y, Schwartz E. Epidemiology of travel-related hospitalization. *J Travel Med* 2005;12(3):136–41.

13 Fahey T, Stocks N, Thomas T. Systematic review of the treatment of upper respiratory tract infection. *Arch Dis Child* 1998;79(3):225–30.

14 Carter MJ. Enterically infecting viruses: pathogenicity, transmission and significance for food and waterborne infection. *J Appl Microbiol* 2005;98(6):1354–80.

15 Camps M, Vilella A, Marcos MA, Letang E, Muñoz J, Salvadó E, et al. Incidence of respiratory viruses among travelers with a febrile syndrome returning from tropical and subtropical areas. *J Med Virol* 2008;80(4):711–15.

16 Luna LK, Panning M, Grywna K, Pfefferle S, Drosten C. Spectrum of viruses and atypical bacteria in intercontinental air travelers with symptoms of acute respiratory infection. *J Infect Dis* 2007;195(5):675–9.

17 Darling CA. The epidemiology and bacteriology of influenza. *Am J Public Health (N Y)* 1918;8(10):751–4.

18 Brownstein JS, Wolfe CJ, Mandl KD. Empirical evidence for the effect of airline travel on inter-regional influenza spread in the United States. *PLoS Med* 2006;3(10):e401.

19 Balkhy HH, Memish ZA, Bafaqeer S, Almuneef MA. Influenza a common viral infection among Hajj pilgrims: time for routine surveillance and vaccination. *J Travel Med* 2004;11(2):82–6.

20 Rashid H, Shafi S, Haworth E, El Bashir H, Memish ZA, Sudhanva M, et al. Viral respiratory infections at the Hajj: comparison between UK and Saudi pilgrims. *Clin Microbiol Infect* 2008;14(6):569–74.

21 Mutsch M, Tavernini M, Marx A, Gregory V, Lin YP, Hay AJ, et al. Influenza virus infection in travelers to tropical and subtropical countries. *Clin Infect Dis* 2005;40(9):1282–7.

22 Brotherton JM, Delpech VC, Gilbert GL, Hatzi S, Paraskevopoulos PD, McAnulty JM; Cruise Ship Outbreak Investigation Team. A large outbreak of influenza A and B on a cruise ship causing widespread morbidity. *Epidemiol Infect* 2003;130(2):263–71.

23 Leder K, Sundararajan V, Weld L, Pandey P, Brown G, Torresi J; GeoSentinel Surveillance Group. Respiratory tract infections in travelers: a review of the GeoSentinel surveillance network. *Clin Infect Dis* 2003;36(4):399–406.

24 O'Brien DP, Leder K, Matchett E, Brown GV, Torresi J. Illness in returned travelers and immigrants/refugees: the 6-year experience of two Australian infectious diseases units. *J Travel Med* 2006;13(3):145–52.

25 Shankar EM, Kumarasamy N, Vignesh R, Balakrishnan P, Solomon SS, Murugavel KG, et al. Epidemiological studies on pulmonary pathogens in HIV-positive and -negative subjects with or without community-acquired pneumonia with special emphasis on Mycoplasma pneumoniae. *Jpn J Infect Dis* 2007;60(6):337–41.

26 Scott JA, Hall AJ, Muyodi C, Lowe B, Ross M, Chohan B, et al. Aetiology, outcome, and risk factors for mortality among adults with acute pneumonia in Kenya. *Lancet* 2000;355(9211):1225–30.

27 Nicodemo AC. An open label, multicenter, non-comparative study of the efficacy and safety of oral gatifloxacin in the treatment of community-acquired pneumonia: a Brazilian study in five centers. *Braz J Infect Dis* 2003;7(1):62–8.

28 Ta TH, Jiménez B, Navarro M, Meije Y, González FJ, Lopez-Velez R. Q Fever in returned febrile travelers. *J Travel Med* 2008;15(2):126–9.

29 Potasman I, Rzotkiewicz S, Pick N, Keysary A. Outbreak of Q fever following a safari trip. *Clin Infect Dis* 2000;30(1):214–15.

30 Cardeñosa N, Sanfeliu I, Font B, Muñoz T, Nogueras MM, Segura F. Short report: seroprevalence of human infection by *Coxiella burnetii* in Barcelona (northeast of Spain). *Am J Trop Med Hyg* 2006;75(1):33–5.

31 Ansart S, Pajot O, Grivois JP, Zeller V, Klement E, Perez L, et al. Pneumonia among travelers returning from abroad. *J Travel Med* 2004;11(2):87–91.

32 Felmingham D, Cantón R, Jenkins SG. Regional trends in beta-lactam, macrolide, fluoroquinolone and telithromycin resistance among *Streptococcus pneumoniae* isolates 2001–2004. *J Infect* 2007;55(2):111–18.

33 Morice AH, McGarvey L, Pavord I; British Thoracic Society Cough Guideline Group. Recommendations for the management of cough in adults. *Thorax* 2006;61 Suppl 1:i1–i24.

34 Anstey NM, Jacups SP, Cain T, Pearson T, Ziesing PJ, Fisher DA, et al. Pulmonary manifestations of uncomplicated falciparum and vivax malaria: cough small airways obstruction, impaired gas transfer, and increased pulmonary phagocytic activity. *J Infect Dis* 2002;185(9):1326–34.

35 Su CP, Chen YC, Chang SC. Changing characteristics of typhoid fever in Taiwan. *J Microbiol Immunol Infect* 2004;37(2):109–14.

36 Tattevin P, Léveiller G, Flicoteaux R, Jauréguiberry S, Le Tulzo Y, Dupont M, et al. Respiratory manifestations of leptospirosis: a retrospective study. *Lung* 2005;183(4):283–9.

37 Mandell LA, Wunderink RG, Anzueto A, Bartlett JG, Campbell GD, Dean NC, et al. Infectious Diseases Society of America; American Thoracic Society. Infectious Diseases Society of America/American Thoracic Society consensus guidelines on the management of community-acquired

pneumonia in adults. *Clin Infect Dis* 2007;44 Suppl 2:S27–S72.

38 British Infection Society; British Thoracic Society; Health Protection Agency. Pandemic flu: clinical management of patients with an influenza-like illness during an influenza pandemic. Provisional guidelines from the British Infection Society, British Thoracic Society, and Health Protection Agency in collaboration with the Department of Health. *Thorax* 2007;62 Suppl 1:1–46.

39 Lowen AC, Steel J, Mubareka S, Palese P. High temperature (30 degrees C) blocks aerosol but not contact transmission of influenza virus. *J Virol* 2008;82(11):5650–52.

40 Rothberg MB, Haessler SD, Brown RB. Complications of viral influenza. *Am J Med* 2008;121(4):258–64.

41 Wechsler ME. Pulmonary eosinophilic syndromes. *Immunol Allergy Clin North Am* 2007;27(3):477–92.

42 Schwartz E. Pulmonary schistosomiasis. *Clin Chest Med* 2002;23(2):433–43.

43 Beigel Y, Greenberg Z, Ostfeld I. Clinical problem-solving. Letting the patient off the hook. *N Engl J Med* 2000;342(22):1658–61.

44 Leshem E, Maor Y, Meltzer E, Assous M, Schwartz E. Acute schistosomiasis outbreak: clinical features and economic impact. *Clin Infect Dis* 2008;47(12):1499–506.

45 Meltzer E, Percik R, Shatzkes J, Sidi Y, Schwartz E. Eosinophilia among returning travelers: a practical approach. *Am J Trop Med Hyg* 2008;78(5):702–9.

46 Kretsinger K, Broder KR, Cortese MM, Joyce MP, Ortega-Sanchez I, Lee GM, et al.; Centers for Disease Control and Prevention; Advisory Committee on Immunization Practices; Healthcare Infection Control Practices Advisory Committee. Preventing tetanus, diphtheria, and pertussis among adults: use of tetanus toxoid, reduced diphtheria toxoid and acellular pertussis vaccine recommendations of the Advisory Committee on Immunization Practices (ACIP) and recommendation of ACIP, supported by the Healthcare Infection Control Practices Advisory Committee (HICPAC), for use of Tdap among health-care personnel. *MMWR Recomm Rep* 2006;55(RR-17):1–37.

47 Wilder-Smith A, Earnest A, Ravindran S, Paton NI. High incidence of pertussis among Hajj pilgrims. *Clin Infect Dis* 2003;37(9):1270–2.

48 Ricketts KD, Joseph CA; European Working Group for *Legionella* Infections. Legionnaires' disease in Europe 2003–2004. *Euro Surveill* 2005;10(12):256–9.

49 Ricketts K, McNaught B, Joseph C; European Working Group for *Legionella* Infections. Travel-associated legionnaires disease in Europe: 2005. *Euro Surveill* 2007;12(1).

50 Centers for Disease Control and Prevention (CDC). Surveillance for travel-associated legionnaires disease—United States, 2005–2006. *MMWR Morb Mortal Wkly Rep* 2007;56(48):1261–3.

51 Centers for Disease Control and Prevention (CDC). Cruise-ship-associated Legionnaires disease, November 2003–May 2004. *MMWR Morb Mortal Wkly Rep* 2005;54(45):1153–5.

52 Beyrer K, Lai S, Dreesman J, Lee JV, Joseph C, Harrison T, et al. Legionnaires' disease outbreak associated with a cruise liner, August 2003: epidemiological and microbiological findings. *Epidemiol Infect* 2007;135(5):802–10.

53 Murdoch DR. Diagnosis of *Legionella* infection. *Clin Infect Dis* 2003;36(1):64–9.

54 Payne L, Andersson Y, Ledet Muller L, Blystad H, Nguyen Tran Minh TM, Ruutu P, et al. Outbreak of Legionnaires' disease among tourists staying at a hotel in Phuket, Thailand. *Euro Surveill* 2007;12(1):E070111.2.

55 Prapphal N, Suwanjutha S, Durongkaveroj P, Lochindarat S, Kunakorn M, Deerojanawong J, et al. Prevalence and clinical presentations of atypical pathogens infection in community acquired pneumonia in Thailand. *J Med Assoc Thai* 2006;89(9):1412–19.

56 Phares CR, Wangroongsarb P, Chantra S, Paveenkitiporn W, Tondella ML, Benson RF, et al. Epidemiology of severe pneumonia caused by *Legionella longbeachae*, *Mycoplasma pneumoniae*, and *Chlamydia pneumoniae*: 1-year, population-based surveillance for severe pneumonia in Thailand. *Clin Infect Dis* 2007;45(12):e147–55.

57 Inglis TJ, Rolim DB, Sousa Ade Q. Melioidosis in the Americas. *Am J Trop Med Hyg* 2006;75(5):947–54.

58 Elliott JH, Anstey NM, Jacups SP, Fisher DA, Currie BJ. Community-acquired pneumonia in northern Australia: low mortality in a tropical region using locally-developed treatment guidelines. *Int J Infect Dis* 2005;9(1):15–20.

59 Reechaipichitkul W, Lulitanond V, Tantiwong P, Saelee R, Pisprasert V. Etiologies and treatment outcomes in patients hospitalized with community-acquired pneumonia (CAP) at Srinagarind Hospital, Khon Kaen, Thailand. *Southeast Asian J Trop Med Public Health* 2005;36(1):156–61.

60 Anuntagool N, Naigowit P, Petkanchanapong V, Aramsri P, Panichakul T, Sirisinha S. Monoclonal antibody-based rapid identification of *Burkholderia pseudomallei* in blood culture fluid from patients with community-acquired septicaemia. *J Med Microbiol* 2000;49(12):1075–8.

61 Wuthiekanun V, Chierakul W, Langa S, Chaowagul W, Panpitpat C, Saipan P, et al. Development of antibodies to *Burkholderia pseudomallei* during childhood in melioidosis-endemic northeast Thailand. *Am J Trop Med Hyg* 2006;74(6):1074–5.

62 Clayton AJ, Lisella RS, Martin DG. Melioidosis: a serological survey in military personnel. *Mil Med* 1973;138(1):24–6.

63 Lee R, Cross JH, Irving GS, Lane C, Watten RH. Surveillance of some infectious diseases among aircrew personnel in Southeast Asia. *Aviat Space Environ Med* 1975;46(9):1152–4.

64 Thin RN. Melioidosis antibodies in Commonwealth soldiers. *Lancet* 1976;1(7949):31–3.

65 Maccanti O, Pardelli R, Tonziello A, Gracci G, Vivaldi I, Bolognesi L, et al. Melioidosis in a traveller from Thailand: case report. *J Chemother* 2004;16(4):404–7.

66 Schwarzmaier A, Riezinger-Geppert F, Schober G, Karnik R, Valentin A. Fulminant septic melioidosis after a vacation in Thailand. *Wien Klin Wochenschr* 2000;112(20):892–5.

67 Wilks D, Jacobson SK, Lever AM, Farrington M. Fatal melioidosis in a tourist returning from Thailand. *J Infect* 1994;29(1):87–90.

68 Visca P, Cazzola G, Petrucca A, Braggion C. Travel-associated *Burkholderia pseudomallei* infection (melioidosis) in a patient with cystic fibrosis: a case report. *Clin Infect Dis* 2001;32(1):E15–E16.

69 Shibuya H, Taniguchi Y, Tashiro N, Hara K, Hisada T. A Japanese case of melioidosis presenting as multiple organ lesions accompanied by sepsis and disseminated intravascular coagulation, after a visit to Thailand. *Kansenshogaku Zasshi* 2007;81(3):297–301.

70 Riecke K, Wagner S, Eller J, Lode H, Schaberg T. Pulmonary melioidosis in a German Southeast Asia tourist. *Pneumologie* 1997;51(5):499–502.

71 Sauerwein RW, Lammers JW, Horrevorts AM. Ceftazidime monotherapy for pulmonary melioidosis in a traveler returning from Thailand. *Chest* 1992;101(2):555–7.

72 Hassanein MM, Croall J, Ewins DL, Worth RC. An unusual cause of diabetic ketoacidosis and fulminant septicaemia. *Diabet Med* 2003;20(3):242–4.

73 Ngauy V, Lemeshev Y, Sadkowski L, Crawford G. Cutaneous melioidosis in a man who was taken as a prisoner of war by the Japanese during World War II. *J Clin Microbiol* 2005;43(2):970–72.

74 Jung P, Banks RH. Tuberculosis risk in US Peace Corps Volunteers, 1996 to 2005. *J Travel Med* 2008;15(2):87–94.

75 Cobelens FG, van Deutekom H, Draayer-Jansen IW, Schepp-Beelen AC, van Gerven PJ, van Kessel RP, et al. Risk of infection with *Mycobacterium tuberculosis* in travellers to areas of high tuberculosis endemicity. *Lancet* 2000;356(9228):461–5.

76 Leder K, Tong S, Weld L, Kain KC, Wilder-Smith A, von Sonnenburg F, et al.; GeoSentinel Surveillance Network. Illness in travelers visiting friends and relatives: a review of the GeoSentinel surveillance network. *Clin Infect Dis* 2006;43(9):1185–93.

77 Ansart S, Perez L, Vergely O, Danis M, Bricaire F, et al. Illnesses in travelers returning from the tropics: a prospective study of 622 patients. *J Travel Med* 2005;12(6):312–18.

78 Matteelli A, Beltrame A, Saleri N, Bisoffi Z, Allegri R, Volonterio A, et al. Respiratory syndrome and respiratory tract infections in foreign-born and national travelers hospitalized with fever in Italy. *J Travel Med* 2005;12(4):190–6.

79 Thomas JH, Morgan DB, Davies TW. Primary tuberculosis of the lung. *Br Med J* 1954; 2(4900): 1325–9.

80 Morrison JB. Natural history of segmental lesions in primary pulmonary tuberculosis: long-term review of 383 patients. *Arch Dis Child* 1973;48(2):90–8.

81 Fitzgerald D, Haas DW. Chapter 248 – Mycobacterium tuberculosis. In: Mandell GL, Bennett JE, Dolin R, editors. *Mandell, Bennett, & Dolin: Principles and Practice of Infectious Diseases*, 6th ed. Philadelphia: Churchill Livingstone, Elsevier; 2005.

82 Jülg B, Elias J, Zahn A, Köppen S, Becker-Gaab C, Bogner JR. Bat-associated histoplasmosis can be transmitted at entrances of bat caves and not only inside the caves. *J Travel Med* 2008;15(2):133–6.

83 Advisory Committee on Immunization Practices. Recommended Adult Immunization Schedule—United States, October 2007–September 2008. *MMWR Morb Mortal Wkly Rep* 2007;56:Q1–4 [cited 2008 April 27]. Available from URL: http://www.cdc.gov/mmwr/pdf/wk/mm5641-Immunization.pdf.

84 Mustafa AN, Gessner BD, Ismail R, Yusoff AF, Abdullah N, Ishak I, et al. A case-control study of influenza vaccine effectiveness among Malaysian pilgrims attending the Haj in Saudi Arabia. *Int J Infect Dis* 2003;7(3):210–14.

85 Qureshi H, Gessner BD, Leboulleux D, Hasan H, Alam SE, Moulton LH. The incidence of vaccine preventable influenza-like illness and medication use among Pakistani pilgrims to the Haj in Saudi Arabia. *Vaccine* 2000;18(26):2956–62.

86 WHO. Health conditions for travellers to Saudi Arabia for the pilgrimage to Mecca (Hajj). *Wkly Epidemiol Rec* 2006;81(44):417–24.

87 Centers for Disease Control and Prevention. Health Information for International Travel 2008 (CDC "Yellow Book"). 2007 [cited 2008 August 1]. Available from URL: http://wwwn.cdc.gov/travel/contentYellowBook.aspx.

88 Ortiz JR, Wallis TR, Katz MA, Berman LS, Balish A, Lindstrom SE, et al. No evidence of avian influenza A (H5N1) among returning US travelers. *Emerg Infect Dis* 2007;13(2):294–7.

89 Thomas RE. Preparing patients to travel abroad safely. Part 2: Updating vaccinations. *Can Fam Physician* 2000;46:646–52, 655–6.

# 42 Neurological Signs and Symptoms in Travelers

Einar P. Wilder-Smith and Annelies Wilder-Smith

National University of Singapore, Singapore

## Introduction and approach

This chapter addresses newly presenting neurological symptoms and signs in returning travelers. The emphasis is on symptoms and signs of infectious diseases of the nervous system that are geographically restricted and thus may not be well known in the country of the traveler's origin. Therefore, this chapter does not aim to cover all possible types of causation and also does not address management issues. We address the issue of imported neurological disorders via the characteristics of neurological symptoms and signs and identify clues provided by the geographical distribution.

## Neurological signs and symptoms in the returning traveler

Neurological signs and symptoms in the returning traveler are mainly headache, with or without meningism and with or without fever, altered consciousness, epileptic seizures, peripheral motor or sensory abnormalities, and other focal neurological deficits (Table 42.1).

### Headache and fever

Any systemic febrile illness in travelers can be associated with headache. Symptoms of meningitis or encephalitis are fever and headache that is often severe and may be accompanied by nausea/vomiting. In examining the patient, it is important to look specifically for the clinical clues of meningeal irritation, photophobia, phonophobia, osmophobia (hypersensitivity to smell), neck stiffness, and

*Tropical Diseases in Travelers*, 1st edition. Edited by F. Schwartz.
© 2009 by Blackwell Publishing, ISBN: 978-1-4051-8441-0.

hypersensitivity of trigeminal exit points (V1 and V2). Altered or reduced consciousness is an additional important sign of meningoencephalitis but often occurs when the meningoencephalitis has progressed, in the elderly or in the presence of a particularly virulent pathogen. When a CNS infection is suspected, it is important to ascertain whether the etiology is bacterial, viral, parasitic, or fungal. Clinical features are limited in helping elucidate this, and there are few reliable features allowing such a distinction to be made. Generally, however, those suffering from a bacterial etiology are more severely and acutely ill. A petechial rash, which is seen predominantly over the extensor surfaces of the limbs and can progress to become necrotic, is typical of meningococcal disease. A further characteristic feature of meningococcal meningoencephalitis is the rapid deterioration, requiring immediate treatment. Meningococcal disease in the context of travel has mainly been described in Hajj pilgrims [1], but sporadic cases in general travelers have also been reported [2].

Features of meningoencephalitis accompanied by septic arthritis should prompt a search for Group B streptococcal meningoencephalitis, and pneumonia together with meningoencephalitis a search for *Streptococcus pneumoniae*.

Arthropod-borne viruses are important causes of diseases of the CNS that can affect travelers, and have been reviewed by Dobler [3]. All flavivirus infections are systemic viral infections and all can affect the CNS to some degree. Even in dengue infections—frequent in travelers—encephalopathy has been described [4]. Very rarely, transverse myelitis may occur in dengue infections [5]. Flavivirus infections that commonly affect the nervous system are West Nile encephalitis, Japanese encephalitis, and tick-borne encephalitis (TBE). Although not specific, meningoencephalitis with Parkinson-like

**Table 42.1** Some features and characteristics of neurological diseases that can affect travelers.

| | Symptoms | Etiology | Remarks |
|---|---|---|---|
| Brain | Headache, epilepsy—without fever | Neurocysticercosis | Long incubation time (years) |
| | | Schistosomiasis (mainly *S. japonicum* or *S. mansoni*) | Exposure to freshwater lakes in Africa and Asia; long incubation time (months to years) |
| | Headache, epilepsy, and fever | Cerebral malaria | Positive parasitemia for *Plasmodium falciparum* |
| | | Meningitis; encephalitis | Long list of bacterial, and viral causes |
| | | Neurobrucellosis | Food history for unpasteurized milk products |
| | Headache, fever, and somnolence | African trypanosomiasis | Travel to game parks in Africa |
| | Headache and fever plus CSF eosinophilia | Angiostrongyliasis; gnathostomiasis | Food history for uncooked seafood, unwashed lettuce |
| | Headache, fever, hyperpneic breathing, and movement disorder | Japanese encephalitis | Travel to Southeast Asia |
| | Headache, fever, facial palsy, reduced consciousness | Tick-borne encephalitis | Tick bite; walking in forests |
| Spinal cord | Paraparesis | Schistosomiasis | Untreated schistosomiasis |
| | | Neurocysticercosis | Long incubation time |
| | | HTLV | Mainly seen in immigrants |
| | Segmental paresthesia (with meningitis) | *Angiostrongylus cantonensis* | Ingestion of undercooked seafood |
| Peripheral nerves | Guillian–Barré | Post Dysentery | |
| | Facial palsy (± encephalopathy) | Lyme | Tick bite |
| | | Neurobrucellosis | |
| | Deafness (8th nerve damage) | | Very rare in travelers |
| | Leprosy | | |

features and tremors is often seen in patients with Japanese encephalitis (JE) [6]. Permanent neurological deficits with impaired intellectual capacity, hemi- or tetraparesis, Parkinson-like features, or dystonias are the most common neurological problems following JE infection (see Chapter 9). In the returning traveler with a facial palsy in addition to features of meningoencephalitis (or occasionally on its own), the possibility of Lyme disease or TBE should be entertained. No clinical features can reliably distinguish Lyme stage 2 disease (a bacterial disease)

meningopolyradiculitis from TBE (a viral disease), although the latter is associated with more encephalopathic signs, such as disorientation, decreased vigilance, and seizures. The two diseases have similar incubation periods (up to 1 month). However, the clinical spectrum of Lyme disease is far more varied than that of TBE and includes other cranial nerve palsies, radicular syndromes, and myelopathy. In contrast to other CNS infections, fever is often mild or even absent. It is also not unusual for clinical signs of meningeal irritation to be mild. Lyme disease, which is a spirochetal disease, runs a chronological course similar to that of syphilis, with stage 2 disease spontaneously regressing to become dormant even in the absence of treatment. The third stage of the disease occurs much later and is, therefore, often not included in the differential diagnosis of the diverse neurological pictures the disease can present with and is easily missed in countries where Lyme disease is rare. In its third stage, Lyme disease can be difficult to differentiate from multiple sclerosis. Tick-borne encephalitis poses a growing health problem in many European countries and parts of Northern Asia. Vaccination has been employed successfully for many years in endemic countries [7].

Rabies may begin with local paresthesias at the site of the bite. The initial symptoms of rabies resemble those of other systemic viral infections, including fever, headache, malaise, and disorders of the upper respiratory and gastrointestinal tracts. Initial neurological symptoms may include subtle changes in personality and cognition. This prodrome can last for 4–10 days. Human rabies infections are divided into two forms: furious and paralytic rabies (see Chapter 14). The furious form presents with hydrophobia, delirium, and agitation until coma supervenes. Death occurs an average of 18 days after the onset of symptoms, but the range is broad. The paralytic form is characterized by spinal cord and brain stem abnormalities. The initial findings suggest an ascending paralysis, resembling Guillain–Barré syndrome (GBS).

In returning travelers from the tropics and subtropics who present with high fever, meningism, and altered consciousness, usually associated with metabolic acidosis, hypoglycemia, and sometimes status epilepticus, cerebral malaria always needs to be excluded. Parasite sequestration is generally considered to be critical to the pathogenesis of cerebral malaria.

Primary HIV infection in the returning traveler can also present with severe headache accompanied by flu-like illness, lymphadenopathy, or gastrointestinal disturbances [8]. Nonspecific meningoencephalitic features occur in up to 20% of patients with primary HIV infection and may be associated with a more rapid progression of HIV. HIV positive travelers with low CD4 counts may also present with opportunistic infections that affect the CNS, such as toxoplasmosis and cryptococcal meningitis. Cryptococcal meningitis can also affect immunocompetent travelers. *Cryptococcus gatti* risk has been reported in tourists to Vancouver Island, Canada [9].

Brucellosis is a zoonosis, and virtually all infections derive directly or indirectly from exposure to animals. Neurobrucellosis occurs in fewer than 5% of cases. Neurobrucellosis includes meningitis, encephalitis, myelitis–radiculoneuronitis, brain abscess, epidural abscess, granuloma, and demyelinating and meningovascular syndromes. Acute or chronic meningitis is the most frequent nervous system complication.

## Headache, fever, and CSF eosinophilia

Meningitis with high eosinophilia count in the CSF is called "eosinophilic meningitis." Eosinophilic meningitis is defined by the presence of 10 or more eosinophils per microliter or eosinophilia of at least 10% of the total CSF leukocyte count. It is rarely found in Western countries, where it is sometimes seen in association with tuberculosis, syphilis, and coccidioidomycosis. Worldwide, the most common cause of eosinophilic meningitis is helminthic parasites, in particular *Angiostrongylus cantonesis* and *Gnathostoma spinigerum*.

Most cases of *Angiostrongylus* infection occur in Southeast Asia and throughout the Pacific basin, but travelers have also been infected in the Caribbean and in South America [10]. International travel has increased the possibility of exposure to these parasites and has led to further dissemination via ship-borne dispersal of infected rat vectors [11]. Humans become infected by consuming raw snails or slugs, vegetables contaminated with the mollusks' slime, or carrier (transport) hosts such as land crabs and freshwater shrimp that have eaten infected mollusks. Larvae penetrate the intestinal mucosa and migrate to the CNS, burrowing into the neural tissue and inciting an inflammatory response. The nematode does not complete its life cycle in humans and usually dies in the CNS. The correspondent clinical manifestations of angiostrongyliasis are predominantly signs and symptoms relating to the CNS. Acute severe headache is the most significant symptom and is most likely due to elevated intracranial pressure. Neurologic findings are absent in half the cases. Other symptoms include nausea, vomiting, somnolence, lethargy, fever, malaise, anorexia, constipation, and abdominal pain. Clinical signs include meningism, exaggerated deep tendon reflexes, extraocular muscle palsies, and hepatomegaly.

Paresthesias are the most distinctive neurological findings in adults with angiostrongyliasis. Infective larvae can migrate to the eye, causing retinal detachment and hemorrhage leading to blindness. The prognosis is usually very good, with a case mortality rate of less than 0.5%.

Because migrating larvae eventually die in the CNS, the accompanying inflammation subsides and the disease is self-limiting. Progressive improvement during a period of 3–6 weeks is typical, with rare cases having persistent minor deficits (paresthesia, persistent headache, cognitive deficits). The diagnosis of angiostrongyliasis is often clinical—as serologic tests are not commercially available—and is based on an appropriate epidemiological history combined with the characteristic clinical symptomatology and CSF findings. CSF eosinophilia exceeds 10% in 95% of cases and is usually in the range of 20–70%. Blood eosinophilia occurs in two-thirds of cases. CSF protein levels are often slightly elevated, and the CSF glucose level is usually normal. Symptoms of angiostrongyliasis usually develop within 1 month of returning home.

Gnathostomiasis is a less frequent cause of encephalomyelitis than *A. cantonensis*. Eosinophilic meningitis due to *G. spinigerum* is endemic in Southeast Asia, but infections have also been imported by travelers to Latin America, Spain, India, China, Japan, and even Africa [12, 13]. The clinical presentation of cerebral gnathostomiasis is more fulminant than that of angiostrongyliasis. The most distinctive clinical manifestations are radiculitis, paralysis, and myelitis, bloody or xanthochromic CSF, and sudden impairment of the sensorium caused by cerebral hemorrhage. Cutaneous symptoms are more frequent than neurological and there is a characteristic syndrome of intermittent, nonpitting edematous swellings of subcutaneous tissues associated with eosinophilia, caused by the migration of the *Gnathosoma* larva.

### Headache and somnolence

*Trypanosoma gambiense* and *T. rhodesiense* usually invade and replicate in the CNS, causing sleeping sickness. *T. cruzi* preferentially damages cells of the peripheral autonomic nervous system by replicating in the supporting Schwann cells, causing cardiac rhythm disturbances. Trypanosomiasis has been reported in travelers to Africa, mainly as East African trypanosomiasis in tourists who had visited game parks in East Africa [14]. The onset of symptoms in East African trypanosomiasis usually occurs a few days after the patient has been bitten by an infected tsetse fly. Patients present with fever, malaise, and headache. In some patients death may occur even before CNS disease develops. The meningoencephalitis disease of African trypanosomiasis is characterized by headache, daytime somnolence, personality changes, and extrapyramidal signs. The course of the East African trypanosomiasis is much more fulminant than that of West African trypanosomiasis (see Chapter 26).

### Epileptic seizures

An epileptic fit is a feature of neuronal cell dysfunction and can present either as a generalized fit (due to all of the brain's neurons discharging together) or as a focal fit (due to a restricted number of neurons discharging). A first time epileptic fit should prompt the physician to identify the underlying cause. Travel-related risks include all types of CNS infections presenting with a *febrile* episode, as previously discussed.

Among nonfebrile illnesses, the tropical disease that most frequently results in epileptic seizures is neurocysticercosis. Neurocysticercosis is the term used for human CNS involvement with *Taenia solium* cysts (see Chapter 28). Infection may involve any part of the CNS, but symptomatic disease is most often related to intracerebral lesions causing seizures or mass effects, intraventricular cysts causing hydrocephalus, subarachnoid lesions causing chronic meningitis, and spinal cord lesions causing cord compression syndromes. The MRI appearance can be characteristic, with single or multiple cysts and varying degrees of wall enhancement and surrounding edema, depending on the stage of the life cycle of the larva and its associated cyst [15]. Intraparenchymal cerebral cysts enlarge slowly, causing minimal symptoms until years or decades after the onset of infection, when the cysts begin to die. They may also leak antigenic material that provokes a severe inflammatory response that also contributes to symptoms of focal or generalized seizures, sensorimotor deficits, intellectual impairment, psychiatric disorders, and symptoms of hydrocephalus. Occlusion of the small cortical or penetrating vessels at the base of the brain caused by arteriopathy can result in susceptibility to stroke, particularly among young and middle-aged patients [16].

CNS schistosomiasis is most common with *Schistosoma japonicum* infection, occurring in as many as 2–5% of infections and accounting for high rates of epilepsy in endemic areas. Occasionally, CNS involvement may also occur with *S. mansoni*, but virtually never with *S. hematobium*. Symptoms are focal or generalized seizures, focal neurological deficits, signs of increased intracranial pressure due to the mass effect, and diffuse encephalitis.

### Spinal cord syndromes

Ectopic egg deposition from aberrant migration of adult worms or embolization of eggs from distant sites is common with all species of schistosomes and can therefore also affect the neurological system. Neurological disease develops in those in which acute infection was not treated. Acute transverse myelitis and subacute myelo-radiculopathy is the most common neurological complication of *S. mansoni* infection. Schistosomal myelopathy tends to occur early after infection and is more likely to be symptomatic than cerebral schistosomiasis. The conus medullaris and cauda equina are the most common sites of involvement [17]. In transverse myelitis, patients typically present with rapidly evolving weakness and sensory disturbance of both lower limbs, typically associated with bladder-emptying problems. The lumbar region seems to be more commonly involved, sparing the arms from involvement. Diagnosis is achieved by detecting blood eosinophilia and CSF pleocytosis (with or without eosinophilia) and by MRI of the spine showing cord swelling.

Neurocysticercosis can also result in spinal cord syndrome, but is usually associated with other CNS involvement [15].

## Peripheral neuropathy

In the traveler presenting with progressive bilateral lower limb weakness, GBS should be considered. This acute inflammatory neuritis occurs 1–3 weeks after gastrointestinal or other nonspecific febrile illnesses, and also without any obvious underlying causes. *Campylobacter* is the most common association. Initially sensory symptoms are predominant, with dysesthesia and sometimes frank pain over the feet and hands. These are followed by progressive weakness with a distal-to-proximal gradient. Important clinical signs are absent tendon reflexes and facial nerve palsy. If GBS is suspected, urgent hospital referral for further investigation is mandatory, as paralysis can rapidly progress and involve the respiratory muscles.

Leprosy is the most common infectious cause of peripheral neuropathy worldwide. However, leprosy requires a very long time of close exposure because it is not highly transmissible. Therefore, the risk to general travelers is close to zero. One case of leprosy has been reported in a backpacker [18]. Leprosy should also always be part of the differential diagnosis in immigrants from countries where leprosy is still endemic. In the southern and southeastern USA, the nine-banded armadillo is an important reservoir for *Mycobacterium leprae*, the causative agent of leprosy. One woman living in Georgia was diagnosed with borderline tuberculoid leprosy; she had worked for many years in a garden where armadillos burrowed or were buried. There was no history of foreign travel or known exposure to a person with leprosy [19].

Peripheral sensory nerve damage is the leading cause of functional morbidity in people infected by leprosy and is characteristic of both multibacillary and paucibacillary disease. The peripheral nerve damage in leprosy that affects motor, sensory, and autonomic neurons can be mediated both by *M. leprae* itself and by the immune response to *M. leprae* [20].

## Clues to neurological signs and symptoms from the travel history

### Incubation time

Ascertaining the travel history and taking into account the incubation time can give important clues to the underlying etiology of neurological signs and symptoms. Most febrile diseases with CNS involvement have an incubation time of less than 1 month. In these cases, the association of the disease with the travel is more obvious. A special situation arises when illness related to travel presents after a long delay, which notably happens in schistosomiasis (transverse myelitis) and *T. solium* (neurocysticercosis presenting with epileptic seizures), which may occur several years after exposure.

### Geographical areas

Several CNS infections often have certain geographical patterns. JE can be acquired across the whole Southeast Asian region, West Nile encephalitis in the USA, and the Middle East; TBE is acquired across much of Central Europe and the former Soviet Union. Eosinophilic meningitis is commonly acquired in Southeast Asia and the Pacific basin, but well documented outbreaks have occurred with parties holidaying in the Caribbean [10].

### Food history

It is important to take a food history. *A. cantonensis* is typically associated with the ingestion of undercooked seafood, in particular fish, prawns, and even frogs. Other foods known to transmit disease are snails or lettuce, the latter contaminated by animal waste. Brucellosis (neuroborreliosis) and *Listeria* meningitis are associated with intake of unpasteurized milk or soft cheeses, which are particularly popular food entities in South America and the Mediterranean basin.

### Travel activities

A history of activities during travel needs to be taken. Schistosomiasis is associated with swimming in certain *Schistosoma*-infected freshwater lakes and rivers, mainly in Africa and also in Southeast Asia. Walking in forests in Eastern Europe is associated with TBE.

## Travel purpose

The purpose for travel needs to be ascertained; for example, meningococcal disease is mainly related to participation in highly crowded events such as the Hajj pilgrimage in Saudi Arabia.

## Exposure to ticks, flies, or mosquitoes

Taking a history for exposure to ticks is another clue. Lyme disease, a multistage acute or chronic infectious disease that commonly affects the CNS, is acquired via the bite of infected hard ticks harboring *Borrelia burgdorferi* in North America, Europe, and Central Asia. However, a tick bite is remembered in only 50% of cases.

Exposure to tsetse flies may lead to sleeping sickness (trypanosomiasis). The tsetse bite is very noticeable and can be very painful.

## Noninfectious neurological problems in travelers

With long haul travel, the risk of simple nerve entrapment needs to be considered, as cramped space restricts the normal movements that occur in sleep, which are partly there to help relieve nerve ischemia with prolonged or excessive pressure. Alcohol and sleeping tablets, commonly taken on long haul flights, increase the risk of pressure palsies. In the upper limb, the ulnar and radial nerves are most easily compressed. Ulnar nerve dysfunction results in numbness of the fifth and fourth digit with or without hand weakness, radial nerve palsy in wrist numbness and wrist drop. In the lower limb, the peroneal nerve is most commonly damaged, with resultant foot numbness and drop. The less common sciatic nerve compression can result in weakness of all muscles and numbness below the knee.

Many returning travelers suffer from tension headaches or experience exacerbation of migraines. Travel and jet lag commonly exacerbate these types of headache. Tension headache typically is mild to moderate in intensity, squeezing in nature, and located on top of the head, without any other focal neurology or nausea, vomiting, or photo/phonophobia. Migraine is generally more severe, throbbing in nature, and associated with nausea/vomiting and photo/phonophobia.

Seizures in the returning traveler can occur in the context of sleep deprivation, which in itself has proconvulsive properties. Those with known epilepsy may be particularly prone to develop fits during the time of adjustment to jet lag. For this reason, the traveler with epilepsy should be counseled on catching up with sleep in a consistent manner both during and after travel.

## References

1 Wilder-Smith A. Meningococcal disease: risk for international travellers and vaccine strategies. *Travel Med Infect Dis* 2008;6:182–6.

2 Wilder-Smith A, Gon KT. W-135 meningococcal disease in a traveler: a case report. *J Travel Med* 2003;10:59–60.

3 Dobler G. Arboviruses causing neurological disorders in the central nervous system. *Arch Virol Suppl* 1996;11:33–40.

4 Wilder-Smith A, Schwartz E. Dengue in travelers. *N Engl J Med* 2005;353:924–32.

5 Seet RC, Lim EC, Wilder-Smith E. Acute transverse myelitis following dengue virus infection. *J Clin Virol* 2006;35:310–12.

6 Diagana M, Preux PM, Dumas M. Japanese encephalitis revisited. *J Neurol Sci* 2007;262:165–70.

7 Rendi-Wagner P. Advances in vaccination against tick-borne encephalitis. *Expert Rev Vaccines* 2008;7:589–96.

8 Boufassa F, Bachmeyer C, Carre N, et al. Influence of neurologic manifestations of primary human immunodeficiency virus infection on disease progression. SEROCO Study Group. *J Infect Dis* 1995;171:1190–5.

9 Lindberg J, Hagen F, Laursen A, Stenderup J, Boekhout T. *Cryptococcus gattii* risk for tourists visiting Vancouver Island, Canada. *Emerg Infect Dis* 2007;13:178–9.

10 Slom TJ, Cortese MM, Gerber SI, et al. An outbreak of eosinophilic meningitis caused by *Angiostrongylus cantonensis* in travelers returning from the Caribbean. *N Engl J Med* 2002;346:668–75.

11 Lim JM, Lee CC, Wilder-Smith A. Eosinophilic meningitis caused by *Angiostrongylus cantonensis*: a case report and literature review. *J Travel Med* 2004;11:388–90.

12 Gorgolas M, Santos-O'Connor F, Unzu AL, et al. Cutaneous and medullar gnathostomiasis in travelers to Mexico and Thailand. *J Travel Med* 2003;10:358–61.

13 Hale DC, Blumberg L, Frean J. Case report: gnathostomiasis in two travelers to Zambia. *Am J Trop Med Hyg* 2003;68:707–9.

14 Jelinek T, Bisoffi Z, Bonazzi L, et al. Cluster of African trypanosomiasis in travelers to Tanzanian national parks. *Emerg Infect Dis* 2002;8:634–5.

15 Creasy JL, Alarcon JJ. Magnetic resonance imaging of neuro-cysticercosis. *Top Magn Reson Imaging* 1994;6:59–68.

16 Alarcon F, Hidalgo F, Moncayo J, Vinan I, Duenas G. Cerebral cysticercosis and stroke. *Stroke* 1992;23:224–8.

17 Carod-Artal FJ. Neurological complications of *Schistosoma* infection. *Trans R Soc Trop Med Hyg* 2008;102:107–16.

18 Brickell K, Frith R, Ellis-Pegler R. Leprosy in a backpacker. *J Travel Med* 2005;12:161–3.

19 Lane JE, Walsh DS, Meyers WM, Klassen-Fischer MK, Kent DE, Cohen DJ. Borderline tuberculoid leprosy in a woman from the state of Georgia with armadillo exposure. *J Am Acad Dermatol* 2006;55:714–16.

20 Wilder-Smith A, Wilder-Smith E. Electrophysiological evaluation of peripheral autonomic function in leprosy patients, leprosy contacts and controls. *Int J Lepr Other Mycobact Dis* 1996;64:433–40.

# 43 Closing Remarks

Eli Schwartz

Chaim Sheba Medical Center, Tel Hashomer, Israel and Sackler School of Medicine, Tel Aviv University, Tel Aviv, Israel

The explosion of global travel in recent decades includes leisure tourists and businesspersons traveling from industrialized countries to the tropics and other developing countries. The movement of documented and undocumented immigrants, of labor-seeking foreign workers looking for better lives and opportunities, traveling from developing countries to the industrialized world, also contributes to a shrinking globe from the medical perspective. The world is now a small village and physicians may encounter diseases that they have never seen in their own backyards. The increasing number of cases of tropical diseases in Western countries is a clear reflection of this influx, with varied compositions of these subgroups within each Western country. It should be kept in mind that some of these diseases are life-threatening, some may impact public health, but more important, the majority cause patients to suffer, sometimes for extended periods of time. However, most of these diseases are curable.

Infectious diseases historically, until the first half of the twentieth century, were the major cause of human morbidity and mortality, yet subsequently have become much less important, currently accounting for about 5% of death in the industrialized countries. The main focus now in the industrialized countries is on chronic diseases, many of which are incurable or require lifelong treatment. The imported tropical diseases are largely infectious diseases, curable within a few days of treatment. In some cases, such as malaria, prompt treatment will save lives. In other situations, treatment may alleviate protracted symptoms of several months or sometimes years, for example, in the case of untreated parasitic infections.

Thus, with the effects of globalization on everyday clinical practice, it is important for physicians to be equipped with knowledge of imported tropical diseases, particularly those that may be life-threatening or result in chronic misery and suffering (and may in fact be very easy to treat). It is imperative that medical schools and residency programs in family and internal medicine include this aspect of travel medicine as a part of their curriculum. The purpose of this book is to increase awareness among clinicians who see returning travelers and to share with them the clinical experience of experts worldwide who have been treating these patients for decades.

This awareness of the existence of tropical diseases in our backyard is a first step in expanding differential diagnosis among physicians who may see symptomatic returning travelers. However, even when cognizant of the possible infections, clinicians often encounter problems with both diagnosis and treatment.

There is clearly a need for better diagnostic tests to accurately and promptly diagnose tropical diseases or, in fact, infectious diseases, both in endemic countries and in industrialized countries. Timely diagnosis and treatment could save lives and, as in the case of malaria, could prevent unnecessary workups and therapeutic trials. For example, in cases of viral infections such as dengue fever where specific treatment is lacking, a severely ill patient will often have to endure an extensive workup because a diagnosis cannot be made during the early phase of the disease. Hepatitis E, another infection also emerging in industrialized countries, is difficult to diagnose in that there are no readily available tools to diagnose it in many Western countries. For infectious diseases that rely on a serological diagnosis, there is no approach to definitive diagnosis during the acute phase of illness. We instead must wait for immunoglobulin (most often IgM) to be produced in response to the infection, a response that takes about a week after the onset of symptoms. This occurs in other viral infections, such as chikungunya and West Nile fever. It is also the case with bacterial infections, such as leptospirosis and rickettsial infection, and takes even longer in parasitic infections, such as acute schistosomiasis.

*Tropical Diseases in Travelers*, 1st edition. Edited by E. Schwartz.
© 2009 by Blackwell Publishing, ISBN: 978-1-4051-8441-0.

Initiatives to develop rapid diagnostic tools to diagnose, for example, tuberculosis or African trypanosomiasis in developing countries have been supported by organizations such as the Foundation for Innovative New Diagnostics (FIND), through the WHO, and grants from the Bill & Melinda Gates Foundation (see www.finddiagnostics .org). These important undertakings could be beneficial in the diagnosis of a myriad of infectious diseases, not only in the tropics. It should be noted that even in Western countries, the ability to perform rapid diagnosis is often lacking. Antigen detection methods are very much needed, and the PCR as a method of diagnosis is available only in research laboratories and not routinely obtainable.

Despite the fact that the Western countries have the advantages of modern medical technology as well as financial resources, ironically they often lack treatment modalities that are available in developing countries. Arguably, it may be more straightforward to be sick with malaria in Africa rather than in a Western country because antimalarial drugs are often more accessible in Africa. There are huge investments in, for example, artemisinin-based combination treatments for malaria in Africa, and yet these same treatments are not readily available in places such as the USA. Intravenous quinine/quinide, which is the drug of choice for severe malaria, and hence a life-saving drug, has been successfully used for many years, including in the Western countries, and is very low cost. However, currently, this drug is either unavailable or very difficult to procure in many Western countries. It is often stored in a government-regulated pharmaceutical center, to be purchased as needed. This process can be both lengthy and confusing for physicians who are not familiar with the process or completely unaware of the drug's availability. It seems clear that there should be a mandate in place to have IV quinine/quinide or artesunate available in every major medical center as a life-saving drug.

In the last 20 years, orphan drug legislation has been adopted in several Western countries around the world and has successfully promoted investments to develop new pharmaceutical products for the treatment of rare diseases. For economic reasons, the development of medicines for the treatment of tropical diseases is lagging behind and, without these incentives, new drugs would not be developed and produced.

However, the situation in the Western countries is more ironic. Many of the drugs used to treat tropical diseases have been around for many years, used by millions of people, and are, as a rule, not experimental. They have been used in the West as well, and have been registered in the West. However, the renewal registration procedure is costly and many pharmaceutical companies do not want to invest in drugs that do not render a profit, with no patent rights, and relatively few consumers. Thus, for example, primaquine, which is the only drug for the radical cure of vivax malaria, is not available in many countries. The same holds true for praziquantel or albendazole— important anthelminths—both of which are not available in many countries. Quinacrine, an excellent anti-*Giardia* therapy, has vanished from the markets. Paradoxically, the current regulations formulated to improve the care of patients are now potentially harmful to patients who seek treatment for tropical diseases. These orphan drugs need parents; in addition, a procedure and protocol, with special regulations at the governmental level in each country, are also needed.

Tropical diseases should no longer be neglected in Western countries. They are now a common occurrence and probably will continue to be seen more frequently in the future. It is a sad state of affairs to see many individuals enduring diseases, unable to find relief in Western countries where so much money is invested in the quality of health care.

Initiatives should be geared toward easy availability of drugs for those who suffer from tropical diseases that are in fact often easily curable.

# Appendix A: Drugs for Parasitic Infections

With increasing travel, immigration, use of immunosuppressive drugs and the spread of AIDS, physicians anywhere may see infections caused by parasites. The table below lists first-choice and alternative drugs for most parasitic infections. The table on safety of antiparasitic drugs in pregnancy summarizes the known prenatal risks of antiparasitic drugs. Drugs in pregnancy are listed on page 459, and brand names and manufacturers of the drugs are listed on page 462.

| Infection | | Drug | Adult dosage | Pediatric dosage |
|-----------|---|------|--------------|------------------|
| *ACANTHAMOEBA* keratitis | | | | |
| Drug of choice: | | See footnote 1 | | |
| **AMEBIASIS** (*Entamoeba histolytica*) | | | | |
| **Asymptomatic** | | | | |
| Drug of choice: | | Iodoquinol[2] | 650 mg PO tid × 20d | 30–40 mg/kg/d (max. 2g) PO in 3 doses × 20d |
| | OR | Paromomycin[3] | 25–35 mg/kg/d PO in 3 doses × 7d | 25–35 mg/kg/d PO in 3 doses × 7d |
| | OR | Diloxanide furoate[4,*] | 500 mg PO tid × 10d | 20 mg/kg/d PO in 3 doses × 10d |
| **Mild to moderate intestinal disease** | | | | |
| Drug of choice[5]: | | Metronidazole | 500–750 mg PO tid × 7–10d | 35–50 mg/kg/d PO in 3 doses × 7–10d |
| | OR | Tinidazole[6] | 2 g once PO daily × 3d | ≥ 3yrs: 50 mg/kg/d (max. 2g) PO in 1 dose × 3d |
| | | **either followed by** | | |
| | OR | Iodoquinol[2] | 650 mg PO tid × 20d | 30–40 mg/kg/d (max. 2g) PO in 3 doses × 20d |
| | | Paromomycin[3] | 25–35 mg/kg/d PO in 3 doses × 7d | 25–35 mg/kg/d PO in 3 doses × 7d |
| **Severe intestinal and extraintestinal disease** | | | | |
| Drug of choice: | | Metronidazole | 750 mg PO tid × 7–10d | 35–50 mg/kg/d PO in 3 doses × 7–10d |
| | OR | Tinidazole[6] | 2 g once PO daily × 5d | ≥ 3yrs: 50 mg/kg/d (max. 2g) PO in 1 dose × 3d |
| | | **either followed by** | | |

\* Availability problems. See table on manufacturers of drugs used to treat parasitic infections, page 464.

[1] Topical 0.02% chlorhexidine and polyhexamethylene biguanide (PHMB, 0.02%), either alone or in combination, have been used successfully in a large number of patients. Treatment with either chlorhexidine or PHMB is often combined with propamidine isethionate (*Brolene*) or hexamidine (*Desmodine*). None of these drugs is commercially available or approved for use in the US, but they can be obtained from compounding pharmacies (see footnote 2). Leiter's Park Avenue Pharmacy, San Jose, CA (800-292-6773; www.leiterrx.com) is a compounding pharmacy that specializes in ophthalmic drugs. Propamidine is available over the counter in the UK and Australia. Hexamidine is available in France. The combination of chlorhexidine, natamycin (pimaricin), and debridement also has been successful (Kitagawa K et al., *Jpn J Ophthalmol* 2003;47:616). Debridement is most useful during the stage of corneal epithelial infection. Most cysts are resistant to neomycin; its use is no longer recommended. Azole antifungal drugs (ketoconazole, itraconazole) have been used as oral or topical adjuncts (Shuster FL and Visvesvara GS, *Drug Resist Update* 2004;7:41). Use of corticosteroids is controversial (Hammersmith K, *Curr Opinions Ophthal* 2006;17:327; Awwad ST et al., *Eye Contact Lens* 2007;33:1).

*Source*: Appendix A is reproduced with permission from Treatment Guidelines, *The Medical Letter* 2007;5 (suppl).

| Infection | Drug | Adult dosage | Pediatric dosage |
|---|---|---|---|
| **AMEBIASIS** (*Entamoeba histolytica*) (continued) | | | |
| OR | Iodoquinol[2] | 650 mg PO tid × 20d | 30–40 mg/kg/d (max. 2g) PO in 3 doses × 20d |
| | Paromomycin[3] | 25–35 mg/kg/d PO in 3 doses × 7d | 25–35 mg/kg/d PO in 3 doses × 7d |

**AMEBIC MENINGOENCEPHALITIS, primary and granulomatous**
*Naegleria*

| | | | |
|---|---|---|---|
| Drug of choice: | Amphotericin B[7,8] | 1.5 mg/kg/d IV in 2 doses × 3d, then 1 mg/kg/d × 6d plus 1.5 mg/d intrathecally × 2d, then 1 mg/d every other day × 8d | 1.5 mg/kg/d IV in 2 doses × 3d, then 1 mg/kg/d × 6d plus 1.5 mg/d intrathecally × 2d, then 1 mg/d every other day × 8d |
| **plus** | Miconazole[7,8,*] | 350 mg/m$^2$ of body-surface area daily IV in 3 doses × 9d plus 10 mg/d intrathecally × 2d then 10 mg intrathecally every other day × 8d | 350 mg/m$^2$ of body-surface area daily IV in 3 doses × 9d plus 10 mg/d intrathecally × 2d then 10 mg intrathecally every other day × 8d |

*Acanthamoeba*

| | |
|---|---|
| Drug of choice: | See footnote 9 |

**Balamuthia mandrillaris**

| | |
|---|---|
| Drug of choice: | See footnote 10 |

*Sappinia diploidea*

| | |
|---|---|
| Drug of choice: | See footnote 11 |

---

[*] Availability problems. See table on manufacturers of drugs used to treat parasitic infections, page 464.

[2] Iodoquinol should be taken after meals.

[3] Paromomycin should be taken with a meal.

[4] Not available commercially. It may be obtained through compounding pharmacies, such as Panorama Compounding Pharmacy, 6744 Balboa Blvd. Van Nuys, CA 91406 (800-247-9767) or Medical Center Pharmacy, New Haven, CT (203-688-6816). Other compounding pharmacies may be found through the National Association of Compounding Pharmacies (800-687-7850) or the Professional Compounding Centers of America (800-331-2498, www.pccarx.com).

[5] Nitazoxanide may be effective against a variety of protozoan and helminth infections (Bobak DA, *Curr Infect Dis Rep* 2006;8:91; Diaz E et al., *Am J Trop Med Hyg* 2003;68:384). It was effective against mild to moderate amebiasis, 500 mg bid × 3d, in a recent study (Rossignol JF et al., *Trans R Soc Trop Med Hyg* 2007 Oct;101:1025, e pub 2007 July 20). It is FDA-approved only for treatment of diarrhea caused by *Giardia* or *Cryptosporidium* (*Med Lett Drugs Ther* 2003;45:29). Nitazoxanide is available in 500-mg tablets and an oral suspension; it should be taken with food.

[6] A nitroimidazole similar to metronidazole, tinidazole appears to be as effective as metronidazole and better tolerated (*Med Lett Drugs Ther* 2004;46:70). It should be taken with food to minimize GI adverse effects. For children and patients unable to take tablets, a pharmacist can crush the tablets and mix them with cherry syrup (*Humco*, and others). The syrup suspension is good for 7 days at room temperature and must be shaken before use (Fung HB and Doan TL et al., *Clin Ther* 2005;27:1859). Omidazole, a similar drug, is also used outside the US.

[7] Not FDA-approved for this indication.

| Infection | Drug | Adult dosage | Pediatric dosage |
|---|---|---|---|
| **ANCYLOSTOMA caninum** (Eosinophilic enterocolitis) | | | |
| Drug of choice: | Albendazole[7,12] | 400 mg PO once | 400 mg PO once |
| OR | Mebendazole | 100 mg PO bid × 3d | 100 mg PO bid × 3d |
| OR | Pyrantel pamoate[7,13,*] | 11 mg/kg (max. 1g) PO × 3d | 11 mg/kg (max. 1g) PO × 3d |
| OR | Endoscopic removal | | |

*Ancylostoma duodenale*, see HOOKWORM

**ANGIOSTRONGYLIASIS** (*Angiostrongylus cantonensis, Angiostrongylus costaricensis*)

| | | | |
|---|---|---|---|
| Drug of choice: | See footnote 14 | | |

**ANISAKIASIS** (*Anisakis* spp.)

| | | | |
|---|---|---|---|
| Treatment of choice:[15] | Surgical or endoscopic removal | | |

**ASCARIASIS** (*Ascaris lumbricoides, roundworm*)

| | | | |
|---|---|---|---|
| Drug of choice[4]: | Albendazole[7,12] | 400 mg PO once | 400 mg PO once |
| OR | Mebendazole | 100 mg bid PO × 3d or 500 mg once | 100 mg PO bid × 3d or 500 mg once |
| OR | Ivermectin[7,16] | 150–200 mcg/kg PO once | 150–200 mcg/kg PO once |

* Availability problems. See table on manufacturers of drugs used to treat parasitic infections, page 464.

[8] Although regimens have included rifampin, *Medical Letter* consultants believe the rifampin is unnecessary (Visvesvara GS et al., *FEMS Immunol Med Microbiol* 2007;50:1, epub 2007 Apr 11.) Other successful treatment courses have included amphotericin B, ornidazole, and rifampin (Jain R et al., *Neurol India* 2002;50:470) and amphotericin B, fluconazole, and rifampin (Vargas-Zepeda J et al., *Arch Med Research* 2005;36:83). Case reports of other successful therapy have been published (Sehuster FL and Visvesvara GS, *Int J Parasitiol* 2004;34:1001).

[9] Several patients with granulomatous amebic encephalitis (GAE) have been successfully treated with combinations of pentamidine, sulfadiazine, flucytosine, and either fluconazole or itraconazole (Visvesvara GS et al., *FEMS Immunol Med Microbiol* 2007;50:1, epub Apr 11). GAE in an AIDS patient was treated successfuly with sulfadiazine, pyrimethamine and fluconazole combined with surgical resection of the CNS lesion (Seijo M Martinez et al., *J Clin Microbiol* 2000;38:3892). Chronic *Acanthamoeba* meningitis was successfully treated in two children with a combination of oral trimethoprim/sulfamethoxazole, rifampin, and ketoconazole (Singhal T et al., *Pediatr Infect Dis J* 2001;20:623). Disseminated cutaneous infection in an immunocompromised patient was treated successfully with IV pentamidine, topical chlorhexidine and 2% ketoconazole cream, followed by oral itraconazole (Slater CA et al., *N Engl J Med* 1994;331:85) and with voriconazole and amphotericin B lipid complex (Walia R et al., *Transplant Infect Dis* 2007;9:51). Other reports of successful therapy have been described (Schuster FL and Visvesvara GS, *Drug Resistance Updates* 2004;7:41). Susceptibility testing of *Acanthamoeba* isolates has shown differences in drug sensitivity between species and even among strains of a single species; antimicrobial susceptibility testing is advisable (Schuster FL and Visvesvara GS, *Int J Parasitiol* 2004;34:1001).

[10] *B. mandrillaris* is a free-living ameba that causes subacute to fatal granulomatous amebic encephalitis (GAE) and cutaneous disease. Two cases of *Balamuthia* encephalitis have been successfully treated with flucytosine, pentamidine, fluconazole, and sulfadiazine plus either azithromycin or clarithromycin (phenothiazines were also used) combined with surgical resection of the CNS lesion (Deetz TR et al., *Clin Infect Dis* 2003;37:1304). Another case was successfully treated with pentamidine, fluconazole, sulfadiazine, and clarithromycin (Jung S et al., *Arch Pathol Lab Med* 2004;128:466).

| Infection | Drug | Adult dosage | Pediatric dosage |
|---|---|---|---|
| **BABESIOSIS** (*Babesia microti*) | | | |
| Drug of choice[17]: | Clindamycin[7,18] | 1.2 g bid IV or 600 mg tid PO × 7–10d | 20–40 mg/kg/d PO in 3 doses × 7–10d |
| | **plus** Quinine[7,19] | 650 mg PO tid × 7–10d | 30 mg/kg/d PO in 3 doses × 7–10d |
| OR | Atovaquone[7,20] | 750 mg PO bid × 7–10d | 20 mg/kg/d PO in 2 doses × 7–10d |
| | **plus** Azithromycin[7] | 600 mg PO daily × 7–10d | 12 mg/kg/d PO × 7–10d |

*Balamuthia mandrillaris*, see AMEBIC MENINGOENCEPHALITIS, PRIMARY

| Infection | Drug | Adult dosage | Pediatric dosage |
|---|---|---|---|
| **BALANTIDIASIS** (*Balantidium coli*) | | | |
| Drug of choice: | Tetracycline[7,21] | 500 mg PO qid × 10d | 40 mg/kg/d (max. 2 g) PO in 4 doses × 10d |
| Alternative: | Metronidazole[7] | 750 mg PO tid × 5d | 35–50 mg/kg/d PO in 3 doses × 5d |
| OR | Iodoquinol[2,7] | 650 mg PO tid × 20d | 30–40 mg/kg/d (max 2 g) PO in 3 doses × 20d |

[*] Availability problems. See table on manufacturers of drugs used to treat parasitic infections, page 464.

[11] A free-living ameba once thought not to be pathogenic to humans. *S. diploidea* has been successfully treated with azithromycin, pentamidine, itraconazole, and flucytosine combined with surgical resection of the CNS lesion (Gelman BB et al., *J Neuropathol Exp Neurol* 2003;62:990).

[12] Albendazole must be taken with food; a fatty meal increases oral bioavailability.

[13] Pyrantel pamoate suspension can be mixed with milk or fruit juice.

[14] *A. cantonensis* causes predominantly neurotropic disease. *A. costaricensis* causes gastrointestinal disease. Most patients infected with either species have a self-limited course and recover completely. Analgesics, corticosteroids and careful removal of CSF at frequent intervals can relieve symptoms from increased intracranial pressure (Re V Lo III and Gluckman SJ, *Am J Med* 2003;114:217). Treatment of *A. cantonensis* is controversial and varies across endemic areas. No antihelminthic drug is proven to be effective and some patients have worsened with therapy (Slom TJ et al., *N Engl J Med* 2002;346:668). Mebendazole and a corticosteroid, however, appear to shorten the course of infection (Tsai H-C et al., *Am J Med* 2001;111:109; Chotmongkol V et al., *Am J Trop Med Hyg* 2006;74:1122). Albendazole has also relieved symptoms of angiostrongyliasis (Chen XG et al., *Emerg Infect Dis* 2005;11:1645).

[15] Repiso Ortega A et al., *Gastroenterol Hepatol* 2003;26:341. Successful treatment of *Anisakiasis* with albendazole 400 mg PO bid × 3-5d has been reported, but the diagnosis was presumptive (Moore DA et al., *Lancet* 2002;360:54; Pacios E et al., *Clin Infect Dis* 2005;41:1825).

[16] Safety of ivermectin in young children (<15 kg) and pregnant women remains to be established. Ivermectin should be taken on an empty stomach with water.

[17] Exchange transfusion has been used in severely ill patients and those with high (>10%) parasitemia (Powell VI and Grima K, *Transfus Med Rev* 2002;16:239). In patients who were not severely ill, combination therapy with atovaquone and azithromycin was as effective as clindamycin and quinine and may have been better tolerated (Krause PJ et al., *N Engl J Med* 2000;343:1454). Longer treatment courses may be needed in immunosuppressed patients and those with asplenia. Patients are commonly co-infected with Lyme disease (*Med Lett Drugs Ther* 2007;49:49; Steere AC et al., *Clin Infect Dis* 2003;36:1078).

[18] Oral clindamycin should be taken with a full glass of water to minimize esophageal ulceration.

[19] Quinine should be taken with or after a meal to decrease gastrointestinal adverse effects.

[20] Atovaquone is available in an oral suspension that should be taken with a meal to increase absorption.

[21] Use of tetracyclines is contraindicated in pregnancy and in children <8 years old. Tetracycline should be taken 1 hour before or 2 hours after meals and/or with dairy products.

| Infection | Drug | Adult dosage | Pediatric dosage |
|---|---|---|---|
| **BAYLISASCARIASIS** (*Baylisascaris procyonis*) | | | |
| Drug of choice: | See footnote 22 | | |
| **BLASTOCYSTIS hominis** infection | | | |
| Drug of choice: | See footnote 23 | | |
| **CAPILLARIASIS** (*Capillaria philippinensis*) | | | |
| Drug of choice: | Mebendazole[7] | 200 mg PO bid × 20d | 200 mg PO bid × 20d |
| Alternative: | Albendazole[7,12] | 400 mg PO daily × 10d | 400 mg PO daily × 10d |
| **Chagas' disease**, see TRYPANOSOMIASIS | | | |
| *Clonorchis sinensis*, see FLUKE infection | | | |
| **CRYPTOSPORIDIOSIS** (*Cryptosporidium*) | | | |
| **Non-HIV infected** | | | |
| Drug of choice: | Nitazoxanide[5] | 500 mg PO bid × 3d | 1–3yrs: 100 mg PO bid × 3d<br>4–11yrs: 200 mg PO bid × 3d<br>>12yrs: 500 mg PO q12h × 3d |
| **HIV infected** | | | |
| Drug of choice: | See footnote 24 | | |
| **CUTANEOUS LARVA MIGRANS** (creeping eruption, dog and cat hookworm) | | | |
| Drug of choice[25]: | Albendazole[7,12] | 400 mg PO daily × 3d | 400 mg PO daily × 3d |
| OR | Ivermectin[7,16] | 200 mcg/kg PO daily × 1–2d | 200 mcg/kg PO daily × 1–2d |

---

[*] Availability problems. See table on manufacturers of drugs used to treat parasitic infections, page 464.

[22] No drug has been demonstrated to be effective. Albendazole 25 mg/kg/d PO × 20d started as soon as possible (up to 3 days after possible infection) might prevent clinical disease and is recommended for children with known exposure (ingestion of raccoon stool or contaminated soil) (Murray WJ and Kazacos KR, *Clin Infect Dis* 2004;39:1484). Mebendazole, levamisole, or ivermectin could be tried if albendazole is not available. Steroid therapy may be helpful, especially in eye and CNS infections (Gavin PJ et al., *Clin Microbiol Rev* 2005;18:703). Ocular baylisascariasis has been treated successfully using laser photocoagulation therapy to destroy the intraretinal larvae (Garcia CA et al., *Eye* 2004;18:624).

[23] Clinical significance of these organisms is controversial; metronidazole 750 mg PO tid × 10d, iodoquinol 650 mg PO tid × 20d or trimethoprim/sulfamethoxazole 1 DS tab PO bid × 7d have been reported to be effective (Stenzel DJ and Borenam PFL, *Clin Microbiol Rev* 1996;9:563; Ok UZ et al., *Am J Gastroenterol* 1999;94:3245). Metronidazole resistance may be common in some areas (Haresh K et al., *Trop Med Int Health* 1999;4:274). Nitazoxanide has been effective in clearing organism and improving symptoms (Diaz E et al., *Am J Trop Med Hyg* 2003;68:384; Rossignol JF, *Clin Gastroenterol Hepatol* 2005;18:703).

[24] No drug has proven efficacy against cryptosporidiosis in advanced AIDS (Abubakar I et al., *Cochrane Database Syst Rev* 2007;1:CD004932). Treatment with HAART is the mainstay of therapy. Nitazoxanide (Rossignol JF, *Aliment Pharmacol Ther* 2006;24:807), paromomycin (Maggi P et al., *Clin Infect Dis* 2000;33:1609), or a combination of paromomycin and azithromycin (Smith NH et al., *J Infect Dis* 1998;178:900) may be tried to decrease diarrhea and recalcitrant malabsorption of antimicrobial drugs, which can occur with chronic cryptosporidiosis.

| Infection | Drug | Adult dosage | Pediatric dosage |
|---|---|---|---|
| **CYCLOSPORIASIS** (*Cyclospora cayetanensis*) | | | |
| Drug of choice[26]: | Trimethoprim/ sulfamethoxazole[7] | TMP 160 mg/SMX 800 mg (1 DS tab) PO bid × 7–10d | TMP 5 mg/kg/SMX 25 mg/kg/d PO in 2 doses × 7–10d |

**CYSTICERCOSIS**, see **TAPEWORM** infection

| *DIENTAMOEBA fragilis* infection[27] | | | |
|---|---|---|---|
| Drug of choice: | Iodoquinol[2,7] | 650 mg PO tid × 20d | 30–40 mg/kg/d (max. 2g) PO in 3 doses × 20d |
| OR | Paromomycin[3,7] | 25–35 mg/kg/d PO in 3 doses × 7d | 25–35 mg/kg/d PO in 3 doses × 7d |
| OR | Tetracycline[7,21] | 500 mg PO qid × 10d | 40 mg/kg/d (max. 2g) PO in 4 doses × 10d |
| OR | Metronidazole[7] | 500–750 mg PO tid × 10d | 35–50 mg/kg/d PO in 3 doses × 10d |

*Diphyllobothrium latum*, see TAPEWORM infection

**DRACUNCULUS medinensis** (guinea worm) infection
Drug of choice: See footnote 28

Echinococcus, see **TAPEWORM** infection

*Entamoeba histolytica*, see **AMEBIASIS**

* Availability problems. See table on manufacturers of drugs used to treat parasitic infections, page 464.

[25] Albanese G et al., *Int J Dermatol* 2001;40:67; Malvy D. et al., *J Travel Med* 2006;13:244.

[26] HIV-infected patients may need higher dosage and long-term maintenance. Successful use of nitazoxanide (see footnote 4) has been reported in one patient with sulfa allergy (Zimmer SM et al., *Clin Infect Dis* 2007;44:466).

[27] Norberg A et al., *Clin Microbiol Infect* 2003;9:65; Vandenberg O et al., *Int J Infect Dis* 2006;10:255.

[28] No drug is curative against *Dracunculus*. A program for monitoring local sources of drinking water to eliminate transmission has dramatically decreased the number of cases worldwide (Barry M, *N Engl J Med* 2007;356:25). The treatment of choice is slow extraction of worm combined with wound care and pain management (Greenaway C, *CMAJ* 2004;170:495).

[29] Since family members are usually infected, treatment of the entire household is recommended.

[30] Antihistamines or corticosteroids may be required to decrease allergic reactions to components of disintegrating microfilariae that result from treatment especially in infection caused by *Loa loa*. Endosymbiotic *Wolbachia* bacteria may have a role in filarial development and host response, and may represent a potential target for therapy. Addition of doxycycline 100 or 200 mg/d PO × 6–8wks in lymphatic filariasis and onchocerciasis has resulted in substantial loss of *Wolbachia* and decrease in both micro- and macrofilariae (Taylor MJ et al., *Lancet* 2005;365:2116; Debrah AY et al., *Plos Pathog* 2006;e92:0829); but use of tetracyclines is contraindicated in pregnancy and in children <8 yrs old.

| Infection | | Drug | Adult dosage | Pediatric dosage |
|---|---|---|---|---|
| **ENTEROBIUS** vermicularis (pinworm) infection | | | | |
| Drug of choice[29]: | | Mebendazole | 100 mg PO once; repeat in 2wks | 100 mg PO once; repeat in 2wks |
| | OR | Pyrantel pamoate[13],* | 11 mg/kg base PO once (max. 1 g); repeat in 2wks | 11 mg/kg base PO once (max. 1 g); repeat in 2wks[22b] |
| | OR | Albendazole[7, 12] | 400 mg PO once; repeat in 2wks | 400 mg PO once; repeat in 2wks |

**Fasciola hepatica**, see FLUKE infection

| **FILARIASIS**[30] | | | | |
|---|---|---|---|---|
| **Wuchereria bancrofti, Brugia malayi, Brugia timori** | | | | |
| Drug of choice[31]: | | Diethylcarbamazine* | 6 mg/kg/d PO in 3 doses × 12d[32,33] | 6 mg/kg/d PO in 3 doses × 12d[32,33] |
| **Loa loa** | | | | |
| Drug of choice[34]: | | Diethylcarbamazine* | 6 mg/kg/d PO in 3 doses × 12d[32,33] | 6 mg/kg/d PO in 3 doses × 12d[32,33] |

* Availability problems. See table on manufacturers of drugs used to treat parasitic infections, page 464.

[31] Most symptoms are caused by adult worm. A single-dose combination of albendazole (400 mg PO) with either ivermectin (200 mcg/kg PO) or diethylcarbamazine (6 mg/kg PO) is effective for reduction or suppression of *W. bancrofti* microfilaria, but the albendazole/ivermectin combination does not kill all the adult worms (Addiss D et al., *Cochrane Database Syst Rev* 2004;CD003753).

[32] For patients with microfilaria in the blood, Medical Letter consultants start with a lower dosage and scale up: d1: 50 mg; d2: 50 mg tid; d3: 100 mg tid; d4–14: 6 mg/kg in 3 doses (for *Loa Loa* d4–14:9 mg/kg in 3 doses). Multidose regimens have been shown to provide more rapid reduction in microfilaria than single-dose diethylcarbamazine, but microfilaria levels are similar 6–12 months after treatment (Andrade LD et al., *Trans R Soc Trop Med Hyg* 1995;89:319; Simonsen PE et al., *Am J Trop Med Hyg* 1995;53:267). A single dose of 6 mg/kg is used in endemic areas for mass treatment (Figueredo-Silva J et al., *Trans R Soc Trop Med Hyg* 1996;90:192; Noroes J et al., *Trans R Soc Trop Med Hyg* 1997;91:78).

[33] Diethylcarbamazine should not be used for treatment of *Onchocerca volvulus* due to the risk of increased ocular side effects including blindness associated with rapid killing of the worms. It should be used cautiously in geographic regions where *O. volvulus* coexists with other filariae. Diethylcarbamazine is contraindicated during pregnancy. See also footnote 38.

[34] In heavy infections with *Loa loa*, rapid killing of microfilariae can provoke encephalopathy. Apheresis has been reported to be effective in lowering microfilarial counts in patients heavily infected with *Loa loa* (Ottesen EA, *Infect Dis Clin North Am* 1993;7:619). Albendazole may be useful for treatment of loiasis when diethylcarbamazine is ineffective or cannot be used, but repeated courses may be necessary (Klion AD et al., *Clin Infect Dis* 1999;29:680; Tabi TE et al., *Am J Trop Med Hyg* 2004;71:211). Ivermectin has also been used to reduce microfilaremia, but albendazole is preferred because of its slower onset of action and lower risk of precipitating encephalopathy (Klion AD et al., *J Infect Dis* 1993;168:202; Kombila M et al., *Am J Trop Med Hyg* 1998;58:458). Diethylcarbamazine, 300 mg PO once/wk has been recommended for prevention of loiasis (Nutman TB et al., *N Engl J Med* 1988;319:752).

| Infection | Drug | Adult dosage | Pediatric dosage |
|---|---|---|---|
| **FILARIASIS** (continued)[30] | | | |
| *Mansonella ozzardi* | | | |
| Drug of choice: | See footnote 35 | | |
| *Mansonella perstans* | | | |
| Drug of choice: | Albendazole[7,12] | 400 mg PO bid × 10d | 400 mg PO bid × 10d |
| OR | Mebendazole[7] | 100 mg PO bid × 30d | 100 mg PO bid × 30d |
| *Mansonella streptocerca* | | | |
| Drug of choice[36]: | Diethylcarbamazine* | 6 mg/kg/d PO × 12d[33] | 6 mg/kg/d PO × 12d[33] |
| OR | Ivermectin[7,16] | 150 mcg/kg PO once | 150 mcg/kg PO once |
| **Tropical Pulmonary Eosinophilia** (TPE)[29,37] | | | |
| Drug of choice: | Diethylcarbmazine* | 6 mg/kg/d in 3 doses × 12–21d[33] | 6 mg/kg/d in 3 doses × 12–21d[33] |
| *Onchocerca volvulus* (River blindness) | | | |
| Drug of choice: | Ivermectin[16,38] | 150 mcg/kg PO once; repeated every 6–12mos until asymptomatic | 150 mcg/kg PO once; repeated every 6–12mos until asymptomatic |
| **FLUKE**, hermaphroditic, infection | | | |
| *Clonorchis sinensis* (Chinese liver fluke) | | | |
| Drug of choice: | Praziquantel[39] | 75 mg/kg/d PO in 3 doses × 2d | 75 mg/kg/d PO in 3 doses × 2d |
| OR | Albendazole[7,12] | 10 mg/kg/d PO × 7d | 10 mg/kg/d PO × 7d |
| *Fasciola hepatica* (sheep liver fluke) | | | |
| Drug of choice[40]: | Triclabendazole* | 10 mg/kg PO once or twice[41] | 10 mg/kg PO once or twice[41] |
| Alternative: | Bithionol* | 30–50 mg/kg on alternate days × 10–15 doses | 30–50 mg/kg on alternate days × 10–15 doses |
| OR | Nitazoxanide[5,7] | 500 mg PO bid × 7d | 1–3yrs: 100 mg PO q12h × 7d 4–11yrs: 200 mg PO q12h × 7d >12yrs: 500 mg PO q12h × 7d |

* Availability problems. See table on manufacturers of drugs used to treat parasitic infections, page 464.

[35] Diethylcarbamazine has no effect. A single dose of ivermectin 200 mcg/kg PO reduces microfilaria densities and provides both short- and long-term reductions in *M. ozzardi* microfilaremia (Gonzalez AA et al., *W Indian Med J* 1999;48:231).

[36] Diethylcarbamazine is potentially curative due to activity against both adult worms and microfilariae. Ivermectin is active only against microfilariae.

[37] Boggild AK et al., *Clin Infect Dis* 2004;39:1123. Relapses occur and can be treated with a repeated course of diethylcarbamazine.

[38] Diethylcarbamazine should not be used for treatment of this disease because rapid killing of the worms can lead to blindness. Periodic treatment with ivermectin (every 3–12 months). 150 mcg/kg PO can prevent blindness due to ocular onchocerciasis (Udall DN, *Clin Infect Dis* 2007;44:53). Skin reactions after ivermectin treatment are often reported in persons with high microfilarial skin densities. Ivermectin has been inadvertently given to pregnant women during mass treatment programs; the rates of congenital abnormalities were similar in treated and untreated women. Because of the high risk of blindness from onchocerciasis, the use of ivermectin after the first trimester is considered acceptable according to the WHO. Doxycycline (100 mg/day PO for 6wks), followed by a single 150 mcg/kg PO dose of ivermectin, resulted in up to 19 months of amicrofilaridermia and 100% elimination of *Wolbachia* species (Hoerauf A et al., *Lancet* 2001;357:1415).

| Infection | Drug | Adult dosage | Pediatric dosage |
|---|---|---|---|
| *Fasciolopsis buski,* *Heterophyes heterophyes* *Metagonimus yokogawal* (intestinal flukes) | | | |
| Drug of choice: | Praziquantel[7,39] | 75 mg/kg/d PO in 3 doses × 1d | 75 mg/kg/d PO in 3 doses × 1d |
| *Metorchis conjunctus* (North American liver fluke) | | | |
| Drug of choice: | Praziquantel[7,39] | 75 mg/kg/d PO in 3 doses × 1d | 75 mg/kg/d PO in 3 doses × 1d |
| *Nanophyetus salmincola* | | | |
| Drug of choice: | Praziquantel[7,39] | 60 mg/kg/d PO in 3 doses × 1d | 60 mg/kg/d PO in 3 doses × 1d |
| *Opisthorchis viverrini* (Southeast Asian liver fluke) | | | |
| Drug of choice: | Praziquantel[39] | 75 mg/kg/d PO in 3 doses × 2d | 75 mg/kg/d PO in 3 doses × 2d |
| *Paragonimus westermani* (lung fluke) | | | |
| Drug of choice: | Praziquantel[7,39] | 75 mg/kg/d PO in 3 doses × 2d | 75 mg/kg/d PO in 3 doses × 2d |
| Alternative[42]: | Bithionol* | 30–50 mg/kg on alternate days × 10–15 doses | 30–50 mg/kg on alternate days × 10–15 doses |
| **GIARDIASIS** (*Giardia duodenalis*) | | | |
| Drug of choice: | Metronidazole[7] | 250 mg PO tid × 5–7d | 15 mg/kg/d PO in 3 doses × 5–7d |
| OR | Tinidazole[6] | 2 g PO once | 50 mg/kg PO once (max. 2 g) |
| OR | Nitazoxanide[5] | 500 mg PO bid × 3d | 1–3yrs: 100 mg PO q12h × 3d 4–11yrs: 200 mg PO q12h × 3d >12yrs: 500 mg PO q12h × 3d |
| Alternative[43]: | Paromomycin[3,7,44] | 25–35 mg/kg/d PO in 3 doses × 5–10d | 25–35 mg/kg/d PO in 3 doses × 5–10d |
| OR | Furazolidone* | 100 mg PO qid × 7–10d | 6 mg/kg/d PO in 4 doses × 7–10d |
| OR | Quinacrine[4,45,*] | 100 mg PO tid × 5d | 2 mg/d PO in 3 doses × 5d (max. 300 mg/d) |

* Availability problems. See table on manufacturers of drugs used to treat parasitic infections, page 464.

[39] Praziquantel should be taken with liquids during a meal.

[40] Unlike infections with other flukes, *Fasciola hepatica* infections may not respond to praziquantel. Triclabendazole (*Egaten–Novartis*) appears to be safe and effective, but data are limited (Aksoy DY et al., *Clin Microbiol Infect* 2005;11:859). It is available from Victoria Pharmacy, Zurich, Switzerland (www.pharmaworld.com; 41-1-211-24-32) and should be given with food for better absorption. Nitazoxanide also appears to have efficacy in treating fascioliasis in adults and in children (Favennec L et al., *Aliment Pharmacol Ther* 2003;17:265; Rossignol JF et al., *Trans R Soc Trop Med Hyg* 1998;92:103; Kabil SM et al., *Curr Ther Res* 2000;61:339).

[41] Kaiser J et al., *Expert Opin Investig Drugs* 2005;14:1513.

[42] Triclabendazole may be effective in a dosage of 5 mg/kg PO once/d × 3d or 10 mg/kg PO bid × 1d (Calvopina M et al., *Trans R Soc Trop Med Hyg* 1998;92:566). See footnote 40 for availability.

| Infection | Drug | Adult dosage | Pediatric dosage |
|---|---|---|---|
| **GNATHOSTOMIASIS** (*Gnathostoma spinigerum*)[46] | | | |
| Treatment of choice[37]: | Albendazole[7,12] | 400 mg PO bid × 21d | 400 mg PO bid × 21d |
| OR | Ivermectin[7,16] | 200 mcg/kg/d PO × 2d | 200 mcg/kg/d PO × 2d |
| | **either** | | |
| ± | Surgical removal | | |
| **GOGYLONEMIASIS** (*Gongylonema* sp.)[47] | | | |
| Treatment of choice: | Surygical removal | | |
| OR | Albendazole[7,12] | 400 mg/d PO × 3d | 400 mg/d PO × 3d |
| **HOOKWORM** infection (*Ancylostoma duodenale, Necator americanus*) | | | |
| Drug of choice: | Albendazole[7,12] | 400 mg PO once | 400 mg PO once |
| OR | Mebendazole | 100 mg PO bid × 3d or 500 mg once | 100 mg PO bid × 3d or 500 mg once |
| OR | Pyrantel pamoate[7,13,*] | 11 mg/kg (max. 1g) PO × 3d | 11 mg/kg (max. 1g) PO × 3d |

**Hydatid cyst**, see TAPEWORM infection
*Hymenolepis nana*, see TAPEWORM infection

| | | | |
|---|---|---|---|
| **ISOSPORIASIS** (*Isospora belli*) | | | |
| Drug of choice[48]: | Trimethoprim-sulfamethoxazole[7] | TMP 160 mg/SMX 800 mg (1 DS tab) PO bid × 10d | TMP 5 mg/kg/d/SMX 25 mg/kg/d PO in 2 doses × 10d |

* Availability problems. See table on manufacturers of drugs used to treat parasitic infections, page 464.

[43] Another alternative is albendazole 400 mg/d PO × 5d in adults and 10 mg/kg/d PO × 5d in children (Yereli K et al., *Clin Microbiol Infect* 2004;10:527; Karabay O et al., *World J Gastroenterol* 2004;10:1215). Combination treatment with standard doses of metronidazole and quinacrine × 3wks has been effective for a small number of refractory infections (Nash TE et al., *Clin Infect Dis* 2001;33:22). In one study, nitazoxanide was used successfully in high doses to treat a case of *Giardia* resistant to metronidazole and albendazole (Abboud P et al., *Clin Infect Dis* 2001;32:1792).

[44] Poorly absorbed; may be useful for treatment of giardiasis in pregnancy.

[45] Quinacrine should be taken with liquids after a meal.

[46] Nontasat P et al., *Southeast Asian J Trop Med Pub Health* 2005;36:650; Gergolas M de et al., *J Travel Med* 2003;10:358. All patients should be treated with medication whether surgery is attempted or not.

[47] Wilson ME et al., *Clin Infect Dis* 2001;32:1378; Molavi G et al., *J Helminth* 2006;80:425.

[48] Usually a self-limited illness in immunocompetent patients. Immunosuppressed patients may need higher doses, longer duration (TMP/SMX qid × 10d, followed by bid × 3wks), and long-term maintenance. In sulfonamide-sensitive patients, pyrimethamine 50–75 mg daily in divided doses (plus leucovorin 10–25 mg/d) has been effective.

| Infection | | Drug | Adult dosage | Pediatric dosage |
|---|---|---|---|---|
| **LEISHMANIA**<br>**Visceral**[49,50] | | | | |
| Drug of choice: | | Liposomal amphotericin B[51] | 3 mg/kg/d IV d 1–5, 14 and 21[52] | 3 mg/kg/d IV d 1–5, 14 and 21[52] |
| | OR | Sodium stibogluconate* | 20 mg Sb/kg/d IV or IM × 28d | 20 mg Sb/kg/d IV or IM × 28d |
| | OR | Miltefosine[53],* | 2.5 mg/kg/d PO (max. 150 mg/d) × 28d | 2.5 mg/kg/d PO (max 150 mg/d) × 28d |
| Alternative: | | Meglumine antimonate* | 20 mg Sb/kg/d IV or IM × 28d | 20 mg Sb/kg/d IV or IM × 28d |
| | OR | Amphotericin B[7] | 1 mg/kg IV daily × 15–20d or every second day for up to 8wks | 1 mg/kg IV daily × 15–20d or every second day for up to 8 wks |
| | OR | Paromomycin[7,13,54],* | 15 mg/kg/d IM × 21d | 15 mg/kd/d IM × 21d |

* Availability problems. See table on manufacturers of drugs used to treat parasitic infections, page 464.

[49] To maximize effectiveness and minimize toxicity, the choice of drug, dosage, and duration of therapy should be individualized based on the region of disease acquisition, a likely infecting species, and host factors such as immune status (Herwaldt BL, *Lancet* 1999;354:1191). Some of the listed drugs and regimens are effective only against certain *Leishmania* species/strains and only in certain areas of the world (Arevalo J et al., *Clin Infect Dis* 2007;195:1846). Medical Letter consultants recommend consultation with physicians experienced in management of this disease.

[50] Visceral infection is most commonly due to the Old World species *L. donovani* (kala-azar) and *L. infantum* and the New World species *L. chagasi*.

[51] Liposomal amphotericin B (*AmBisome*) is the only lipid formulation of amphotericin B FDA-approved for treatment of visceral leishmania, largely based on clinical trials in patients infected with *L. infantum* (Meyerhoff A, *Clin Infect Dis* 1999;28:42). Two other amphotericin B lipid formulations, amphotericin B lipid complex (*Abelcet*) and amphotericin B cholesteryl sulfate (*Amphotec*) have been used, but are considered investigational for this condition and may not be as effective (Bern C et al., *Clin Infect Dis* 2006;43:917).

[52] The FDA-approved dosage regimen for immunocompromised patients (e.g., HIV infected) is 4 mg/kg/d IV on days 1–5, 10, 17, 24, 31, and 38. The relapse rate is high; maintenance therapy (secondary prevention) may be indicated, but there is no consensus as to dosage or duration.

[53] Effective for both antimony-sensitive and -resistant *L. donovani* (Indian); miltefosine (*Impavido*) is manufactured in 10- or 50-mg capsules by Zentaris (Frankfurt, Germany at info@zentaris.com) and is available through consultation with the CDC. The drug is contraindicated in pregnancy; a negative pregnancy test before drug initiation and effective contraception during and for 2 months after treatment is recommended (Murray H et al., *Lancet* 2005;366:1561). In a placebo-controlled trial in patients ≥ 12 years old, oral miltefosine 2.5 mg/kg/d × 28d was also effective for treatment of cutaneous leishmaniasis due to *L.(V.) panamensis* in Colombia, but not *L.(V.) braziliensis* or *L. mexicana* in Guatemala (Soto J et al., *Clin Infect Dis* 2004;38:1266). "Motion sickness," nausea, headache, and increased creatinine are the most frequent adverse effects (Soto J and Soto P, *Expert Rev Anti Infect Ther* 2006;4:177).

[54] Paromomycin IM has been effective against leishmania in India; it has not yet been tested in South America or the Mediterranean, and there is insufficient data to support its use in pregnancy (Sundar S et al., *N Engl J Med* 2007;356:2371). Topical paromomycin should be used only in geographic regions where cutaneous leishmaniasis species have low potential for mucosal spread. A formulation of 15% paromomycin/12% methylbenzethonium chloride (*Leshcutan*) in soft white paraffin for topical use has been reported to be partially effective against cutaneous leishmaniasis due to *L. major* in Israel and *L. mexicana* and *L.(V.) braziliensis* in Guatemala, where mucosal spread is very rare (Arana BA et al., *Am J Trop Med Hyg* 2001;65:466). The methylbenzethonium is irritating to the skin; lesions may worsen before they improve.

| Infection | | Drug | Adult dosage | Pediatric dosage |
|---|---|---|---|---|
| ***LEISHMANIA*** (continued) | | | | |
| **Cutaneous**[49,55] | | | | |
| Drugs of choice: | | Sodium stibogluconate* | 20 mg Sb/kg/d IV or IM × 20d | 20 mg Sb/kg/d IV or IM × 20d |
| | OR | Meglumine antimonate* | 20 mg Sb/kg/d IV or IM × 20d | 20 mg Sb/kg/d IV or IM × 20d |
| | OR | Miltefosine[53,*] | 2.5 mg/kg/d PO (max. 150 mg/d) × 28d | 2.5 mg/kg/d PO (max. 150 mg/d) × 28d |
| **Alternative**[56]: | | Paromomycin[7,13,54,*] | Topically 2x/d × 10–20d | Topically 2x/d × 10–20d |
| | OR | Pentamidine[7] | 2–3 mg/kg IV or IM daily or every second day × 4–7 doses[57] | 2–3 mg/kg IV or IM daily or every second day × 4–7 doses[57] |
| **Mucosal**[49,58] | | | | |
| Drug of choice: | | Sodium stibogluconate* | 20 mg Sb/kg/d IV or IM × 28d | 20 mg Sb/kg/d IV or IM × 28d |
| | OR | Meglumine antimonate* | 20 mg Sb/kg/d IV or IM × 28d | 20 mg Sb/kg/d IV or IM × 28d |
| | OR | Amphotericin B[7] | 0.5–1 mg/kg IV daily or every second day for up to 8wks | 0.5–1 mg/kg IV daily or every second day for up to 8wks |
| | OR | Miltefosine[53,*] | 2.5 mg/kg/d PO (max. 150 mg/d) × 28d | 2.5 mg/kg/d PO (max 150 mg/d) × 28d |

| Infection | | Drug | Adult dosage | Pediatric dosage |
|---|---|---|---|---|
| **LICE** infestation (*Pediculus humanus, P. capitis, Phthirus pubis*)[59] | | | | |
| Drug of choice: | | 0.5% Malathion[60] | Topically | Topically |
| | OR | 1% Permethrin[61] | Topically | Topically |
| Alternative: | | Pyrethrins with piperonyl butoxide[61] | Topically | Topically |
| | OR | Ivermectin[7,16,62] | 200 mcg/kg PO | ≥15kg: 200 mcg/kg PO |

* Availability problems. See table on manufacturers of drugs used to treat parasitic infections, page 464.

[55] Cutaneous infection is most commonly due to the Old World species *L. major* and *L. tropica* and the New World species *L. mexicana, L. (Viannia) braziliensis,* and others.

[56] Although azole drugs (fluconazole, ketoconazole, itraconazole) have been used to treat cutaneous disease, they are not reliably effective and have no efficacy against mucosal disease (Magill AJ, *Infect Dis Clin North Am* 2005;19:241). For treatment of *L. major* cutaneous lesions, a study in Saudi Arabia found that oral fluconazole, 200 mg once/d × 6wks appeared to speed healing (Alrajhi AA et al., *N Engl J Med* 2002;346:891). Thermotherapy may be an option for cutaneous *L. tropica* infection (Reithinger R et al., *Clin Infect Dis* 2005;40:1148). A device that generates focused and controlled heating of the skin has been approved by the FDA for this indication (*ThermoMed*—ThermoSurgery Technologies Inc., Phoenix, AZ, 602-264-7300; www.thermosurgery.com).

[57] At this dosage pentamidine has been effective in Colombia predominantly against *L.(V.) panamensis* (Soto-Mancipe J. et al., *Clin Infect Dis* 1993;16:417; Soto J et al., *Am J Trop Med Hyg* 1994;50:107). Activity against other species is not well established.

[58] Mucosal infection is most commonly due to the New World species *L.(V.) braziliensis, L.(V.) panamensis,* or *L.(V.) guyanensis.*

| Infection | Drug | Adult dosage | Pediatric dosage |
|---|---|---|---|
| *Loa loa*, see FILARIASIS | | | |

**MALARIA, Treatment of** *(Plasmodium falciparum,*[63] *P. vivax,*[64] *P. ovale, and P. malariae*[65] *)*
**ORAL**[66]
*P. falciparum* or
unidentified species acquired
in areas of chloroquine-
resistant *P. falciparum*[63]

| Infection | Drug | Adult dosage | Pediatric dosage |
|---|---|---|---|
| Drug of choice[67]: | Atovaquone/ proguanil[68] | 2 adult tabs bid[69] or 4 adult tabs once/d × 3d | <5kg: not indicated 5–8kg: 2 peds tabs once/d × 3d 9–10kg: 3 peds tabs once/d × 3d 11–20kg: 1 adult tab once/d × 3d 21–30kg: 2 adult tabs once/d × 3d 31–40kg: 3 adult tabs once/d × 3d >40kg: 4 adult tabs once/d × 3d |

*Availability problems. See table on manufacturers of drugs used to treat parasitic infections, 464.

[59] Pediculocides should not be used for infestations of the eyelashes. Such infestations are treated with petrolatum ointment applied 2–4x/d × 8–10d. Oral TMP/SMX has also been used (Meinking TL and Taplin D, *Curr Probl Dermatol* 1996;24:57). For pubic lice, treat with 5% permethrin or ivermectin as for scabies (see page 452). TMP/SMX has also been effective when used together with permethrin for head lice (Hipolito RB et al., *Pediatrics* 2001;107:E30).

[60] Malathion is both ovicidal and pediculocidal; two applications at least 7 days apart are generally necessary to kill all lice and nits.

[61] Permethrin and pyrethrin are pediculocidal; retreatment in 7.–10 days is needed to eradicate the infestation. Some lice are resistant to pyrethrins and permethrin (Meinking TL et al., *Arch Dermatol* 2002;138:220).

[62] Ivermectin is pediculocidal, but more than one dose is generally necessary to eradicate the infestation (Jones KN and English JC 3rd, *Clin Infect Dis* 2003;36:1355). The number of doses and interval between doses has not been established, but in one study of body lice, three doses administered at 7-day intervals were effective (Fouault C et al., *J Infect Dis* 2006;193:474).

[63] Chloroquine-resistant *P. falciparum* occurs in all malarious areas except Central America (including Panama north and west of the Canal Zone), Mexico, Haiti, the Dominican Republic, Paraguay, northern Argentina, North and South Korea, Georgia, Armenia, most of rural China, and some countries in the Middle East (chloroquine resistance has been reported in Yemen, Oman, Saudi Arabia, and Iran). For treatment of multiple-drug-resistant *P. falciparum* in Southeast Asia, especially Thailand, where mefloquine resistance is frequent atovaquone/proguanil, quinine plus either doxycycline or clindamycin, or artemether/lumefantrine may be used.

[64] *P. vivax* with decreased susceptibility to chloroquine is a significant problem in Papua-New Guinea and Indonesia. There are also a few reports of resistance from Myanmar, India, the Solomon Islands, Vanuatu, Guyana, Brazil, Colombia, and Peru (Baird JK et al., *Curr Infect Dis Rep* 2007;9:39).

[65] Chloroquine-resistant *P. malariae* has been reported from Sumatra (Maguire JD et al., *Lancet* 2002;360:58).

[66] Uncomplicated or mild malaria may be treated with oral drugs. Severe malaria (e.g., impaired consciousness, parasitemia >5%, shock, etc.) should be treated with parenteral drugs (Griffin KS et al., *JAMA* 2007;297:2264).

[67] Primaquine is given for prevention of relapse after infection with *P. vivax* or *P. ovale*. Some experts also prescribe primaquine phosphate 30 mg base/d (0.6 mg base/kg/d for children) for 14 days after departure from areas where these species are endemic (Presumptive Anti-Relapse Therapy [PART], "terminal prophylaxis"). Because this is not always effective as prophylaxis (Schwartz E et al., *N Engl J Med* 2003;349:1510), others prefer to rely on surveillance to detect cases when they occur, particularly when exposure was limited or doubtful. See also footnote 79.

| Infection | | Drug | Adult dosage | Pediatric dosage |
|---|---|---|---|---|
| **MALARIA, Treatment of** (continued) | | | | |
| | OR | Quinine sulfate **plus** | 650 mg q8h × 3 **or** 7d[70] | 30 mg/kg/d in 3 doses × 3 **or** 7d[70] |
| | | doxycycline[7,21,71] **or plus** | 100 mg bid × 7d | 4 mg/kg/d in 2 doses × 7d |
| | | tetracycline[7,21] **or plus** | 250 mg qid × 7d | 6.25 mg/kg/d in 4 doses × 7d |
| | | clindamycin[7,18,72] | 20 mg/kg/d in 3 doses × 7d[73] | 20 mg/kg/d in 3 doses × 7d |
| Alternative[67]: | | Mefloquine[74,75] | 750 mg followed 12 hrs later by 500 mg | 15 mg/kg followed 12 hrs later by 10 mg/kg |
| | OR | Artemether/ lumefantrine[76,77,*] | 6 doses over 3d (4 tabs/dose at 0, 8, 24, 36, 48 and 60 hs) | 6 doses over 3d at same intervals as adults; |
| | | | | <15kg: 1 tab/dose |
| | | | | 15–25kg: 2 tabs/dose |
| | | | | 25–35kg: 3 tabs/dose |
| | | | | >35kg: 4 tabs/dose |

* Availability problems. See table on manufacturers of drugs used to treat parasitic infections, page 464.

[68] Atovaquone/proguanil is available as a fixed-dose combination tablet: adult tablets (*Malaroner*, 250 mg atovaquone/100 mg proguanil) and pediatric tablets (*Malarone Pediatric*; 62.5 mg atovaquone/25 mg proguanil). To enhance absorption and reduce nausea and vomiting, it should be taken with food or a milky drink. Safety in pregnancy is unknown; outcomes were normal in 24 women treated with the combination in the second and third trimester (McGready R et al., *Eur J Clin Pharmacol* 2003;59:545). The drug should not be given to patients with severe renal impairment (creatinine clearance <30mL/min). There have been isolated case reports of resistance in *P. falciparum* in Africa, but *Medical Letter* consultants do not believe there is a high risk for acquisition of *Malarone*-resistant disease (Schwartz E et al., *Clin Infect Dis* 2003;37:450; Farnert A et al., *BMJ* 2003;326:628; Kuhn S et al., *Am J Trop Med Hyg* 2005;72:407; Happi CT et al., *Malaria Journal* 2006;5:82).

[69] Although approved for once-daily dosing, Medical Letter consultants usually divide the dose in two to decrease nausea and vomiting.

[70] Available in the US in a 324-mg capsule; second capsules suffice for adult dosage. In Southeast Asia, relative resistance to quinine has increased and treatment should be continued for 7 days. Quinine should be taken with or after meals to decrease gastrointestinal adverse effects.

[71] Doxycycline should be taken with adequate water to avoid esophageal irritation. It can be taken with food to minimize gastrointestinal adverse effects.

[72] For use in pregnancy and in children <8 years.

[73] Lell B and Kremsner PG, *Antimicrob Agents Chemother* 2002;46:2315; Ramharter M et al., *Clin Infect Dis* 2005; 40:1777.

[74] At this dosage, adverse effects include nausea, vomiting, diarrhea and dizziness. Disturbed sense of balance, toxic psychosis and seizures can also occur. Mefloquine should not be used for treatment of malaria in pregnancy unless there is no other treatment option because of increased-risk for stillbirth (Nosten F et al., *Clin Infect Dis* 1999;28:808). It should be avoided for treatment of malaria in persons with active depression or with a history of psychosis or seizures and should be used with caution in persons with any psychiatric illness. Mefloquine can be given to patients taking β-blockers it they do not have an underlying arrhythmia; it should not be used in patients with conduction abnormalities. Mefloquine should not be given together with quinine or quinidine, and caution is required in using quinine or quinidine to treat patients with malaria who have taken mefloquine for prophylaxis. Mefloquine should not be taken on an empty stomach; it should be taken with at least 8 oz of water.

| Infection | Drug | Adult dosage | Pediatric dosage |
|---|---|---|---|
| | OR    Artesunate[76],* **plus** see footnote 78 | 4 mg/kg/d × 3d | 4 mg/kg/d × 3d |
| *P. vivax* acquired in areas of chloroquine-resistant *P. vivax*[64] | | | |
| Drug of choice[67]: | Mefloquine[74] | 750 mg PO followed 12 hrs later by 500 mg | 15 mg/kg PO followed 12 hrs later by 10 mg/kg |
| OR | Atovaquone/ proguanil[68] | 2 adult tabs bid[69] or 4 adult tabs once/d × 3d | <5kg: not indicated<br>5–8kg: 2 peds tabs once/d × 3d<br>9–10kg: 3 peds tabs once/d × 3d<br>11–20kg: 1 adult tab once/d × 3d<br>21–30kg: 2 adult tabs once/d × 3d<br>31–40kg: 3 adult tabs once/d × 3d<br>>40kg: 4 adult tabs once/d × 3d |
| | **either followed by** primaquine phosphate[79] | 30 mg base/d PO × 14d | 0.6 mg/kg/d PO × 14d |
| Alternative[67]: | Chloroquine phosphate[80] | 25 mg base/kg PO in 3 doses over 48 hrs[81] | 25 mg base/kg PO in 3 doses over 48 hrs[81] |
| OR | Quinine sulfate **plus** | 650 mg PO q8h × 3–7d[70] | 30 mg/kg/d PQ in 3 doses × 3–7d[70] |
| | doxycycline[7,21,71] | 100 mg PO bid × 7d | 4 mg/kg/d PO in 2 doses × 7d |
| | **either followed by** primaquine phosphate[79] | 30 mg base/d PO × 14d | 0.6 mg/kg/d PO × 14d |
| All *Plasmodium* species except chloroquine-resistant *P. falciparum*[63] and chloroquine-resistant *P. vivax*[64] | | | |
| Drug of choice[67]: | Chloroquine phosphate[80] | 1 g (600 mg base) PO, then 500 mg (300 mg base) 6 hrs later, then 500mg (300 mg base) at 24 and 48 hrs[81] | 10 mg base/kg (max. 600 mg base) PO, then 5 mg base/kg 6 hrs later, then 5 mg base/kg at 24 and 48 hrs[81] |

* Availability problems. See table on manufacturers of drugs used to treat parasitic infections, page 464.

[75] *P. falciparum* with resistance to mefloquine is a significant problem in the malarious areas of Thailand and in areas of Myanmar and Cambodia that border on Thailand. It has also been reported on the borders between Myanmar and China, Laos and Myanmar, and in Southern Vietnam. In the US, a 250-mg tablet of mefloquine contains 228 mg mefloquine base. Outside the US, each 275-mg tablet contains 250 mg base.

[76] The artemisinin-derivatives, artemether and artesunate, are both frequently used globally in combination regimens to treat malaria. Both are available in oral, parenteral, and rectal formulations, but manufacturing standards are not consistent (Karunajeewa HA et al., *JAMA* 2007;297:2381; Ashley EA and White NJ, *Curr Opin Infect Dis* 2005;18:531). In the US, only the IV formulation of artesunate is available; it can be obtained through the CDC under an IND for patients with severe disease who do not have timely access, cannot tolerate, or fail to respond to IV quinidine (www.cdc.gov/malaria/features/artesunate_now_available.htm). To avoid development of resistance, monotherapy should be avoided (Duffy PE and Sibley CH, *Lancet* 2005;366:1908). Artemisinins are contraindicated during the first trimester of pregnancy and should be used with caution during the second and third trimester. Based on the few studies available, they have been relatively safe during pregnancy (Dellicour S et al., *Malaria Journal* 2007;6:15).

| Infection | | Drug | Adult dosage | Pediatric dosage |
|---|---|---|---|---|
| **PARENTERAL**[66] | | | | |
| All *Plasmodium* species (Chloroquine-sensitive and resistant) | | | | |
| Drug of choice[67,82]: | | Quinidine gluconate[83] | 10 mg/kg IV loading dose (max. 600 mg) in normal saline over 1–2 hrs, followed by continuous infusion of 0.02 mg/kg/min until PO therapy can be started | 10 mg/kg IV loading dose (max. 600 mg) in normal saline over 1–2 hrs, followed by continuous infusion of 0.02 mg/kg/min until PO therapy can be started |
| | OR | Quinine dihydro chloride[83,*] | 20 mg/kg IV loading dose in 5% dextrose over 4 hrs, followed by 10 mg/kg over 2–4 hrs q8h (max. 1800 mg/d) until PO therapy can be started | 20 mg/kg IV loading dose in 5% dextrose over 4 hrs, followed by 10 mg/kg over 2–4 hrs q8h (max. 1800 mg/d) until PO therapy can be started |
| | OR | Artesunate[76,*] | 2.4 mg/kg/dose IV × 3d at 0, 12, 24, 48, and 72 hrs | 2.4 mg/kg/dose IV × 3d at 0, 12, 24, 48, and 72 hrs |
| | | **plus** see footnote 78 | | |
| **MALARIA, Prevention of**[84] | | | | |
| All *Plasmodium* species in chloroquine-sensitive areas[63,64,65] | | | | |
| Drug of choice[67,85]: | | Chloroquine phosphate[80,86] | 500 mg (300 mg base) PO once/wk[87] | 5 mg/kg base PO once/wk, up to adult dose of 300 mg base[87] |

* Availability problems. See table on manufacturers of drugs used to treat parasitic infections, page 464.

[77] Artemether/lumefantrine is available as a fixed-dose combination tablet (*Coartem* in countries with endemic malaria, *Riamet* in Europe and countries without endemic malaria); each tablet contains 20 mg artemether and 120 mg lumefantrine (van Vugt M et al., *Am J Trop Med Hyg* 1999;60:936). It is contraindicated during the first trimester of pregnancy; safety during the second and third trimester is not known. The tablets should be taken with food. Artemether/lumefantrine should not be used in patients with cardiac arrhythmias, bradycardia, severe cardiac disease, or QT prolongation. Concomitant use of drugs that prolong the QT interval or are metabolized by CYP2D6 is contraindicated.

[78] Adults treated with artesunate should also receive oral treatment doses of either atovaquone/proguanil, doxycycline, clindamycin, or mefloquine; children should take either atovaquone/proguanil, clindamycin, or mefloquine (Nosten F et al., *Lancet* 2000;356:297; van Vugt M, *Clin Infect Dis* 2002;35:1498; Smithuis F et al., *Trans R Soc Trop Med Hyg* 2004;98:182). If artesunate is given IV, oral medication should be started when the patient is able to tolerate it (SEAQUAMAT group, *Lancet* 2005;366:717).

[79] Primaquine phosphate can cause hemolytic anemia, especially in patients whose red cells are deficient in G-6-PD. This deficiency is most common in African, Asian, and Mediterranean peoples. Patients should be screened for G-6-PD deficiency before treatment. Primaquine should not be used during pregnancy. It should be taken with food to minimize nausea and abdominal pain. Primaquine-tolerant *P. vivax* can be found globally. Relapses of primaquine-resistant strains may be retreated with 30 mg (base) × 28d.

[80] Chloroquine should be taken with food to decrease gastrointestinal adverse effects. If chloroquine phosphate is not available, hydroxychloroquine sulfate is as effective; 400 mg of hydroxychloroquine sulfate is equivalent to 500 mg of chloroquine phosphate.

[81] Chloroquine combined with primaquine was effective in 85% of patients with *P. vivax* resistant to chloroquine and could be a resonable choice in areas where other alternatives are not available (Baird JK et al., *J Infect Dis* 1995;171:1678).

| Infection | | Drug | Adult dosage | Pediatric dosage |
|---|---|---|---|---|
| All *Plasmodium* species in chloroquine-resistant areas[63,64,65] | | | | |
| Drug of choice[67]: | | Atovaquone/ proguanil[68] | 1 adult tab/d[88] | 5–8kg: $\frac{1}{2}$ peds tab/d[68,88] |
| | | | | 9–10kg: $\frac{3}{4}$ peds tab/d[68,88] |
| | | | | 11–20kg: 1 peds tab/d[68,88] |
| | | | | 21–30kg: 2 peds tabs/d[68,88] |
| | | | | 31–40kg: 3 peds tabs/d[68,88] |
| | | | | >40kg: 1 adult tab/d[68,88] |
| | OR | Doxycycline[7,21,71] | 100 mg PO daily[89] | 2 mg/kg/d PO, up to 100 mg/d[89] |
| | OR | Mefloquine[74,75,90] | 250 mg PO once/wk[91] | 5–10kg: $\frac{1}{8}$ tab once/wk[91] |
| | | | | 11–20kg: $\frac{1}{4}$ tab once/wk[91] |
| | | | | 21–30kg: $\frac{1}{2}$ tab once/wk[91] |
| | | | | 31–45kg: $\frac{3}{4}$ tab once/wk[91] |
| | | | | >45kg: 1 tab once/wk[91] |
| Alternative[92]: | | Primaquine[7,79] phosphate | 30 mg base PO daily[93] | 0.6 mg/kg base PO daily[93] |

**MALARIA, Prevention of relapses: *P. vivax* and *P. ovale*[67]**

| | | | | |
|---|---|---|---|---|
| Drug of choice: | | Primaquine phosphate[79] | 30 mg base/d PO × 14d | 0.6 mg base/kg/d PO × 14d |

**MALARIA, Self-Presumptive Treatment[94]**

| | | | | |
|---|---|---|---|---|
| Drug of Choice: | | Atovaquone/ proguanil[7,68] | 4 adult tabs once/d × 3d[69] | <5kg: not indicated |
| | | | | 5–8kg: 2 peds tabs once/d × 3d |
| | | | | 9–10kg: 3 peds tabs once/d × 3d |
| | | | | 11–20kg: 1 adult tab once/d × 3d |
| | | | | 21–30kg: 2 adult tabs once/d × 3d |
| | | | | 31–40kg: 3 adult tabs once/d × 3d |
| | | | | >40kg: 4 adult tabs once/d × 3d[69] |
| | OR | Quinine sulfate **plus** | 650 mg PO q8h × 3 or 7d[70] | 30 mg/kg/d PO in 3 doses × 3 or 7d[70] |
| | | doxycycline[7,21,71] | 100 mg PO bid × 7d | 4 mg/kg/d PO in 2 doses × 7d |
| | OR | Artesunate[76,*] **plus** see footnote 78 | 4 mg/kg/d PO × 3d | 4 mg/kg/d PO × 3d |

* Availability problems. See table on manufacturers of drugs used to treat parasitic infections, page 464.

[82] Exchange transfusion is controversial, but has been helpful for some patients with high-density (>10%) parasitemia, altered mental status, pulmonary edema, or renal complications (Powell VI and Grima K, *Transfus Med Rev* 2002;16:239; Riddle MS et al., *Clin Infect Dis* 2002;34:1192).

[83] Continuous EKG, blood pressure, and glucose monitoring are recommended, especially in pregnant women and young children. For problems with quinidine availability, call the manufacturer (Eli Lilly, 800-821-0538) or the CDC Malaria Hotline (770-488-7788). Quinidine may have greater antimalarial activity than quinine. The loading dose should be decreased or omitted in patients who have received quinine or mefloquine. If more than 48 hours of parenteral treatment is required, the quinine or quinidine dose should be reduced by 30–50%.

[84] No drug guarantees protection against malaria. Travelers should be advised to seek medical attention if fever develops after they return. Insect repellents, insecticide-impregnated bed nets, and proper clothing are important adjuncts for malaria prophylaxis (*Med Lett Drugs Ther* 2005;47:100). Malaria in pregnancy is particularly serious for both mother and fetus; prophylaxis is indicated if exposure cannot be avoided.

| Infection | Drug | Adult dosage | Pediatric dosage |
|---|---|---|---|

**MICROSPORIDIOSIS**

**Ocular** *(Encephalitozoon hellem, E.cuniculi, Vittaforma corneae [Nosema corneum])*

| | | | |
|---|---|---|---|
| Drug of choice: | Albendazole[7,12] | 400 mg PO bid | |
| | **plus** fumagillin[95,*] | | |

**Intestinal** *(E. bieneusi, E. [Septata] intestinalis)*

**E. bieneusi**

| | | | |
|---|---|---|---|
| Drug of choice: | Fumagillin[96,*] | 20 mg PO tid × 14d | |

**E. intestinalis**

| | | | |
|---|---|---|---|
| Drug of choice: | Albendazole[7,12] | 400 mg PO bid × 21d | |

**Disseminated** *(E. hellem, E. cuniculi, E. intestinalis, Pleistophora* sp., *Trachipleistophora* sp. and *Brachiola vesicularum)*

| | | | |
|---|---|---|---|
| Drug of choice[97]: | Albendazole[7,12,*] | 400 mg PO bid | |

---

**Mites**, see SCABIES

---

**MONILIFORMIS** *moniliformis* infection

| | | | |
|---|---|---|---|
| Drug of choice: | Pyrantel pamoate[7,13,*] | 11 mg/kg PO once; repeat twice, 2wks apart | 11 mg/kg PO once, repeat twice, 2wks apart |

---

* Availability problems. See table on manufacturers of drugs used to treat parasitic infections, page 464.

[85] Alternatives for patients who are unable to take chloroquine include atovaquone/proguanil, mefloquine, doxycycline, or primaquine dosed as for chloroquine-resistant areas.

[86] Has been used extensively and safely for prophylaxis in pregnancy.

[87] Beginning 1–2 weeks before travel and continuing weekly for the duration of stay and for 4 weeks after leaving.

[88] Beginning 1–2 days before travel and continuing for the duration of stay and for 1 week after leaving. In one study of malaria prophylaxis, atovaquone/proguanil was better tolerated than mefloquine in nonimmune travelers (Overbosch D et al., *Clin Infect Dis* 2001;33:1015). The protective efficacy of *Malarone* against *P. vivax* is variable ranging from 84% in Indonesian New Guinea (Ling J et al., *Clin Infect Dis* 2002;35:825) to 100% in Colombia (Soto J et al., *Am J Trop Med Hyg* 2006;75:430). Some Medical Letter consultants prefer alternate drugs if traveling to areas where *P. vivax* predominates.

[89] Beginning 1–2 days before travel and continuing for the duration of stay and for 4 weeks after leaving. Use of tetracyclines is contraindicated in pregnancy and in children <8 years old. Doxycycline can cause gastrointestinal disturbances, vaginal moniliasis and photosensitivity reactions.

[90] Mefloquine has not been approved for use during pregnancy. However, it has been reported to be safe for prophylactic use during the second and third trimester of pregnancy and possibly during early pregnancy as well (CDC Health Information for International Travel, 2008, page 228; Smoak BL et al., *J Infect Dis* 1997;176:831). For pediatric doses $<\frac{1}{2}$ tablet, it is advisable to have a pharmacist crush the tablet, estimate doses by weighing, and package them in gelatin capsules. There is no data for use in children <5 kg, but based on dosages in other weight groups, a dose of 5 mg/kg can be used. Not recommended for use in travelers with active depression or with a history of psychosis or seizures, and should be used with caution in persons with psychiatric illness. Mefloquine can be given to patients taking β-blockers if they do not have an underlying arrhythmia; it should not be used in patients with conduction abnormalities.

[91] Beginning 1–2 weeks before travel and continuing weekly for the duration of stay and for 4 weeks after leaving. Most adverse events occur within three doses. Some *Medical Letter* consultants favor starting mefloquine 3 weeks prior to travel and monitoring the patient for adverse events, this allows time to change to an alternative regimen if mefloquine is not tolerated.

| Infection | Drug | Adult dosage | Pediatric dosage |
|---|---|---|---|
| ***Naegleria* species**, see AMEBIC MENINGOENCEPHALITIS, PRIMARY | | | |
| ***Necator americanus***, see HOOKWORM infection | | | |
| ***OESOPHAGOSTOMUM*** bifurcum | | | |
| Drug of choice: | See footnote 98 | | |
| ***Onchocerca volvulus***, see FILARIASIS | | | |
| ***Opisthorchis viverrini***, see FLUKE infection | | | |
| ***Paragonimus westermani***, see FLUKE infection | | | |
| ***Pediculus capitis, humanus, Phthirus pubis***, see LICE | | | |
| **Pinworm**, see ENTEROBIUS | | | |

* Availability problems. See table on manufacturers of drugs used to treat parasitic infections, page 464.

[92] The combination of weekly chloroquine (300 mg base) and daily proguanil (200 mg) is recommended by the World Health Organization (www.WHO.int) for use in selected areas; this combination is no longer recommended by the CDC. Proguanil (*Paludrine*–AstraZeneca, United Kingdom) is not available alone in the US but is widely available in Canada and Europe. Prophylaxis is recommended during exposure and for 4 weeks afterwards. Proguanil has been used in pregnancy without evidence of toxicity (Phillips-Howard PA and Wood D, *Drug Saf* 1996;14:131).

[93] Studies have shown that daily primaquine beginning 1d before departure and continued until 3–7 days after leaving the malarious area provides effective prophylaxis against chloroquine-resistant *P. falciparum* (Baird JK et al., *Clin Infect Dis* 2003;37:1659). Some studies have shown less efficacy against *P. vivax*. Nausea and abdominal pain can be diminished by taking with food.

[94] A traveler can be given a course of medication for presumptive self-treatment of febrile illness. The drug given for self-treatment should be different from that used for prophylaxis. This approach should be used only in very rare circumstances when a traveler would not be able to get medical care promptly.

[95] Chan CM et al., *Ophthalmology* 2003;110:1420. Ocular lesions due to *E. hellem* in HIV-infected patients have responded to fumagillin eyedrops prepared from *Fumidil-B* (bicyclohexyl ammonium fumagillin) used to control a microsporidial disease of honey bees (Garvey MJ et al., *Ann Pharmacother* 1995;29:872), available from Leiter's Park Avenue Pharmacy (see footnote 1). For lesions due to *V. corneae*, topical therapy is generally not effective and keratoplasty may be required (Davis RM et al., *Ophthalmology* 1990;97:953).

[96] Oral fumagillin (*Flisint*—Sanofi-Aventis, France) has been effective in treating *E. bieneusi* (Molina J-M et al., *N Engl J Med* 2002;346:1963), but has been associated with thrombocytopenia and neutropenia. Highly active antiretroviral therapy (HAART) may lead to microbiologic and clinical response in HIV-infected patients with microsporidial diarrhea. Octreotide (*Sandostatin*) has provided symptomatic relief in some patients with large-volume diarrhea.

[97] Molina J-M et al., *J Infect Dis* 1995;171:245. There is no established treatment for *Pleistophora*. For disseminated disease due to *Trachipleistophora* or *Brachiola*, itraconazole 400 mg PO once/d plus albendazole may also be tried (Coyle CM et al., *N Engl J Med* 2004;351:42).

| Infection | Drug | Adult dosage | Pediatric dosage |
|---|---|---|---|
| **PNEUMOCYSTIS JIROVECI** (formerly *carinii*) pneumonia (PCP)[99] | | | |
| Drug of choice: | Trimethoprim/ sulfamethoxazole | TMP 15 mg/SMX 75 mg/kg/d, PO or IV in 3 or 4 doses × 21d | TMP 15 mg/SMX 75 mg/kg/d, PO or IV in 3 or 4 doses × 21d |
| Alternative: | Primaquine[7,79] **plus** clindamycin[7,18] | 30 mg base PO daily × 21d 600 mg IV q6h × 21d, or 300–450 mg PO q6h × 21d | 0.3 mg/kg base PO daily × 21d 15–25 mg/kg IV q6h × 21d, or 10 mg/kg PO q6h × 21d |
| OR | Trimethoprim[7] **plus** dapsone[7] | 5 mg/kg PO tid × 21d 100 mg daily × 21d | 5 mg/kg PO tid × 21d 2 mg/kg/d PO × 21d |
| OR | Pentamidine | 3–4 mg/kg IV daily × 21d | 3–4 mg/kg IV daily × 21d |
| OR | Atovaquone | 750 mg PO bid × 21d | 1–3mos: 30 mg/kg/d PO × 21d 4–24mos: 45 mg/kg/d PO × 21d >24mos: 30 mg/d PO × 21d |
| **Primary and secondary prophylaxis**[100] | | | |
| Drug of Choice: | Trimethoprim/ sulfamethoxazole | 1 tab (single or double strength) daily or 1 DS tab PO 3d/wk | TMP 150 mg/SMX 750 mg/m$^2$/d PO in 2 doses 3d/wk |
| Alternative: | Dapsone[7] | 50 mg PO bid or 100 mg PO daily | 2 mg/kg/d (max. 100 mg) PO or 4 mg/kg (max. 200 mg) PO each wk |
| OR | Dapsone[7] **plus** pyrimethamine[101] | 50 mg PO daily or 200 mg PO each wk 50 mg PO or 75 mg PO each wk | |
| OR | Pentamidine | 300 mg aerosol inhaled monthly via *Respirgard II* neublizer | ≥5yrs: 300 mg inhaled monthly via *Respirgard II* nebulizer |
| OR | Atovaquone[7,20] | 1500 mg PO daily | 1-3mos: 30 mg/kg/d PO 4–24mos: 45 mg/kg/d PO >24mos: 30 mg/kg/d PO |

**River Blindness**, see FILARIASIS

**Roundworm**, see ASCARIASIS

*Sappinia diploidea*, See AMEBIC MENINGOENCEPHALITIS, PRIMARY

| **SCABIES** (*Sarcoptes scabiei*) | | | |
|---|---|---|---|
| Drug of choice: | 5% Permethrin | Topically once[102] | Topically once[102] |
| Alternative[103]: | Ivermectin[7,16,104] | 200 mcg/kg PO once[102] | 200 mcg/kg PO once[102] |
| | 10% Crotamiton | Topically once/d × 2 | Topically once/d PO × 2 |

* Availability problems. See table on manufacturers of drugs used to treat parasitic infections, page 464.

[98] Albendazole or pyrantel pamoate may be effective (Ziem JB et al., *Ann Trop Med Parasitol* 2004;98:385).

[99] Pneumocystis has been reclassified as a fungus. In severe disease with room air PO$_2$ ≤ 70 mmHg or Aa gradient ≥ 35 mmHg, prednisone should also be used (Gagnon S et al., *N Engl J Med* 1990;323:1444; Caumes E et al., *Clin Infect Dis* 1994;18:319).

[100] Primary/secondary prophylaxis in patients with HIV can be discontinued after CD4 count increases to >200 × 10$^6$/L for >3mos.

| Infection | Drug | Adult dosage | Pediatric dosage |
| --- | --- | --- | --- |
| **SCHISTOSOMIASIS** (*Bilharziasis*) | | | |
| ***S. haematobium*** | | | |
| Drug of choice: | Praziquantel[39] | 40 mg/kg/d PO in 2 doses × 1d | 40 mg/kg/d PO in 2 doses × 1d |
| ***S. Japonicum*** | | | |
| Drug of choice: | Praziquantel[39] | 60 mg/kg/d PO in 3 doses × 1d | 60 mg/kg/d PO in 3 doses × 1d |
| ***S. mansoni*** | | | |
| Drug of choice: | Praziquantel[39] | 40 mg/kg/d PO in 2 doses × 1d | 40 mg/kg/d PO in 2 doses × 1d |
| Alternative: | Oxamniquine[105,*] | 15 mg/kg PO once[106] | 20 mg/kg/d PO in 2 doses × 1d[106] |
| ***S. mekongi*** | | | |
| Drug of choice: | Praziquantel[39] | 60 mg/kg/d PO in 3 doses × 1d | 60 mg/kg/d PO in 3 doses × 1d |

**Sleeping sickness**, see TRYPANOSOMIASIS

| | | | |
| --- | --- | --- | --- |
| **STRONGYLOIDIASIS** (*Strongyloides stercoralis*) | | | |
| Drug of choice[107]: | Ivermectin[16] | 200 mcg/kg/d PO × 2d | 200 mcg/kg/d PO × 2d |
| Alternative: | Albendazole[7,12] | 400 mg PO bid × 7d | 400 mg PO bid × 7d |

* Availability problems. See table on manufacturers of drugs used to treat parasitic infections, page 464.

[101] Plus leucovorin 25 mg with each dose of pyrimethamine. Pyrimethamine should be taken with food to minimize gastrointestinal adverse effects.

[102] Treatment may need to be repeated in 10–14 days. A second ivermectin dose taken 2 weeks later increases the cure rate to 95%, which is equivalent to that of 5% permethrin (Usha V et al., *J Am Acad Dermatol* 2000;42:236; Chosidow O, *N Engl J Med* 2006;354:1718; Heukelbach J and Feldmeier H, *Lancet* 2006;367:1767).

[103] Lindane (γ-benzene hexachloride) should be reserved for treatment of patients who fail to respond to other drugs. The FDA has recommended it not be used for immunocompromised patients, young children, the elderly, pregnant and breast-feeding women, and patients weighing <50 kg.

[104] Ivermectin, either alone or in combination with a topical scabicide, is the drug of choice for crusted scabies in immunocompromised patients (del Giudice P, *Curr Opin Infect Dis* 2004;15:123).

[105] Oxamniquine, which is not available in the US, is generally not as effective as praziquantel. It has been useful, however, in some areas in which praziquantel is less effective (Ferrari ML et al., *Bull World Health Organ* 2003;81:190; Harder A, *Parasitol Res* 2002;88:395). Oxamniquine is contraindicated in pregnancy. It should be taken after food.

[106] In East Africa, the dose should be increased to 30 mg/kg, and in Egypt and South Africa to 30 mg/kg/d × 2d. Some experts recommend 40–60 mg/kg over 2–3 days in all of Africa (Shekhar KC, *Drugs* 1991;42:379).

[107] In immunocompromised patients or disseminated disease, it may be necessary to prolong or repeat therapy, or to use other agents. Veterinary parenteral and enema formulations of ivermectin have been used in severely ill patients with hyperinfection who were unable to take or reliably absorb oral medications (Orem J et al., *Clin Infect Dis* 2003;37:152; Tarr PE, *Am J Trop Med Hyg* 2003;68:453; Marty FM et al., *Clin Infect Dis* 2005;41:e5). In disseminated strongyloidiasis, combination therapy with albendazole and ivermectin has been suggested (Lim S et al., *CMAJ* 2004;171:479).

| Infection | Drug | Adult dosage | Pediatric dosage |
|---|---|---|---|
| **TAPEWORM** infection | | | |
| **—Adult** (intestinal stage) | | | |
| ***Diphyllobothrium latum* (fish), *Taenia saginata* (beef), *Taenia solium* (pork), *Dipylidium caninum* (dog)** | | | |
| Drug of choice: | Praziquantel[7,39] | 5–10 mg/kg PO once | 5–10 mg/kg PO once |
| Alternative: | Niclosamide[108,*] | 2 g PO once | 50 mg/kg PO once |
| ***Hymenolepis nana* (dwarf tapeworm)** | | | |
| Drug of choice: | Praziquantel[7,39] | 25 mg/kg PO once | 25 mg/kg PO once |
| Alternative: | Nitazoxanide[5,7] | 500 mg PO once/d or bid × 3d[109] | 1–3yrs: 100 mg PO bid × 3d[109] |
| | | | 4–11yrs: 200 mg PO bid × 3d[109] |
| **—Larval** (tissue stage) | | | |
| ***Echinococcus granulosus*** (hydatid cyst) | | | |
| Drug of choice[110]: | Albendazole[12] | 400 mg PO bid × 1–6mos | 15 mg/kg/d (max. 800 mg) × 1–6mos |
| ***Echinococcus multilocularis*** | | | |
| Treatment of choice: | See footnote 111 | | |
| ***Taenia solium*** (*Cysticercosis*) | | | |
| Treatment of choice: | See footnote 112 | | |
| Alternative: | Albendazole[12] | 400 mg PO bid × 8–30d; can be repeated as necessary | 15 mg/kg/d (max. 800 mg) PO in 2 doses × 8–30d; can be repeated as necessary |
| OR | Praziquantel[7,39] | 100 mg/kg/d PO in 3 doses × 1 day; then 50 mg/kg/d in 3 doses × 29d | 100 mg/kg/d PO in 3 doses × 1d; then 50 mg/kg/d in 3 doses × 29d |

**Toxocariasis**, see VISCERAL LARVA MIGRANS

---

* Availability problems. See table on manufacturers of drugs used to treat parasitic infections, page 464.

[108] Niclosamide must be chewed thoroughly before swallowing and washed down with water.

[109] Juan JO et al., *Trans R Soc Trop Med Hyg* 2002;96:193; Chero JC et al., *Trans R Soc Trop Med Hyg* 2007;101:203; Diaz E et al., *Am J Trop Med Hyg* 2003;68:384.

[110] Patients may benefit from surgical resection or percutaneous drainage of cysts. Praziquantel is useful preoperatively or in case of spillage of cyst contents during surgery. Percutaneous aspiration-injection-reaspiration (PAIR) with ultrasound guidance plus albendazole therapy has been effective for management of hepatic hydatid cyst disease (Smego RA, Jr et al., *Clin Infect Dis* 2003;37:1073; Nepalia S et al., *J Assoc Physicians India* 2006;54:458; Zerem E and Jusufovic R, *Surg Endosc* 2006;20:1543).

[111] Surgical excision is the only reliable means of cure. Reports have suggested that in nonresectable cases use of albendazole (400 mg bid) can stabilize and sometimes cure infection (Craig P, *Curr Opin Infect Dis* 2003;16:437; Lidove O et al., *Am J Med* 2005;118:195).

[112] Initial therapy for patients with inflamed parenchymal cysticercosis should focus on symptomatic treatment with anti-seizure medication (Yancey LS et al., *Curr Infect Dis Rep* 2005;7:39; del Brutto AH et al., *Ann Intern Med* 2006;145:43). Patients with live parenchymal cysts who have seizures should be treated with albendazole together with steroids (dexamethasone 6 mg/d or prednisone 40–60 mg/d) and an anti-seizure medication (Garcia HH et al., *N Engl J Med* 2004;350:249). Patients with subarachnoid cysts or giant cysts in the fissures should be treated for at least 30d (Proaño JV et al., *N Engl J Med* 2001;345:879). Surgical intervention (especially neuroendoscopic removal) or CSF diversion followed by albendazole and steroids is indicated for obstructive hydocephaius. Arachnoiditis, vasculitis or cerebral edema is treated with prednisone 60 mg/d or dexamethasone 4–6 mg/d together with albendazole or praziquantel (White AC, Jr, *Annu Rev Med* 2000;51:187). Any cysticercocidal drug may cause irreparable damage when used to treat ocular or spinal cysts, even when corticosteroids are used. An ophthalmic exam should always precede treatment to rule out intraocular cysts.

| Infection | Drug | Adult dosage | Pediatric dosage |
|---|---|---|---|
| **TOXOPLASMOSIS** (*Toxoplasma gondii*) | | | |
| Drug of choice[113]: | Pyrimethamine[114] **plus** sulfadiazine[116] | 25–100 mg/d PO × 3–4wks 1–1.5 g PO qid × 3–4wks | 2 mg/kg/d PO × 2d, then 1 mg/kg/d (max. 25 mg/d) × 4wks[115] 100–200 mg/kg/d PO × 3–4wks |
| **TRICHINELLOSIS** (*Trichinella spiralis*) | | | |
| Drug of choice: | Steroids for severe symptoms **plus** Albendazole[7,12] | 400 mg PO bid × 8–14d | 400 mg PO bid × 8–14d |
| Alternative: | Mebendazole[7] | 200–400 mg PO tid × 3d, then 400–500 mg tid × 10d | 200–400 mg PO tid × 3d; then 400–500 mg tid × 10d |
| **TRICHOMONIASIS** (*Trichomonas vaginalis*) | | | |
| Drug of choice[117]: | Metronidazole | 2 g PO once or 500 mg bid × 7d | 15 mg/kg/d PO in 3 doses × 7d |
| OR | Tinidazole[6] | 2 g PO once | 50 mg/kg once (max. 2 g) |

\* Availability problems. See table on manufacturers of drugs used to treat parasitic infections, page 464.

[113] To treat CNS toxoplasmosis in HIV-infected patients, some clinicians have used pyrimethamine 50–100 mg/d (after a loading dose of 200 mg) with sulfadiazine and, when sulfonamide sensitivity developed, have given clindamycin 1.8–2.4 g/d in divided doses instead of the sulfonamide. Treatment is usually given for at least 4–6 weeks. Atovaquone (1500 mg PO bid) plus pyrimethamine (200 mg loading dose, followed by 75 mg/d PO) for 6 weeks appears to be an effective alternative in sulfa-intolerant patients (Chirgwin K et al., *Clin Infect Dis* 2002;34:1243). Atovaquone must be taken with a meal to enhance absorption. Treatment is followed by chronic suppression with lower dosage regimens of the same drugs. For primary prophylaxis in HIV patients with <100 × 10⁶/L CD4 cells, either trimethoprim-sulfamethoxazole, pyrimethamine with dapsone, or atovaquone with or without pyrimethamine can be used. Primary or secondary prophylaxis may be discontinued when the CD4 count increases to >200 × 10⁶/L for >3mos (*MMWR Morb Mortal Wkly Rep* 2004;53 [RR15]:1. In ocular toxoplasmosis with macular involvement, corticosteroids are recommended in addition to antiparasitic therapy for an anti-inflammatory effect. In one randomized single-blind study, trimethoprim/sulfamethoxazole was reported to be as effective as pyrimethamine/sulfadiazine for treatment of ocular toxoplasmosis (Soheilian M et al., *Ophthalmology* 2005;112:1876). Women who develop toxoplasmosis during the first trimester of pregnancy should be treated with spiramycin (3–4 g/d). After the first trimester, if there is no documented transmission to the fetus, spiramycin can be continued until term. If transmission has occurred *in utero*, therapy with pyrimethamine and sulfadiazine should be started (Montoya JG and Liesenfeld O, *Lancet* 2004;363:1965). Pyrimethamine is a potential teratogen and should be used only after the first trimester.

[114] Plus leucovorin 10–25 mg with each dose of pyrimethamine. Pyrimethamine should be taken with food to minimize gastrointestinal adverse effects.

[115] Congenitally infected newborns should be treated with pyrimethamine every 2 or 3 days and a sulfonamide daily for about 1 year (Remington JS and Desmonts G in: Remington JS and Klein JO, eds, *Infectious Disease of the Fetus and Newborn Infant*, 6th ed, Philadelphia:Saunders, 2006, page 1038).

[116] Sulfadiazine should be taken on an empty stomach with adequate water.

[117] Sexual partners should be treated simultaneously with same dosage. Metronidazole-resistant strains have been reported and can be treated with higher doses of metronidazole (2–4 g/d × 7–14d) or with tinidazole (*MMWR Morb Mortal Wkly Rep* 2006;55 [RR11]:1).

| Infection | | Drug | Adult dosage | Pediatric dosage |
|---|---|---|---|---|
| **TRICHOSTRONGYLUS** infection | | | | |
| Drug of choice: | | Pyrantel pamoate[113],* | 11 mg/kg base PO once (max. 1 g) | 11 mg/kg PO once (max. 1 g) |
| Alternative: | | Mebendazole[7] | 100 mg PO bid × 3d | 100 mg PO bid × 3d |
| | OR | Albendazole[7,12] | 400 mg PO once | 400 mg PO once |
| **TRICHURIASIS** (*Trichuris trichiura*, whipworm) | | | | |
| Drug of choice: | | Mebendazole | 100 mg PO bid × 3d or 500 mg once | 100 mg PO bid × 3d or 500 mg once |
| Alternative: | | Albendazole[7,12] | 400 mg PO × 3d | 400 mg PO × 3d |
| | OR | Ivermectin[7,16] | 200 mcg/kg PO daily × 3d | 200 mcg/kg/d PO × 3d |
| **TRYPANOSOMIASIS**[118] | | | | |
| ***T. cruzi*** (American trypanosomiasis, Chagas' disease) | | | | |
| Drug of choice: | | Nifurtimox* | 8–10 mg/kg/d PO in 3–4 doses × 90–120d | 1–10yrs: 15–20 mg/kg/d PO in 4 doses × 90–120d <br> 11–16yrs: 12.5–15 mg/kg/d in 4 doses × 90–120d |
| | OR | Benznidazole[119],* | 5–7 mg/kg/d PO in 2 doses × 30–90d | ≤12yrs: 10 mg/kg/d PO in 2 doses × 30–90d <br> >12 yrs: 5–7 mg/kg/d in 2 doses × 30–90d |
| ***T. brucei gambiense*** (West African trypanosomiasis, sleeping sickness) hemolymphatic stage | | | | |
| Drug of choice[120]: | | Pentamidine[7] | 4 mg/kg/d IM × 7d | 4 mg/kg/d IM × 7d |
| Alternative: | | Suramin* | 100–200 mg (test dose) IV; then 1 g IV on days 1, 3, 7, 14, and 21 | 20 mg/kg on d 1, 3, 7, 14, and 21 |

---

* Availability problems. See table on manufacturers of drugs used to treat parasitic infections, page 464.

[118] Barrett MP et al., *Lancet* 2003;362:1469. Treatment of chronic or indeterminate Chagas' disease with benznidazole has been associated with reduced progression and increased negative seroconversion (Viotti R et al., *Ann Intern Med* 2006;144:724).

[119] Benznidazole should be taken with meals to minimize gastrointestinal adverse effects. It is contraindicated during pregnancy.

[120] Pentamidine and suramin have equal efficacy, but pentamidine is better tolerated.

[121] Eflornithine is highly effective in *T.b. gambiense*, but not in *T.b. rhodesiense* infections. In one study of treatment of CNS disease due to *T.b. gambiense*, there were fewer serious complications with eflornithine than with melarsoprol (Chappuis F et al., *Clin Infect Dis* 2005;41:748). Eflornithine is available in limited supply only from the WHO and the CDC. It is contraindicated during pregnancy.

| Infection | Drug | Adult dosage | Pediatric dosage |
|-----------|------|--------------|------------------|
| **Late disease with CNS involvement** | | | |
| Drug of Choice: | Eflornithine[121],* | 400 mg/kg/d IV in 4 doses × 14d | 400 mg/kg/d IV in 4 doses × 14d |
| OR | Melarsoprol[122] | 2.2 mg/kg/d IV × 10d | 2.2 mg/kg/d IV × 10d |
| ***T. b. rhodesiense*** (East African trypanosomiasis, sleeping sickness) | | | |
| Hemolymphatic stage | | | |
| Drug of choice: | Suramin* | 100–200 mg (test dose) IV; then 1 g IV on d 1,3,7,14 and 21 | 20 mg/kg on d 1,3,7,14, and 21 |
| **Late disease with CNS involvement** | | | |
| Drug of choice: | Melarsoprol[122] | 2–3.6 mg/kg/d IV × 3d; after 7d 3.6 mg/kg/d × 3d; repeat again after 7d | 2–3.6 mg/kg/d × 3d; after 7d 3.6 mg/kg/d × 3d; repeat again after 7d |

| | | | |
|-----------|------|--------------|------------------|
| **VISCERAL LARVA MIGRANS**[123] (*Toxocariasis*) | | | |
| Drug of choice: | Albendazole[7,12] | 400 mg PO bid × 5d | 400 mg PO bid × 5d |
| OR | Mebendazole[7] | 100–200 mg PO bid × 5d | 100–200 mg PO bid × 5d |

**Whipworm**, see TRICHURIASIS

***Wuchereria bancrofti***, see FILARIASIS

---

* Availability problems. See table on manufacturers of drugs used to treat parasitic infections, page 464.

[122] Schmid E et al., *J Infect Dis* 2005;191:1922. Corticosteroids have been used to prevent arsenical encephalopathy (Pepin J et al., *Trans R Soc Trop Med Hyg* 1995;89:92). Up to 20% of patients with *T.b. gambiense* fail to respond to melarsoprol (Barrett MP, *Lancet* 1999;353:1113). In one study, a combination of low-dose melarsoprol (1.2 mg/kg/d IV) and nifurtimox (7.5 mg/kg PO bid) × 10d was more effective than standard-dose melarsoprol alone (Bisser S et al., *J Infect Dis* 2007;195:322).

[123] Optimum duration of therapy is not known; some *Medical Letter* consultants would treat × 20d. For severe symptoms or eye involvement, corticosteroids can be used in addition (Despommier D, *Clin Microbiol Rev* 2003;16:265).

## Safety of Antiparasitic Drugs in Pregnancy

| Drug | Toxicity in Pregnancy | Recommendations |
|---|---|---|
| Albendazole (*Albenza*) | Teratogenic and embryotoxic in animals | Caution* |
| Amphotericin B (*Fungizone*, and others) | None known | Caution* |
| Amphotericin B liposomal (*AmBisome*) | None known | Caution* |
| Artemether/lumefantrine (*Coartem, Riamet*)[1] | Unknown | Contraindicated during 1st trimester; caution 2nd and 3rd trimesters* |
| Artesunate[1] | Embryocidal and teratogenic in rats | Contraindicated during 1st trimester; caution 2nd and 3rd trimesters* |
| Atovaquone (*Mepron*) | Maternal and fetal toxicity in animals | Caution* |
| Atovaquone/proguanil (*Malarone*)[2] | Maternal and fetal toxicity in animals | Caution* |
| Azithromycin (*Zithromax*) | None known | Probably safe |
| Benznidazole (*Rochagan*) | Unknown | Contraindicated |
| Chloroquine (*Aralen*, and others) | None known with doses recommended for malaria prophylaxis | Probably safe in low doses |
| Clarithromycin (*Biaxin*) | Teratogenic in animals | Contraindicated |
| Clindamycin (*Cleocin*, and others) | None known | Caution* |
| Crotamiton (*Eurax*) | Unknown | Caution* |
| Dapsone | None known; carcinogenic in rats and mice; hemolytic reactions in neonates | Caution*, especially at term |
| Diethylcarbamazine (DEC; *Hetrazan*) | Not known; abortifacient in one study in rabbits | Contraindicated |
| Diloxanide (*Furamide*) | Safety not established | Caution* |
| Doxycycline (*Vibramycin*, and others) | Tooth discoloration and dysplasia, inhibition of bone growth in fetus; hepatic toxicity and azotemia with IV use in pregnant patients with decreased renal function or with overdosage | Contraindicated |
| Eflornitine (*Ornidyl*) | Embryocidal in animals | Contraindicated |
| Fluconazole (*Diflucan*) | Teratogenic | Contraindicated for high dose; caution* for single dose |
| Flucytosine (*Ancoban*) | Teratogenic in rats | Contraindicated |
| Furazolidone (*Furoxone*) | None known; carcinogenic in rodents; hemolysis with G-6-PD deficiency in newborn | Caution*; contraindicated at term |
| Hydroxychloroquine (*Plaquenil*) | None known with doses recommended for malaria prophylaxis | Probably safe in low doses |
| Itraconazole (*Sporanox*, and others) | Teratogenic and embryotoxic in rats | Caution* |

| Drug | Toxicity in Pregnancy | Recommendations |
|---|---|---|
| Iodoquinel (*Yodoxin*, and others) | Unknown | Caution* |
| Ivermectin (*Stromectol*) | Teratogenic in animals | Contraindicated |
| Ketoconazole (*Nizoral*, and others) | Teratogenic and embryotoxic in rats | Contraindicated; topical probably safe |
| Lindane | Absorbed from the skin; potential CNS toxicity in fetus | Contraindicated |
| Malathion, topical (*Ovide*) | None known | Probably safe |
| Mebendazole (*Vermox*) | Teratogenic and embryotoxic in rats | Caution* |
| Mefloquine (*Lariam*)[3] | Teratogenic in animals | Caution* |
| Meglumine (*Glucantine*) | Not known | Caution* |
| Metronidazole (*Flagyl*, and others) | None known—carcinogenic in rats and mice | Caution* |
| Miconazole (*Monistat i.v.*) | None known | Caution* |
| Miltefosine (*Impavido*) | Teratogenic in rats and induces abortions in animals | Contraindicated; effective contraception must be used for 2mon after the last dose |
| Niclosamide (*Niclocide*) | Not absorbed; no known toxicity in fetus | Probably safe |
| Nitazoxanide (*Alinia*) | None known | Caution* |
| Oxamniquine (*Vansil*) | Embryocidal in animals | Contraindicated |
| Paromomycin (*Humatin*) | Poorly absorbed; toxicity in fetus unknown | Oral capsules probably safe |
| Pentamidine (*Pentam 300*, *NebuPent*, and others) | Safety not established | Caution* |
| Permethrin (*Nix*, and others) | Poorly absorbed; no known toxicity in fetus | Probably safe |
| Praziquantel (*Biltricide*) | Not known | Probably safe |
| Primaquine | Hemolysis in G-6-PD deficiency | Contraindicated |
| Pyrantel pamoate (*Antiminth*, and others) | Absorbed in small amounts; no known toxicity in fetus | Probably safe |
| Pyrethrins and piperonyl butoxide (*RID*, and others) | Poorly absorbed; no known toxicity in fetus | Probably safe |
| Pyrimethamine (*Daraprim*)[4] | Teratogenic in animals | Caution*; contraindicated during 1st trimester |
| Quinacrine (*Atabrine*) | Safety not established | Caution* |
| Quinidine | Large doses can cause abortion | Probably safe |
| Quinine (*Qualaquin*) | Large doses can cause abortion; auditory nerve hypoplasia, deafness in fetus; visual changes, limb anomalies, visceral defects also reported | Caution* |
| Sodium stibogluconate (*Pentostam*) | Not known | Caution* |
| Sulfonamides | Teratogenic in some animal studies; hemolysis in newborn with G-6-PD deficiency; increased risk of kernicterus in newborn | Caution*; contraindicated at term |
| Suramin sodium (*Germanin*) | Teratogenic in mice | Caution* |

| Drug | Toxicity in Pregnancy | Recommendations |
|------|----------------------|-----------------|
| Tetracycline (*Sumycin*, and others) | Tooth discoloration and dysplasia, inhibition of bone growth in fetus; hepatic toxicity and azotemia with IV use in pregnant patients with decreased renal function or with overdosage | Contraindicated |
| Tinidazole (*Tindamax*) | Increased fetal mortality in rats | Caution* |
| Trimethoprim (*Proloprim*, and others) | Folate antagonism; teratogenic in rats | Caution* |
| Trimethoprim-sulfamethoxazole (*Bactrim*, and others) | Same as sulfonamides and trimethoprim | Caution*; contraindicated at term |

* Use only for strong clinical indication in absence of suitable alternative.

[1] See also footnote 76 on page 450.

[2] See also footnote 68 on page 449.

[3] See also footnotes 74 on page 449 and 90 on page 453.

[4] See also footnote 113 on page 458.

## Manufacturers of drugs used to treat parasitic infections

albendazole: *Albenza* (GlaxoSmithKline)

*Albenza* (GlaxoSmithKline): albendazole

*Alinia* (Romark): nitazoxanide

*AmBisome* (Gilead): amphotericin B, liposomal

amphotericin B: *Fungizone* (Apothecon), others

amphotericin B, liposomal: *AmBisome* (Gilead)

*Ancobon* (Valeant): flucytosine

§ *Antiminth* (Pfizer): pyrantel pamoate

● *Aralen* (Sanofi): chloroquine HCI and chloroquine phosphate

§ artemether: *Artenam* (Arenco, Belgium)

§ artemether/lumefantrine: *Coartem, Riamet* (Novartis)

§ *Artenam* (Arenco, Belgium): artemether

§ artesunate: (Guilin No. 1 Factory, People's Republic of China)

atovaquone: *Mepron* (GlaxoSmithKline)

atovaquone/proguanil: *Malarone* (GlaxoSmithKline)

azithromycin: *Zithromax* (Pfizer), others

● *Bactrim* (Roche): TMP/Sulfa

§ benznidazole: *Rochagan* (Brazil)

● *Biaxin* (Abbott): clarithromycin

§ *Biltricide* (Bayer): praziquantel

† bithionol: *Bitin* (Tanabe, Japan)

† *Bitin* (Tanabe, Japan): bithionol

*Brolene* (Aventis, Canada): propamidine isethionate

chloroquine HCI and chloroquine phosphate: *Aralen* (Sanofi), others

clarithromycin: *Biaxin* (Abbott), others

● *Cleocin* (Pfizer): clindamycin

clindamycin: *Cleocin* (Pfizer), others

*Coartem* (Novartis): artemether/lumefantrine

crotamiton: *Eurax* (Westwood-Squibb) dapsone: (Jacobus)

§ *Daraprim* (GlaxoSmithKline): pyrimethamine USP

† diethylcarbamazine citrate (DEC): *Hetrazan*

● *Diflucan* (Pfizer): fluconazole

§ diloxanide furoate: *Furamide* (Boots, United Kingdom)

doxycycline: *Vibramycin* (Pfizer), others

† eflornithine (Difluoromethylornithine, DFMO): *Ornidyl* (Aventis)

§ *Egaten* (Novartis): triclabendazole

*Elimite* (Allergan): permethrin

*Ergamisol* (Janssen): levamisole

*Eurax* (Westwood-Squibb): crotamiton

● *Flagyl* (Pfizer): metronidazole

§ *Flisint* (Sanofi-Aventis, France): fumagillin

fluconazole: *Diflucan* (Pfizer), others

flucytosine: *Ancobon* (Valeant)

§ fumagillin: *Flisint* (Sanofl-Aventis, France)

● *Fungizone* (Apothecon): amphotericin

§ *Furamide* (Boots, United Kingdom): diloxanide furoate

§ furazolidone: *Furozone* (Roberts)

§ *Furozone* (Roberts): furazolidone

† *Germanin* (Bayer, Germany): suramin sodium

§ *Glucantime* (Aventis, France): meglumine antimonate

† *Hetrazan*: diethylcarbamazine citrate (DEC)

*Humatin* (Monarch): paromomycin

§ *Impavido* (Zentaris, Germany): miltefosine

iodoquinol: *Yodoxin* (Glenwood), others

itraconazole: *Sporanox* (Janssen-Ortho), others

ivermectin: *Stromectol* (Merck)

ketoconazole: *Nizoral* (Janssen), others

† *Lampit* (Bayer, Germany): nifurtimox

*Lariam* (Roche): mefloquine

§ *Leshcutan* (Teva, Israel): topical paromomycin

levamisole: *Ergamisol* (Janssen)

lumefantrine/artemether: *Coartem, Riamet* (Novartis)

*Malarone* (GlaxoSmithKline): atovaquone/proguanil

malathion: *Ovide* (Medicis)

mebendazole: *Vermox* (McNeil), others

mefloquine: *Lariam* (Roche)

§ meglumine antimonate: *Glucantime* (Aventis, France)

† melarsoprol: *Mel-B*

† *Mel-B*: melarsoprol

*Mepron* (GlaxoSmithKline): atovaquone

metronidazole: *Flagyl* (Pfizer), others

§ miltefosine: *Impavido* (Zentaris, Germany)

*NebuPent* (Fujisawa): pentamidine isethionate

*Neutrexin* (US Bioscience): trimetrexate

§ niclosamide: *Yomesan* (Bayer, Germany)

† nifurtimox: *Lampit* (Bayer, Germany)

nitazoxanide: *Alinia* (Romark)

● *Nizoral* (Janssen): ketoconazole

*Nix* (GlaxoSmithKline): permethrin

§ ornidazole: *Tiberal* (Roche, France)

† *Ornidyl* (Aventis): eflornithine (Difluoromethylornithine, DFMO)

*Ovide* (Medicis): malathion

§ oxamniquine: *Vansil* (Pfizer)

§ *Paludrine* (AstraZeneca, United Kingdom): proguanil

paromomycin: *Humatin* (Monarch); *Leshcutan* (Teva, Israel; (topical formulation not available in US)
*Pentam 300* (Fujisawa): pentamidine isethionate
pentamidine isethionate: *Pentam 300* (Fujisawa), *NebuPent* (Fujisawa)

† *Pentostam* (GlaxoSmithKline, United Kingdom): sodium stibogluconate
permethrin: *Nix* (GlaxoSmithKline), *Elimite* (Allergen)

§ praziquantel: *Biltricide* (Bayer)
primaquine phosphate USP

§ proguanil: *Paludrine* (AstraZeneca, United Kingdom)
proguanil/atovaquone: *Malarone* (GlaxoSmithKline)

§ propamidine isethionate: *Brolene* (Aventis, Canada)

§ pyrantel pamoate: *Antiminth* (Pfizer)
pyrethrins and piperonyl butoxide: *RID* (Pfizer), others

§ pyrimethamine USP: *Daraprim* (GlaxoSmithKline)
*Qualaquin*: quinine sulfate (Mutual Pharmaceutical Co/AR Scientific)

* quinidine gluconate (Eli Lilly)

§ quinine dihydrochloride
quinine sulfate: *Qualaquin* (Mutual Pharmaceutical Co/AR Scientific)
*Riamet* (Novartis): artemether/lumefantrine

- *RID* (Pfizer): pyrethrins and piperonyl butoxide
- *Rifadin* (Aventis): rifampin
  rifampin: *Rifadin* (Aventis), others
§ *Rochagan* (Brazil): benznidazole
* *Rovamyclne* (Aventis): spiramycin
† sodium stibogluconate: *Pentostam* (GlaxoSmithKline, United Kingdom)
* spiramycin: *Rovamycine* (Aventis)
- *Sporanox* (Janssen-Ortho): itraconazole
  *Stromectol* (Merck): ivermectin sulfadiazine: (Eon)
† suramin sodium: *Germanin* (Bayer, Germany)
§ *Tiberal* (Roche, France): ornidazole
  *Tindamax* (Mission): tinidazole
  tinidazole: *Tindamax* (Mission)
  TMP/Sulfa: *Bactrim* (Roche), others
§ triclabendazole: *Egaten* (Novartis)
  trimetrexate: *Neutrexin* (US Bioscience)
§ *Vansil* (Pfizer): oxamniquine
- *Vermox* (McNeil): mebendazole
- *Vibramycin* (Pfizer): doxycycline
- *Yodoxin* (Glenwood): iodoquinol
§ *Yomesan* (Bayer, Germany): niclosamide
- *Zithromax* (Pfizer): azithromycin

---

* Available in the US only from the manufacturer.
§ Not available in the US; may be available through a compounding pharmacy (see footnote 4).
† Available from the CDC Drug Service, Centers for Disease Control and Prevention, Atlanta, Georgia 30333; 404-639-3670 (evenings, weekends, or holidays: 404-639-2888).
• Also available generically.

# Appendix B: Laboratory Tests for Tropical Diseases

The following list of tests, laboratories, and contact information may be useful to clinicians who see patients with various tropical diseases. This list should be considered a preliminary list and any additional information about other laboratories or other tests is welcomed by the author.

This collection of sites includes laboratories in several continents, as well as their locations and contact persons. To verify any conditions for submission, it is recommended that one communicate with the lab before submitting specimens.

## Parasitic infections

| Disease | Laboratory | Organism | Test | Acceptable specimens |
|---------|-----------|----------|------|----------------------|
| Amebiasis | CDC, Atlanta, **USA**[1] | *Entamoeba histolytica* | Enzyme immunoassay (EIA) | Serum |
| Amebiasis | McGill University, **Canada**[2] | *Entamoeba histolytica* | ELISA | Serum |
| Amebiasis | Hospital for Tropical Diseases, **London**[3] | *Entamoeba histolytica* | (IFAT) (CIE) (CAP) Latex Agglutination | Serum |
| Babesiosis | CDC, Atlanta, **USA**[1] | *Babesia microti* *Babesia* sp. WA1 | Immunofluorescence (IFA) | Serum |
| Babesia | Hospital for Tropical Diseases, **London**[3] | *Babesia* sp | IFAT | Serum |
| Chagas Disease | CDC, Atlanta, **USA**[1] | *Trypanosoma cruzi* | IFA, PCR | Serum |
| Cysticercosis | CDC, Atlanta, **USA**[1] | Larval *Taenia solium* | Immunoblot (Blot) | Serum or CSF |
| Cysticercosis | McGill University, **Canada**[2] | *Taenia solium* | Western Blot | Serum |
| Cysticercosis | Hospital for Tropical Diseases, **London**[3] | *Taenia solium* | EITB (Immunoblot) | Serum |
| Echinococcosis | CDC, Atlanta, **USA**[1] | *Echinococcus granulosus* | EIA, Blot | Serum |
| Echinococcosis | McGill University, **Canada**[2] | *Echinococcus granulosus* | ELISA Immunoblot | Serum |

| Disease | Laboratory | Organism | Test | Acceptable specimens |
|---|---|---|---|---|
| Echinococcosis | Hospital for Tropical Diseases, **London**[3] | *Echinococcus species* | ELISA | Serum |
| Fasciolasis | Hospital for Tropical Diseases, **London**[3] | *Fasciola hepatica* | IFAT | Serum |
| Filariasis | McGill University, **Canada**[2] | | ELISA | Serum |
| Filariasis | NIH, **USA**[4] | | IgG and IgG4, PCR | Serum |
| Filariasis | Hospital for Tropical Diseases, **London**[3] | | ELISA | Serum |
| Giardiasis | Hospital for Tropical Diseases, **London**[3] | *Giardia lamblia* | IFAT | Serum |
| Gnathostomiasis | Mahidol University, Bangkok, **Thailand**[9] | *Gnathostoma spinigerum* | Immunoblot (Western blot) | Serum |
| Gnathostomiasis | McGill University, **Canada**[2] | | Immunoblot (done in Mahidol Univ. BKK, Thailand) | Serum |
| Histoplasmosis | S. Africa[5] | | | Serum |
| Histoplasmosis | Australia[6] | | | Serum |
| Histoplasmosis | CDC, Atlanta, **USA**[1] | | | Serum |
| Leishmanisais | CDC, Atlanta, **USA**[1] | *Leishmania braziliensis* *L. donovani* *L. tropica* | IFA, PCR | Skin lesion, Serum, bone marrow |
| Leishmanisais | Hospital for Tropical Diseases, **London**[3] | | rK39 rapid diagnostic test (RDT) Direct Agglutination Test (DAT) | |
| Malaria | CDC, Atlanta, **USA**[1] | *Plasmodium falciparum* *P. malariae* *P. ovale* *P. vivax* | IFA | Serum |
| Malaria | McGill University, **Canada**[2] | | Immunofluorescence, PCR | Serum, blood |
| Malaria | Hospital for Tropical Diseases, **London**[3] | | IFAT/ELISA | Serum |

| Disease | Laboratory | Organism | Test | Acceptable specimens |
|---|---|---|---|---|
| Paragonimiasis | CDC, Atlanta, **USA**[1] | *Paragonimus westermani* | Western Blot | Serum |
| Schistosomiasis | CDC, Atlanta, **USA**[1] | *Schistosoma* sp. *S. mansoni* *S. haematobium* *S. japonicum* | FAST-ELISA Immunoblot | Serum |
| Schistosomiasis | McGill University, **Canada**[2] | *Schistosoma* sp. *S. mansoni* *S. haematobium* *S. japonicum* | ELISA Immunoblot | Serum |
| Schistosomasis | Hospital for Tropical Diseases, **London**[3] | | ELISA | Serum |
| Strongyloidiasis | CDC, Atlanta, **USA**[1] | *Strongyloides stercoralis* | EIA | Serum |
| Strongyloidiasis | McGill University, **Canada**[2] | *Strongyloides stercoralis* | ELISA | Serum |
| Strongyloidiasis | Hospital for Tropical Diseases, **London**[3] | *Strongyloides stercoralis* | ELISA | Serum |
| Toxocariasis | CDC, Atlanta, **USA**[1] | *Toxocara canis* | EIA | Serum or vitreous fluid |
| Toxocariasis | McGill University, **Canada**[2] | *Toxocara canis* | ELISA | Serum |
| Toxocarasis | Hospital for Tropical Diseases, **London**[3] | | ELISA | Serum |
| Toxoplasmosis | CDC, Atlanta, **USA**[1] | *Toxoplasma gondii* | IFA-IgG, EIA-IgM | Serum |
| Toxoplasmosis | McGill University, **Canada**[2] | *Toxoplasma gondii* | PCR, EIA IgG EIA IgM Immunocapture ISAGA IgM | Serum |
| Trichinosis | CDC, Atlanta, **USA**[1] | *Trichinella spiralis* | EIA | Serum |
| Trichinosis | McGill University, **Canada**[2] | *Trichinella spiralis* | ELISA | Serum |
| Trichinosis | Hospital for Tropical Diseases, **London**[3] | | IFAT | Serum |
| Trypanosomiasis | McGill University, **Canada**[2] | African trypanosomiasis | CATT, PCR | Serum |
| Trypanosomiasis (Chagas Disease) | CDC, Atlanta, **USA**[1] | *Trypanosoma cruzi* | Immunofluorescence, PCR | Serum |

| Disease | Laboratory | Organism | Test | Acceptable specimens |
|---------|-----------|----------|------|---------------------|
| Trypanosomiasis | Hospital for Tropical Diseases, **London**[3] | *Trypanosoma brucei* | IFAT | Serum |
| Trypanosomiasis | Hospital for Tropical Diseases, **London**[3] | *Trypanosoma cruzi* | IFAT/ELISA | Serum |

[1] **USA-CDC:** The Centers for Disease Control in the USA can be contacted for information regarding testing
tel: 770 488-4431;email: dpdx@cdc.gov.

[2] **Canda:** McGill University Centre for Tropical Diseases, Canada
http://www.medicine.mcgill.ca/tropmed/txt/services.htm.

[3] The Department of Clinical Parasitology, The Hospital for Tropical Diseases, Mortimer Market, Capper Street, London WC1E 6AU
tel: ++44 (0) 207 383 0482; fax ++44 (0) 207 388 8985
email: Monika.Kettelhut@btinternet.com.

[4] **USA:** National Institutes of Health (NIH)
Helminth Immunology Section and Clinical Parasitology Unit, Laboratory of Parasitic Diseases Bldg 4 Room B1-03, 4 Center Drive, Bethesda, MD 20892-0425
tel: 301-496-5398; fax: 301-480-3757
e-mail: tnutman@niaid.nih.
Contact: Thomas B. Nutman, M.D.

In addition to the above-mentioned sites, one can try to enquire at the institutes below:

[5] **South Africa:** National Institute for Communicable Diseases–South Africa at http://www.nicd.ac.za/.

[6] **Australia:** Central Sydney Laboratory Service–Sydney at http://www.cs.nsw.gov.au/csls/.

[7] **Belgium Antwerp:** Prins Leopold Instituut voor Trop. Geneeskunde, Centraal Laboratorium, voor Klinische Biologie
http://www.itg.be
Dr Marjan Van Esbroeck at mvesbroeck@itg.be.

[8] **Germany:** Bernhard Nocht Institute for Tropical Medicine
http://www15.bni-hamburg.de/bni/bni2/neu2/getfile.acgi?area_engl=diagnostics&pid=411

[9] **Thailand:** Mahidol University Bangkok
Immunodiagnostic Unit for Helminthic Infections, Dept. of Helminthology, Faculty of Tropical Medicine, Mahidol University
Bangkok 10400, Thailand
tel: 662-354-9100 to 19, ext 1820; fax: 662-643-5600
email: tmpdk@mahidol.ac.th
Contact: Dr. Paron Dekumyoy (Trop.Med.)
For logistic information, visit web pages:
http://www.tm.mahidol.ac.th/eng/tmhm/tmhm_service_sero.htm
http://www.tm.mahidol.ac.th/eng/special_lab/sp_immunodiag.htm

## Rickettsial infections

| Disease | Laboratory | Organism | Test | Acceptable specimens |
|---|---|---|---|---|
| Bartonelloses | Marseille, **France** | *Bartonella bacilliformi* | Serology, PCR | Serum |
| Ehrlichioses | Marseille, **France** | *Ehrlichia* | Serology, PCR | Serum |
| Q fever | Marseille, **France** | *Coxiella burnettii* | Serology, PCR | Serum |
| Rickettsioses | Marseille, **France** | All pathogens in "Spotted fever group" and "Typhus group" | Serology, PCR | Serum, skin biopsies, ticks, |

[1] France: Unité des Rickettsies, WHO Collaboratice Center for Rickettsial Diseases and Other Arthropod Borne Bacterial Diseases, Faculté de Medecine 27 Boulevard Jean Moulin, 13385 Marseille, France
tel.: 33 (0) 491 32 43 75; fax: 33 (0) 491 38 77 72
email: didier.raoult@gmail.com.
[2] Also done in **Australia:** Central Sydney Laboratory Service–Sydney
http://www.cs.nsw.gov.au/csls/
*CDC accepts specimens for Tickborne Rickettsial Diseases (TBRD) for TBRD testing from state health department public health laboratories. For questions regarding specimen submission, contact your state health department laboratory.

## Viral infections

| Disease | Laboratory | Test | Acceptable specimens |
|---|---|---|---|
| Barmah Forest virus | Australia[1] | Serology | Serum |
| Ross River virus | Australia[1] | Serology | Serum |
| Dengue fever | Australia[1] | Serology | Serum |
| Dengue fever | CDC-US[2] | Serology | Serum |
| Japanese encephalitis | Australia[1] | Serology | Serum, CSF |
| Japanese encephalitis | CDC-US[2] | Serology | Serum |
| Yellow Fever | Australia[1] | Serology | Serum |
| Yellow Fever | CDC-US[2] | Serology | Serum |
| West Nile Fever | Australia[1] | Serology | Serum |
| West Nile Fever | CDC-US[2] | Serology | Serum |
| West Nile Fever | Israel[3] | Serology, PCR | Serum |
| Viral Hemorrhagic Fevers | Australia[1] | Serology, PCR | Serum |
| Viral Hemorrhagic Fevers | CDC-US[2] | Serology | Serum |
| Viral Hemorrhagic Fevers | S. Africa[4] | Serology, PCR, | Serum, tissue culture |

[1] **Australia**: Central Sydney Laboratory Service–Sydney at http://www.cs.nsw.gov.au/csls/.

[2] **USA**: Division of Vector-Borne Infectious Diseases (DVBID), specimen submission instructions and arboviral reagent ordering system at http://www.cdc.gov/ncidod/dvbid/ misc/specimen-submission.htm.
Centers for Disease Control and Prevention
National Center for Zoonotic, Vector-borne and Enteric Diseases (NCZVED)
Division of Vector Borne Infectious Diseases (DVBID)
3150 Rampart Road, Fort Collins, CO 80521
tel: 1 (800) CDC-INFO (232-4636); tty: 1 (888) 232-6348; fax: (770) 488-4760
email: cdcinfo@cdc.gov.

[3] **Israel**: National Center for Zoonotic Diseases
Central Virology Laboratory, Sheba Medical Center
Ramat Gan, 52621, Israel
tel/fax: +972-3-530-5268
email: hannab@sheba.health.gov.il

[4] **South Africa**: National Institute for Communicalble Diseases–South Africa at http://www.nicd.ac.za/.

In addition to the sites mentioned above, one can try to enquire at the following institutes:

[5] **Germany**: Bernhard Nocht Institute for Tropical Medicine
http://www15.bni-hamburg.de/bni/bni2/neu2/getfile.acgi?area_engl=diagnostics&pid=411.

[6] **Australia**: Victorian Infectious Diseases Reference Laboratory–Melbourne at http://www.vidrl.org.au/.

[7] A very useful network of all European reference diagnostic laboratories for viral diseases: http://www.enivd.org//.

[8] **USA**: CDC, Special Pathogens Branch at http://www.cdc.gov/ncidod/dvrd/Spb/contactus.htm.
Special Pathogens Branch
National Center for Infectious Diseases, Division of Viral and Rickettsial Diseases MS A-26, Centers for Disease Control and Prevention
1600 Clifton Road Atlanta, GA 30333
tel: 404-639-1510; fax: 404-639-1509
email: dvd1spath@cdc.gov.

# Index